Sports Medicine Essentials

Sports Medicine Essentials

Edited by Ellis Baker

SYRAWOOD PUBLISHING HOUSE
New York

Published by Syrawood Publishing House,
750 Third Avenue, 9th Floor,
New York, NY 10017, USA
www.syrawoodpublishinghouse.com

Sports Medicine Essentials
Edited by Ellis Baker

International Standard Book Number: 978-1-68286-689-4 (Hardback)

Cataloging-in-Publication Data

Sports medicine essentials / edited by Ellis Baker.
p. cm.
Includes bibliographical references and index.
ISBN 978-1-68286-689-4
1. Sports medicine. 2. Sports sciences. 3. Physical education and training.
I. Baker, Ellis.
RC1210 .S66 2019
617.102 7--dc23

Printed in China.

TABLE OF CONTENTS

PREFACE

This book has been a concerted effort by a group of academicians, researchers and scientists, who have contributed their research works for the realization of the book. This book has materialized in the wake of emerging advancements and innovations in this field. Therefore, the need of the hour was to compile all the required researches and disseminate the knowledge to a broad spectrum of people comprising of students, researchers and specialists of the field.

Sports medicine is the integration of sports science and medicine for the study of treatment and prevention of physical injuries related to sports such as knee injury, exercise-induced asthma, fractures, etc. Sports medicine though not a specialty in itself, is a vast field and is essential to the development of a number of significant areas of science such as sports nutrition, sports science, physiatry, etc. This book is a compilation of fundamental theories and concepts central to sports medicine and provides detailed information about the essential techniques and methods of the field. This book elucidates new techniques and their applications in a multidisciplinary approach. Sports medicine practioners, experts, researchers and students who want to broaden the expanse of their knowledge will be greatly benefited by this book.

At the end of the preface, I would like to thank the authors for their brilliant chapters and the publisher for guiding us all-through the making of the book till its final stage. Also, I would like to thank my family for providing the support and encouragement throughout my academic career and research projects.

Editor

How Effective are Injections of Platelet-Rich Plasma (PRP) for the Treatment of Sports Injuries: a Critical Review of the Literature

JL Ziltener*, L Allet, P Sclison and M Grosclaude

Geneva University Hospital, Geneva, Switzerland

Abstract

Acute soft-tissue lesions and chronic overuse injuries in the sports medicine field are very frequent and in most cases, difficult to treat. Tissue repair in musculoskeletal lesions is often too slow and sometimes incomplete for a given athlete. The fastest, most complete recovery is of primary importance, and keeping the delay until return-to-field as brief as possible, a priority. Many bioactive proteins and growth factors amongst others influence healing processes. Administration of Platelet Rich Plasma enables the production, from the patient's own blood, of natural, high concentrations of autologous growth factors. Basic research and animal studies are promising, but evidence-based studies examining the treatment of human musculoskeletal lesions by Platelet Rich Plasma are still lacking. Nevertheless, such treatment is increasingly used in sports medicine clinical practice and much is expected of growth factor injections. The aim of this non exhaustive review is to analyze the existing literature published in the fields of sports medicine. The results of this analysis do not permit us to recommend the systematic and generalized use of Platelet Rich Plasma injections in the management of sport injuries. Nevertheless, a few promising results have to be mentioned, but high-quality studies are needed to provide scientific evidence about these injections' effectiveness.

Introduction

Acute and chronic musculoskeletal injuries are common during physical activities, are frequently problematic for an athlete, and always represent a therapeutic challenge for the clinician. Tissue healing after such injuries may be slow and sometimes incomplete. Nevertheless, optimal treatment for these injuries is mandatory and should be as safe, quick and cost-effective as possible, in order to restore athletes' pre-injury level in sports participation.

Physiologically, the healing of an injury progresses in overlapping phases and is characterized by a cascade of events triggered by the injured tissues. The three classic phases are: inflammation, proliferation and remodeling.

There are several treatment strategies with which to address musculoskeletal injuries. One novel approach is intra-lesion, autologous blood injection. Several products are available: Autologous Conditioned Serum (ACS), Platelet-Rich Plasma (PRP), Plasma Rich in Growth Factors (PRGF) and other derivatives. The large variety of products speaks for their different possible compositions with diverse biological effects. Other variables such as modalities of PRP activation, presence or not of white blood cells, local anesthesia or not, use of non-steroidal anti-inflammatory drugs, post-injection rehabilitation protocols, and many others, are confounding factors in studies, explaining the diversity of the experimental, but most of all clinical results [1,2].

PRP is a simple and minimally invasive means of obtaining the concentration of autologous growth factors. It is defined as a fraction of blood plasma, containing higher concentration of platelets than normal plasma, and consequently, a source of growth factors. Blood platelets consist of fifty to eighty alpha granula per unit. Each granula has more than thirty bioactive proteins, including platelet-derived growth factor (PDGF), transforming growth factor (TGF-Beta), vascular endothelial growth factor (VEGF), fibroblastic growth factor (FGF), epidermal growth factor (EGF), and insulin-like growth factor 1 (IGF-1). The different effects these factors have on human tissues have been extensively discussed in numerous papers, synthesized in two recent reviews [3,4]

PRP is directly injected in the lesion, mostly under echo graphic control. PRP thus supports tissue regeneration by acting as a biological catalyst. In addition, it seems to show antibacterial characteristics [5].

PRP is neither considered as medication, nor as a therapeutic substance. Hence, the rules of its application remain vague. Furthermore, its use is no longer banned by the world anti-doping agency, regardless of the chosen application procedure. Administration of PRP has been rapidly increasing since 2005 (the year the first clinical study involving injured athletes was published), probably due to its low price and efforts by the chemical industry. The world of sports is interested in any therapeutic approach that may promote the speedy recovery of injured athletes. In order to specify the clinical use of PRP, an international consensus covering all domains of sports medicine has been published by the International Olympic Committee [3].

Basic research and animal studies on the subject are relatively promising. Nevertheless, there is still ample discussion about the effectiveness of platelet-rich plasma injections for the treatment of human acute, or chronic, musculoskeletal injuries. This paper provides a critical, but not exhaustive, overview of the effect of platelet-rich plasma injections on tendon, muscle or ligament lesions, described in experimental and animal studies. We focused in particular in human *in-vivo* investigations.

Methodology

To assess current evidence for autologous plasma injections in the management of not surgically treated musculoskeletal injuries, a literature search using EMBASE and MEDLINE databases was conducted. We didn't extend our search to other databases, for example those including non-English articles. The key words were (autologous conditioned serum OR platelet-rich plasma) AND

***Corresponding author:** Jean Luc Ziltener, Geneva University Hospital, Geneva, Switzerland, E-mail: Jean-Luc.Ziltener@hcuge.ch

(animals OR Fundamentals OR Human studies) AND (soft tissues-muscle-ligament-tendon injuries). All titles were checked for the presence of a reference to autologous plasma injections. All articles with the said reference were then classified, based on their abstract, into fundamental or non fundamental studies, the latter group being subdivided in animal or human studies. At this time of selection, we identified 74 studies, 52 concerning animal research and 22 for human trials. Two persons read the articles and selected the studies considered methodologically acceptable following the Judet criteria.

As a particular focus was paid on human investigations we were interested in the quality of these trials. Among all identified human trials, only seven articles reached an evidence level type I or II (three studies referred to anterior cruciate ligament and four other were concerning tendon injuries). The quality of these studies was evaluated with the Pedro Scale. The quality ranged between 6/10 and 9/10 points. Given the paucity of high-level evidence based articles (level I and II) concerning soft tissue injuries, we finally decided to check the references of recent literature reviews on the subject. However, no additional article could be identified.

This article provides an overview and update destined to primary care physicians and sports medicine specialists. It should help them to better evaluate the risks and benefits inherent to PRP injections.

Platelet-Rich Plasma and Fundamental Sciences – Animal Studies

PRP and tendon

PRP is a relatively well established treatment option for the management of chronic tendon injuries, and its beneficial effects have been demonstrated in various animal studies listed in several recent reviews [2,3,6].

A Japanese study tested the effect of PRP in rats with a patella tendon lesion. In this paper, fibroblast cells and bone marrow stem cells in, and around the lesion were found to increase. Additionally, cell proliferation was twice as high, seven days post injection, as three days post injection. The group treated with PRP also showed a significant increase in collagen type I and III compared to the control group [7].

Another study conducted *in-vitro* cultures of equine tenocytes. Tendons that had been placed in a culture of PRP showed an increase in the genetic expression of mRNA for collagen type I and III, without an increase of metalloproteinase concentration or of catabolic proteins (MMP-13, MMP-3). An optimal concentration of PRP seems to be the determinant factor for increasing the expression of pro-collagen factors, but not the genetic expression of pro-inflammatory factors [8].

PRP increased cellular proliferation and the production of collagen in human tenocytes *in vitro*. The tenocytes in a PRP culture also increased the receptor expression for Vascular Endothelial Growth Factor A *(*VEGF-A*)*. VEGF concentration was at its peak during the phases of proliferation and remodeling, and led to angiogenesis - an important process of tissue healing. The Transforming Growth Factor-beta (TGF-B), highly concentrated in presence of PRP, played a predominant role in the tendon healing process. In the presence of a lesion, the number of TGF-B receptors on the tenocyte surface of rats (*in vitro*) had increased, which demonstrates the production of collagen Type I and III [9].

PRP and ligaments

Application of PRP is relatively well described for the anterior cruciate knee ligament in experimental and animal studies.

For example, *in-vitro* treatment of cells of the anterior cruciate ligament with PRP showed an increase of cells and collagen production [10].

Recently, in another *in-vitro* study conducted in mice, the association of basic Fibroblast Growth Factor (bFGF) and Growth Differentiation Factor 5 (GDF-5) increased cell proliferation, fibroblast migration, and the genetic expression of collagen Type I. The same study identified a better alignment of the medial collateral ligaments (MCL) collagen fibers compared to a control group [11].

It also has been shown that PDGF may play a significant role in the early stages of healing. Injected in the ruptured medial collateral ligament (MCL) of rabbits, PDGF improved biomechanical parameters such as ultimate load to failure, energy absorbed to failure and ultimate elongation of the MCL at 6 weeks [12].

A study conducted in rats found a 73% higher MCL ligament strength, compared to a control group who had no injection, at 12 days [13].

However, a study investigating the effect of PDGF on injured medial collateral ligament of rats, showed a significant decrease in its effectiveness when administered more than 24 hours after injury. This would suggest administering PRP preparation in the early phase for optimal healing [14].

Thus, basic science shows that the application of PRP stimulates the early healing of acute ligament injuries while improving the structure of injured ligaments.

PRP and muscle

Only a few experimental, *in-vivo* studies demonstrated the importance of growth factors for the healing process of muscle lesions, in terms of muscle regeneration and myogenesis. IGF-1, PDGF, NGF, FGF-2, HGF, and TGF-Beta seem to play an important role in muscle tissue healing. The last three, FGF-2, HGF, and TGF-beta, are particularly useful for the activation of satellite cells and are potent stimulators of the proliferation and fusion of myoblasts [15]. For example, the injection of anti FGF-2 decreased the number and diameter of myofibers, and delayed the fusion activation of satellite cells [16].

Extrinsic muscle lesions in animals (shock-induced gastrocnemius muscle contusion in mice), if placed in an environment rich in growth factors, in particular FGF-2 and TGF-Beta, were shown to react positively. The application of autologous conditioned serum (ACS) activated satellite cells and triggered the proliferation and differentiation of myoblasts, with fusion in myotubes. Wright-Carpenter et al. observed an increase in mature myofibers by day seven in a group that was treated with growth factors, compared to the control group. However, no significant difference could be identified by day fourteen, which only indicates an initial healing effect on muscle tissue, but not on muscle function, in the treated group [17].

More recently, PRP applied to a model of multiple, eccentrically loaded small muscle strains in rats, and caused a significant decrease in the total recovery time in the treated group, compared to non-treated rats. Functional improvement was significant in the PRP group from day seven and later at day 14. In the same study with a model of a large strain injury, moderate functional improvement appeared at day three after injection, but not later on. Hence, in animal models of small eccentric muscle strains, PRP could improve muscle regeneration, but in presence of larger intrinsic muscle strains, results seem more doubtful [18].

PRP in Human Chronic Tendinopathies

Chronic tendinopathy is one of the most frequent lesions in musculoskeletal, sports injuries. Tendon problems are reputed to represent 30 to 50 % of all sports injuries in both professional and hobby athletes. The tendons affected by lesions are primarily sport-specific.

Chronic tendinopathy is characterized by pain, edema and tendon weakness. Its origin is multi factorial. The repetition of micro traumas due to exercise, can lead to degenerative intra tendon lesions, micro ruptures, and sometimes to poor healing [19]. Histo-pathologically, these lesions present non-inflammatory cell proliferation (in particular fibroblasts), vascular hyperplasia (neo-vascularization), and disorganized collagen fibers, without any sign of inflammation [20,21].

In the tendon area, only a very few randomized controlled trials have been conducted in humans. Most of the studies are either cohort studies or case series. In this critical, non-exhaustive review, we focus on the three tendons most frequently affected in sports lesions: the Achilles tendon, patellar tendon, and tendons around the elbow ("epicondylitis"). These also happen to be the structures for which the PRP effect has been most investigated. It might be that we missed some interesting studies with our limited literature search strategy. However, the main reviews on the topic [5,22,23] mention similar conclusions as we did.

Achilles tendinopathy

Only one double blind randomized controlled trial exists on this topic. PRP injections were compared with a saline isotonic solution in 54 patients that presented symptoms for at least two months. Concurrently, the subjects were admitted to a three month-long, eccentric exercise program. As a result of the treatment, pain decreased, and functional scores, such as VISA-A, improved significantly in both groups. Even if results in the PRP group were somewhat higher, no statistical significance was found after six months. There was also no difference in patient satisfaction or in the time taken to return to sport. Importantly, no relevant side effects were identified. The limitations of this study were the unique injection of the PRP, limited follow up time, the relatively old age of the participants, and the lack of a control group without an eccentric program [24].

The same investigators subsequently extended the follow up to one year, without finding any supplementary PRP benefit. Localized bleeding caused by the injecting syringe might have triggered the tissue healing process. A positive response could also be due to a placebo effect, as invasive procedures lead to higher expectancy of good results [25]. Finally, in both groups, ultrasound showed that tendon structure and neo-vascularization improved significantly, without any group differences after six and twelve months. One of the main reasons for the absence of group differences is certainly the fact that standardized eccentric exercise training has already been shown to improve actual tendon structure [26].

Another article, a prospective case series with fourteen patients, showed a significant improvement of functional scores for up to eighteen months after PRP injections. Echography further confirmed an improvement of structural anomalies. This study supports previous results, indicating a potentially beneficial effect of PRP. Nevertheless, the absence of a control group does not permit any final conclusion [27].

Patellar tendinopathy (jumper's knee)

Only three articles of moderate quality (level of evidence III and IV) investigated knee extensor lesions in a recent review on the subject [28].

The first study was performed on eight elite athletes in 2007. Participants received a single injection of PRP and were observed for four months, but only seven patients received a follow up examination. Nevertheless, the authors found a significant improvement of the VISA score and of the radiological aspects in magnetic resonance (tendon abnormal signal and pre-insertion edema) [29].

The second article, a pilot study, included twenty athletes who experienced recurrent patellar tendinopathy symptoms, over a twenty-month period. Participants received three PRP injections within one month. Pain was evaluated on a visual analog scale, sports activity on the Tegner scale. Results showed a significant improvement at six months, compared to baseline. At the end of the study, most athletes returned to the same competition level as before. No relevant side effects were noted, except for pain at the time of injection. The rehabilitation protocol after the infiltration was systematically structured, an element underscored by the authors as a key factor for the success described. These investigators claim that such standardization should be a pre-requisite for all future studies. This study confirms the importance of the combination of growth factors and mechanical stimuli. Perhaps mechanical stimulation acts synergically with biological treatment and also modifies the micro-environment influencing tissue repair, independently of the presence of growth factors [2,30].

The most recent study followed 15 patients with a jumper's knee resistant to conservative treatment. Participants' symptoms lasted for a mean of 24 months. All received multiple PRP injections. This population was then compared to 16 controls with moderate tendinopathy symptoms (mean duration of symptoms: six months), who had been admitted to a classical physiotherapy treatment program. Follow-up took place after six months. No difference in pain, patient satisfaction with management and time to return to sport was observed between both groups. However, the 2 groups were not randomized and the characteristics (severity and duration of symptoms) of the control group were not comparable with those of the intervention group. Those limitations should be taken into account when interpreting the study's results. Nevertheless, patients with refractory jumper's knee, resistant to conventional treatment, may respond to PRP injections as positively as patients with less severe pathologies and classically treated [31].

Elbow tendinopathy

Since 2003, only a few single case studies and case series reports were published on epicondylopathy, with encouraging results [5].

A prospective, pilot, cohort study investigated the effect of PRP infiltration in 15 patients with chronic elbow tendinopathies. PRP was administered under local anesthesia. The test group was compared to a control group of five patients receiving local anesthesia only. The patients were observed for 24 months. Unfortunately, by week eight, all of the small control group participants left the study because of the persistence of pain. At that time, 60% of the subjects who had been injected with PRP, but only 16% of those not treated with PRP, showed a significant decrease of pain. At six months, 80 of patients in the PRP group still showed a decrease in pain, and 93 at 24 months. Functional improvement was similar according to the Mayo elbow score. In addition, 94 of the participants returned to work or restarted their sports activities after 24 months [32].

These findings were confirmed in a recent, randomized, double blind controlled trial that included 51 patients in a PRP group, and 49 patients in a group that received local infiltrations of corticosteroids. Pain (VAS) and a functional score of the upper extremity (DASH score) improved significantly compared to baseline values in both groups without any significant difference between groups during the first weeks after injections. From week 12, pain decreased and DASH significantly improved in the PRP group only, and for up to one year. This confirms the potentially early effect of corticosteroids in insertion injuries during the first weeks after injection, but maybe also their subsequent, negative influence on the tendon healing process [33].

Recently, a double blinded, randomized trial investigated two types of blood injections. A group of 150 patients with elbow symptoms resistant to conventional treatment received either PRP injections or autologous conditioned plasma. The injections were repeated twice and both groups were compared. Unfortunately, there was no placebo control group. The authors of this study planned a follow up after six months. In both groups, they reported marked reduction in pain and increase in function, but without any significant difference between groups. This raises the question of which concentration of platelets and growth factors is the best. "Less might be better", and the fact that the tissue healing response could be saturated after a certain concentration of growth factors locally should be taken into account. The number of platelets and the concentration of growth factors applied to the lesion site are probably determinant factors. Also, after a certain stage of healing, other factors may start influencing the process [34].

PRP in Acute Human Ligament Injuries

Studies on ligaments have mainly been conducted on animals, as seen before, but there are also some case reports in humans some years ago. The complex process of normal tissue healing is only partially known. In addition, the temporal expression of cells and molecules during spontaneous healing has been barely studied and thus, the timing for optimal PRP administration is not yet known. No human studies are available about timing. A recent systematic review identifying articles with the keywords "PRP" and "ligament" included only three human studies on ACL reconstruction which fulfilled criteria for an evidence level I or II [23]. No statistically significant differences with regard to clinical outcomes, tunnel widening, and graft integration have been identified between control and PRP groups.

In general, studies on ACL reconstruction focus more on the osteo-integration of ACL grafts and less on the graft itself. However, a prospective, single blinded MRI study has recently shown a 48% reduction in the time needed to present a complete, homogeneous graft signal with PRP injection versus controls, after surgical ACL reconstruction [35].

As this article should particularly help primary care physicians and sports medicine specialists in the clinical decision making we kept attention on conservative treatment of ligament injuries. Forster et al. [6] evaluated professional soccer players (n = 22) with grade II acute medial collateral ligament injuries. A group of 22 was treated with a single PRP injection within 72 hours of injury and compared to a control group treated with standard rest and rehabilitation. The return-to-play time was shortened by 27% in the PRP treated group compared to the control group.

More recently, a published case report evaluated the effect of two consecutive injections of a preparation rich in growth factors (PRGF) on an acute rupture of the medial collateral ligament of the elbow of a judoka. The authors reported an early return to full contact training at 3 months after injury and faster MRI recovery images at 6 weeks follow-up, compared to "classical" MRI outcome of those injuries [36].

Thus, human studies other than those concerning ACL surgery are inconclusive regarding any clearly positive effect of PRP on ligament injuries. Further investigations are needed to assess the effectiveness of PRP injections in the treatment of such lesions.

PRP in Acute Human Muscle Injuries

Physiologically, muscle injuries undergo distinct but overlapping healing phases, and the proper timing of PRP application is still unclear. The speed of recovery depends on the severity of the lesion, the treatment applied after injury, and the patient's ability to heal soft tissue lesions. At the time of trauma, myofiber ruptures and capillary lesions result in hematoma that fills the gap, with the release of cytokines and growth factors. The inflammatory phase thus starts from the first day on, involves a number of inflammatory responses and after one week, leads to the regenerative process. During this time and up to four to six weeks, the muscle gap is progressively replaced by fibrotic tissue which provides early support for new muscle tissue, involving in particular fibroblasts. Capillary neo-formation occurs to reestablish the nutrition of the area. The proliferation and differentiation of muscle precursor cells then permit the fusion of differentiated cells, leading to the formation of new, multinucleated myotubes. After week three, the remodeling phase begins, leading to the increase of the muscle's functional capacities.

Regeneration frequently does not fully restore muscle tissue to its previous level. The two processes of healing and fibrosis compete with each other, impairing full regeneration. Thus, the most important issue in muscle regeneration could be to prevent the development of fibrosis, thereby avoiding the apparition of a fibrotic tissue scar. PRP, with its high TGF-Beta1 level, might be deleterious to muscle healing by inducing fibrotic, muscle scar formation, possibly leading to increased risk of re-injury [37,38].

Moreover, the presence of neutrophils in some PRP preparations raises the problem of the potential release of pro-inflammatory proteases and reactive oxygen species by the said cells, leading to secondary damage to muscle tissue [18].

Despite the relatively promising results in animal models, literature on humans is much less clear. No randomized controlled studies conducted in humans could be identified and only three other studies were performed on small samples with only few valuable controls. Therefore, statistical power to support clinical evidence in humans is generally weak, due to this lack of methodologically robust studies.

The first description in humans did not strictly use PRP, but rather autologous conditioned serum (ACS). Eighteen professional athletes suffering from muscle strains were treated by ACS muscle injection and compared with 11 athletes with similar injuries and previously treated by Actovegin or Traumeel injections. Primary outcome was the time to return to competitive sport. The study reported a significant reduction in return-to-field days (16 versus 22), but presented numerous limitations: small sample size, no-blinded, atypical controls, variable injury sites, absence of long-term follow-up [39].

Two other case-reports were published. The first one by Loo et al. [40] presented a 35-year-old male bodybuilder with an adductor longus strain injury confirmed by echography. A weekly intra-muscle injection for three consecutive weeks permitted the return to competitive training, only one week after the last injection. Nevertheless, there were no details about the grade of injury, additional treatments, and follow-up.

The second paper described a 42-year-old active male with a sudden history of grade II medial hamstring muscle strain (semi-membranous), confirmed by an MRI scan. PRP was injected once in the muscle, with an ultra-sound guided technique. Seventeen days after injury, the athlete had full ROM, was pain-free during muscle contractions and was able to perform all his recreational sporting activities. MRI performed at the same time revealed complete resolution of the signal enhancement, which was clearly different to the usual MRI outcome, with a signal intensity remaining positive for at least six weeks after injury. Long-term follow-up at twelve months did not reveal any negative outcomes [41].

Some unpublished case-series were also presented in different Sports Medicine congresses, but all the presentations were retrospective, without control groups, and comparisons were based on expected return-to-play delays according to previously published series [42].

Concluding Remarks

The role of PRP in tissue healing could open a new field in sports medicine, but a significant amount of research is still needed to understand the effect of PRP on the regenerative and healing processes of a given soft tissue.

Many basic science or animal studies assessed the effect of PRP on the musculoskeletal system during the last decade. In general results are promising. However, this is not yet the case for human studies, especially in the area of sports medicine. Only a few human studies could be identified and a paucity of RCTs providing level I or II evidence for the efficacy of this intervention method exists. Furthermore, several questions remain unanswered. First of all, there is no consensus about the PRP preparations. A large diversity exists without knowing which one to adopt as the clinical best practice. There are no recommendations concerning the number of injections that should be administered, a single one or serial injections. We further do not know if pre-injection anesthetic affects the outcome. No standardized procedure for the administration of the injections exist (ultrasound guidance or not for example) and no precise information about ideal timing to administer PRP, depending on the lesions. No standardized follow-up can be found, especially concerning the use of non-steroidal anti-inflammatory drugs. A comprehensive rehabilitation planning is actually unavailable, in terms of what kind of activities should be permitted or avoided and during how much time.

However, studies agree on the absence of side effects or complications, albeit with limited duration of follow-up. Thus, the usefulness of autologous blood injections (growth factor preparations) for the treatment of acute or chronic injuries of the human musculoskeletal system, in particular among athletes, but also for people who play sport as a hobby, is still controversial. An analysis of the existing literature in human research reveals a weak evidence for the effect of PRP applications in soft tissue injuries. At this time, robust studies, with a good methodological quality and representative sample size are urgently needed and should be conducted. The authors are however confident that new studies will emerge in the near future.

Primary care physicians and sports medicine specialists should, with respect to current medical ethics, be cautious with the use of PRP to treat athletic or sporting injuries. Nevertheless, this field of treatment seems promising in the arsenal of non-operative management of sport injuries and particularly the cost-benefit ratio could be in favor of such procedures.

References

1. Creaney L, Hamilton B (2008) Growth factor delivery methods in the management of sports injuries: the state of play. Br J Sports Med 42: 314-320.
2. Kon E, Filardo G, Di Martino A, Marcacci M (2011) Platelet-rich plasma (PRP) to treat sports injuries: evidence to support its use. Knee Surg Sports Traumatol Arthrosc 19: 516-527.
3. Engebretsen L, Steffen K, Alsousou J, Anitua E, Bachl N, et al. (2010) IOC consensus paper on the use of platelet-rich plasma in sports medicine. Br J Sports Med 44: 1072-1081.
4. Borrione P, Di Gianfrancesco A, Pereira MT, Pigozzi F (2010) PRP in muscle healing. Am J Phys Med Rehabil 89: 854-861.
5. Kampa RJ, Connell DA (2010) Treatment of tendinopathy: is there a role for autologous whole blood and PRP injection? Int J Clin Pract 64: 1813-1823.
6. Foster TE, Puskas BL, Mandelbaum BR, Gerhardt MB, Rodeo SA (2009) Platelet rich plasma: from basic science to clinical applications. Am J Sports Med 37: 2259-2272.
7. Kajikawa Y, Morihara T, Sakamoto H, Matsuda K, Oshima Y, et al. (2008) Platelet-Rich plasma enhances the initial mobilization of circulation-derived cells for tendon healing. J Cell Physiol 215: 837-845.
8. Schnabel LV, Mohammed HO, Miller BJ, McDermott WG, Jacobson MS, et al. (2007) Platelet rich plasma (PRP) enhances anabolic gene expression patterns in flexor digitorum superficialis tendons. J Orthop Res 25: 230-240.
9. Klein MB, Yalamanchi N, Pham H, Longaker MT, Chang J (2002) Flexor tendon healing *in vitro*: Effects of TGF-beta on tendon cell collagen production. J Hand Surg Am 27: 615-620.
10. Fallouh L, Nakagawa K, Sasho T, Arai M, Kitahara S, et al. (2010) Effects of autologous platelet-rich plasma on cell viability and collagen synthesis in injured human anterior cruciate ligament. J Bone Joint Surg Am 92: 2909-2916.
11. Saiga K, Furumatsu T, Yoshida A, Masuda S, Takihira S, et al. (2010) Combined use of bFGF and GDF-5 enhances the healing of medial collateral ligament injury. Biochem Biophys Res Commun 402: 329-334.
12. Hildebrand KA, Woo SL, Smith DW, Allen CR, Deie M, et al. (1998) The Effects of Platelet-Derived Growth Factor-BB on Healing of the Rabbit Medial Collateral Ligament. An *in Vivo* Study. Am J Sports Med 26: 549-554.
13. Letson AK, Dahners LE (1994) The Effect of Combinations of Growth Factors on Ligament Healing. Clin Orthop Relat Res 308: 207-212.
14. Batten ML, Hansen JC, Dahners LE (1996) Influence of Dosage and Timing of Application of Platelet-Derived Growth Factor on Early Healing of the Rat Medial Collateral Ligament. J Orthop Res 14: 736-741.
15. Kasemkijwattana C, Menetrey J, Bosch P, Somogyi G, Moreland MS, et al. (2000) Use of growth factors to improve muscle healing after strain injury. Clin Orthop Relat Res 370: 272-285.
16. Lefaucheur JP, Gjata B, Lafont H, Sebille A (1996) Angiogenic and inflammatory responses following skeletal muscle injury are altered by immune neutralization of endogenous basic fibroblast growth factor, insulin-like growth factor and transforming growth factor-beta 1. J Neuroimmunol 70: 37-44.
17. Wright-Carpenter T, Opolon P, Appell HJ, Meijer H, Wehling P, et al. (2004) Treatment of muscle injuries by local administration of autologous conditioned serum: Animal experiments using a muscle contusion model. Int J Sports Med 25: 582-587.
18. Hammond JW, Hinton RY, Curl LA, Muriel JM, Lovering RM (2009) Use of autologous PRP to treat muscle injuries. Am J Sports Med 37: 1135-1142.
19. Sharma P, Maffulli N (2005) Tendon injury and tendinopathy: healing and repair. J Bone Joint Surg Am 87: 187-202.
20. Maffulli N, Longo UG, Denaro V (2010) Novel approaches for the management of tendinopathy. J Bone Joint Surg Am 92: 2604-2613.
21. Andia I, Sanchez M, Maffulli N (2010) Tendon healing and PRP therapies. Expert Opin Biol Ther 10: 1415-1426.
22. De Vos RJ, Van Veldhoven PL, Moen MH, Weir A, Tol JL, et al. (2010) Autologous growth factor injections in chronic tendinopathy: a systematic review. Br Med Bull 95: 63-77.
23. Taylor DW, Petrera M, Hendry M, Theodoropoulos JS (2011) A Systematic Review of the Use of Platelet-Rich Plasma in Sports Medicine as a New Treatment for Tendon and Ligament Injuries. Clin J Sport Med 21: 344-352.

24. De Vos RJ, Weir A, Verhaar J, Weinans H, Tol JL, et al. (2010) Platelet-rich plasma injection for chronic Achilles tendinopathy. JAMA 303: 144-149.

25. De Jonge S, De Vos RJ, Weir A, Verhaar J, Weinans H, et al. (2011) One year follow-up of PRP treatment in chronic Achilles tendinopathy. Am J Sports Med 39: 1623-1629.

26. De Vos RJ, Weir A, Tol JL, Verhaar J, Weinans H, et al. (2011) No effects of PRP on ultrasonographic tendon structure and neovascularisation in chronic midportion Achilles tendinopathy. Br J Sports Med 45: 387-392.

27. Gaweda K, Tarczynska M, Kryzanowski W (2010) Treatment of Achilles tendinopathy with PRP. Int J Sports Med 31: 577-583.

28. Van Ark M, Zwerver J, Akker-Scheek I (2011) Injection treatments for patellar tendinopathy. Br J Sports Med 45: 1068-1076.

29. Volpi P, Marinoni L, Bait C, De Girolamo L, Schoenhuber H (2007) Treatment of chronic patellar tendinosis with buffered PRP: a preliminary study. Med Sport 60: 595-603.

30. Kon E, Filardo G, Delcogliano M, Russo a, Bondi A, et al. (2009) Platelet-rich plasma: new clinical application. A pilot study for treatment of jumper's knee. Injury 40: 598-603.

31. Filardo G, Kon E, Della Villa S, Vincentelli F, Fornasari PM, et al. (2010) Use of platelet-rich plasma for the treatment of refractory jumper's knee. Int Orthop 34: 909-915.

32. Mishra A, Pavelko T (2006) Treatment of chronic elbow tendinosis with buffered platelet-rich plasma. Am J Sports Med 34: 1774-1778.

33. Peerbooms JC, Sluimer J, Bruijn DJ, Gosens T (2010) Positive effects of an autologous platelet concentrate in lateral epicondylitis in a double- blind randomized controlled trial: PRP versus corticosteroid injection with 1 year follow-up. Am J Sports Med 38: 255-262.

34. Creaney L, Wallace A, Curtis M, Connell D (2011) Growth factor-based therapies provide additional benefit beyond physical therapy in resistant elbow tendinopathy: a prospective randomized trial of autologous blood injections versus PRP injections. Br J Sports Med 45: 966-971.

35. Radice F, Yanez R, Gutierrez V, Rosales J, Pinedo M, et al. (2010) Comparison of Magnetic Resonance Imaging Findings in Anterior Cruciate Ligament Grafts with and Without Autologous Platelet-Derived Growth Factors. Arthroscopy 26: 50-57.

36. Mei-Dan O, Carmont M, Kots E, Barchilon V, Nyska M, et al. (2010) Early Return to Play following Complete Rupture of the Medial Collateral Ligament of the Elbow Using Preparation Rich in Growth Factors: A Case Report. J Shoulder Elbow Surg 19: e1-5.

37. Chan YS, Li Y, Foster W, Fu FH, Huard J (2005) The use of suramin, an antifibrotic agent, to improve muscle recovery after strain injury. Am J Sports Med 33: 43-51.

38. Sampson S, Gerhardt M, Mandelbaum B (2008) Platelet rich plasma injection grafts for musculoskeletal injuries: A review. Curr Rev Musculoskelet Med 1: 165-174.

39. Wright-Carpenter T, Klein P, Schafferhof P, Appell HJ, Mir LM, et al. (2004) Treatment of muscle injuries by local administration of autologous conditioned serum: a pilot study on sportsmen with muscle strains. Int J Sports Med 25: 588-593.

40. Loo W, Lee D, Soon M (2009) Plasma rich in growth factors to treat Adductor Longus tear. Ann Acad Med 38: 733-734.

41. Hamilton BH, Knez W, Eirale C, Chalabi H (2010) Platelet enriched plasma for acute muscle injury. Acta Orthop Belg 76: 443-448.

42. Hamilton BH, Best TM (2011) Platelet enriched plasma and muscle strain injuries: challenges imposed by the burden of proof. Clin J Sport Med 21: 31-36.

Genetic Predictors of Adenosine Monophosphate Deaminase Deficiency

Lawrence D Hayes[1,2], Fraser E Houston[3] and Julien S Baker[1*]

[1]Institute of Clinical Exercise and Health Science, University of the West of Scotland, Scotland
[2]School of Human Sciences, London Metropolitan University, UK
[3]Center for Exercise Science, University of Florida, USA

Abstract

In the majority of the population, during high intensity exercise, Adenosine Monohosphate Deaminase (AMPD) Converts Adenosine Monophosphate (AMP) to Inosine Monophosphate (IMP), with the liberation of ammonia in the process. The AMPD reaction displaces the adenylate kinase equilibrium in the direction of ATP formation during exercise, providing additional energy and preventing a large increase in ADP. AMPD deficiency has been proposed to result in faster fatigue development and earlier inhibition of muscle contractions. This review considers a number of genetic mutations that lead to skeletal muscle AMPD deficiency, their pathology and likely symptoms of the disorder.

Keywords: Exercise intolerance; ADP; AMP; AMPD; ATP

Introduction

During high intensity exercise, Adenosine Triphosphate (ATP) hydrolysis exceeds the rate of Adenosine Diphosphate (ADP) rephosphorylation in the muscle cell, leading to excessive formation of the latter. This results in a shift in the adenylate kinase equilibrium (2 ADP ↔ ATP + AMP) towards increased Adenosine Monophosphate (AMP) content. In the majority of the population, such conditions activate the enzyme Adenosine Monophosphate Deaminase (AMPD) also known as myoadenylate deaminase. AMPD converts AMP to Inosine Monophosphate (IMP), with the liberation of ammonia in the process. The AMPD reaction displaces the adenylate kinase equilibrium in the direction of ATP formation during exercise, providing additional energy and preventing a large increase in ADP. Together with adenylosuccinate synthase and adenylosuccinate lyase, it forms the purine nucleotide cycle which produces fumarate, an intermediate of the Krebs cycle, and therefore yields energy (Figure 1). As AMP deamination displaces the adenylate kinase equilibrium toward ATP resynthnesis, a proposed role for AMPD is to alleviate the exercise-induced decrease in the ATP/ADP ratio and its inhibitory effect on muscle contraction [1].

The aforementioned accumulation of ADP has been shown in rabbit and rodent skeletal muscle to reduce maximal shortening velocity and slow relaxation time [3-4]. Therefore, AMPD deficiency has been proposed to result in faster fatigue development and earlier inhibition of muscle contractions. Support for this proposal derives from reports of exercise-related symptoms such as early fatigue, muscle cramps and pain in AMPD deficient individuals [5]. Nevertheless, the combination of symptomatic variability and high incidence has resulted in some authors referring to AMPD deficiency as a "harmless genetic variant" [6]. In contrast, Isackson et al. reported symptoms of AMPD deficiency to include German measles, restless leg syndrome, cramps, abdominal discomfort, increasing joint hypermobility, chronic muscle pain, lack of aerobic stamina, chronic fatigue and deep burning in muscles with any repetitive movement [7]. These authors recognise that AMPD deficiency can potentially be a debilitating and crippling disease resulting in exercise intolerance. Skeletal muscle AMPD activities are varied across a wide array of neuromuscular disorders, owing to a combination of genetic and pathological factors that influence the expression of this enzyme [8]. Approximately 1-2% of the general Caucasian population exhibits a skeletal muscle AMPD deficiency however, only a few develop symptoms [9].

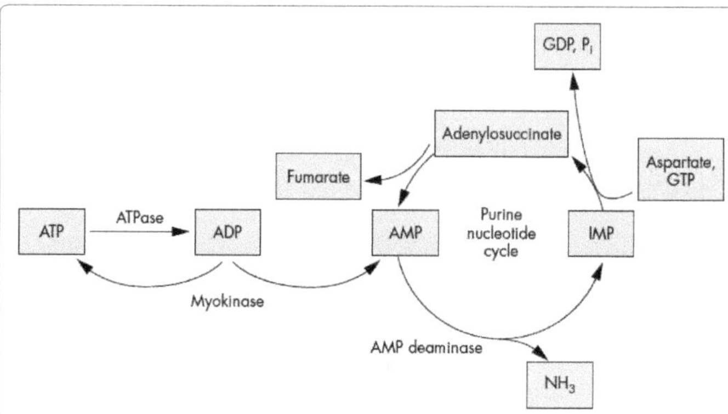

Figure 1: The purine nucleotide cycle (adapted from Lucia et al. [2]).

AMPD deficiency was first reported by Fishbein et al. [5]. There are no specific diagnostic criteria, and no clinical or biochemical definition for this disorder [10]. However, AMPD deficiency should be considered with any presented exercise-induced muscular symptoms especially premature fatigue and/or cramps [11]. The subsequent diagnosis would be based on the biochemical detection of AMPD deficiency in a muscle biopsy or detection of a disease-inducing genetic mutation. The disorder exclusively affects skeletal muscle as the disorder is a specific lack of the skeletal muscle type of AMPD activity. Unfortunately, there is no medical cure for this disorder. The only treatment possibility is the administration of D-ribose which is easily absorbed in the gut and rapidly cleared by metabolic pathways [12]. It serves as an additional energy source and is only effective as long as it is present in the blood. Due to its short half-life, it must be taken constantly to be beneficial. 0.1- 0.15 mg·kg^{-1} body mass must be taken per hour for the treatment to be beneficial. Any less yields no effect and doses above this result in diarrhoea. These limitations suggest it is only reasonable to take ribose at times of increased workload. Ribose is not approved by any organisation for the treatment of patients and must be bought from the chemical industry. So far, there is no explanation for the clinical

***Corresponding author:** Julien S Baker, Professor, Institute of Clinical Exercise and Health Science, University of the West of Scotland, Lanarkshire, Scotland
E-mail: jsbaker@uws.ac.uk

symptomatic variability of AMPD deficient individuals. Presumably, there are alternative pathways for energy production in asymptomatic homozygote patients however, these have not been established.

The muscle-specific isoform AMPD is coded by the *AMPD1* gene and the majority of AMPD deficient cases are due to a C to T transition at nucleotide 34 in exon 2 of the gene, creating a nonsense codon that prematurely terminates translation [7,13]. The frequency of the mutant allele is 8–11% in sedentary Caucasians, with only 2% of the population being homozygous for this mutation (20% are heterozygous) [14]. AMPD muscle activity is greatly diminished even in heterozygous individuals, reaching only ~39% activity of healthy controls [11]. Furthermore, in some heterozygotes, AMPD activity has been reported to be as low as 16% of its normal activity [15]. As a result, deleterious effects on exercise capacity associated with the C34T mutation have been reported, even in heterozygotes. For instance, Norman reported that young heterozygotes for the c.34C>T mutation had reduced capacity to deplete ATP and accumulate IMP during high intensity exercise, demonstrated by higher and lower concentrations of ATP and IMP (+18% and -32% respectively) when compared to normal homozygotes [15].

A number of studies have examined different performance parameters or markers of muscle metabolism in relation to the expression of *AMPD1* with varied findings [14-18]. Fischer et al. examined metabolic differences across *AMPD1* genotypes and the influence on muscle power [9]. It was hypothesised that AMPD deficient individuals would have an earlier onset of fatigue during the Wingate test (30 second (s) cycle ergometer sprint). Blood samples for DNA isolation were collected and genotyped for three different *AMPD1* mutations: c.468G>T, c.34C>T, and c.404delT. The c.404delT was described for the first time in two of three siblings. Investigators then analysed the newly identified c.404delT and previously described c.468G>T mutations in DNA samples from the Swedish population (*n* = 704), finding one c.404delT allele. Notably, this individual was compound heterozygous for the common c.34C>T mutation. AMPD assays performed using skeletal muscle biopsies showed that both compound heterozygotes for the c.404delT mutation lacked enzymatic activity. Fischer et al [9]. sampled 139 participants, of which 89 homozygous for the normal C34 allele (CC), 38 were heterozygotes (CT) and 9 were homozygotes for the mutant c.34C>T allele (TT). Due to their lack of AMPD activity, the three heterozygotes harbouring the c.34C>T and c.404delT mutations were included in the latter group and were referred to collectively as TT+. No differences were observed in anthropometric data or training index across genotypes.

The TT+ group were older than the CC group; however a regression analysis showed that age did not contribute significantly to any of the power variables measured. Figure 2 shows relative power outputs for the different *AMPD1* genotypes during the 30s Wingate.

Power output profiles normalized for Body weight (Bw) (means ± SE) during 30 2 wingate cycling in different *AMPD1* genotypes; CC, normal homozygotes; CT, heterozygotes; TT+, mutant homozygotes and compound heterozygotes. TT+ group consists of nine subjects that are homozygous for the exon 2c.34C>T mutation and three subjects that are compound heteozygotes for the c.34C>T mutation in exon 2 and c.40delT mutation in exon 5. *A*: men and women; *B*: men; *C*: women. *P* value for the interactopm term (genotype x time) in the ANOV analysis indicates level of significance for the comparison of performance between genotypes

There appeared to be no difference in Peak Power (PP) across genotypes, however a premature decrease in power in TT+ individuals

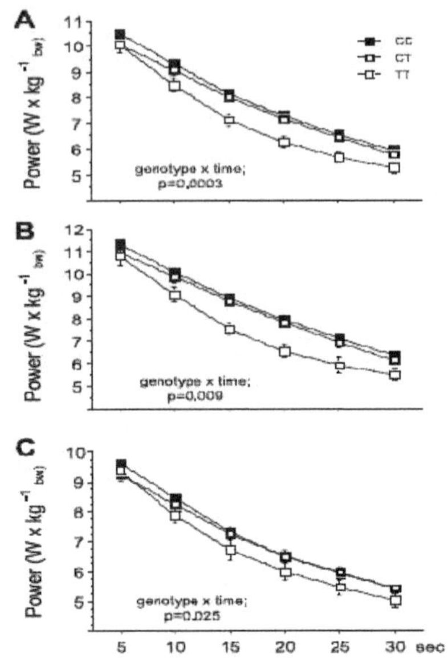

Figure 2: From Fischer et al. [9].

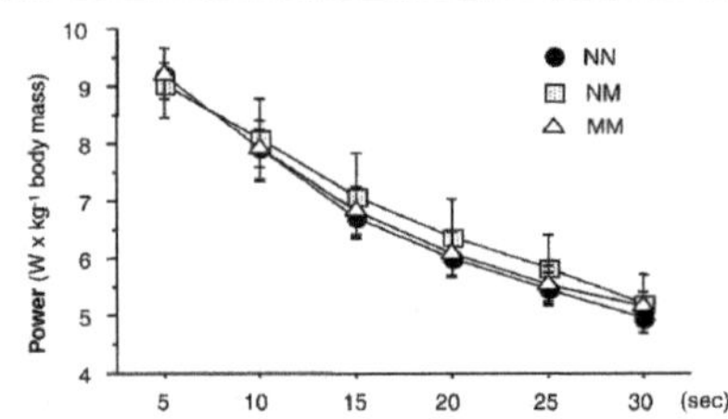

Figure 3: From Norman, Sabina and Jansson [15].

resulted in a difference in Mean Power (MP) across the genotypes (*P*=0.020). The decrease in power output at 15s was significantly greater in the TT+ group compared to the CT and CC groups (*P*=0.0006). This difference remained after 30s but was not as pronounced (*P*=0.046) and was more apparent in males. With regards to metabolic responses, the TT+ group showed almost no increase in plasma ammonia after completion of the Wingate test, which is consistent with a lack of AMPD activity. Fischer et al. concluded that AMPD deficiency was associated with diminished Wingate performance in otherwise healthy individuals and although the MP was only decreased by approximately 10% in TT+ individuals, this indicates a clear functional role for AMPD in skeletal muscle. Fischer et al. failed to detail the mechanism for deleterious effects of AMPD deficiency, and were unclear on how a small subset of the AMPD deficient population experience exercise-related cramping. Fischer et al. were successful in reporting significant findings despite the inherent difficulties when examining AMPD deficiency i.e. the small sample size and magnitude of expected differences.

Norman, also investigated AMPD deficient patients during a Wingate cycle ergometer sprint with contrasting findings to Fischer et al. [9,15]. As shown in Figure 3, no differences in power were observed between genotypes for the *AMPD1* gene unlike the Fischer et al. study.

Power output profiles (mean ± SD) during 30s Wingate cycling normalized for body weight in Normal Homozygotes (NN), Heterozygotes (NM), and Mutant Homozygotes (MM). Mutant allele = c.34C>T mutation in exon 2. In fact, no differences were observed in fiber type, peak power, mean power or ADP, AMP, lactate or creatine phosphate concentrations between groups. There was a pronounced difference between AMPD activity as expected; with normal homozygotes exhibiting the highest values and homozygotes for the mutation, the lowest. Unlike the other genotypes, the mutant homozygotes did not exhibit a decrease in ATP levels after exercise compared to baseline. Other metabolic discrepancies between genotypes include homozygotes for the mutant allele not showing any significant post-exercise increase in venous plasma ammonia, which is constant with the absence of IMP accumulation. Energy charge exhibited no change in the mutant homozygotes whereas both other genotypes experienced a decrease. Norman et al. summarised by suggesting that due to the high incidence of asymptomatic cases, AMPD deficiency does not commonly cause exercise intolerance. This is consistent with the prediction that, when individuals present severe exercise intolerance and are found to have an isolated deficiency in AMPD, the disorder may not be due to this enzymatic deficiency alone [17]. It is unclear as to why Fischer et al. and Norman et al. reported conflicting findings as the basic characteristics of the subjects (age, height, mass and training status) as well as the sample size were similar between studies. One characteristic of AMPD deficiency is the symptomatic variability. This, coupled with small sample sizes may have caused the discrepancy in findings. A difference in statistical analysis between papers may have caused differences in the findings. Norman et al. conducted an ANCOVA with fibre type as the nuisance variable as this factor is known to affect metabolism despite finding no significant difference between genotypes for fibre type [17]. Contrastingly, Fishcer et al. conducted an ANOVA, which would not take into consideration inconsistencies in fiber type between genotypes despite none being found.

Ruiter et al. also analysed muscle function in individuals homozygous for the C34T mutation [16]. However, Ruiter et al. reported that all AMPD deficient individuals were symptomatic; reporting muscle aches and early fatigue during and after intense exertion. The main methodical difference between the Ruiter et al. paper and the two previously mentioned is that unlike the previous two studies, Ruiter et al. attempted to exclude the influence of central fatigue by maximally stimulating the ulnar nerve electrically and measuring force output at the thumb [9,15]. In accordance with the previous findings by Norman et al. and Fischer et al. PP showed a greater rate of decrease in AMPD deficient individuals (Figure 4).

Change in power during repetitive contractions. Peak power (γ-axis) of 60 repetitive isovelocity (153°·s) concentric contractions (χ-axis) with occluded blood flow is shown for AMPD deficient (clear circle) and control (filled square) human adductor pollicis muscle. Note that the unusual unit for power (N°·s) is the result of multiplying shortening velocity (°·s) and force applied by the thumb at the transducer (N).

However, there were no observed differences between genotypes for

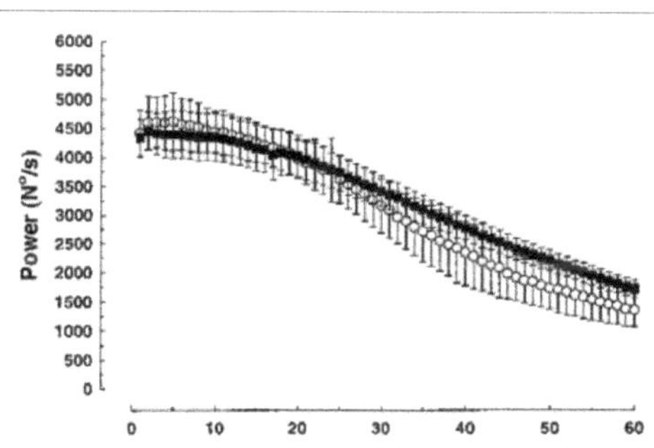

Figure 4: From Ruiter et al. [16].

maximal shortening velocity (V_{max}), maximal isometric force (F_{max}) or optimal shortening velocity (V_{opt}) defined as the velocity of shortening giving the highest power output on the velocity/power curve. Therefore, Ruiter et al. concluded that changes in contractile properties of the human adductor pollicis muscle in response to 60 electrically induced shortening contractions were similar for AMPD deficient individuals and the control group. In other words, the absence of AMPD appeared to have no functional consequences despite the decrease in PP [16].

Although the C34T mutation in exon 2 of *AMPD1* is the most common mutation causing AMPD deficiency, Isackson et al. and Gross et al. have described rarer genetic mutations [7,19]. Isackson et al. examined two Caucasian brothers with AMPD deficiency reporting exercise intolerance and muscle cramps who did not exhibit the common mutations (C34T in exon 2 or C143T in exon 3) in the *AMPD1* gene. However, both brothers were compound heterozygotes for a previously unreported deletion within intron 2 (IVS2-(4-7) del-CTTT) and an A860T mutation in exon 7. The IVS2-(4-7) delCTTT appeared to be accountable for the presence of numerous aberrantly spliced *AMPD1* mRNA species. In the IVS2-(4-7) delCTTT mutation, four pyrimidine bases (bold) were deleted from the middle of the pyrimidine-rich tract (cctc**ttt**tagA). Genetta et al. identified two regions in the centre of intron 2 that are necessary for splicing to generate the predominant *AMPD1* transcript apparent in skeletal muscle that includes exon 2 [18]. The IVS2-(4-7) delCTTT mutation, at the 3' end of intron 2, did not fall inside either of those regions and exon 2 was present in all transcripts required. Isackson et al. noted that although both brothers were absent in the common C34T mutation of the *AMPD1* gene, AMPD activity was still reduced to 20% of the reference mean (137 Caucasian adults). Although the precise nature of the changes in AMPD activity resulting from these two mutations is unidentified, exercise intolerance in both brothers along with the decreased enzymatic activity observed in one of the brothers suggests that the impact of heterozygosity is similar to that observed with homozygosity for the common co-segregating Q12X/P48l mutations. Additional genetic mutations probably contributed to the symptomatic problems of these brothers relative to the asymptomatic AMPD deficient members of the general population. In addition, the more severe symptoms of one sibling suggest further genetic variation may be present in this patient in view of his complex phenotype. One limitation of the above study and the conclusions drawn from it is the small sample size (n=2) expressing the IVS2-(4-7) delCTTT mutation. However, this is unavoidable as the intronic deletion has not previously been reported, with the size of the control group suggesting IVS2-(4-7) delCTTT to be a rare mutation and therefore not commonly expressed. This characteristic would make the intronic deletion problematic to investigate as finding other heterozygotes would require large sampling. Studying any possible linkage with other genetic mutations would prove very challenging.

Despite AMPD deficiency being shown to limit exercise capacity (albeit inconsistently) and the physiology of the disorder suggesting muscle metabolism is inhibited, there are reports of AMPD deficient individuals achieving sporting excellence. One such example of this is a case report by Lucia et al. who studied the case of an elite Spanish white runner, who was in the top eight in the 5,000 m at the Word Championships despite being heterozygous for the common C34T mutation in *AMPD1* [2]. Lucia et al. reported the test subject to have lower ammonia and lactate concentrations than the control group (four world class elite East-African runners and five of the best Spanish runners) [2]. His VO_2 cost of running was higher at all three velocities measured than the control group yet he still managed to compete at the highest level of athletics. This was suggested to be due to a number of compensatory mechanisms (which have been reported in other carriers), for example, a higher oxidative capacity as a result of higher adenosine concentrations stimulating enhanced blood flow. Lucia et al. also suggested more research into the area of central fatigue in AMPD deficient individuals is necessary, as during prolonged endurance exercise, increased blood ammonia concentrations result in increased cerebral uptake of this metabolite, leading to central fatigue [2]. In summary, the paper by Lucia et al. suggests that endurance running at world class competition can be achieved despite partial deficiency in AMPD activity [2]. One criticism of the Lucia et al. study in particular was that although the subject was indeed heterozygous for the mutant allele C34T, AMPD activity was not actually quantified. Rubio et al. sampled a group of top-level Caucasian Spanish endurance athletes (runners and cyclists) and found that the expression of the C34T mutant allele was significantly lower ($P<0.05$) in the athlete group that the control group (4.3% vs 8.5%) with no individuals homozygous for the mutant allele [14]. However, when comparing performance measures within the group of athletes, no significant differences were found in VO_{2max} or ventilation threshold between genotypes. Rubio et al. concluded by suggesting that the C34T *AMPD1* genotype was expressed less in elite endurance athletes compared to controls, however, once elite status has been achieved, this mutation does not appear to affect endurance performance [14].

Conclusion

In conclusion, the often asymptomatic nature of AMPD deficiency makes it a difficult disorder to investigate. The disorder can limit exercise capacity and cause physical pain, as shown by the study of Isackson et al. [7]. However, elite endurance athlete status can be achieved despite a decreased level of AMPD enzyme activity, due to physiological adaptations [2]. The differences in the severity of the disorder have been attributed to additional genetic defects that influence muscle metabolism [7]. To better understand the genetic predictors of AMPD deficiency, additional research could focus on any potential linkage between mutations or additional mutations that determine the symptomatic variance.

References

1. Lowenstein JM (1990) The purine nucleotide cycle revisited [corrected]. Int J Sports Med 11 Suppl 2: S37-46.
2. Lucia A, Martin MA, Esteve-Lanao J, San Juan AF, Rubio J, et al. (2006) C34T mutation of the AMPD1 gene in an elite white runner. Br J Sports Med 40: e7.
3. Westerblad H, Dahlstedt AJ, Lännergren J (1998) Mechanisms underlying reduced maximum shortening velocity during fatigue of intact, single fibres of mouse muscle. J Physiol 510: 269-277.
4. Westerblad H, Lännergren J (1994) Changes of the force-velocity relation, isometric tension and relaxation rate during fatigue in intact, single fibres of Xenopus skeletal muscle. J Muscle Res Cell Motil 15: 287-298.
5. Fishbein WN, Armbrustmacher VW, Griffin JL (1978) Myoadenylate deaminase deficiency: a new disease of muscle. Science 200: 545-548.
6. Verzijl HT, van Engelen BG, Luyten JA, Steenbergen GC, van den Heuvel LP, et al. (1998) Genetic characteristics of myoadenylate deaminase deficiency. Ann Neurol 44: 140-143.
7. Isackson PJ, Bujnicki H, Harding CO, Vladutiu GD (2005) Myoadenylate deaminase deficiency caused by alternative splicing due to a novel intronic mutation in the AMPD1 gene. Mol Genet Metab 86: 250-256.
8. Komi PV, Karlsson J (1978) Skeletal muscle fibre types, enzyme activities and physical performance in young males and females. Acta Physiol Scand 103: 210-218.
9. Fischer H, Esbjörnsson M, Sabina RL, Strömberg A, Peyrard-Janvid M, et al. (2007) AMP deaminase deficiency is associated with lower sprint cycling performance in healthy subjects. J Appl Physiol 103: 315-322.
10. Gross M (1997) Clinical heterogeneity and molecular mechanisms in inborn muscle AMP deaminase deficiency. J Inherit Metab Dis 20: 186-192.
11. Norman B, Glenmark B, Jansson E (1995) Muscle AMP deaminase deficiency in 2% of a healthy population. Muscle Nerve 18: 239-241.
12. Gross M, Reiter S, Zöllner N (1989) Metabolism of D-ribose administered continuously to healthy persons and to patients with myoadenylate deaminase deficiency. Klin Wochenschr 67: 1205-1213.
13. Sabina RL, Fishbein WN, Pezeshkpour G, Clarke PR, Holmes EW (1992) Molecular analysis of the myoadenylate deaminase deficiencies. Neurology 42: 170-179.
14. Rubio JC, Martín MA, Rabadán M, Gómez-Gallego F, San Juan AF, et al. (2005) Frequency of the C34T mutation of the AMPD1 gene in world-class endurance athletes: does this mutation impair performance? J Appl Physiol 98: 2108-2112.
15. Norman B, Sabina RL, Jansson E (2001) Regulation of skeletal muscle ATP catabolism by AMPD1 genotype during sprint exercise in asymptomatic subjects. J Appl Physiol 91: 258-264.
16. De Ruiter CJ, Van EDE HAANngelen BG, Wevers RA, De Haan A (2000) Muscle function during fatigue in myoadenylate deaminase-deficient Dutch subjects. Clin Sci (Lond) 98: 579-585.
17. Norman B, Mahnke-Zizelman DK, Vallis A, Sabina RL (1998) Genetic and other determinants of AMP deaminase activity in healthy adult skeletal muscle. J Appl Physiol 85: 1273-1278.
18. Vladutiu GD (2000) Complex phenotypes in metabolic muscle diseases. Muscle Nerve 23: 1157-1159.
19. Gross M, Rötzer E, Kölle P, Mortier W, Reichmann H, et al. (2002) A G468-T AMPD1 mutant allele contributes to the high incidence of myoadenylate deaminase deficiency in the Caucasian population. Neuromuscul Disord 12: 558-565.

3

Effect of Accommodation Training on Visual Function of Visual Inspection Workers and Middle-Aged People

Masumi Takada[1], Masaru Miyao[2], Motohiko Satoh[1], Kazuki Yoshikawa[3], Yasuyuki Matsuura[3] and Hiroki Takada[1,3]*

[1]Graduate School of Medicine, Aichi University of Medicine, Nagakute 480-1195, Japan
[2]Graduate School of Information Science, Nagoya University, Japan
[3]Graduate Schools of Engineering, University of Fukui, Fukui 910-8507, Japan

Abstract

By relaxing the contracted focus-adjustment muscles around the eyeball, such as the ciliary and extraocular muscles, improvement of the pseudo-myopia is expected. This understanding has led to the accommodation training in which the visual target is given by stereoscopic video clips. In this study, we verify short-term effects of the apparatus on eyesight of visual inspection workers (22 females) suffering from eye fatigue and 12 middle-aged persons. In the Measurement 1, the workers were trained in 3 days. Moreover, the middle-aged were investigated on several trials of the eyesight recovering apparatus in the Measurement 2. As a result, the visual acuity was statistically improved by continuous accommodation training which will promote a ciliary muscle-stretching effect.

Keywords*:* Myopia; Presbyopia; Spherical diopter (SPH); Visual acuity; Stereoscopic images; Ciliary muscle; Accommodation

Introduction

With the development of computers and widespread use of the internet, near visual tasks, such as Visual Display Terminal (VDT) activities have increased in young to elderly persons, causing social problems. Near visual tasks for a prolonged time strain the ciliary muscle, which may cause abnormalities in the accommodative function of the lens. This condition is called pseudomyopia, considered to be a part of refractive myopia. Prolonged near visual tasks have been reported to possibly induce cervico-omo-brachial syndrome and psychoneurotic symptoms [1]. The main cause of these vision problems is an accommodative function error. Therefore, we assume that it is possible to improve an abnormal accommodative function of the lens by activating the muscles by alternately repeating negative and positive accommodation. By improving the abnormal accommodative function, we can improve or prevent these vision problems. We call this operation "accommodation training." In Japan, an apparatus called MD-SS was developed [2]. This apparatus works by using a Landolt ring drawn on a flat plate that moves back and forth over a distance of 2 m in order to encourage alternately repeating negative and positive accommodation in the observers. However, the moving distance of the target object is very short. Therefore, the back-and-forth motion of the objects might have no effect on the observers. In order to solve the above mentioned problems, we suggest that the accommodation training is accomplished by gazing at an image in 3D movies, which simulate the back-and-forth motion in a stereoscopic space by using a computer and a Liquid Crystal Display (LCD).

For pseudomyopia, stretching exercise of the ciliary muscle, involved in accommodation of the lens, by alternately repeating negative and positive accommodation alleviates strain of the ciliary muscle. Miyao et al. experimentally showed that the lens was accommodated by following stereoscopic images when gazing at them displayed on a CRT or LCD [3,4].

Presbyopia represents senile impairment of near vision due to a reduced accommodative function of the lens with aging. The major cause of the reduction of accommodative function is thickening of the lens with aging, increasing the radius of the frontal curvature of the lens. In addition to this increase in lens volume, the elasticity of the lens capsule decreases, which results in an insufficient increase in the lens curvature even when the ciliary zonule is relaxed by ciliary muscle contraction, reducing the amplitude of accommodation [5]?

Stereoscopic videos utilizing binocular stereoscopic vision often cause unpleasant symptoms of asthenopia, such as headache and vomiting, depending on the audiovisual condition [6]. Ataxia in simulator-induced sickness has been reported. The influence of video-induced motion sickness on the body has been measured employing subjective scales, such as the Simulator Sickness Questionnaire (SSQ) [7], and by quantitatively investigating the relationship between external factors and internal conditions using physiological indices [8-11], such as respiratory function, electrocardiogram, skin electrical activity, fluctuation of the center of gravity, and electrogastrogram.

A new 3D video construction method has recently been developed to prevent video-induced motion sickness [12,13]. Humans perceive 3-dimensional objects by simultaneous convergence and accommodation of the lens, but stereoscopic videos generally consist of unnatural images perceived along a fixed visual line, negating such convergence and accommodation. Stereoscopic images using the POWER3D method (Olympus Visual Communications Co., Ltd.) prepared in order to reduce inconsistency between experience and the actual senses [14]. Some preceding studies showed that the degree of sickness was reduced by viewing stereoscopic videos prepared using this method [15,16]. We focused on stereoscopic videos prepared using this method. An LCD displaying the stereoscopic videos and visual acuity recovery device utilizing liquid crystal shutter eyeglasses (DR.REX Eye Care Program [14]) include several stereoscopic video contents (Figure 1), which induce near and distant visual conditions. The alternating presentation of these with appropriate intervals is expected to improve and prevent myopia and presbyopia.

In this study, we investigated the short-term effect of the accommodation training with the device utilizing stereoscopic videos

***Corresponding author:** Hiroki TAKADA, Graduate Schools of Engineering, University of Fukui, Fukui 910-8507, Japan
E-mail: takada@u-fukui.ac.jp

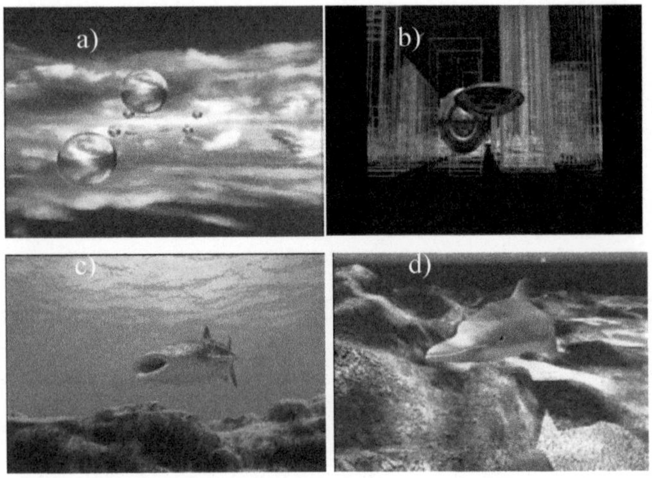

Figure 1: DR.REX Eye Care Program [14] includes several stereoscopic video contents: Sky vision a), Cyber vision b), Under the sea c), Dolphin d).

on visual inspection workers suffering from eye fatigue and middle-aged subjects becoming aware of presbyopia.

Material and Method

The objective and contents of the study and consideration of protection of personal information were explained to all subjects before the experiment, and written informed consent was obtained. The measurement was performed in a dimly lit room (about 260 lx) air-conditioned at 25°C. Before (Pre) and after (Post) the accommodation training stated below, the tests:

1) Simulator Sickness Questionnaire (SSQ)
2) Visual Analog Scale (VAS)
3) Objective refractometry
4) Visual acuity test (distant vision)
5) Visual acuity test (near vision)

were performed in this order. The auto visual acuity meter NV-300 (NIDEK) was used for the visual acuity tests that were employed for binocular and monocular visions. Time-course changes in the VAS, the Best Visual Acuity (BVA) at a distance, and that from near were investigated. Findings on Pre and Post values were compared employing the Wilcoxon signed-rank test, setting the significance level to 0.05.

Measurement 1

The subjects of the experiment were 22 female visual inspection workers, aged 37 ± 6 years. These subjects were also divided into two groups. One group underwent the accommodation training, in which they viewed a stereoscopic video (Figure 1a) for 6 min after the visual inspection work, and the other group was not given any task to perform during the first three consecutive days. Thereafter, the groups switched tasks, and the experiment was performed in a similar manner to collect data without the influence of task order. The above -mentioned items (1)-(5) were performed before the visual inspection work on the first day morning and after the task every experimental day.

Measurement 2

The subjects were 12 middle-aged persons aged 46.6 ± 3.5 years (6 males and 6 females). The accommodation training was performed, in which the subjects viewed 4 contents of the DR.REX Eye Care Program (Figure 1) for 6 minutes each in a random order. Before the accommodation training and after viewing each content, the tests (1)-(5) were performed in this order. The subjects then viewed the 4 contents in the same order for 6 minutes each, and the above-mentioned tests (1)-(5) were repeated.

Results

Measurement 1

The VAS for the evaluation of the visual fatigue significantly increased after their work (Figure 2a) although the other subjective indices (SSQ sub scores) did not significantly increase.

Variations in the BVA at a distance and from near with the experimental dates are shown in Figure 3a-4a, respectively. The gravitational mean BVA of the 22 subjects increased with the date. Irrespective of the subjects undergoing the accommodation training, when the Wilcoxon signed-rank test was used to compare the BVA before and after the initiation of this experiment, a significant difference in the visual acuity was observed ($p < 0.05$). The monocular vision test yielded a similar statistical significance. Although in comparison to the values obtained from the previous test, the visual acuity after the visual inspection work increased significantly on the experimental days ($p < 0.05$), the dioptric mean did not increase throughout this period.

Measurement 2

Subjective indices did not significantly increase with viewing frequency. The time-course changes in the VAS were shown in Figure 2b. The degree of asthenopia tended to decrease at 5th and 7th Post viewing than that measured at Pre viewing ($p<0.10$).

Changes in the binocular near and distant visual acuities with the frequency of video viewing are shown in Figure 3b. The gravitational mean binocular near and distant visual acuities of the 12 subjects

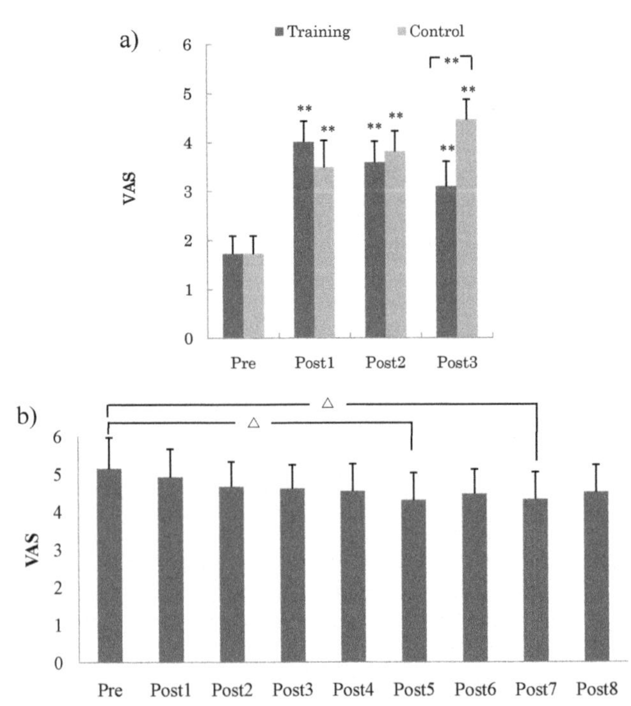

Figure 2: Time-course changes in the VAS for evaluating visual fatigue, in the measurement 1 a), in the measurement 2 b) (**p<0.01, Δp<0.10).

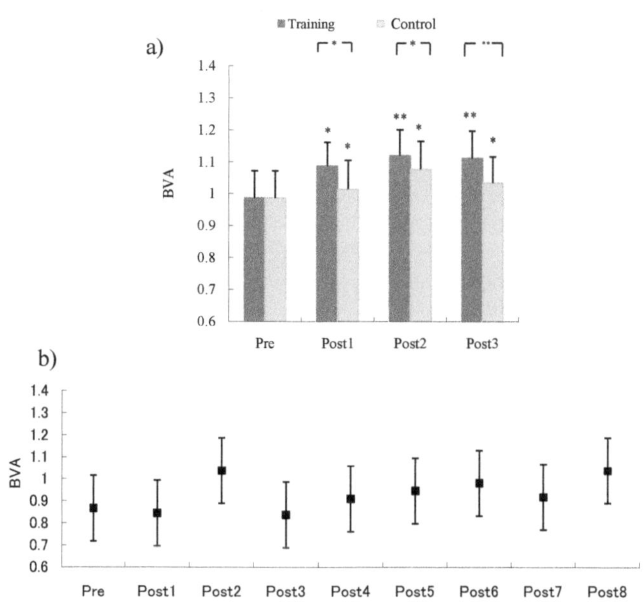

Figure 3: Time-course changes in binocular BVA at a distance, in the measurement 1 a), in the measurement 2 b) (**p<0.01, *p<0.05).

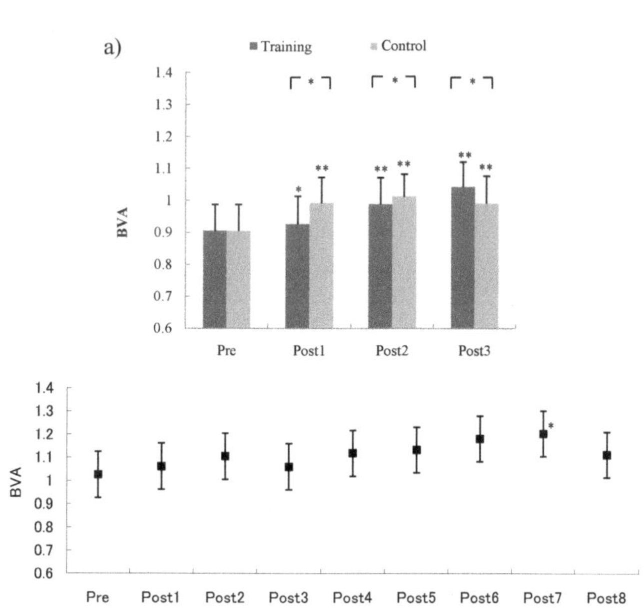

Figure 4: Time-course changes in binocular BVA from near, in the measurement 1 a), in the measurement 2 b) (**p<0.01, *p<0.05).

increased with the viewing frequency from the 1st to the 8th viewing, although there was some variation. On comparison of the uncorrected near visual acuity between the Pre and after the 7th video viewing employing the Wilcoxon signed-rank test, a significant difference was noted ($p<0.05$).

Discussion

In this study, we presented a movie using the POWER 3D method as the movie for the accommodation training, and a short-term effect of the accommodation training was investigated in visual inspection workers suffering from eye fatigue and middle-aged people. In both measurements, the motion sickness could not be induced by viewing 3D video clips in accordance with subjective tests, and the visual acuity was improved by continuous training.

In measurement 1, we showed that the visual inspection workers suffered from eye fatigue after their work as shown in Figure 2a. Although the dioptric comparison between the control and the training groups showed that there was no significant difference between the values for the groups ($p < 0.05$), the binocular BVA increased in 13 of the 22 visual inspection workers (59.1%) [17].

As shown in Figure 2a-3a, the visual acuity of the control group without the accommodation training showed an improvement. The myopic tendency had increased due to the visual inspection work. Moreover, it was possible that the subjects became skilled in the vision test. However, the results obtained from the Wilcoxon signed-rank test showed that the distant visual acuity in the training group had increased considerably compared to that in the control group ($p < 0.05$). As compared to the near visual acuity in the control group, that in the training group had increased significantly on day 3 ($p < 0.05$).

The VAS in the training group had also increased significantly on day 3 as compared to that in the control group (Figure 5). There seemed to be not only visual acuity improving effect but also reduction of the visual fatigue by the accommodation training for more than 3 consecutive days.

The authors have verified a middle-term effect of accommodation training that uses the strategy of presenting a stereoscopic movie to 32 myopic youth (20 ± 1 years). The movie consists of one to five balls moving back and forth in the stereoscopic sky background. At a viewing distance of 60 cm, the stereoscopic ball is viewed to move from 30 cm (forward) to infinity (backward). This ball completes a round-trip movement more than 25 times in 3 min. The uncorrected distant visual acuity increased in 17 of the 32 subjects (53.1%) participating in this study. Although there were some variations, the visual acuity improved in the accommodation training group and not in the control group. Upon comparing the value obtained on each measurement day using the Wilcoxon signed ranks test, we found that the visual acuity on day 11 was considerably higher in the accommodation group than in the control group ($p < 0.05$). This result suggests that the accommodation training using a stereoscopic movie has a cumulative positive effect on eyesight and prevents the deterioration of visual acuity. Although the myopic tendency improved slightly in the accommodation training group, there was only slight progress in the control group. These results suggested that the accommodation training using the stereoscopic movie did not deform the lens, thus not improving myopia fundamentally [18].

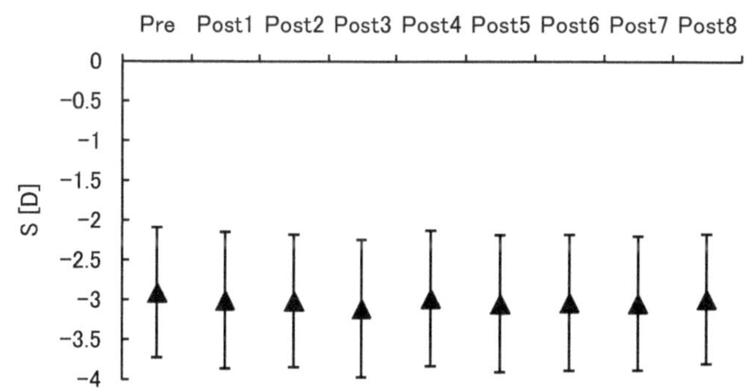

Figure 5: Time-course changes in SPH.

We assumed that these effects of the accommodation training were temporary, but the findings suggest that the continuous accommodation training will promote a ciliary-muscle-stretching effect, leading to an improvement in visual acuity. Accommodation reflex for near vision may be defined as the mechanism of working the ciliary muscle. This may also inhibit a reduction in the visual acuity.

In measurement 2, both the binocular near and distant visual acuities were improved, suggesting that the viewing of the stereoscopic video reduced strain and increased the flexibility of the ciliary muscle, which temporarily recovered the visual acuity. In contrast, findings on objective refractometry at Pre and post viewing stereoscopic videos were compared employing the Wilcoxon signed-rank test, setting the significance level to 0.05 [19]. Changes in the spherical diopter (SPH) of individual eyes with the frequency of video viewing are shown in Figure 5. The mean SPH was about −3 diopters in both eyes, showing no significant changes with the viewing frequency. Therefore, diopteric measurements did not change in either eye. The duration of the accommodation training may have been too short to modify the eyeball (lens) structure. It was suggested that the short-term repeated use of the accommodation training increased the near visual acuity, for which the improvement and prevention of presbyopia may be expected.

Conclusions

The visual acuity-improving effect of the visual acuity recovery device utilizing stereoscopic videos was investigated in visual inspection workers suffering from eye fatigue and middle-aged subjects becoming aware of presbyopia, and the visual acuity was improved by the continuous accommodation training for a short-term period. We are planning to investigate the effect of the device employed for a prolonged period.:

References

1. Nakazawa T, Okubo Y, Suwazono Y, Kobayashi E, Komine S, et al. (2002) Association between duration of daily VDT use and subjective symptoms. Am J Ind Med 42: 421-426.
2. Kobayashi S (1994) Eye sight recovering apparatus. Japan Patent H6 – 339501.
3. Miyao M, Ishihara SY, Saito S, Kondo TA, Sakakibara H, et al. (1996) Visual accommodation and subject performance during a stereoscopic object task using liquid crystal shutters. Ergonomics 39: 1294-1309.
4. Omori M, Watanabe T, Takai J, Takada H, Miyao M (2003) An attempt at preventing asthenopia among VDT workers. Int J Occup Saf Ergon 9: 453-462.
5. Fukuda T (1991) Aging and visual fuctions. ITEJ technical report 15: 1-8.
6. Ukai K, Howarth PA (2008) Visual fatigue caused by viewing stereoscopic motion images: Background, theories, and observations. Displays 29: 106-116.
7. Kennedy RS, Lane NE, Berbaum KS, Lilienthal MG (1993) Simulator Sickness Questionnaire: An Enhanced Method for Quantifying Simulator Sickness. Int J Aviation Psychology 3: 203-220.
8. Holomes SR, Griffin MJ (2001) Correlation between heart rate and the severity of motion sickness caused by optokinetic stimulation. J Psychophysiology 15: 35-42.
9. Himi N, Koga T, Nakamura E, Kobashi M, Yamane M, et al. (2004) Differences in autonomic responses between subjects with and without nausea while watching an irregularly oscillating video. Auton Neurosci 116: 46-53.
10. Yokota Y, Aoki M, Mizuta K, Ito Y, Isu N (2005) Motion sickness susceptibility associated with visually induced postural instability and cardiac autonomic responses in healthy subjects. Acta Otolaryngol 125: 280-285.
11. Scibora LM, Villard S, Bardy B, Stoffregen TA (2007) Wider stance reduces body sway and motion sickness. in Proc. the First International Symposium on Visually Induced Motion Sickness, Fatigue, and Photosensitive Epileptic Seizures. Hong Kong 18-23.
12. Yasui R, Matsuda I, Kakeya H (2006) Combining volumetric edge display and multiview display for expression of natural 3D images. SPIE 6055: 315-323.
13. Kakeya H (2007) MOEVision:simple multiview display with clear floating image. SPIE 6490: 1-8.
14. Nishihira T, Tahara H (2008) Apparatus for recovering eyesight utilizing stereoscopic video and method for displaying stereoscopic video. US7 404 639 B2.
15. Takada H, Fujikake K, Omori M, Hasegawa S, Watanabe T, et al. (2009) Reduction of body sway can be evaluated by sparse density during exposure to movies on Liquid Cristal Displays. IFMBE Proceedings 23: 987-991.
16. Takada H, Fujikake K, Watanabe T, Hasegawa S, Omori M, et al. (2009) A method for evaluating motion sickness induced by watching stereoscopic images on head-mounted display. SPIE 7237: 1-8.
17. Takada M, Miyao M, Shiozawa T, Matsuura Y, Omori M et al. (2010) Effect of eyesight-recovering stereoscopic movie system on visual acuity and fatigue of visual inspection workers. IADIS Visual Communications 494-497.
18. Takada H, Yamamoto T, Sugiura S, Miyao M (2009) Effect of an Eyesight Recovering Stereoscopic Movie System on Visual Acuity of middle-aged and Myopic Young People. IFMBE Proceedings 25: 331-334.
19. Sugiura A, Miyao M, Yamamoto T, Takada H (2011) Effect of strategic accommodation training by wide stereoscopic movie presentation on myopic young people of visual acuity and asthenopia. Displays 32: 219-224.

4

A Rapid and Sensitive LC – MS/MS Assay for the Quantitation of Bromantane in Human Plasma

Igor I Miroshnichenko, Svetlana A Sergeeva, Angelina I Platova* and Lyudmila M Krasnykh

Mental Health Research Center of RAMS, Moscow, Russia

Abstract

The purpose of this study was to develop and validate a high-performance liquid chromatographic–tandem mass spectrometric (LC–MS/MS) method for analysis of the bromantane in human plasma. The analyte and Internal Standard (IS), selenox, were extracted from human plasma by solid-phase extraction and separated on a Zorbax SB-C18 column using methanol–0.2% formic acid as mobile phase. Detection was performed using an atmospheric pressure chemical ionization source and mass spectrometric positive Multi-Reaction-Monitoring-Mode (+MRM) at an ion voltage of +2000 V. The assay was linear over the concentration range 1–500 ng/mL with the Lowest Limit of Quantification (LLOQ) of 1 ng/mL. The method also afforded satisfactory results in terms of the sensitivity, specificity, precision (intra- and inter-day, CV<10%), accuracy, recovery as well as the stability of the analyte under various conditions. The method can be applied to pharmacokinetic and toxicological studies.

Keywords: Bromantane; Liquid Chromatography–Mass Spectrometry (LC–MS/MS); APCI; Plasma

Introduction

Bromantane, N-(4-bromophenyl) adamantan-2-amine, is a drug with anxiolytic and immunostimulatory actions and elements of actoprotective activity [1-3]. Bromantane is not potentially addictive and does not exert effects of hypnosedation or neuromuscular relaxation. The use of the drug, in contrast to the action of a typical psycho stimulant, is not associated with the phenomenon of hyper stimulation and causes no consequences such as functional exhaustion of the body [4]. These properties of drug stipulated its using as a doping agent [5]. According to World Anti-Doping Agency classification, Bromantane belongs to S6; a class of prohibited substances [6].

The therapeutic action of Bromantane in patients with asthenic and anxiety-asthenic disorders is exhibited from first day of application, which is expressed by a marked reduction of asthenic symptoms, signs of emotional tension, and somatoautonomic manifestations; the drug works by restoring performance and enhancing the endurance of the body. Its mechanism of action is associated with the release of reinforcing dopamine from the presynaptic terminal [7], blockade of its reuptake, and enhancement of biosynthesis and induced tyrosine hydroxylase gene expression, as well as with a modulatory effect on the Benzodiazepine-GABA-receptor-chloride ion channel complex, up-regulating the stress-induced decrease of benzodiazepine reception. Bromantane increases GABAergic transmission, reduces gene expression, and regulates the synthesis of GABA-mediators, which act as reuptake transmitters. Bromantane has low toxicity (LD50 in rats is higher than 10000 mg/kg, exceeding the effective dose by 100 times).

Appropriate analytical method is an urgent need to study bromantane pharmacokinetic properties. The gas chromatography approach for content determination has been applied to a pharmacokinetic study of Bromantane [8]. However, this method was not quite appropriate for clinic pharmacokinetic studies of bromantane. LC/MS spectrometry based techniques are now the mainstay for such pharmacokinetic studies because of sensitivity, selectivity, speed and cost effectiveness [9]. Recently some papers devoted LC-MS/MS method for the quantitative estimation of amantadine (1-adamantylamine) [10] and memantine appeared in press [11,12].

The most commonly used sample preparation methods for blood plasma samples are Liquid–Liquid Extraction (LLE) and Solid-Phase Extraction (SPE). SPE is growing in use, and it offers certain advantages over LLE, including better specificity, the ability to obtain cleaner samples, good reproducibility, and a substantial reduction in the volume of solvent required [13].

However, we do not find HPLC–MS/MS methods reported in the literature for quantification of bromantane in biological samples. This paper reports on a rapid and sensitive LC–MS/MS method for the determination of bromantane in human plasma using SOLA cartridges. The method employs using 9-phenyl-sym-octahydroselenoxanthene (selenox) as internal standard and is completed in a run time of 6 min.

Experimental

Chemicals and reagents

Bromantane was kindly supplied by the Pharmacology Institute of RAMS, Moscow, 9-phenyl-sym-octahydroselenoxanthene synthesized by "Medbiopharm", Obninsk, and Kaluga region. Formic acid (Sigma Inc., USA), methanol and acetonitrile (Lab-Scan, Poland) were HPLC-grade. Deionized water was prepared from distilled water using Simplicity UV System (Millipore, USA). All other chemicals and solvents were analytical grade and used as received. The SOLA reversed phase extraction cartridges were purchased from Thermo Fisher Scientific Inc. (USA).

LC–MS/MS conditions

The HPLC–MS/MS system consisted of an Agilent 1200 series binary pump, an auto sampler connected to Agilent 6410-2K Triple Quad LC-MS (Agilent Technologies, Palo Alto, CA, USA) using a atmospheric pressure chemical ionization (APCI). The instrument was interfaced to a computer running Agilent Mass Hunter B.01.04. Software.

***Corresponding author:** Angelina I Platova, Mental Health Research Center of RAMS, Moscow, Russia, E-mail: Platova6283@mail.ru

Bromantane and IS were separated a Zorbax SB-C18 column (3.5 μm, 100 mm × 4.6 mm I.D., Agilent, USA) through a 12.5 mm × 4.6 mm Zorbax SB-C18 precolumn maintained 20°C. The mobile phase consisted of methanol–0.2% formic acid (95:5, v/v). The flow rate throughout the chromatographic analysis was 0.8 mL/min, and the total run time was 6 minutes. The injection volume was 5 μL. The retention times were 3.2 min for bromantane and 5.1 min for IS.

The detector was operated at unit resolution in the positive Multiple-Reaction Monitoring-Mode (+MRM) mode using the transitions of the protonated molecular ions of bromantane (308.1 → 135.2 *m/z*), IS (331.0 → 250.0 *m/z*). MS parameters were optimized by syringe pump infusing of standard solution containing analyte and IS. The spray voltage was set at 2000 V. Corona discharge was 4 μA. Nitrogen was used as nebulizer gas and pressure was set at 20 psi. Desolvation gas (nitrogen) was heated to 350°C and delivered at a flow rate of 5 L/min. For Collision-Induced Dissociation (CID), high purity nitrogen was used at a pressure of 0.15 MPa. During the data acquisition, dwell time was 200 ms. The fragmentation energy of Q1 and collision energy were 135 V and 25 V (bromantane), 90 V and 5 V (IS), respectively.

Preparation of calibration standards and quality control samples

A stock solution of bromantane was prepared in methanol at a concentration of 1.0 mg/mL. Standard solutions (10, 25, 50, 100, 500, 1000, 5000 ng/mL) were prepared by serial dilution of the stock solution with methanol. Low, medium and high concentration Quality Control (QC) solutions (4, 45, 125 ng/mL) were prepared in the similar way. The stock solution of I.S. (1.0 mg/mL) was also prepared in methanol and then diluted with methanol to a final concentration of 10 μg/mL. All solutions were stored at 4°C and used within one month after preparation. Calibration standards and QC samples were prepared by adding 50 μL standard and 50 μL IS or QC solution to 500 μL blank human plasma.

Sample preparation

A sample (500 μL) of human plasma was transferred to a 5.0 mL glass tube, 50 μL methanol or 50 μL standard of bromantane and 50 μL IS solutions were added. If needed (sample not transparent), the mixture was ultra-sonicated. SPE was conducted by using SOLA RP extraction cartridges. The cartridges were conditioned sequentially with 500 μL of ethanol and with 500 μL of water, and 500 μL of plasma sample diluted equal volume of water was then loaded. The loaded cartridges were washed with 500 μL 5% ethanol in water, and subsequently the analyte was eluted with ethanol. The elution was then evaporated to dryness under N2 stream at 50°C, reconstituted with 200 μL of methanol, and vortex mixed for 10 s. Finally, the solution was transferred to the autosampler vials, and 5 μL was injected into HPLC/MS/MS system.

Method validation

The method validation assays were carried out according to the currently accepted US Food and Drug Administration (FDA) bioanalytical method validation guidance [14].

The method's specificity was tested by screening six different batches of healthy human blank plasma. Each blank sample was tested for interference using the proposed extraction procedure and chromatographic/spectroscopic conditions and compared with those obtained with an aqueous solution of the analyte at a concentration near to the LLOQ.

The matrix effect on the ionization of analytes was evaluated by comparing the peak area of analytes resolved in blank sample (the final solution of blank plasma after extraction and reconstitution) with that resolved in mobile phase.

Three different concentration levels of bromantane (4, 45 and 125 ng/mL) were evaluated by analyzing five samples at each level. The blank plasma used in this study was five different batches of healthy human blank plasma. If the ratio <85 or >115%, an exogenous matrix effect was implied.

For the calibration standards, peak area ratios (the analyte/IS) were plotted against nominal plasma concentrations, and fitted by weighted ($1/y^2$) least-squares linear regression. Plasma calibration curves were prepared and assayed in triplicate on three separate days. In addition, blank plasma was also analyzed to confirm absence of interferences.

The intra-day precision and accuracy of the assay was measured by analyzing five spiked samples of bromantane at each QC level (4, 45 and 125 ng/mL). The inter-day precision and accuracy was determined over three consecutive days by analyzing 15 QC samples. The acceptance criteria for precision and accuracy deviation values should be within 15% of the actual values. The extraction yield (or absolute recovery) was determined by comparing the bromantane/IS peak area ratios obtained following the outlined extraction procedure (the procedure was a little different from the outlined extraction procedure for QC, calibration curve and clinical plasma samples, that is IS was added to the organic layer after the extraction of bromantane) and the result compared with those obtained from samples which contained the same amount of bromantane in extracted plasma but not be extracted after addition of the drug. This procedure was repeated for the three different concentrations of bromantane added, namely 4, 45 and 125 ng/mL.

For sensitivity determination, the LLOQ was defined as the lowest concentration in the calibration curve at which both precision and accuracy were less than or equal to 20%, and signal/noise (S/N) >10. The 1 ng/mL concentration was investigated as the lower limit of quantification. Reproducibility and precision were also determined.

To evaluate stability on repeat analysis of samples, freeze-thaw stability was determined for three concentrations of bromantane in plasma. QC plasma samples were tested after three freeze (–20°C) and thaw (room temperature) cycles.

Results and Discussion

LC/MS/MS conditions

Certain classes of compounds are traditionally very difficult to ionize or tend to show low sensitivity in LC/MS/MS techniques. Although electrospray ionization is often used as an LC-MS interface, APCI, another type of atmospheric pressure ionization, is more applicable to low polarity compounds [15]. In APCI, the corona discharge can provide a source of electrons in the gas-phase. This can be an advantage for such non polar compounds as adamantanes.

The LC–MS/MS operation parameters for determination of bromantane and IS were carefully optimized. Selenox was selected as the IS because its chromatographic behavior and extraction efficiency were similar to those of analyte. Both analyte and IS responded best to the positive ionization mode, with the protonated molecular ions $[M+H]^+$ as the major species. Full scan ion spectrum of Bromantane was shown in figure 1. The MRM acquisitions were performed at unit resolution using the transition 308.1 → 135.2 *m/z* for bromantane and 331.0 → 250.0 *m/z* for IS respectively (Figure 2). The transition 308.1 → 135.2 *m/z* was used for quantification of bromantane because of its stabilized ions response

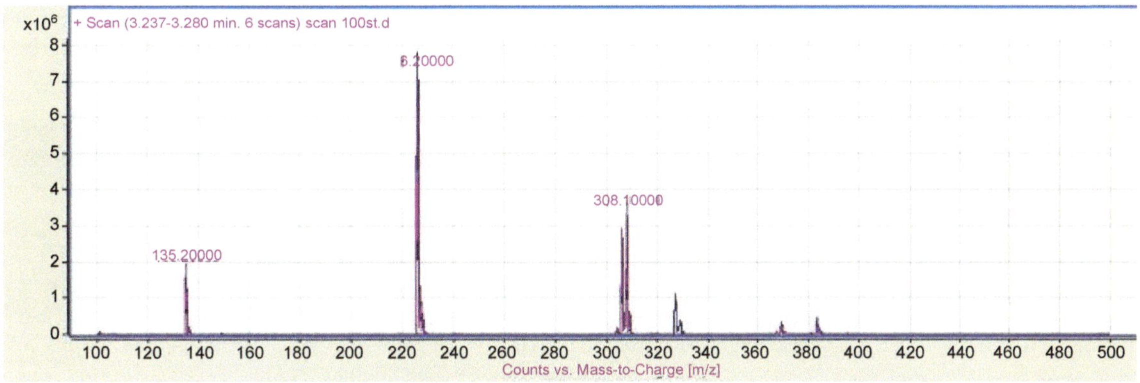

Figure 1: Full scan positive ion turbolonspray Q1 mass spectrum of Bromantane.

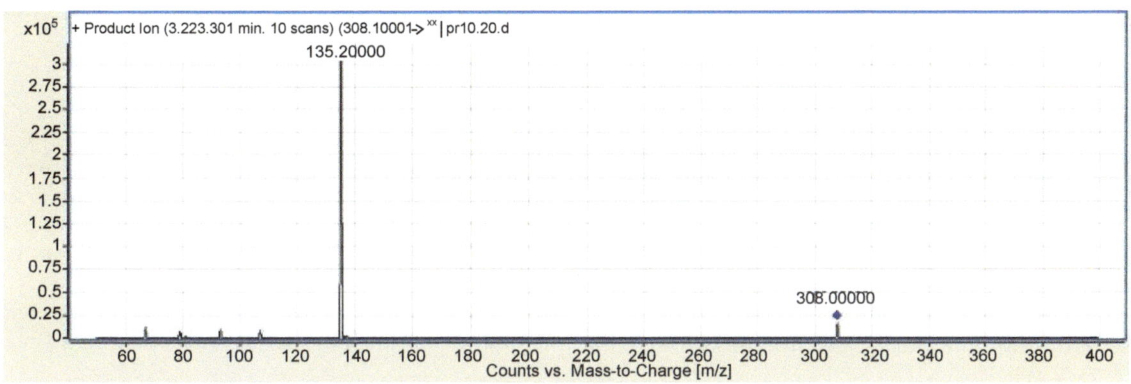

Figure 2: MS/MS spectrum of the m/z = 308.1 parent ion, exhibiting the product ions of Bromantane at m/z =135.2.

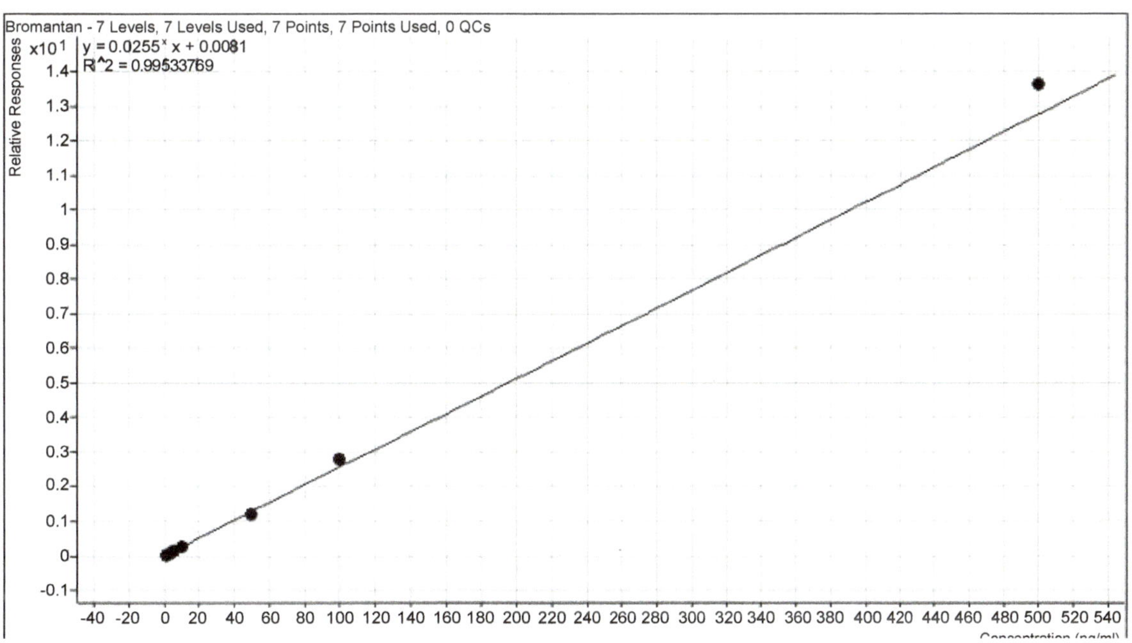

Figure 3: Regression line for the determination of Bromantane in human plasma.

and no endogenous interference. The mass parameters were optimized by observing the maximum response obtained for the product ions. The intensities of its protonated molecules were compared at fragmentor voltages of 90, 100, 120, 130, 135, 140 and 150 V in order to determine the optimal collision energy. The results showed that the highest sensitivities could be obtained by using a 135 V fragmentor voltage.

Furthermore, the mobile phase system was optimized through several trials to achieve satisfactory chromatographic behavior and the ionization responses of bromantane and IS. The ionization of bromantane and IS was affected by the composition of mobile phase. In the preliminary experiments, methanol, acetonitrile, ammonium acetate and formic acid in various proportions were tested. Methanol, rather than acetonitrile, was chosen as the organic modifier because it leads to the good peak shape of bromantane and satisfactory retention time. When ammonium acetate was added in the mobile phase, the response of the analyte was distinctly decreased. Both the analyte and IS were found to have higher response and better peak shapes in the mobile phase containing 0.5% formic acid. Finally, in terms of peak shape, retention time and sensitivity, we employed methanol -0.5% formic acid (95:5, v/v), as the mobile phase.

Assay validation

The linearity for bromantane was investigated by linear regression of peak area ratios against concentrations (Figure 3). The regression equation for the calibration plot was y=0.081+0.0255*x, with a coefficient of correlation (*r*) of 0.995 (where y – the ratio of the peak areas of bromantane to the peak area of the internal standard; x – bromantane concentration, ng/mL). The calibration curves of bromantane showed good linearity in the ranges of 1-500 ng/mL (Table 1). LLOQ for bromantane in plasma was proved to be 1 ng/mL (S/N=9.5) (Figure 4).

Our investigations have confirmed the fact of negligible matrix effects coupled to APCI [16]: the ratios of the peak responses for bromantane were 99.0%, 98.9%, and 100.3% at 4, 45 and 135 ng/mL, respectively (Figure 5). The results indicated that co-eluting endogenous substances hardly inhibited the ionization of bromantane, and the ion suppression from human plasma matrix was consistent for this analytical method and would not interfere with the measurement of analyte. Thus, no ion suppression was observed.

The extraction recovery determined for bromantane was shown to be consistent, precise and reproducible. The absolute recoveries of bromantane from the rat plasma at the three concentrations were about 89%. There was no significant difference in the extraction efficacy of the present assay over the range of concentrations studied.

The intra-day and inter-day precision (CV, $n = 5$) for bromantane were satisfactory at the three concentrations studied. Data on precision, accuracy are shown in table 2. The results of freeze–thaw stability indicated that the analyte is stable in plasma for three freeze–thaw cycles, when stored at–20°C and thawed to room temperature. Long-term stability indicates that storage of bromantane plasma samples at −20°C is adequate when stored for 30 days and no stability related problems would be expected during routine analysis for the pharmacokinetic or abuse control studies.

Conclusion

The proposed method of analysis provided a sensitive and specific assay for bromantane determination in human plasma. No significant interference caused by endogenous compounds was observed. The method was rapid, selective and highly sensitive with a LLOQ of 1 ng/mL for bromantane. Simple liquid–liquid extraction procedure and short run time can provide a short analysis time that is important for large sample batches. The developed method was completely validated showing satisfactory data for all the method validation parameters

Spike Conc.	RT	Final Conc.	Accuracy	Area	S/N	Area IS
1	3.21	1.02	102.3	661	9.5	19337
2.5	3.22	2.53	101.4	1321	16.0	18147
5	3.22	4.67	93.4	2305	26.7	18105
10	3.22	9.63	96.3	3841	16.3	15123
50	3.22	47.52	95.0	19068	82.6	15611
100	3.22	109.02	109.0	44764	143.2	16035
500	3.22	533.34	106.7	246547	209.4	18096

Table 1: The linearity of Bromantane determination.

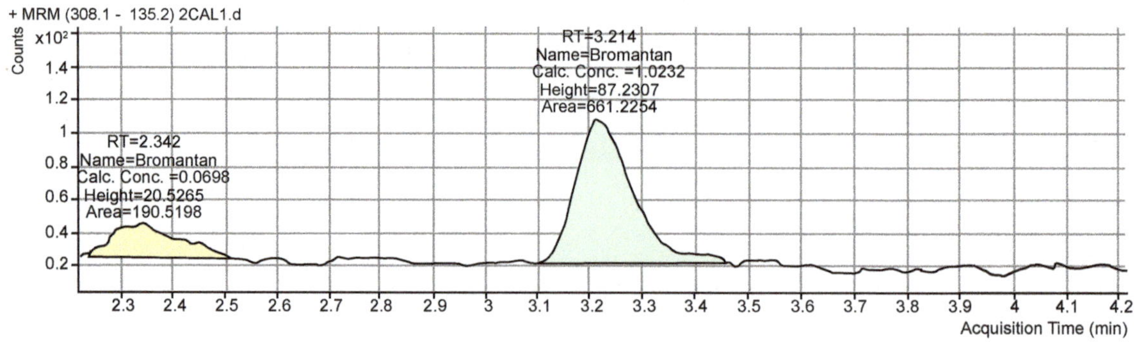

Figure 4: MRM mass chromatograms of LLOQ (1 ng/mL) of Bromantane.

Calculated *C* (ng/ml)	Found *C* (ng/ml)	Intra-day precision R.S.D. (%)	Inter-day precision R.S.D. (%)	Accuracy RE (%)
4	4.26	7.5	8.6	6.5
45	44.26	9.4	8.9	-1.6
135	138	5.1	7.3	1.9

Table 2: Accuracy and precision of the assay for determination of Bromantane in plasma (n=5).

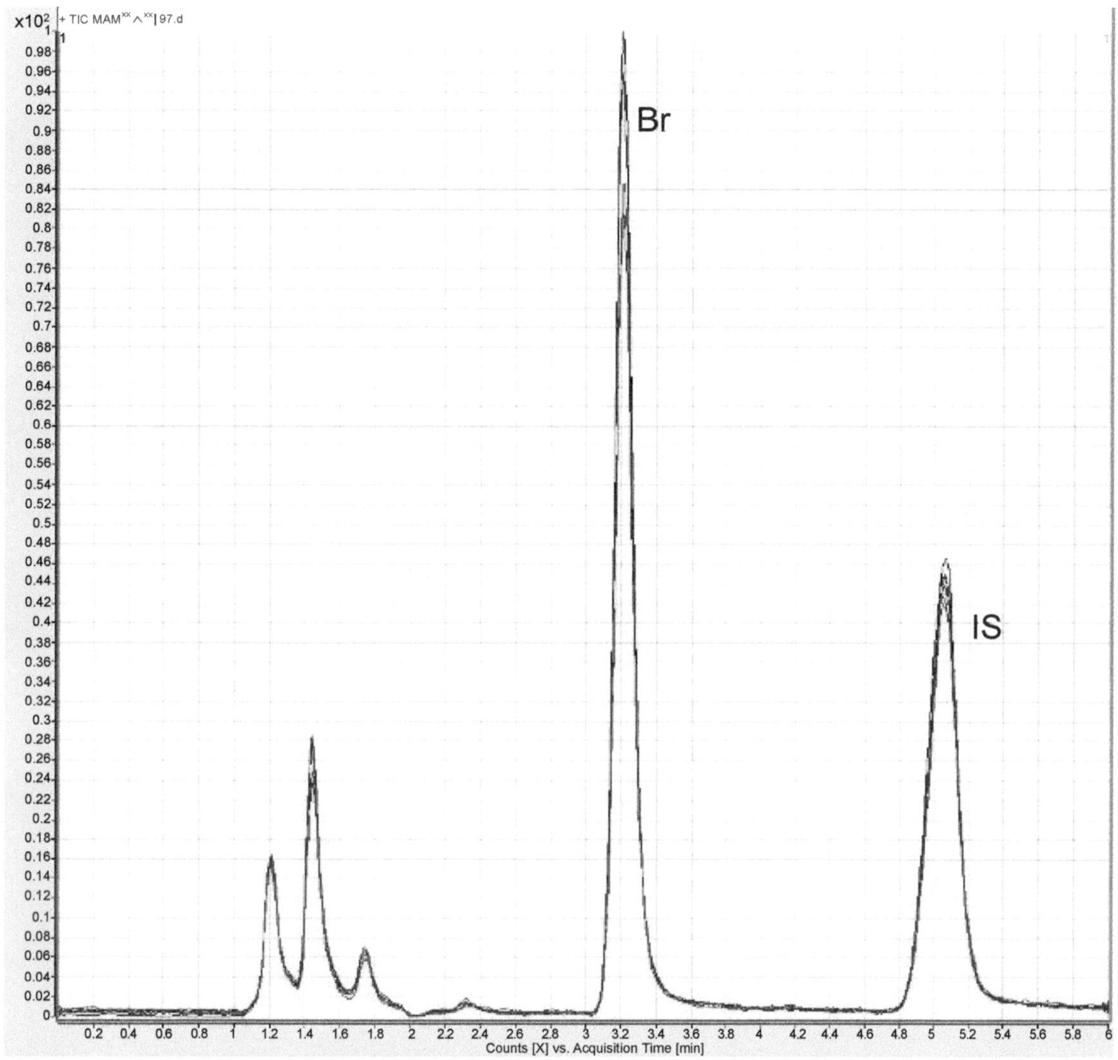

Figure 5: Typical mass chromatograms of plasma spiked with Bromantane (45 ng/mL) and the IS (1 µg/mL), validation of Bromantane Quantitation.

tested. It was shown that this method is suitable for the analysis of bromantane in plasma samples collected for pharmacokinetic, bioavailability, bioequivalence studies or doping control.

Acknowledgments

The authors are thankful to prof. N.N. Zolotov from the Institute of Pharmacology Russian Academy of Medical Sciences for providing sample of Bromantane for the research work.

References

1. Krapivin SV, Sergeeva SA, Morozov IS (1993) A quantitative pharmaco-electroencephalographic analysis of the action of bromantane. Biull Eksper Biolog Med 116: 515-518.
2. Grekhova TV, Gaĭnetdinov RR, Sotnikova TD, Krasnykh LM, Kudrin VS, et al. (1995) The effect of bromantane, a new immunostimulant with psychostimulating action, on release and metabolism of dopamine in the dorsal striatum of freely moving rats: a microdialysis study. Biull Eksper Biol Med 119: 302-304.
3. Kudrin VS, Sergeeva SA, Krasnykh LM, Miroshnichenko II, Grekhova TV, et al. (1995) The effect of bromantane on the dopamin- and serotoninergic systems of the rat brain. Eksper Klin Farmak 58: 8-11.
4. Morozov IS, Petrov V I, Sergeeva SA (2001) The Pharmacology of Adamantanes. Volgograd State Medical Academy, Volgograd.
5. Burnat P, Payen A, Le Brumant-Payen C, Hugon M, Ceppa F (1997) Bromontan, a new doping agent. Lancet 350: 963-964.
6. Bowers LD (2009) The analytical chemistry of drug monitoring in athletes. Annu Rev Anal Chem 2: 485–507.
7. Morozov IS, Pukhova GS, Avdulov NA, Sergeeva SA, Spasov AA, et al. (1999) The mechanisms of the neurotropic action of bromantan. Eksper Klin Farmak 62: 11-14.
8. Gui K, Wu M, Liu X, Zhang Y, Wang S (1999) Study on the metabolites of bromantane in urine using GC/MS and GC/Tandem MS/MS. In: Schanzer W, Geyer H, Gotzmann A, Mareck-Engelke U (Eds.), Recent advances in doping analysis. Sport and Buch Straus, Koln: 375-390.
9. Niwa M (2012) Chemical derivatization as a tool for optimizing MS response in sensitive LC-MS/MS bioanalysis and its role in pharmacokinetic studies. Bioanalysis 4: 213-220
10. Arndt T, Guessregen B, Hohl A, Reis J (2005) Determination of serum amantadine by liquid chromatography-tandem mass spectrometry. Clin Chim Acta 359: 125-131.
11. Almeida AA, Campos DR, Bernasconi G, Calafatti S, Barros FA, et al. (2007) Determination of memantine in human plasma by liquid chromatography-electrospray tandem mass spectrometry: application to a bioequivalence study. J Chromatogr B 848: 311–316.

12. Konda RK, Challa BR, Chandu BR, Chandrasekhar KB (2012) Bioanalytical method development and validation of memantine in human plasma by high performance liquid chromatography with tandem mass spectrometry: application to bioequivalence study. J Anal Methods Chem 2012: 1-8.

13. Meadows K, Liddicoat T, Oliver M (2012) Revolutionizing SPE for improved bioanalysis. Bioanalysis 4: 2661–2663.

14. Guidance for Industry, Bioanalytical Method Validation (2001) US Department of Health and Human Services, Food and Drug Administration, Center for Drug Evaluation and Research (CDER).

15. Hourani N, Kuhnert N (2012) High molecular weight non-polar hydrocarbons as pure model substances and in motor oil samples can be ionized without fragmentation by atmospheric pressure chemical ionization mass spectrometry. Rapid Commun Mass Spectrom 26: 2365-2371.

16. Ackermann BL, Berna MJ, Eckstein JA, Ott LW, Chaudhary AK (2008) Current applications of liquid chromatography/mass spectrometry in pharmaceutical discovery after a decade of innovation. Annu Rev Anal Chem 1: 357–396.

Levels of Professionalism among Physical Therapists in India- A National Cross-Sectional Survey

Senthil P Kumar[1]*, Vaishali Sisodia[2] and Ernest Jacob[3]

[1]*Associate Professor in Musculoskeletal and Manual Therapy, Dept of Physiotherapy, Kasturba Medical College, Manipal University, Mangalore, India*
[2]*Department of Physiotherapy, Career Institute of Medical Sciences, Bhopal, India*
[3]*Assistant Professor, Dr. M.V.Shetty College of Physiotherapy, Mangalore, India*

Abstract

Background and purpose: The American Physical Therapy Association (APTA) developed the core values of leadership, administration, management and professionalism for physical therapists. The aim of this study was to assess the levels of professionalism among physical therapists in India.

Materials and methods: This cross-sectional study was done using a survey questionnaire- Professionalism In Physical Therapy- Core Values (PPTCV) instrument that consisted of sample indicators for each of the seven core values- accountability (10 indicators), altruism (5 indicators), compassion/caring (11 indicators), excellence (11 indicators), integrity (12 indicators), professional duty (7 indicators), and social responsibility (12 indicators). Each sample indicator was to be rated using a 5-point Likert scale from 'never, rarely, occasionally, frequently and rarely.' 771 eligible questionnaires out of 889 participants with a response rate of 91.33% were analyzed and computed based upon individual- and profession-related variables. Descriptive analysis was done using SPSS version 11.5 (SPSS Inc, IL) at 95% confidence interval.

Results: Overall, high levels of professionalism was reported by post-graduate students, followed by researchers and teaching faculty. Younger male physical therapy students were more likely to report high levels of professionalism. Individually, accountability was high among teaching faculty, altruism, compassion/caring and social responsibility among clinician-therapists, and integrity and professional duty was high among researchers. No single professional category showed high levels of professionalism in all seven core values.

Conclusion: Overall levels of professionalism among Indian physical therapists were moderate, and altruism and compassion levels were also low. Other indicators of professionalism were fairly evenly distributed among the students and therapists, and between genders. The study findings are of importance to develop curricular and educational modifications to improve levels of professionalism among physical therapists in India and future studies are warranted around the world.

Keywords: Professionalism; Leadership; Administration; Management; Professional development

Introduction

Professionalism may be defined as; "the qualities or typical features of a profession or of professionals, especially competence, skills and code of behavior that maintains the ethics and dignity of the profession [1]. Professionalism in physical therapy includes those aspects of the occupational control of work which are in the best interests of customers, clients and patients, as well as in the advice-giving, lobbying and sometimes oppositional aspects of professions' relations with states, legislative bodies, and regional and local administrative agencies [2]. The other related term is professionalization that is often appropriately understood as development of profession while professionalism is development of professionals per se. Professionalization is a series of diverse and variable, social and historical processes of development, of how work sometimes becomes an occupation, and how occupations achieve various forms of occupational control of work sometimes called professional [3].

The earliest mentioning of professionalism in medicine was in the Hippocratic oath and ever since then, had been evolving through a series of milestones from 1847 when American Medical Association (AMA) code of medical ethics was established until 2002 when the physician's charter was formed [4]. The profession of physical therapy evolved from a medically directed clinical decision-making in treating patients to an autonomous direct-access service [5]. With growth in practice autonomy, there is an increased need for professional accountability which improves quality of provided care [6,7].

In 2003, the American physical therapy association developed the core values definition and included it as part of credentials and requirements for entry-level PT programmes [8]. In 2004, the eleven ethical principles were established by American Physical Therapy Association (APTA) as the Guide for professional conduct that involved the core values necessary for professional autonomy and interprofessional care [9]. Understanding the current levels of professionalism not only provides a baseline information upon which to further develop using educational and professional development strategies, but also to facilitate enhanced professionalization by addressing individual- and professional-related factors. The objective of the present study was to assess the levels of professionalism and core values among physical therapists in India.

Materials and Methods

The study design was an assessor-blinded cross-sectional study. The study was conducted at Dept of Physiotherapy; Kasturba Medical College (Manipal University), Mangalore and data was collected from

***Corresponding author:** Senthil P Kumar, Associate Professor in Musculoskeletal and Manual Therapy, PhD Candidate, Department of Physiotherapy, Kasturba Medical College (Manipal University), Mangalore, India, E-mail: senthil.kumar@manipal.edu

the conference participants at the 48th annual conference of Indian Association Of Physiotherapists (IAP), a national physiotherapy conference organized by Mangalore branch of IAP, from 21-23 January 2010. The APTA core values of professionalism self-evaluation form which were named as professionalism in Physical Therapy- Core Values (PPTCV) instrument was used for the data collection [10]. The survey questionnaire consisted of sample indicators for each of the seven core values- 1) accountability (10 indicators), 2) altruism (5 indicators), 3) compassion/caring (11 indicators), 4) excellence (11 indicators), 5) integrity (12 indicators), 6) professional duty (7 indicators), and 7) social responsibility (12 indicators). Each sample indicator was to be rated using a 5-point Likert scale from 'never, rarely, occasionally, frequently and rarely.' The questionnaire was designed for self-assessment and was validated and used previously.

All participants signed a written informed consent prior to answering the survey. The questionnaires were coded to ensure participant anonymity and privacy and confidentiality of obtained data. The data was collected by physiotherapy students and/or interns who were volunteers in the conference and were blinded from the purpose of the study.

Data synthesis

We considered seven professional categories (profession-related variables): under-graduate or entry-level student (2nd year, 3rd year, final year), intern, post-graduate student, practising therapist (private practitioner, hospital-based), educator/ teacher-faculty (freelancer, institution-based), researcher and administrator. Age and gender were considered as person-related variables. The overall scores and score of each of the seven core values were thus compared across the categories.

Data analysis

The questionnaire involved five-point Likert scaling and we converted the categorical variables into continuous by coding them according to their ascending order of emphasis eg, score-1 for 'never' and score-5 for 'always' as recommended by APTA scoring instructions. Thus we could compute means and standard deviations for the obtained scores for each core value, and total scores. We arbitrarily assigned the total scores and sub-scores categorized into six: < 15%- very low; 16-30%- low; 31-45%- moderate; 46-60%- fair; 61-75%- high; and, >75%- very high. The percentiles were obtained from calculating proportion of obtained scores with respect to total achievable scores. One-way analysis of variance (ANOVA) was used for between-group comparisons (professional and personal-related groups) and between-core value comparisons. Friedman's test was used for all comparisons of categorical variables. All analysis was done using SPSS version 16.0 (SPSS Inc, IL) at 95% confidence interval.

Results

Sample size estimation

There are a total 50,000 physiotherapists and 20,000 physiotherapy students in the country. Annually, the attendance of this conference ranges around 3,000 in which 500 may be students making it 85% physical therapists and 15% students. We arbitrarily anticipated moderate levels of professionalism among the participants at 50%-60% range scores in the questionnaire. Since the total score for the questionnaire is 345, the required score range was from 173-207. Hence using the sample size estimation formula we needed to recruit a minimum of 750 participants at 90% power and 5% type-1 error (alpha) [11]. To get a final number of 750, we needed to consider 1250 participants at a response rate of 60% (Table 1).

$N= Z^2 (1-\infty/2) P (1-P) / e^2$

N- Number of sample

Z^2- $(1.96)^2$ for 95% confidence interval (i.e., a=0.05 or 5%)

P- Best guess for prevalence (eg, ± 0.50)

e- Maximum tolerable/ acceptable error for the prevalence estimate (eg, ± .05 or 5%)

The survey was administered to 889 physical therapists and students, and 812 completed questionnaires were received with a response rate of 91.33%. The participants were selected by convenient sampling. After scrutiny, 771 eligible questionnaires were then analyzed and computed based upon individual- and profession-related variables.

Primary outcomes

The overall scores of PPT-CV for each of its core values are provided in table 2 and comparison between professional categories is given in table 3 and figure 1.

Though the female (145.24 ± 40.94) physical therapists had a higher overall score in PPT-CV than their male counterparts (140.02 ± 39.78), the difference was not statistically significant (p=0.088). Age had a strong positive correlation (r=0.809) with total scores of PPT-CV which was statistically significant (p=0.000).

Variables	Sub-categories		Values- individual	Values- total N (%)
Sample size, N				771
Gender N (%)	Male			319 (41.37%)
	Female			452 (58.63%)
Age (years) Mean ± SD				26.54 ± 4.87
Professional categories	Student/ intern	2nd year	13	376 (48.76%)
		3rd year	78	
		Final year	157	
		Intern	128	
	Professional	PG student	88	395 (51.24%)
		Practising therapist	114	
		Educator	185	
		Researcher	6	
		Administrator	2	

Table 1: Overall demographic characteristic of participants.

Core values	Number of indicators	Total score	Obtained score (overall)	Obtained (%) overall
Accountability	10	50	22.37 ± 9.76	44.74%[a]
Altruism	5	25	12.11 ± 4.16	48.44%[b]
Compassion/ caring	11	55	25.39 ± 8.42	46.16%[b]
Excellence	11	55	23.35 ± 7.68	42.45%[a]
Integrity	12	60	23.31 ± 7.72	38.85%[a]
Professional duty	7	35	14.01 ± 3.10	40.02%[a]
Social responsibility	12	60	22.51 ± 7.22	37.51%[a]
Total score	69	345	143.08 ± 40.52	41.47%[a]

[a]Moderate level of professionalism
[b]Fair level of professionalism

Table 2: Overall scores of PPT-CV for each of its seven subscales.

Professional category	Professionalism in physical therapy- core values (PPT-CV) Sub scores							Total score (PPT-CV)
	Accountability	Altruism	Compassion	Excellence	Integrity	Professional duty	Social responsibility	
2nd year	7.33 ± 1.18	6.07 ± 0.95	13.84 ± 2.11	14.07 ± 1.89	14 ± 2.19	8.15 ± 1.72	13.84 ± 2.11	77.30 ± 6.31
3rd year	10.92 ± 2.30	8.03 ± 0 .95	16.87 ± 1.65	16.85 ± 1.57	16.74 ± 1.7	11.46 ± 1.82	16.21 ± 2.38	97.11 ± 5.85
Final year	13.87 ± 1.68	8.56 ± 0.94	17.92 ± 1.47	17.94 ± 1.47	17.89 ± 1.47	12.47 ± 2.05	17.46 ± 1.21	106.13 ± 3.95
Intern	17 ± 1.70	8.46 ± 1.78	16.96 ± 2.13	16.96 ± 2.13	16.9 ± 2.05	11.86 ± 2.05	17.65 ± 2.37	105.82 ± 6.86
PG student	18.06 ± 1.49	12.54 ± 1.12	32.48 ± 1.88	32.23 ± 1.94	31.86 ± 2.77	13.01 ± 1.8	23.09 ± 1.74	163.30 ± 5.40
Practising the rapist	32.09 ± 2.04	16.29 ± 1.89	36.5 ± 2.86	20.85 ± 6.27	21.14 ± 6.54	16.3 ± 1.85	37.25 ± 2.72	180.45 ± 12.44
Educator	35.12 ± 1.96	16.96 ± 1.26	31.72 ± 2.24	39.16 ± 0.75	32.5 ± 1.97	17.02 ± 1.23	23.75 ± 2.38	189.69 ± 4.74
Researcher	24 ± 2.82	14.5 ± 1.87	26.83 ± 2.92	32.6 ± 1.26	39.66 ± 1.36	24.5 ± 1.04	29 ± 1.41	197.66 ± 2.16
Administrator	28 ± 1.41	8.5 ± 0.70	24 ± 5.65	21.5 ± 3.53	24.5 ± 3.53	14.5 ± 3.53	32.5 ± 3.53	153.50 ± 19.09

Table 3: Scores of sub-scales (core values) compared between nine professional categories.

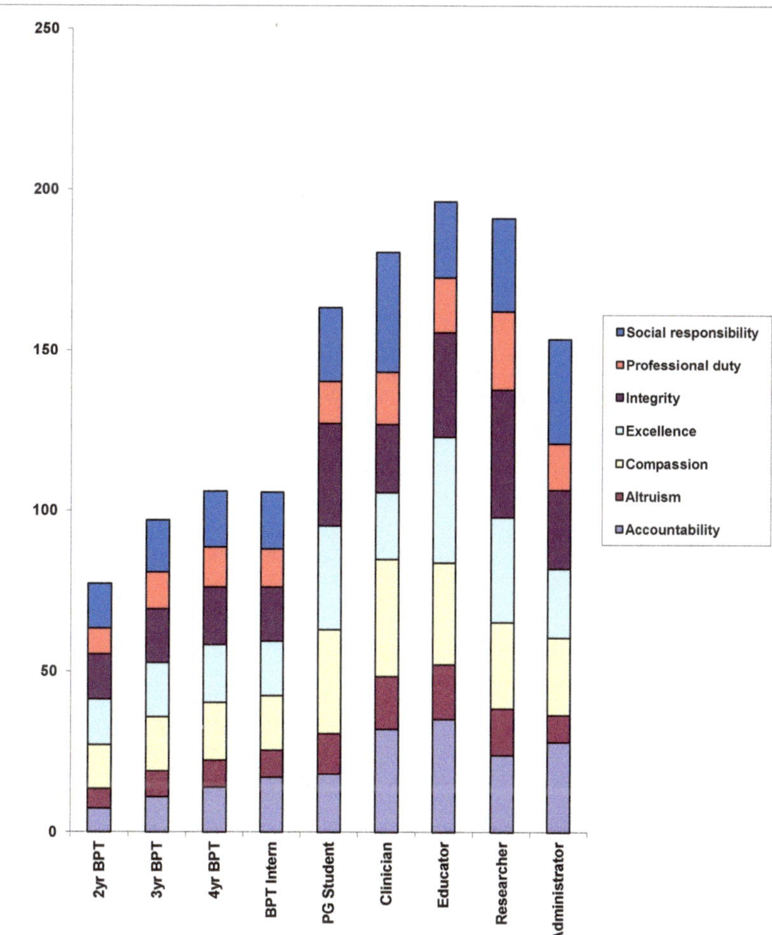

Figure 1: Comparison of scores of seven core values between the nine professional categories.

a < 15%- very low; b 16-30%- low; c 31-45%- moderate; d 46-60%- fair; e 61-75%- high; and, f >75%- very high

Main findings- summary:

Accountability=teaching faculty>clinician-therapists>administrators>researchers>post-graduate students>interns>4BPT>3BPT>2BPT.

Altruism=clinician-therapists>teaching faculty>researchers>interns>post-graduate students>administrators>interns>4BPT>3BPT>2BPT

Compassion/caring=clinician-therapists>teaching faculty>post-graduate students>interns>researchers>administrators>interns>4BPT>3BPT>2BPT

Excellence=researchers>post-graduate students>teaching faculty>clinician-therapists>interns>administrators>4BPT>3BPT>2BPT

Integrity=researchers>teaching faculty>clinician-therapists>post-graduate students>administrators>interns>4BPT>3BPT>2BPT

Professional duty=researchers>clinician-therapists>post-graduate students>teaching faculty>administrators>interns>4BPT>3BPT>2BPT

Social responsibility=clinician-therapists>administrators>researchers>teaching faculty>post-graduate students>interns>4BPT>3BPT>2BPT

Discussion

Factors influencing our findings

Internal and external factors influence the actual or reported levels of professionalism [12]. The internal factors (clinician-related) are knowledge, attitudes, beliefs and behaviors, and external factors (organization-related, public opinion-related, and professional leadership- local and national) inevitably exert a huge influence on the assessed levels of professionalism, and this may hold good among the PTs. Knowledge, not only about theoretical construct related to education, practice and research, but also related to profession and professionalism per se, would exert a huge impact on the reported levels of professionalism [13]. Assessing and facilitating positive attitudes towards professionalism and empathy was often less emphasized/reported in earlier studies. However, the actual behaviors might be different from attributions by individuals [14-16].

Comparison of findings with similar studies

We found higher scores of accountability, altruism, integrity, professional duty and social responsibility for PT interns compared to final/fourth year students, and such findings were reported earlier by Poirier and Gupchup who found increase in scores of accountability, altruism and integrity amongst pharmacy students from their first year to fourth year that the authors attributed to curricular and co-curricular activities in the institution [17,18].

Teachers: have the responsibility to be as role models for students both in classroom and clinical environment. The counter-argument favors professionalism being absorbed and learnt so that it is integrated into one's behavior, and not taught per se [19,20]. Beauchamp opined that teachers have the obligation to educate their residents not only for healing and caring of patients but also for active participation in managing the healthcare system [21]. Saultz suggested four steps to overcome the challenges to improve teaching professionalism that can be taken in the medical education community [22]. First, medical schools should address cost and access to care as first-order intellectual problems and should encourage research programs in these areas. Second, schools should develop programs to humanize science and restore scientific integrity beyond the requirements of compliance programs. Next, medical school leaders should celebrate those who best embody moral leadership in the profession. Finally, the medical education community should acknowledge that the availability of affordable health care to the public depends on the practice choices of medical school graduates and should accept greater responsibility for this outcome. The above suggestions are applicable to PT as well.

List of recommendations put forth by Wear and Kuczewski [23]:

- Each medical school and residency program should be evaluated in terms of efforts to empower residents and medical students to address problems and deficits in the learning environment.
- Educators should enlist medical students and residents in developing a theory of professionalism through reflection on the activities these groups see as important to fostering their professionalism.
- The professionalism of students should be fostered by encouraging positive behaviors in each of the relationships that contribute to patient care and rewarding such behaviors. In other words, we must encourage residents and medical students when they exhibit leadership in professionalism and try to correct problems they see in the patient-care relationships around them.
- Teaching about professionalism must include education relating to social justice. Such justice education must include a macrocosmic picture of the economics of healthcare and a microcosmic picture of how injustice is reflected in the social and cultural barriers encountered daily within the clinic.

Clinical practitioners: Plochg et al. suggested seven strategies to transform professionalism to fit changing health needs: defining professionalism; creating supportive professional bodies; targeting research funding; targeting technology development; modernizing curricula; managing performance; and, developing supportive payment models. The core role of the practitioner was identified as having three components: dynamic practice, professional efficacy and clinical leadership [24,25]. In an era of consumerism in health care, professionalism equally should be emphasized and made to grow through two special initiatives: accountability and efficiency [26].

The moral obligations of a medical practitioner include "professional ethics" that regulate a wide range of professional conduct of which three types are of exceptional importance: preserving the focal values of the medical profession, protecting the Patient-Physician Relationship (PPR), and promoting the patient's best interest [27]. Robert Veatch, an American pioneer bioethicist, proposed four models of the Patient-Physician Relationship (PPR) in 1972: "engineering", "priestly", "collegial", and "contractual" [28]. Emanuel and Emanuel proposed another four PPR models: "paternalistic", "deliberative", "interpretive", and "informative". The roles of physician extend far from being mentors, to being technicians or contractors, or as friends or counselors [28,29].

Professionalism operates on a system of relationships: physician-patient, physician-society, physician-health care system, physician-physician, and physician-to-self [30]. The more recently evolved 'contractual model' and commercialization has lead to demise of medical professionalism by two ways- physician-owned clinical services and managed care payment policies [31]. Clinicians who had undergone continuing professional development programmes had improved levels of professionalism and they chose supervision as a method for self-directed professional development [32].

Suggestions for future studies: Studies' following up the students across a curriculum was done earlier amongst pharmacy students and such studies may be warranted to attribute factors responsible for changes in levels of professionalism [17]. Evaluation methodology for assessment of professionalism should be more quantitative such as Objective Structured Clinical Examination (OSCE) to evaluate separate elements and value conflicts and thereby to resolve them and recognize the contextual nature of professional behaviors and their environmental influences [33]. Professionalism can also be assessed using a combination of observed clinical encounters, multisource feedback, patients' opinions, paper-based tests or simulations, measures of research and/or teaching activities, and scrutiny of self-assessments compared with assessments by others [34].

Future studies are also indicated on assessment centers reported by Deusinger et al. which were implemented by Missouri Physical Therapy Association [35]. Such assessment centers enabled individuals to assess voluntarily their own practice competence and to use the results of the assessment to plan educational pursuits that might enhance professional growth. Bruhn advised three levels of aggressive intervention for improving professionalism among health care professionals- the professional organization, the organization one works for, and the individual- to revitalize good citizenship and professionalism [36].

Hayward and Blackmer found significant changes in PPTCV scores following doctor of physical therapy program in their institute [37]. The authors also found that those with high levels of professionalism had higher work-related self-efficacy and confidence. There is a scope for such interventional studies to be done among Indian PTs. With the ever-continuing growth in research in terms of randomized clinical trials and systematic reviews, and realization to 'think out of the box' into a rehabilitation framework in clinical practice necessitates.

Conclusions

Overall levels of professionalism among Indian physical therapists were moderate, and altruism and compassion levels were also low. Other indicators of professionalism were fairly evenly distributed among the students and therapists, and between genders. A relatively higher level of professionalism was observed with increase in age of the individual.

Implications

Professionalism is central to the survival of our profession. First, professionalism is the therapist's attitude and behavior in the practice of physical therapy. Second, it is a promise to serve not only the patient but also the society in which we practice. Third, it is accepting an unambiguous accountability to the healthcare system. It is a moral obligation. In a society overwhelmed by the spiraling cost of healthcare, we must be responsive to the state and the public which demands for accountability. There is a question of justice. Our own professional autonomy is related to our compliance with the values and needs of our community. On the other hand, it is our duty to resist any action that does not conform to the technical and moral ideal of the profession. There is no reason why anyone should become slaves to the healthcare system, consumers or the healthcare industry. Keeping a balance is not easy and requires courage. Finally, the teaching of professionalism and transmitting the soul of the profession is part of the profession's very long tradition and we have the responsibility to carry on this tradition [21]. The study findings thus are of importance to develop curricular and educational modifications to improve levels of professionalism among physical therapists in India and future studies are warranted around the world.

Future efforts at understanding professionalism, and future methods of evaluating professionalism, must focus on behaviors rather than personality traits or vague concepts of character. Our understanding and evaluation must include context and conflict in order to be relevant and valid. Ideally, methods of evaluation should include elements of peer assessment and self-assessment, which are becoming required elements in the continuing professional development of all practicing physicians. Finally, we should attempt to understand what drives students to demonstrate occasional lapses in professional behavior, in order to develop effective teaching and remediation in this domain [16].

Acknowledgements

The American Physical Therapy Association (APTA) for developing the survey instrument and granting permission for reprint and use in this study and the study participants for taking their valuable time to respond to the survey questionnaire. Prof Ifthikar Ali, organizing secretary of 48th annual conference of Indian Association of Physiotherapists (IAP) and convener- IAP Mangalore branch for granting permission to collect the data.

Related information

The study was presented as a platform presentation in Chartered Society of Physiotherapy (CSP) 2011 Congress conducted on 7-8th October 2011 at BT convention center, Liverpool, UK. The presentation was done by SPK and was funded by Faculty Research Incentives Grant of Manipal University, India.

References

1. Swick HM (2000) Toward a normative definition of medical professionalism. Acad Med 75: 612-616
2. Kumar SP (2011) Physical therapy- a review of realization of the need versus need for realization. Physiotimes 2: 12-15.
3. Marcus ER (1999) Empathy, humanism, and the professionalization process of medical education. Acad Med 74: 1211-1215.
4. Stevens RA (2002) Themes in the history of medical professionalism. Mt Sinai J Med 69: 357-362.
5. Kumar SP (2010) Evolution of professional autonomy in physical therapy practice- a century-long walk through PubMed from 1910-2010. J Phys Ther 2: 1-10.
6. Schneller ES, Wilson NA (2009) Professionalism in 21st century professional practice- autonomy and accountability in orthopaedic surgery. Clin Orthop Relat Res 467: 2561-2569.
7. Pawlson LG, O'Kane ME (2002) Professionalism, regulation and the market: impact on accountability for quality of care- physicians and accreditors need to respond to the market's emerging dominant influence on accountability. Health Aff 21: 200-207.
8. Davis DS (2009) Teaching professionalism: a survey of physical therapy educators. J Allied Health 38: 74-80.
9. Lopopolo RB, Schafer DS, Nosse LJ (2004) Leadership, administration, management, and professionalism (LAMP) in physical therapy: a Delphi study. Phys Ther 84: 137-150.
10. 10. American Physical Therapy Association (2003) Professionalism in physical therapy: core values- self-assessment. Alexandria, Virginia.
11. Sample size calculator (2012). National Statistical Service, Australian Bureau of Statistics, Locked Bag 10, Belconnen ACT 2616, Australia.
12. Ratanawongsa N, Bolen S, Howell EE, Kern DE, Sisson SD (2006) Residents' perceptions of professionalism in training and practice: barriers, promoters, and duty hour requirements. J Gen Intern Med 21: 758-763.
13. Kraemer WJ (2005) The body of knowledge: use and professionalism. J Strength Cond Res 27: 33-35.
14. Jha V, Bekker HL, Duffy SRG, Roberts TE (2007) A systematic review of studies assessing and facilitating attitudes towards professionalism in medicine. Med Educ 41: 822-829.

15. Crandall SJ, Marion GS (2009) Identifying attitudes towards empathy: an essential feature of professionalism. Acad Med 84: 1174-1176.

16. Hickson GB, Pichert JW, Webb LE, Gabbe SG (2007) A complementary approach to promoting professionalism: identifying, measuring, and addressing unprofessional behaviors. Acad Med 82: 1040-1048.

17. Poirier TI, Gupchup GV (2010) Assessment of pharmacy student professionalism across a curriculum. Am J Pharm Educ 74: 62

18. Bennett AJ, Roman B, Arnold LM, Kay J, Goldenhar LM (2005) Professionalism deficits among medical students: models of identification and intervention. Acad Psychiatry 29: 426-432.

19. Harris GD (2004) Professionalism: part I- introduction and being a role model. Family Med 36: 314-315.

20. Hochberg MS, Kalet A, Zabar S, Kachur E, Gillespie C, et al. (2010) Can professionalism be taught? Encouraging evidence. Am J Surg 199: 86-93.

21. Beauchamp G (2004) The challenge of teaching professionalism. Ann Acad Med Singapore 33: 697-705.

22. Saultz JW (2007) Are we serious about teaching professionalism in medicine? Acad Med 82: 574-577.

23. Wear D, Kuczewski MG (2004) The professionalism movement: can we pause? Am J Bioeth 4:1-10.

24. Plochg T, Klazinga NS, Starfield B (2009) Transforming medical professionalism to fit changing health needs. BMC Med 7: 64.

25. Carryer J, Gardner G, Dunn S, Gardner A (2007) The core role of the nurse practitioner: practice, professionalism and clinical leadership. J Clin Nurs 16: 1818-1825.

26. Imanaka Y (1999) Professionalism and consumerism: can they grow together? Int J Qual Health Care 9: 395-397.

27. Hui EC (2005) The physician as a professional and the moral implications of medical professionalism. Hong Kong Med J 11: 67-69.

28. Hui EC (2005) The centrality of patient-physician relationship to medical professionalism: an ethical evaluation of some contemporary models. Hong Kong Med J 11: 222-223.

29. Emanuel EJ, Emanuel LL (1992) Four models of the physician-patient relationship. JAMA 267: 2221-2226.

30. Walker KL, Arnold CL, Miller-Day M, Webb LM (2002) Investigating the physician-patient relationship: examining emerging themes. Health Commun 14: 45-68.

31. Hui EC (2005) The contractual model of the patient-physician relationship and the demise of medical professionalism. Hong Kong Med J 11: 420-422.

32. Tulinius C, Holge-Hazelton B (2010) Continuing professional development for general practitioners: supporting the development of professionalism. Med Educ 44: 412-420.

33. Arnold L (2002) Assessing professional behavior: yesterday, today and tomorrow. Acad Med 77: 502-515.

34. Wilkinson TJ, Wade WB, Knock LD (2009) A blueprint to assess professionalism: results of a systematic review. Academic Medicine 84: 551-558.

35. Deusinger SS, Sindelar B, Stritter FT (1986) Assessment center- a model for professional development and evaluation. Phys Ther 66: 1119-1123.

36. Bruhn JG (2001) Being Good and Doing Good: The Culture of Professionalism in the Health Professions. Health Care Manag 19: 47-58.

37. Hayward LM, Blackmer B (2010) A model for teaching and assessing core values development in doctor of physical therapy students. J Phys Ther Educ 24: 16-26.

Comparison of Cardiorespiratory and Hormonal Responses between Sustained Constant and Alternating Intensity Exercise

Spanoudaki S[1]*, Maridaki M[1], Karatzanos E[2], Bogdanis GC[1], Spanoudaki C[3] and Baltopoulos P[1]

[1]*Department of Sports Medicine & Biology of Physical Activity, Faculty of Physical Education and Sports Science, National & Kapodistrian University of Athens, 41 Ethnikis Antistasis, Dafni, Greece*
[2]*Cardiopulmonary Exercise Testing and Rehabilitation Laboratory, Evgenidio Hospital, School of Medicine, National & Kapodistrian University of Athens, Greece, 20 Papadiamantopoulou Str., 115 28, Athens, Greece*
[3]*Neonatal Intensive Care Unit, General Hospital of Chania, Greece*

Abstract

Background: Cardiorespiratory and hormonal responses were investigated during and after prolonged exercise of constant and alternating exercise intensity.

Methods: Ten healthy males underwent two main cycling exercise trials at the same overall power output, lasting one hour each. During the first trial, exercise intensity was constant at 70±5% VO_{2max}, while during the second trial, exercise intensity was alternated between 47±2% VO_{2max} for 40 s and 120% VO_{2max} for 20 s.

Results: Oxygen uptake (VO_2) and heart rate (HR) were higher in constant compared with alternating intensity exercise (VO_2: 32.5±6.6 vs. 29.8±5.9 ml/kg/min, $p<0.05$; HR: 152 ± 16 vs. 142 ± 15 b/min, $p<0.05$). Pulmonary ventilation, respiratory exchange ratio and blood lactate were similar in both trials. Plasma adrenaline and growth hormone during and 1 hour after exercise were similar in both trials, while nor-adrenaline was higher during constant intensity exercise ($p<0.05$). Significant time effects were found for all cardiorespiratory, lactate and hormonal parameters.

Conclusions: Constant and alternating intensity exercise of the same mean intensity and duration provoked similar changes in terms of stress and blood- lactate, while VO_2 and HR responses and nor-adrenaline concentration were higher when exercise intensity was constant, suggesting that constant exercise impose greater demand on the cardiovascular system.

Keywords: Adrenaline; Noradrenaline; Growth hormone; Blood-lactate

Introduction

Alternating intensity exercise consists of repeated periods of intense exercise followed by periods of less intense exercise. This type of exercise is used in many sports activities and it has the advantage that high intensity can be sustained for longer period of time than during constant exercise, depending on exercise protocols (ratio of exercise- rest, intensity [1,2]. Furthermore, it is well established that alternating intensity training improves performance of athletes and sedentary populations [1]. Comparison of the two exercise patterns are important, as both types are used in sports training in order to facilitate physiological adaptations to improve performance.

A few studies have examined the acute cardiorespiratory and metabolic response in intermittent exercise in comparison to constant exercise. Some of these showed that maximal oxygen uptake (VO_2), pulmonary ventilation (VE), respiratory exchange ratio (R), and heart rate (HR) did not differ between the two exercise protocols [3-5], or found lower values [6-8] or were higher compared to intermittent exercise [9].

Also, there are only a few studies that examined and compared hormonal changes in terms of stress response between constant and intermittent exercise. Catecholamines (adrenaline, nor-adrenaline) are known to regulate important cardiorespiratory and metabolic functions [10]. Nieman et al. [11], showed that adrenaline concentration was the same after both exercise regimes using a cycle ergometer. Moreover, growth hormone (GH) has been found to be either higher with intermittent exercise [12] or similar to constant [13].

Exercise at a high intensity results in an increase of VO_2 and blood lactate concentration in a non – sustainable way. Thus, it may be expected that the hormonal responses to alternating exercise would differ from those observed during constant exercise, even if mean intensity is similar. We hypothesized that alternating intensity exercise would evoke larger cardiorespiratory and hormonal responses than constant exercise, implying that alternating exercise is more stressful and demanding.

To the best of our knowledge, there is no other study that compared cardiorespiratory, stress responses and blood lactate concentration between the two types of exercise, when power output and exercise duration are equal. Thus, the purpose of this study was to compare the cardiorespiratory and hormonal response in constant and alternating intensity exercise of the same duration and average intensity.

Material and Methods

Participants

Ten healthy moderately trained young men volunteered for the study (age: 24.7±4.7 years, body mass: 78.5±8.9 kg, height: 180.8±6 cm, body fat: 9.1±3.1%. Prior to commencement, approval was obtained from the Institutional Ethical Committee and all experimental procedures

***Corresponding author:** Sofia S. Spanoudaki, Department of Sports Medicine & Biology of Physical Activity, Faculty of Physical Education and Sports Science, National & Kapodistrian University of Athens, Valtetsiou St, Vrilissia 15235, Athens, Greece, E-mail: sspanoud@ yahoo.gr

conformed to the Declaration of Helsinki for experimentation with human participants. All participants were informed of all procedures and purposes of the study and gave their written informed consent.

Experimental design

Each participant completed three preliminary tests for a) measurement of VO_{2max}, b)onset of blood lactate accumulation, and c) familiarization with the two main tests: I) constant and II) alternating intensity exercise protocol. These laboratory tests were conducted on five separate occasions. VO_{2max} and lactate threshold tests were conducted at least three days apart and no longer than a week. The two main tests were conducted one week apart in random order and took place at the same time of the day (at 6:00 am), so as to avoid alternations on performance because of circardian rhythm. Participants were fasted overnight and avoided exercise 2 days prior to the main tests. Also, they were asked to write down their food diary for the last 2 days before the first main test, and follow the same diet, so as to consume the same foods in both tests.

All tests (VO_{2max}, submaximal, Constant and Alternating intensity exercise) were conducted on the same modified, friction loaded cycle ergometer (Monark model, Sweden) in which a special alteration was made in order to run the alternating intensity exercise test. Specifically, a mechanical construction was affixed on the handles of the cycle ergometer and had the ability to change the workload of the cycle ergometer instantaneously with a flip of a switch. This operation was conducted manually by an assistant. Also, the cycle ergometer was equipped with a photocell, which monitored the velocity of the flywheel (122 black and white strips placed on the flywheel rim). The signal was amplified (Biopac Systems Inc) and stored on a computer. The calculation of power output was described elsewhere [14]. Shortly, Instantaneous flywheel velocity data were low pass filtered with a cut off frequency of Hz and flywheel acceleration was obtained by digital derivation. Flywheel inertia was calculated from deceleration measurements against different loads and power output was corrected for changes in kinetic energy of the flywheel. Values of power output and pedal rate were averaged over each pedal down stroke.

Protocol of VO_{2max} and onset of blood lactate accumulation

VO_{2max} was determined by continuous incremental cycling test to exhaustion with open circuit – spirometry (MedGraphics CPX/D, USA). The pedaling frequency was set at 70 rpm and was maintained throughout the test. VO_{2max} was defined as the highest VO_2 obtained in 30 seconds. Each participant was verbally encouraged to continue exercise until volitional exhaustion. The test was terminated when the participants met at least three of the following five criteria: a) a plateau in the VO_2 vs. exercise intensity relationship, which has been defined as an increase in VO_2 of less than 2ml/Kg/min with an increase in exercise intensity, b) R greater than 1.1, c) a final heart rate within 10 b/min of the age predicted maximum, d) participants fatigue and e) a rating of perceived exhaustion (RPE) of 19-20 on the Borg scale. Prior to each test, the gas analyzers were calibrated, using gases of known O_2 and CO_2 concentrations.

Maximal Power Output (POmax) was defined as the highest average power output during the last minute of the VO_{2max} protocol.

During the onset of blood lactate accumulation test (OBLA), each subject performed 5 submaximal sets using the cycle ergometer, which each lasting 5 minutes and the frequency was set at 70 rpm. The pedaling frequency was maintained through both tests, with the aid of a digital display adjusted to the bike. In addition, an assistant was verbally giving feedback to the participants, to either speed up, slow down, or maintain the pedaling frequency. At the end of each set, 20μl of blood was taken from the participant's fingertip and diluted with 200μl percloric acid and then stored at -20°C until the analysis was conducted. Determination of the OBLA (based on the 4mmole/l method) was obtained from non-linear plots of exercise intensity (power) against lactate concentration [15]. Four hours before each test participants were told to refrain from consuming food, coffee and alcohol.

Constant- alternating intensity protocol

The duration of each test was 1 hour with the same mean intensity at 105% of the OBLA for both protocols. Alternating intensity exercise was a continuous protocol in which there was no rest period and intensity fluctuated in a repeating pattern. The exercise protocol has been explained in detail previously [16]. Shortly, during constant exercise (CON), participants cycled at a power output corresponding to 105% of the OBLA (69.8±4.7% VO_{2max}). During alternating intensity exercise (ALT), 40 seconds of light exercise, (46.5±1.9% VO_{2max}), was alternated with 20 seconds intervals of hard cycling at 120% of VO_{2max}, so as the mean intensity (power output) was the same. The intensity of both protocols was based on pilot studies in which intensities corresponding from105% - 115% OBLA were tested. The intensity corresponding to 105% OBLA was chosen because all athletes could manage to exercise for at least 1 hour. Supramaximal intensity (120% of VO_{2max}) would recruit energy from both aerobic and anaerobic sources [17], suggesting different metabolic response between the two exercise protocols. Exercise intensity was calculated based on the equation of power (kg) against % of VO_2 in submaximal tests, and from the equation of time spent at 40′′ and 20′′ [(OBLA+ (5%of OBLA x OBLA)-(0.33*40%)]/0.66. The pedaling frequency was set at 70 rpm and maintained through both tests (both the slow and fast parts of the ALT exercise) with the aid of digital display adjusted to the bike. Furthermore, an assistant was verbally giving feedback to the participants.

Both protocols were conducted under the same environmental conditions (temperature of 20°C – 22°C, and relative humidity of 45-50%).

Measurements

Body composition: Percent of body fat was estimated by measuring skinfold thickness at four sites (biceps, triceps, suprailiac, subcapular) using a caliper [18].

Ventilatory parameters: VO_2, VE, and R were measured breath by breath. In both main trials (ALT and CON exercise) the ventilatory parameters were measured continuously during the first 10 minutes of the exercise and then continuously for the last 3 minutes of each of the remaining 10 minute intervals, until the completion of the exercise.

Lactate analysis (La): 20μl capillary blood from fingertips was collected at rest, 5, 10, 15, 20, 30, 40, 50 and 60 minutes for lactate concentration. The analysis of the lactate was made photometrically (Jenway, 3600, UK, [19]).

Heart rate was measured continuously throughout the tests with Polar (Sports Tester, Filand). Each test performed with the same HR monitor.

Borg scale: The subject perception of exertion during each test was referenced with 6-20 scale [15].

Venous blood sampling

Venous blood samples were drawn from an antecubital vein from each participant, in the sitting position, at the following times: prior to test, during the last seconds of 30 and 60 minutes of exercise and 1 hour after the end of exercise. Changes of plasma volume were calculated from Hemoglobin and Hematocrit according to Dill and Costil [20] equations.

Hormones

For Nor- adrenaline (NADR) and adrenaline (ADR) measurement, 2ml of blood for each hormone was collected into EDTA tubes and centrifuged and the plasma stored at -70°C until analysis. The concentration of each catecholamine was measured using the commercially available Elisa Kit (Biosource, Belgium, KAPL 10-200, KAPL 10-0100). The intra- and interassay coefficients of variation have been reported to be less than 5.2% and 7.0%, respectively

For Growth Hormone analysis (GH), serum was separated from whole blood by centrifugation at 1000 g for 10 min at room temperature, then, stored at -70˚C until analysis was conducted. The concentration of growth hormone was measured using the commercially available Elisa Kit (Biosource, Belgium, KAP1081). The intra- and interassay coefficients of variation have been reported to be less than 9.8% and 15%, respectively.

Hematocrit - Hemoglobin: were measured via routine methods (ABBOT, USA).

Statistical analysis

Data are presented as means and ±SD. Differences between the two conditions over time were analyzed using two-way ANOVA with repeated measures. In case a statistical significance was detected, a Tukey - Post Hoc Test was conducted for multiple comparisons. Statistical analysis was performed using Statistica V.8, the level of significance was set at $p<0.05$. Power analysis was conducted by commercial available software (G*Power 3.1, Germany), level was set at 0.8 level.

Results

Performance baseline characteristics of the subjects were: VO_{2max}: 47.9 ± 6.5 ml/kg/min, HRmax: 188 ± 12 b/min, maximal power (POmax): 267 ± 18 Watts and VO_2 at LT: 32.3±5.0 ml/kg/min. Mean PO for CON was 154 ± 17 Watts, (57.8±6.5% POmax), while mean PO for ALT was 158.8 ±20.5 Watts, (59.4± 7.8 % POmax). No difference was found between the two exercise protocols concerning PO, either in relative or absolute values, ($p=0.12$).

Cardiorespiratory and metabolic parameters

Oxygen uptake (VO_2) was affected by the type of exercise, with higher VO_2 in CON compared to ALT exercise, (32.5±6.6 vs. 29.8±5.9 ml/kg/min, $p<0.05$, see Figure 1). VO_2 was also, affected by the time ($p<0.01$, see Figure 1 and increased in both CON and ALT over time). Similarly, HR was overall higher in CON compared to ALT exercise, (152 ± 16 vs. 142 ± 15 b/min, see Figure 2). The type of exercise had no effect on VE ($p=0.55$, see Figure 3) or on the R value ($p=0.42$, see Figure 4). There was a drift in VO_2, HR and VE showing a gradual increase, while R showed a gradual decrease over time (Figures 1-4).

Changes in blood lactate concentration for CON and ALT are shown in Figure 5. Lactate concentration increased over time ($p<0.01$) in both exercise conditions, but there were no significant differences between the two protocols ($p = 0.75$).

Hormonal parameters

There were no significant differences in plasma volume changes between CON and ALT from rest to the 30th minute ($p= 0.11$), from rest to the 60th minute of exercise ($p = 0.33$) and from rest to 1 hour post-exercise ($p = 0.36$). Table 1 shows the changes in hormone

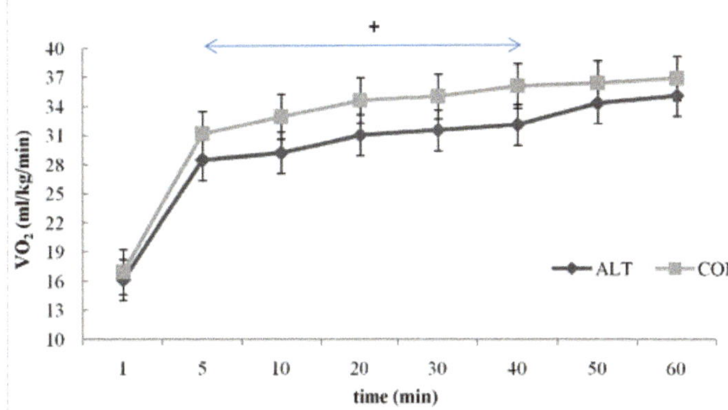

+ significant difference between CON and ALT at 5, 10, 30, and 40 minutes ($p<0.05$).

Figure 1: Changes in VO_2 (mean ± SD) in constant and alternating intensity exercise.

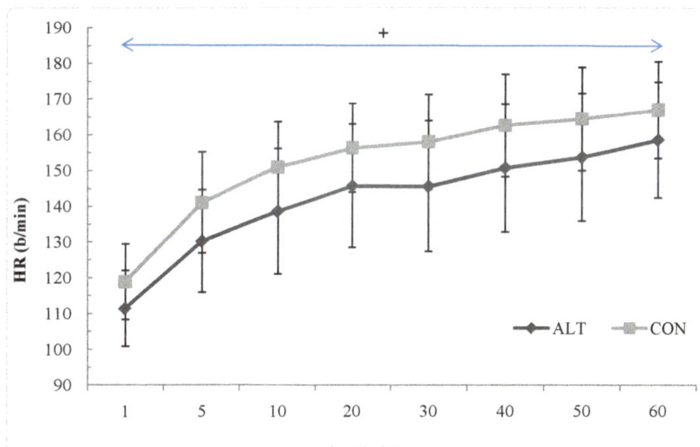

+ significant difference between CON and ALT ($p<0.05$).

Figure 2: Changes in HR (mean ± SD) in constant and alternating intensity exercise.

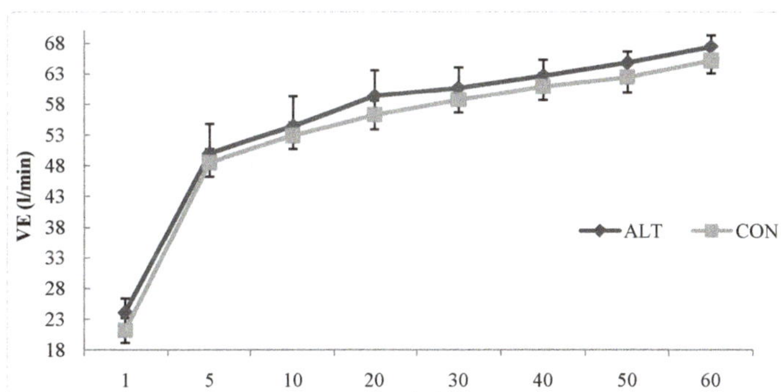

Figure 3: Changes in VE (mean ± SD) in constant and alternating intensity exercise.

concentration in CON and ALT. There was no difference between CON and ALT in the changes of ADR ($p=0.22$), and GH ($p=0.80$), but there were significant main effects for time ($p<0.01$). ADR and GH increased at 30 and 60 minute of exercise and returned to the resting values 1 hour post exercise (Table 1). Changes in NADR concentration were affected by the type ($p=0.05$) of exercise and by time ($p<0.01$) with values in CON being higher than values in ALT. The NADR concentration was increased from rest over time and returned to resting value 1 hour post exercise (Table 1). For all 3 hormones examined, higher values were observed at the 30th and 60th min of exercise in comparison to rest ($p\leq 0.01$), but no differences were observed between rest and 1 hour post exercise ($p> 0.05$). For NADR and GH there were also significant difference between the 30th and 60th min of exercise ($p\leq 0.05$).

In relation to type of exercise and the interaction of 'time by type', power analysis showed that sample size is not a confounding factor (ADR: 0.22; 0.12, GH: 0.06; 0.05, VE: 0.05; 0.25, for type and 'time by type' respectively). This was not the case for La concentration (power: 0.06 for time, 0.56 for time by type) and R (power: 0.12 for type, 0.54 for time by type), for which, power analysis showed that some differences in time by type interaction could be found increasing the sample size.

Borg Scale: We found no differences between the two exercise protocols concerning the type and the time ($p=0.35$, and $p=0.30$ accordingly, see Figure 6).

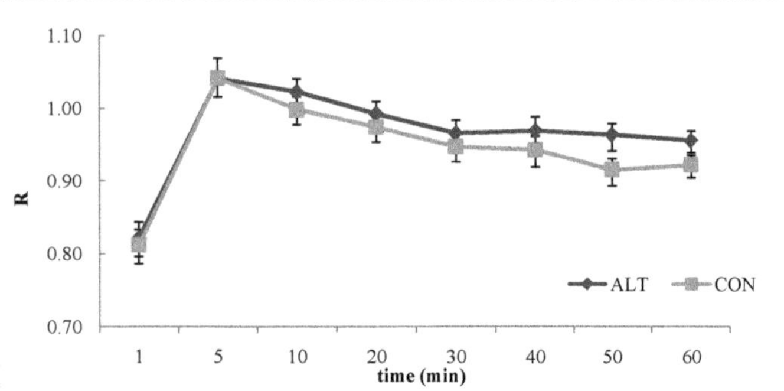

Figure 4: Changes in R (mean ± SD) in constant and alternating intensity exercise.

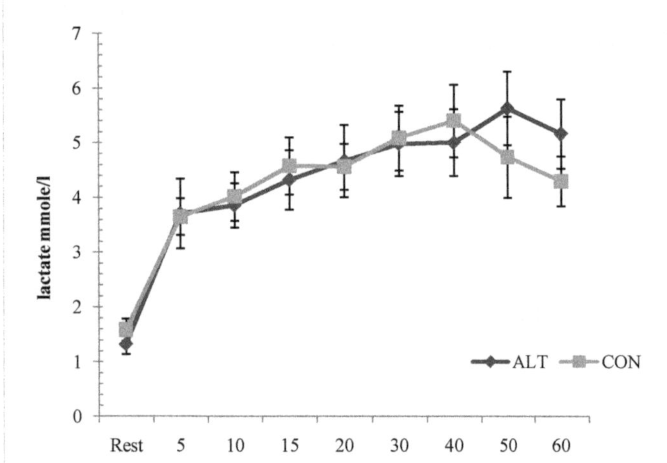

Figure 5: Changes in blood lactate concentration (mean ± SD) in constant and alternating intensity exercise.

Variable	Rest	30'	60'	120'	P
Adrenaline (ng/ml)					
Alternating Intensity	0.03±0.03	0.14±0.07	0.20±0.08	0.05±0.03	<0.01;0.23
Constant Intensity	0.03±0.01	0.14±0.05	0.17±0.10	0.04±0.04	
Nor-Adrenaline (ng/ml)					
Alternating Intensity	0.62±0.48	1.98±1.30	3.30±1.65	0.84±0.57	<0.01;0.05
Constant Intensity	0.79±0.28	3.03±1.05	3.70±2.06	1.21±0.76	
Growth Hormone (ng/ml)					
Alternating Intensity	0.38±0.34	3.62±3.13	7.83±4.34	0.77±0.57	<0.01;0.80
Constant Intensity	0.34±0.37	3.47±3.80	7.50±6.40	0.69±0.81	

The first p value represents the time effect; the second p value represents the type (continuous versus intermittent) x time interaction

Table 1: Plasma catecholamines and serum growth hormone changes (mean ± SD) before, 30 and 60 min of exercise and 1 hour after the end of exercise (ALT-CON).

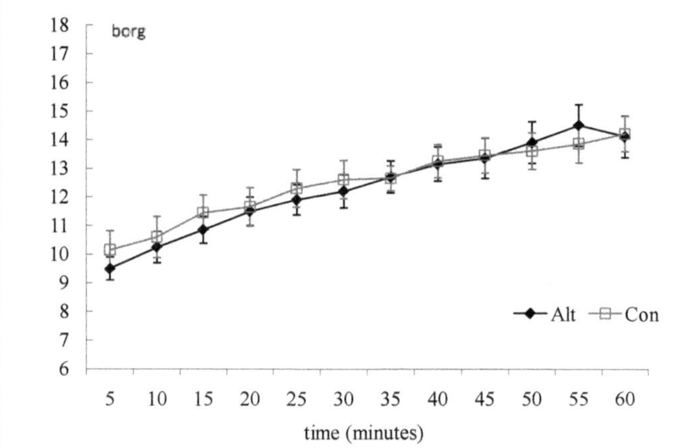

Figure 6: Changes in Borg Scale (mean ± SD) in constant and alternating intensity exercise .

Discussion

The main finding of the present study was that during sustained exercise slightly above the lactate threshold, VO_2, HR and NADR were higher in the CON compared with the ALT condition. In contrast, large fluctuations of exercise intensity (power corresponding to 47%-120% VO_{2max}) did not alter the time course of VE and R value, lactate, ADR and GH concentration from that observed in the CON exercise protocol (power corresponding to 70% VO_{2max}).

Our data differed from the findings of Essen et al. [3,4], who found that cycling for 60 minutes continuously or with alternating intensity (15 sec work – 15 sec rest) with identical average power output and mean intensity corresponding to 50-55% of VO_{2max}, resulted in similar cardiorespiratory response. Also, differed from other studies, who found that R and blood lactate concentration were higher in intermittent compared to continuous exercise, while there were no differences in HR response [21,22]. In these protocols, exercise either lasted 30 minutes with mean intensity corresponding to 90% of the Lactate Threshold, or they cycled for 1 hour to 78% of VO_{2max}. In addition, other investigators showed that interval running (1- to 60 sec work altered with 20 to 120 sec rest) caused lower lactate concentration compared to running continuously to exhaustion with the same amount of work [23], or found no difference on lactate concentration and VO_2 when constant and alternating intensity exercise performed with the same power output corresponding to 90% of critical power and to 75 Watt [24,25].

The controversial results between the previous studies and our study are possibly due to methodological differences in exercise protocol depending on the purpose of each study. There were differences in exercise protocols concerning the type of exercise, cycling vs running, the overall intensity, fluctuating from 50% to 120% of VO_{2max}, exercise duration and ratio of intense exercise and rest/or lower impact exercise. Another explanation could be the different substrate utilization between the studies. Essen et al. [3,4] found that lipid metabolism was higher in intermittent exercise compared to constant. Others [26,27] showed that fat oxidation was 3 times lower in intermittent exercise compared to continuous submaximal exercise, despite similar overall VO_2, when running at 70% of VO_{2max}. Earlier studies, mentioned that ATP- CP and oxygen bound to myoglobin were used predominately in intermittent exercise compared to constant with the same workload [6,7,23].

Energy production through ATP-CP system is unlikely to be the main source of energy in ALT exercise, since 40 seconds of low intensity exercise alternated with 20 seconds of supramaximal exercise may not be enough for complete resynthesization of ATP-CP in ALT [24]. VE for exercise intensities above LT is stimulated by metabolic acidosis resulting in lactate accumulation [28]. We found no difference in lactate concentration between the two types of exercise, explaining why VE didn't differ and suggesting that ALT intensity exercise could not place greater stress on anaerobic energy systems than CON exercise. Possibly, the lower intensity during ALT exercise stimulated lactate removal and as a result metabolic acidosis was avoided [29]. R values, fluctuating between 0.9 and 1, didn't differ between the two exercise protocols, suggesting that in both protocols energy was supplied by carbohydrate. In intense and non steady state exercise there is an underestimation of fat oxidation with Indirect Calorimetry [30]. Since, we didn't measure carbohydrate, fat oxidation and ATP-CP system only speculations we could made. More studies need to be conducted in order to examine the energy source in two exercise regimes. The greater VO_2 in CON exercise could not be explained by environmental condition and water supply during exercises, because both were kept constant in both studies. The variations in VO_2 and HR response between the two types of exercise could be explained by the different kinetics. Morris et al. [8], showed that the slower kinetics of HR and VO_2 in alternating exercise caused lower VO_2, VE and HR values compared to constant exercise. Probably, the lower values in VO_2 and HR response in AL compared to CON may reflect a delay on kinetics from light to supramaximal exercise. On the contrary, Dorado et al. [31], mentioned that active recovery (20% of VO_{2max}) between high intensity intermittent cycling for two minutes and corresponding to 120% of VO_{2max} caused greater contribution of aerobic metabolism due to faster VO_2 kinetics. Our results differ from Dorado et al. [31], because in our protocol the alternating intensity exercise was longer, lasting 1 hour and the alterations between 40′′ of light exercise with only 20′′ of intense exercise may not be enough for changes in VO_2 kinetics.

The higher HR and NADR response in CON exercise suggests greater demand on the cardiovascular system compared to ALT. Despite the significant difference between the two protocols concerning the NADR concentration, more studies need to be conducted in order to examine the NADR response because of the large standard deviation in ALT values at the 30th minute of exercise.

We found that the concentration of ADR and GH did not differ between the two exercise protocols. Our results are in line with the study of Nieman et al. [11], who examined 2 hours cycling at 64% of Wattmax continuously or with 3 minutes rest interspersed every 10 minutes. They showed that the concentration of cortisol and ADR was the same either in constant or alternating intensity cycling. The concentration of GH in intermittent exercise was higher [12], or there was no difference [13] when compared to constant. The differences may be attributed to different exercise protocol. In one study the duration of exercise was 20 minutes, while in the other was 40 minutes, and the intensity was set at 150 watt and 45% of the minimum load which elicit VO_{2max} accordingly (shorter duration and different exercise intensity).

ADR and NADR regulate cardiovascular and metabolic functions, and their blood levels reflect sympatho-adrenal activity [10]. Adrenaline level is supposed to represent emotional stress, while NADR reflects physical stress [32]. The fact that we found no differences in ADR concentration between the two types of exercise maybe explained by the rate of perceived exertion, ALT and CON exercise had similar RPE, indicating that subjects when exercising at the same average intensity did not perceive ALT as more or less stressful. So, the concentration of ADR, GH, and Cortisol [16] did not seem to be influenced by the type of exercise when mean intensity and duration are similar.

Limitations

These results could not be applied in different exercise protocols, (different ratio of intense – light exercise, duration and mean intensity) in which the stress and cardiorespiratory demand could be different.

Conclusions

Our study showed that VO_2 HR response and NADR concentration was higher in CON exercise compared to ALT exercise of the same average intensity and duration, suggesting that CON exercise evoke greater demand on the cardiovascular system. On the other hand, stress hormones, (ADR and GH concentration) did not differ between the two exercise protocols, implying that both protocols are equally stressful. These findings could be applied in designing exercise training programs in various sports and disciplines.

Acknowledgements

We would like to acknowledge Prof. M. Koutsilieri (MD, PhD), Director of Experimental Physiology Laboratory and Anastasio Philipou (PhD) for their technical support on hormonal analysis.

References

1. Laursen PB, Jenkins DG (2002) The scientific basis for high intensity interval training: optimizing training programmes and maximising performance in highly trained endurance athletes. Sports Med 32: 53-73.
2. Zafeiridis A, Sarivasiliou H, Dipla K, Vrabas IS (2010) The effect of heavy continuous versus long and short intermittent aerobic exercise protocol on oxygen consumption, heart rate and lactate responses in adolescents. Eur J Appl Physiol 110: 17-26.
3. Essen B, Hagenfeld L, Kaijser L (1977) Utilization of blood –borne and intramuscular substrates during continuous and intermittent exercise in man. J Physiol 265: 489-506.
4. Essen B (1978) Glycogen depletion of different fibre types in human skeletal muscle during intermittent and continuous exercise. Acta Physiol Scand 103: 446-455.

5. Palmer GS, Borghouts LB, Noakes TD, Hawley JA (1999) Metabolic and performance responses to constant- load vs. variable – intensity exercise in trained cyclists. J Appl Physiol 87: 1186-1196.

6. Astrand I, Astrand PO, Christensen EH, Hedman R (1960) Intermittent Muscular Work. Acta Physiol Scand 48: 448-453.

7. Christensen EH, Hedman R, Saltin B (1960) Intermittent and Continuous Running Acta Physiol Scand 50: 269-286.

8. Morris M, Gass G, Thompson M, Confort D (2003) Physiological responses to intermittent and continuous exercise at the same relative intensity in older men. Eur J Appl Physiol 90: 620-625.

9. Edwards RH, Ekelund LG, Harris RC, Hesser C, Hultman E, et al. (1973) Cardiorespiratory and metabolic costs of continuous and intermittent exercise in man. J Physiol 234: 481-497.

10. Kindermann W, Schnabel A, Schmitt WM, Biro G, Cassens J, et al. (1982) Catecholamines, growth hormones, cortisol, insulin, and sex hormones in anaerobic and aerobic exercise. Eur J Appl Physiol Occup Physiol 49: 389-399.

11. Nieman D, Henson D, Gojanovich G, Davis J, Dumke C, et al. (2007) Immune changes: 2 h of continuous vs Intermittent cycling. Int J Sports Med 28: 625-630.

12. Karagiorgos A, Garcia JF, Brooks GA (1979) Growth hormone response to continuous and intermittent exercise. Med Sci Sports 11: 302-307.

13. Weltman A, Weltman JY, Watson WD, Frick K, Patrie J, et al. (2008) Effects of continuous versus intermittent exercise, obesity, and gender on growth hormone secretion. J Clin Endocrinol Metabol 93: 4711-4720.

14. Bogdanis GC, Papaspyrou A, Theos A, Maridaki M (2007) Influence of resistive Load on power output and fatigue during intermittent sprint cycling exercise in children. Eur J Appl Physiol 101: 313-320.

15. Bird S, Davison R (1997) The British Association of Sport and Exercise Sciences, 3rd Edition. In Physiological Testing Guidelines. Determination of the lactate threshold and the onset of blood lactate accumulation data, (pp 68-70), the use of effort perception, (pp 71-72).

16. Spanoudaki S, Maridaki M, Tsironi M, Baltopoulos G, Bogdanis G, et al. (2010) Immune responses during and after exercise of constant and alternating intensity above the lactate threshold. J Sports Med Phys Fitness 50: 363-370.

17. Hargreaves M, Mckenna MJ, Jenkins DG, Warmington SA, Li JL, et al. (1998) Muscle metabolites and performance during high- intensity, intermittent exercise. J Appl Physiol 84: 1687-1691.

18. Durnin RV, Rahaman MM (1967) The assessment of the amount of fat in the human body for measurements of skinfold thickness. Brit J Nutr 21: 681-689.

19. Maughan RJ, Williams C, Campbell DM, Hepburn D (1978) Fat and carbohydrate metabolism during low intensity exercise: effects of the availability of muscle glycogen. Eur J Appl Physiol Occup Physiol 39: 7-16.

20. Dill DB, Costill DL (1974) Calculation of percentage changes in volumes of blood, plasma and red cells in dehydration. J Appl Physiol 37: 247-248.

21. Suriano R, Vercruyssen F, Bishop D, Brisswalter J (2007) Variable power output during cycling improves subsequent treadmill run time to exhaustion. J Sci Med Sport 10: 244- 251.

22. Liedl M, Swain D, Branch JD (1999) Physiolagical effects of constant versus variable power during endurance cycling. Med Sci Sports Exerc 31: 1472-1477.

23. Fox E, Robinson S, Wiegman DL (1969) Metabolic energy sources during continuous and interval running. J Appl Physiol 27: 174-178.

24. Brickley G, Green S, Jenkins DG, McEinery M, Wishart C, et al. (2007) Muscle Metabolism during constant- and alternating-intensity exercise around critical power. Int J Sports Med 28: 300-305.

25. Kang J, Mangine GT, Ratamess NA, Faigenbau AD, Hoffman JR (2007) Infleunce of intensity fluctuation on exercise metabolism. Eur J Appl Physiol 100: 253-260.

26. Christmass MA, Dawson B, Arthur PG (1999) Effect of work and recovery duration on skeletal muscle oxygenation and fuel use during sustained intermittent exercise. Eur J Appl Physiol Occup Physiol 80: 436-447.

27. Christmass MA, Dawson B, Passeretto P, Arthur PG (1999) Comparison of skeletal muscle oxygenation and fuel use in sustained continuous and intermittent exercise. Eur J Appl Physiol Occup Physiol 80: 423-435.

28. Wassermann K, Beaver WL, Whipp BJ (1990) Gas exchange theory and the lactic acidosis (anaerobic) threshold. Circulation 81: 14-30.

29. Brooks GA, Fahey TD White TP (1996) Exercise Physiology. Mayfield Publishing, Company, Mountain View, CA.

30. Romijn JA, Coyle EF, Hibbert J, Wolfe RR (1992) Comparison of indirect calorimetry and a new breath 13C/12 C ratio method during strenuous exercise. Am J Physiol 263: E64-E71.

31. Dorado C, Sanchis-Moysi J, Calbet JA (2004) Effects of recovery mode on performance O_2 uptake, and O_2 deficit during high- intensity intermittent exercise. Can J Appl Physiol 29: 227-244.

32. Pierce D, Kupprat I, Harry D (1976) Urinary epinephrine and norepinephrine levels in women athletes during training and competition. Eur J Appl Physiol Occup Physiol 36: 1-6.

Acute Resistance Exercise Program Variables and Subsequent Hormonal Response

Lawrence D Hayes[1,2], Gordon F Bickerstaff[3] and Julien S Baker[1*]

[1]*Institute of Clinical Exercise and Health Science, University of the West of Scotland, Scotland*
[2]*School of Human Sciences, London Metropolitan University, Scotland*
[3]*Department of Biology, University of the West of Scotland, Scotland*

Abstract

Resistance Exercise (RE) is a widely practiced activity both in leisure time and in training periods for competitive athletes. Recent advanced in molecular biology and muscle physiology has elucidated some of the mechanisms that regulate muscle growth. However, these molecular advances require application in acute program variables of RE. Therefore, we present an updated paradigm of resistance exercise variables and the effect manipulating these has on signalling pathways and hormonal response to optimise RE adaptations. We herein explore the effect of altering (i) choice of exercise; (ii) order of exercises performed; (iii) load (weight/resistance); (iv) volume (i.e. repetitions x sets x load) and (v) rest period between sets. Manipulating these variables has a consequential effect on signalling pathways, hormone response and neural adaptations that may influence protein synthesis and therefore gradual protein accretion leading to increased muscle size and strength.

Keywords: Resistance exercise; Weight training; Growth hormone; Testosterone; Cortisol

Introduction

Resistance Exercise (RE) is one of the most widely practiced forms of physical activity. This type of exercise is used to enhance athletic performance, augment musculo-skeletal health and alter body aesthetics. The health benefits of RE are primarily as a preventative or countermeasure to circumstances where muscle weakness compromises optimal function (injury or prolonged inactivity, sarcopenia or musculo-skeletal disorders) however, it also has a positive effect on skeletal and metabolic health as well as potential psychological benefits. This review addresses factors that can impact upon RE outcomes and attempts to outline recommendations for favourable physiological adaptations.

Training Design

Acute RE program variables, originally defined by Kraemer characterise the type and magnitude of the RE stimulus [1]. These variables are: (i) choice of exercise; (ii) order of exercises performed; (iii) load (weight/resistance); (iv) volume (i.e. repetitions x sets x load) and (v) rest period between sets.

Choice of exercise: Exercise selection determines the muscle group exercised and the speed of muscle contraction (eccentric, concentric and/or isometric). Multiple-joint exercises such as bench press and squat require complex neural responses and have generally been found most effective for overall strength increases because they allow greater weight to be lifted [2,3]. Exercising large muscle groups provides a larger hormone response than exercising small muscle groups [4,5]. An increased level of hypertrophy in response to RE has previously been reported in the upper body muscles compared to lower extremity muscles [6]. Welle et al. [6] reported Anatomical Cross-Sectional Area (ACSA) of elbow flexors to increase by 9% and 22% in old and young subjects, respectively; whereas, knee extension ACSA increased by only 6% and 4% respectively. Abe et al. [7] found a similar response when assessing muscle thickness by ultrasound. A logical explanation for this is that the lower body musculature is habitually activated and loaded to a higher level during diurnal activities than the upper body musculature [8]. Alternatively, Kadi et al. [9] suggested that intramuscular differences in androgen receptor concentrations may explain the increased potential for upper body hypertrophy.

Muscle contraction velocity is inversely related to the capacity for maximum load [10]. However, isokinetic training has been shown to increase muscular strength specific to the training velocity [11] yet, training at a moderate velocity (180-240$^{\circ}\cdot s^{-1}$) produces the greatest carryover of strength [12]. The velocity of muscular contraction also impacts signalling responses and adaptations to RE [13]. Eccentric contractions noticeably increase the 70 kDa ribosomal protein S6 kinase (p70 S6K) phosphorylation, while maximal concentric and isometric contractions provide smaller effects [14]. Additionally, eccentric muscle actions stimulate mitogen-activated protein kinase (MAPK) signalling [15]. When force is equated, concentric, isometric and eccentric actions produce similar signalling responses [16], however it is well reported that skeletal muscle can generate ~30% more tension during eccentric contractions than during concentric muscle actions [14]. This inequality in muscle tension has been proposed as an explanation for greater signalling response during eccentric contractions [14]. Furthermore, hypertrophy is attenuated after concentric only RE (matched with conventional concentric/eccentric for total work) [17]. Together, these studies suggest that signalling is similar for all muscle contraction velocities. However, force production capacity is greater during eccentric contractions and may be a more potent stimulus for muscle signalling. Although inclusion of eccentric contractions may be beneficial for RE adaptations, excessive eccentric muscle actions may produce excessive muscle damage. However, this myofibrillar disruption may be causally related to hypertrophy but this is still speculative.

Order of Exercises Performed: Exercise order significantly affects

***Corresponding author:** Julien S Baker, Professor, Director, Institute of Clinical Exercise and Health Science, Chair & Head of Sport and Exercise Science Subject Development Group, Exercise Science Research Laboratory, School of Science, Faculty of Science and Technology, University of the West of Scotland, Hamilton, Lanarkshire, ML3 OJB, Scotland
E-mail: jsbaker@uws.ac.uk

the acute expression of muscular strength [18]. Spreuwenberg et al. [18] reported that performing a squat last, as opposed to first during a RE session significantly reduced the number of repetitions performed. Strength and power during multiple joint exercises may be reduced when performed after several other exercises in a RE session [19]. A reduction in muscle activation (measured by electromyography) and metabolic fatigue (reductions in glycogen and/or phosphocreatine) are likely explanations for reduced strength and/or muscular endurance [13,20]. Interestingly, when exercises are sequenced based on agonist/antagonist muscle group relationships, muscle force and power may be potentiated [21]. Considering that multiple-joint exercises have been shown effective for increasing strength and hypertrophy, maximising performance of these exercises early in a workout may be necessary for optimal strength gains [18]. In fact, the American College of Sports Medicine Position Stand recommends that workouts include large muscle groups before small muscle groups, multiple-joint before single-joint exercises, high-intensity before lower-intensity exercises [22]. The same authors offer alternative recommendations; rotation of upper and lower body exercises or agonist-antagonist exercises (commonly known as "supersets").

Load: Load represents the amount of weight lifted or the resistance used during an exercise. Altering this load affects the acute metabolic hormonal neural and cardiovascular responses to RE [23-26]. The maximal load that can be used is heavily dependent on other acute program variables such as exercise order, exercise selection (specifically the muscle action), volume and rest interval length. Load is typically prescribed as a percentage of one repetition maximum (1RM) (e.g. 80% 1RM) or as a weight that allows a certain number of repetitions (e.g. 6RM). Typically in RE, there is an inverse relationship between the load and the volume (i.e. as the load increases the number of repetitions decreases). Loads of below 50% 1RM have been shown to increase dynamic muscular strength in untrained individuals [27,28]. Hakkinen et al. [26] reported that at least 80% 1RM was required to stimulate further neural adaptations and strength during RE in experienced weight lifters. In agreement with these findings, several authors indicated that loads of approximately 5-6RM were optimal for increasing maximal dynamic strength [29-31]. Although significant increases in strength have been reported using loads of 8-12RM [32,33], these loads may be insufficient to stimulate adaptations in experienced weight lifters [26,32,33].

In RE research, rarely is the effect of load on muscular adaptations examined without being affected by confounding variables such as volume. However, Low-Frequency Electrical Stimulation (LFES, simulating low-force contractions) and High-Frequency Electrical Stimulation (HFES, simulating high-force contractions) allow the effect of load on RE adaptations to be analysed [34,35]. LFES increases Adenosine Monophosphate-Activated Protein Kinase (AMPK) activity which promotes glucose and fatty acid oxidisation and inhibits protein synthesis (Figure 1). Simply, AMPK promotes energy release and inhibits energy consumption when cellular energy is low (marked by high Adenosine Monophosphate (AMP) and low glycogen) [13]. HFES stimulates protein kinase B (Akt)-mammalian target of rapamycin (mTOR) signalling. This response is critical for increasing muscle protein synthesis and subsequent hypertrophy [36,37]. mTOR signalling increases protein synthesis by increasing the number of messenger RNA translated per ribosome [38]. According to Henneman's size principal smaller motor units (primarily type I) are recruited prior to larger motor units (primarily type II) until force production is equal to force requirement [39]. Low-force activities recruit primarily type I, slow fatiguing motor units. As the load increases, higher threshold motor units are recruited, encompassing more type II fast-fatiguing fibres until near maximal-loads where the entire spectrum of motor units is activated. As the size principal is related to force, and force=mass×acceleration, rapidly accelerating a load can recruit higher-threshold motor units [40]. Linnamo et al. [41] reported that performing 'explosive' concentric contractions using ~40% of maximal isometric force increased Electromyographic (EMG) activity when compared with the same exercise at ~67% of maximal isometric force at a slow velocity. EMG activity has also been found to increase with the onset of fatigue [42]. This indicates increased contribution of higher threshold motor units to maintain force output as lower threshold units begin to fatigue. Therefore, a heavy weight, 'explosive' contractions, or fatigue may all increase the number of type II motor units recruited. This may affect the adaptations to RE as only motor units recruited respond to RE type II fibres have a greater capacity for hypertrophy and different muscle groups contain varied percentages of type I and type II fibres [43]. RE to maximize hypertrophy typically include moderate to high loads [13,43-45]. These loads allow the volume to be high and the rest periods to be short to maximize hormonal response (Figure 1) [44].

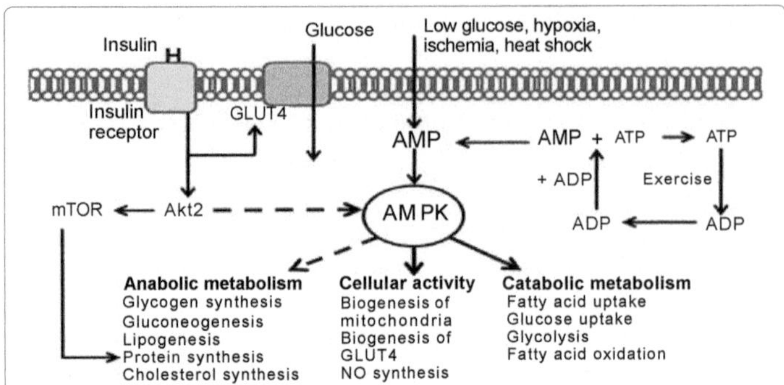

Figure 1: AMPK activity and subsequent metabolic effects.

Traditionally, 1-6RM, 8-12RM and 15+RM loads are recommended to maximize strength, hypertrophy and local muscular endurance, respectively. Campos et al. confirmed these preconceptions by investigating the adaptations following an 8 week RE program in groups using 3-5RM loads (strength protocol), 9-11RM loads (hypertrophy protocol) and 20-28RM loads (muscular endurance protocol) [28]. The investigation revealed a step-wise increase in strength (strength protocol > hypertrophy protocol>muscular endurance protocol), local muscular endurance (muscular endurance protocol>hypertrophy protocol >strength protocol). Increased muscle fiber Cross-Sectional Area (CSA) occurred only in the hypertrophy and strength protocol groups with no significant difference observed between the two. Maximal aerobic power increased solely in the muscular endurance protocol group. Campos et al. however, did not control for volume of training, which has been suggested as a strong indicator for muscular adaptations [28,46].

Research examining periodization has demonstrated a need for variable-intensity loading schemes in RE [45,47]. Rhea et al. reported that daily undulating periodization elicited greater strength gains than the classic linear schedule [48]. An example of daily undulating periodization would be training at 70, 85, and 95% of 1RM on Monday, Wednesday, and Friday, respectively. The mechanisms behind increased strength due solely to periodization are unclear. Selye's General Adaptation Syndrome suggests that a system will adapt to an unaccustomed stress (i.e. overload). Greater volumes and intensities of RE result in strength adaptations to a certain level presumably, due to an overload of the neuromuscular system [46,49]. Therefore, variations in training may increase the neuromuscular overload by continually applying an unaccustomed stress. The American College of Sports Medicine Position Stand recommends that workouts cycle training loads of 80-100% 1RM to maximize muscular strength and 70-100% 1RM to maximize hypertrophy [22].

Volume: Exercise volume is typically described as the total number of repetitions performed during a training session multiplied by the resistance used and is reflective of the duration which muscles are being stressed [50]. Therefore, manipulation of training volume can be achieved by altering the number of exercises per session, the number of sets per exercise, the number of repetitions per set, or the resistance used. Volume has been shown to affect neural hypertrophic metabolic and hormonal responses to RE [22,24,50,51]. For example, multiple-set workouts invoke significantly greater Growth Hormone (GH) and Testosterone (T) responses than single-set programs [52]. Long-term training that employs multiple sets, compared to single sets appears to be superior for strength development and hypertrophy [51]. It is unclear however, whether a dose response exists between volume and RE adaptations. Studies incorporating two three four to five and six or more sets per exercise have all produced significant increases in strength in trained and untrained individuals. Interestingly, similar strength increases have been reported when comparing two and four sets and two and three sets [32,33,53-57]. In contrast to Ostrowski et al. [56], Berger [29] reported that three sets were indeed superior to two sets for the development of strength. The optimal number of sets per exercise still remains an equivocal matter with varied opinions even between review and meta-analytical papers. A recent meta-regression reported that multiple sets were associated with a larger effect size than a single set [58]. In a dose-response manner, two to three sets per exercise were associated with a significantly greater effect size than one set. However, no significant difference between one set per exercise and four to six sets per exercise, or between two to three sets per exercise and four to six sets per exercise was observed. Despite no significant difference observed between one set and four to six sets, a trend for four to six sets to result in greater strength increases existed. This was not significant due to the large standard deviation observed. The authors concluded by advising that two to three sets per exercise are associated with 46% greater strength gains than one set, in both trained and untrained subjects. An alternative view has been proposed by Peterson et al. [46], who reported that approximately eight sets per muscle group produced the largest effect size in athletes. Peterson et al. [46] investigated 177 studies and 1,803 effect sizes and advised the following RE prescription: For athletes, maximal strength gains are elicited at a mean training intensity of 80% of 1RM (agreeing with the American College of Sports Medicine Position Stand) two days per week, with a training volume of eight sets per muscle group [22]. RE trained non-athletes exhibit maximal strength gains with a training intensity of 80% 1RM, 3 days per week, with a training volume of 4 sets per muscle group. Untrained individuals experienced maximal strength gains at 60% 1RM, three days per week and four sets per muscle group. These authors demonstrated that exercise prescription for maximum strength gains should vary between populations. However, trained non athletes commonly train for hypertrophy rather than strength and therefore, the above prescriptions may not be relevant to this population.

Hypertrophy involves a proportionate increase in the net accretion of actin and myosin as well as other structural proteins. Mechanical loading leads to a series of intracellular events that ultimately regulate gene expression and protein synthesis [22]. Protein synthesis in human muscle increases after only one bout of RE and peaks approximately 24 h post exercise [59]. This anabolic environment remains elevated from ~2 h post exercise up through 36-48 h post exercise [60] (depending on training status). For previously untrained individuals neural adaptations dominate early stages of training with muscle hypertrophy occurring within six weeks [61]. Similarly to strength training, hypertrophy has shown to be enhanced with multiple-set over single-set training [23]. In untrained individuals however, as with strength, general nonspecific program design appears to be an adequate overload to stimulate hypertrophy [62]. For more experienced individuals, periodized training schemes appear to be the most effective way to maximize hypertrophy. RE targeting hypertrophy commonly include moderate to very high loading, relatively high volume, and short rest intervals as this design produces a greater elevation in T and GH than a strength program with long rest, high-load and low-volume [22]. Total work, in combination with loading has been implicated for gains in hypertrophy [63]. This result has been supported by greater hypertrophy associated with multiple-set, high-volume programs compared to single-set programs [33,64]. Goto et al. reported that the addition of a high-repetition low-load set to a traditional strength training protocol increased muscle CSA [65]. However, this combination protocol was compared with a strength only protocol and a typical hypertrophy regimen was not analysed. Campos et al. examined eight weeks of a high-load RE protocol and reported that neither type I nor type II muscle fibres exhibited hypertrophy [28]. Therefore, the American College of Sports Medicine Position Stand advised that a combination of strength training and typical hypertrophy training is most effective for advanced hypertrophy training as it compromises a load sufficient to overload the musculature and a volume high enough to elicit an elevated endocrine response [22]. As with many RE variables, volume is difficult to isolate as and therefore most experiments manipulate load and volume concomitantly. It seems logical however, that increased load would affect muscle signalling. High-volume RE would deplete muscle glycogen stores and therefore stimulate AMPK activity [13]. As previously reported AMPK promotes muscular endurance adaptations and inhibits protein synthesis (via inhibition of Akt-mTOR signalling). This relationship between volume, glycogen, and AMPK is supported by research that demonstrates that low muscle glycogen potentiates exercise-induced AMPK activity and attenuates Akt signalling [64-66]. Comparatively, adequate exercise volume appears necessary for optimal gains in muscular strength and size [51]. Therefore, making conclusions and recommendations about RE volume and muscle signalling is difficult and a further research to establish the threshold RE volume at which AMPK begins to inhibit Akt-mTOR signalling is required.

Rest intervals: Rest periods between sets significantly influence the adaptations and responses to RE. Short rest periods are recommended for hypertrophy as short rest periods augment the GH response [67]. However, short rest intervals have a detrimental effect of subsequent sets and over several weeks, attenuate strength increases [42,68]. When training to optimise strength gains, longer rest periods are advised as performance may be compromised with one-min compared to three min rest periods [69]. Strength recovery may not even be complete after 2 mins with several studies suggesting that 3 – 5 min rest interval produce less performance decrements than 30 s - 2 min [23,71,70]. The American College of Sports Medicine Position Stand advised rest periods of at least 2 – 3 min for core exercises using heavy loads (e.g. Olympic lifts) and one – two min for assistance exercises for the development of strength [22]. The authors advised identical rest periods to maximize hypertrophy in advanced RE training. The aim of hypertrophy training is to produce an anabolic environment, which appears to be best done with short rest periods. However, Robinson et al. [72] reported no difference in muscle girths, body mass or skin folds in recreationally trained participants when utilising 30, 90 and 180 s rest intervals. In agreement, Ahtiainen et al. [73] found no difference in muscle CSA after three months of training with 5 min or 2 min rest periods. Intuitively, short rest periods would increase AMPK activity due to the metabolic stress associated with little rest and therefore inhibit protein synthesis following RE, explicating why short rest periods attenuate strength gains [42,69]. However, there is some debate as to whether short rest periods inhibit protein synthesis via AMPK activity as GH is increased with short rest periods, therefore promoting hypertrophy. Also, the importance of increased AMPK activity ~ 1 – 2 h post-exercise remains unclear [13]. Regardless of these indefinites, short rest periods are commonly prescribed when hypertrophy is the aim [13,22].

Resistance training and the endocrine system

Dependent upon RE variables, RE incites an anabolic hormonal response, including T, GH and Insulin-Like Growth Factor-1 (IGF-1), but also Cortisol (C; a catabolic hormone) [22]. The acute program variables discussed in section 1 dictate the magnitude of this hormonal response. Typical hypertrophy protocols (moderate to high load, short rest periods and high volume) recruiting large muscle groups appear to produce the greatest endocrine response (Figure 2) [3].

Testosterone

T is considered to be of high importance in resistance training adaptations in men [74]. T is a steroid hormone secreted from the Leydig cells of the testes under hypothalamic and pituitary control. T has both anabolic and anticatabolic effects on muscle tissue [75]. The direct action of T on muscle is supported by the presence of cytoplasmic receptors for T in skeletal muscle homogenates [76]. T promotes protein synthesis in muscle tissue with the result being increased muscle mass and strength [77]. Kvorning et al. [78] suppressed endogenous production of T with goserelin in healthy young males and reported serum T below 10% of normal levels strongly attenuated the increase in lean mass and muscle strength and actually increased fat mass during a resistance training protocol. The placebo group in the study adapted to the resistance training period by significantly increasing isometric strength and lean leg mass. These results demonstrate a direct link between endogenous T and adaptations to resistance training. Hansen et al. [79] subjected 16 untrained men to nine weeks of training either unilateral arm alone, or unilateral arm and legs. It was reported that the group who training both legs and arm in the same training session exhibited a mean isometric elbow flexion strength gain of 37% compared to 10% in the arm only group after nine weeks. In fact, even the untrained arm showed a significant increase in strength for the legs and arm group over the nine week training program. In contrast, West et al.

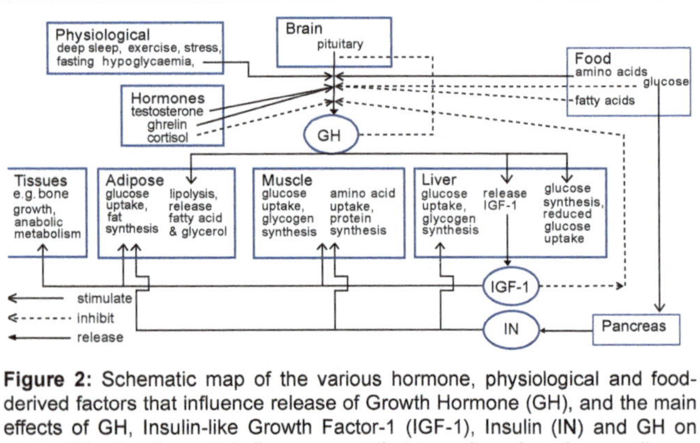

Figure 2: Schematic map of the various hormone, physiological and food-derived factors that influence release of Growth Hormone (GH), and the main effects of GH, Insulin-like Growth Factor-1 (IGF-1), Insulin (IN) and GH on some of the key the metabolic processes that occur in various tissue cells.

[5] conducted a similar study but utilised a within-participants design and noted that despite a higher hormonal response to training, subjects achieved significantly indifferent hypertrophy and strength gains when training one arm and legs compared to one arm alone. These authors summarised by suggesting that acute systemic hormone responses are not responsible for muscle hypertrophy and that local mechanisms are primary in producing gains in strength and hypertrophy. However, West et al. [5] tested strength dynamically, whereas Hansen et al. [79] tested isometric strength and this may explain some difference.

The correlation reported by Ahtiainen et al. [80] between changes in isometric strength and T suggest that T may be an important factor for strength development. Interestingly, participants who exhibited increased acute T response after the training period were able to increase CSA of muscle more than those with a lowered response. However, caution should be exerted when examining T concentrations correlated to strength or hypertrophy as T response to resistance exercise is transient and the accretion of protein leading to hypertrophy and strength increases are accumulative. Although T causes up regulation of androgen receptors, the increase in T is transitory and muscle protein synthetic response can be elevated for ~48 h although this time course is reduced with training [13,81]. The hormone response to resistance training has been repeatedly investigated with the current theory of interaction between endogenous T and androgen receptors in the recovery phase stimulating muscle hypertrophy, protein synthesis and strength [4,74,80]. This is furthermore supported by the fact that exogenous T (via supplementation) significantly increases muscle mass and strength, especially when combined with resistance training [82]. A reduction in T may cause an increased storage of fat via decreased fat oxidation, decreased resting energy expenditure, and increased adiposity [83,84].

Despite many authors suggesting that resistance exercise-induced hypertrophy is attributable to acute hormonal response recent findings have suggested otherwise [4,25,79,85,86]. West et al. [86] found that myofibrillar protein synthesis and phosphorylation of the 70 kDa S6 protein kinase (both thought to be predictors of hypertrophy) exhibited no difference between arm only and arm and legs training. The latter protocol elicited a marked elevation in serum T, GH and insulin-like growth factor-1 (IGF-1) from resting values, whereas the former did not. However, participants were supplemented with 25 g whey protein after both protocols which led West et al. [5] to suggest that high quality protein availability, rather than training designed to elevate hormone levels is crucial for muscle hypertrophy.

T indirectly stimulates secretion of IGF-1 and GH, known to be correlated with the magnitude of type I and type II muscle fiber hypertrophy [87]. Numerous studies have demonstrated that resistance exercise increase circulating T concentrations [5,9,25,85]. T exerts its influence on protein synthesis via androgen receptors in the muscle. T binds to and converts androgen receptors to a sequence-specific DNA binding factor capable of transferring to the nucleus and associating with DNA to regulate androgen-specific gene expression. Blocking of androgen receptors reduces muscle protein accretion, indicating the physiological importance of T-androgen receptor interactions for hypertrophy [88]. Androgen receptors are up regulated by T therefore the higher T concentrations in men likely explains the higher androgen receptor content found in men compared to women [38,89]. Kraemer et al. [90] reported that a resistance training protocol significantly increased resting testosterone concentrations and that this was augmented by essential amino acid supplementation. This would suggest that androgen receptors were up regulated as a result of this and indeed, hypertrophy (as a result of protein accretion) did occur as a result of the 12-week training protocol. While endurance exercise may transiently increase T values the number of muscle fibres recruited is less than during resistance training and androgen receptors are only impacted if the motor unit is activated [91]. Therefore, endurance training is less effective at promoting hypertrophy than resistance exercise as resistance exercise (particularly when working to failure) recruits more muscle fibres [13].

It has previously been reported that T responses to training may affect individual adaptation and the ability to exhibit hypertrophy [25,78,85]. For example, Kraemer et al. [92] reported that protocol-specific acute serum T increases were observed after strength and hypertrophy protocols. However, the direction and amplitude of hormonal responses has been shown to vary even in response to similar resistance training protocols [25,68,85]. Beaven et al. [25] investigated the effect of four different resistance exercise protocols on hormonal response in elite rugby players and reported large inter-individual variability for serum T. None of the four protocols: strength (3 X 5 reps at 85% 1RM), hypertrophy (4 X 10 reps at 70% 1RM), power (3 X 5 reps at 40% 1RM) and strength endurance (5 X 15 reps at 55% 1RM) induced a statistically significant increase in T. This was probably due to the large inter-individual variability within the study. The strength endurance and power protocols in the Beaven et al. [25] study elicited lower T responses than the strength and hypertrophy protocols. However, significance was not reached as there was large variability in hormonal responses to resistance exercise as indicated by large standard errors. The authors noted, however, that individual's hormonal response was pronounced in one or occasionally two of the protocols implemented. Therefore, the protocol considered to be optimal in terms on anabolism (defined by an absolute increase in free T concentration) varied amongst individuals. These investigators were the first to observe this phenomenon and offered it as a potential reason why studies have varied in terms of observed hormonal response to resistance exercise. Beaven et al. [25] reported four groups of responders (hypertrophy: $n = 4$; strength: $n = 5$; strength endurance: $n = 4$; power: $n = 2$). If these findings were representative across a wider population, pooling data would likely elicited skewed results depending on subject homogeneity.

As suggested by Beaven et al. [25] different resistance exercise protocols may result in individualised T responses and as already suggested, a relationship between T response and muscular adaptations has been suggested [78]. Therefore, Beaven et al. [85] assigned a group of amateur rugby players to three weeks of the protocol which elicited the lowest T response (T_{min}), and three weeks to the protocol which elicited the highest T response (T_{max}) in a cross-over design. The protocols were the same as in the earlier investigation [25]. It was reported that body mass, 1RM bench press and leg press all showed significant increases after the period of T_{max} training. When performing the T_{min} period of training, 75% of athletes showed either no change or a significant decline in 1RM performance. The authors concluded by suggesting the ability of a resistance exercise protocol to induce an increase in free T is causatively linked to strength and bodyweight gains. The observation by Beaven et al. [25] that hormone response to certain resistance exercise protocols shows inter-individual variability has many practical implications. Athletes may be able to make further musculoskeletal gains by individually prescribed resistance exercise protocols based on acute T response.

Cortisol: C is a steroid hormone released by the adrenocortical glands under hypothalamic and pituitary control. C has catabolic effects on muscle tissue and has important metabolic functions such as influencing the metabolism of lipids, proteins and glucose [76]. It increases the mobilisation of fatty acids from fat reserves to active tissue and raises blood glucose [93]. Intense physical exercise causes an increase in C which may inhibit protein synthesis and consequently increases in muscle mass by its catabolic effect [93,94]. All protocols investigated by Beaven et al. [25] resulted in a decrease in C concentration with strength, hypertrophy, power and strength endurance protocols decreasing C by 38.2 ± 20.6%, 33.6 ± 20.6%, 44.3 ± 20.6% and 22.2 ± 20.6% respectively. These findings conflict with a number of studies who report acute increases in C in response to resistance exercise [25,68,95]. Beaven et al. [25] attributed these differences to the anticipatory anxious response to stressful events that cause an increase in C and suggested that by investigating individuals with experience of resistance training and using non-invasive saliva-obtained samples, the stress to individuals in the study was reduced. In exercising humans, C increases the availability of metabolic substrates for exercising musculature, protects from an over-reaction of the immune system to the stress of exercise and maintains normal vascular integrity [96]. C also prepares the body for the next bout of exercise explaining why post-exercise levels of C are raised and the return to basal concentrations is prolonged. An important role of the acute C response is to meet the greater metabolic demand of resistance training [97,98]. In previous reports, acute C response has been highest when the overall stress of the training period has been very high and the response has been linked to the volume and/or intensity of total work [68,91,95]. Long-term resistance exercise may lead to an overall reduction of acute C response during exercise in men [32,91]. However, Cadore et al. [24] opposed this by suggesting that untrained and resistance trained men exhibited a similar C response to a resistance exercise stimulus. Nevertheless, an increased T response to resistance exercise in trained individuals was reported. These findings may suggest that the participants were in an increased state of anabolism due to an increase in protein synthesis rather than a reduction in protein degradation. However, this opposes the understanding that untrained individuals embarking on resistance training experience more drastic hypertrophy than trained individuals. This may be due to long-term resistance training attenuating the protein synthetic response to acute resistance exercise, by shortening the duration for which protein synthesis is elevated [59].

The ratio of T/C is being intensively discussed and examined as a possible indicator of the anabolic/catabolic status of athletes. From a physiological view, the formation of such a quotient is problematic, as a number of other hormones also affect the anabolic/catabolic status of the body [99]. Addlercruetz et al. [100] however, suggested the T/C ratio as the most sensitive indicator of physical overload. Defining values of overload using this ratio have proven difficult due to high inter-individual variability [101]. Therefore, the ratio may be useful when investigating within-subjects effects however, caution should be used when applying this ratio to between subjects design. (Figure 3)

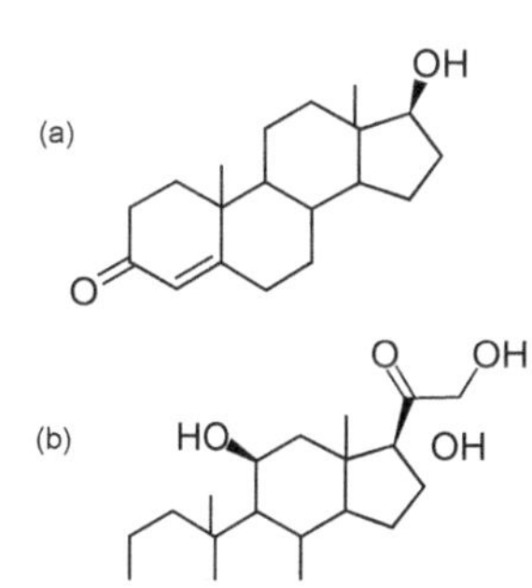

Figure 3: Line diagrams of steroid hormones (a) testosterone and (b) cortisol.

IGF-1: IGF-1 is secreted as it is produced in the liver in response to GH-stimulated DNA synthesis [102] and remains the most prescribed signal for activating the signal transduction necessary for the initiation of protein translation after mechanical loading of the muscle [103]. IGF-1 is a potent activator of the Akt/mTOR signalling pathway with inhibition shown to prevent protein synthesis after RE [104, 105]. RE has been shown to increase concentrations of circulating and muscle IGF-1 although a number of studies have reported no change [106-108]. The lack of change has been attributed to a delayed response of IGF-1 (3-9 h), following GH-stimulated mRNA synthesis with peak values not occurring until 16-28 h post-exercise [77,107]. RE alters concentrations of IGF binding proteins that influence the biological activity of IGF-1 [108,109]. IGF-1 stimulates muscle hypertrophy via phosphatidylinositol-3 kinase-(PI-3K) Akt-mTOR signalling. IGF-1 also increases the proliferation and differentiation of satellite cells to aid hypertrophy [110] and in response to mechanical overload, mechano-growth factor (MGF; a splice variant of IGF-1) stimulates satellite cell activation [76]. IGF-1 is known to stimulate myoblast proliferation and differentiation in vitro as well as muscle protein synthesis [17,111]. Local expression of IGF-1 in skeletal muscle appears to be load dependent and acts independently of changes in serum GH or IGF-1 [112]. However, Wilborn et al. [113] reported increased mRNA expression of IGF-1 for protocols of 60-65% 1RM 4 x 18-20 repetitions and 80-85% 1RM 4 x 8-10 repetitions. No significant effect for RE protocol was reported for IGF-1, IGF-1 receptor or MGF suggesting that these isoforms may not be load dependent. Interestingly, volume was not controlled for by Wilborn et al. [113] and may have contributed to this indifference as the 60-65% 1RM group experienced greater training volume. It would have been interesting if Wilborn et al. [113] had continued this study over a longer period to determine if hypertrophy, like muscle IGF-1, was equal for both protocols over time. Muscle IGF-1 is thought to induce myofiber hypertrophy by autocrine and/or paracrine action [111]. The effectiveness of muscle IGF-1 is dependent not only on its expression but also on its availability, which is controlled by a family of six IGF binding proteins and by the number of the IGF-1 receptor. As already suggested, expression of IGF-1 in muscle is independent of serum GH and IGF-1 and therefore, exogenous supplementation of serum GH or IGF-1 does not appear to stimulate muscular hypertrophy in the absence of applied load [114]. However, administration of IGF-1 directly into skeletal muscle does increase muscle mass suggesting that any increase in muscle IGF-1 availability may lead to hypertrophy [115]. Bamman et al. [108] hypothesised that muscle IGF-1 after a single bout of resistance exercise would be higher after eccentric contractions compared with concentric contractions. However, the results revealed that although MVC was decreased for longer and muscle soreness was perceived higher after eccentric exercise, serum IGF-1 expression showed no significant difference between the muscle actions. Nevertheless, local IGF-1 is independent of serum IGF-1 and therefore IGF-binding protein-4 (known to inhibit IGF-1) mRNA was reduced significantly after eccentric loading which lead to an increase in skeletal IGF-1 mRNA. This would lead to increased IGF-1 availability within the muscle after mechanical loading. Therefore, the authors suggested that IGF-1 was linked to mechanisms involved in tissue regeneration caused by muscle damage. This muscle damage may not lead to hypertrophy however as downhill running and other endurance exercises with large eccentric component cause significant muscle damage, yet endurance exercise is not a potent hypertrophic stimulus [91].

Insulin: Insulin causes cells in the liver, muscle, and adipose tissue to uptake glucose from the blood, storing it as glycogen in the liver and muscle, and stopping use of fat as an energy source. During exercise, insulin secretion is reduced to allow more glucose to the muscle cells. However, it is the aim during RE to minimise this reduction in insulin as it has been shown to have significant effect on muscle protein synthesis when adequate amino acid concentrations are available, by reducing protein catabolism [115]. Exercise-induced mRNA transcription and synthesis of proteins is only fully activated when plasma insulin levels are elevated [116]. Elevations in insulin are expected to inhibit AMPK activity, therefore promoting protein synthesis. Insulin likely exerts its effect on translation through the Akt-mTOR signal transduction pathway [117]. Serum insulin concentrations parallel changes in blood glucose, and the response is enhanced when protein and carbohydrates are ingestion prior to, during, or after a workout [107,115]. A potent anabolic hormone in its normal physiological range; insulin is mostly affected by blood glucose concentrations and dietary intake. Ingestion of carbohydrates, amino acids or a combination of both prior to, during, or after a workout is recommended for maximising insulin's effects on tissue anabolism [91]. Supplementation before or during RE may maximize benefits as a consequence of increased muscular blood flow and subsequent amino acid delivery.

GH: The acidophilic cells of the anterior pituitary secrete molecules that make up the family of GH polypeptides. The most commonly studied GH isoform, the 22kD molecule, consists of 191 amino acids [118]. Other isoforms also exist and appear to function similarly to the 22kD molecule in promoting tissue anabolism. RE has been shown to acutely elevate many of the GH variants [119]. GH binding to its receptor initiates janus kinase 2 (JAK2) signalling. JAK2 signaling activates PI-3K. As PI-3K is proximal to Akt-mTOR signalling, it appears that RE-induced elevations in GH promote translational efficiency and muscle anabolism [13]. Animal studies support this, as GH injection into pigs resulted in enhance translational efficiency and protein synthesis [120,121]. This RE-induced elevation in GH has been shown through 30 min post-exercise [77]. The magnitude of this response appears dependent upon the amount of muscle mass recruited contraction velocity volume intensity and rest intervals [3,21,67,68,80,95]. As with T, greater GH acute responses have been reported with workouts consisting of multiple-sets [68]. GH appears to be highly influenced by the volume of the RE protocol. GH response appears to be most substantial when a protocol elicits a high blood lactate concentration [67]. To evoke a substantial blood lactate response, a RE protocol should include moderate to high load, high volume, short rest intervals and activate large muscle groups. High correlations between serum GH and blood lactate have been reported and Kraemer et al. [77] proposed the accumulation of H^+ produced by lactic acid acidosis as the primary factor influencing GH release [95]. Mulligan et al. [122] supported this hypothesis by suggesting that GH response was attenuated following induced alkalosis during high-intensity cycling. Although endurance exercise may transiently increases many of the anabolic hormones, prolonged endurance exercise is not a potent stimulus of hypertrophy as it does not recruit enough muscle fibres (androgen receptors are only activated if the motor unit is activated), specifically type II fibres (known to be most susceptible to hypertrophy) or stimulate protein synthesis via the Akt-mTOR pathway. Breath-holding, Hypoxia, protein catabolism and acid base shifts have also been reported to influence GH release [77]. Therefore, resistance exercise is a potent stimulus for increasing GH as long as exercise intensity and volume is sufficient [123]. A number of studies have reported a correlation between the total work of a RE protocol and the acute GH response [95,122]. Mostly, these studies compare typical strength protocols (high load, low repetitions, and long rest) with typical hypertrophy protocols (moderate load, moderate repetitions, short rest) or a typical strength endurance protocol (low load, high repetitions and short rest). Commonly the strength endurance protocol results in the greatest

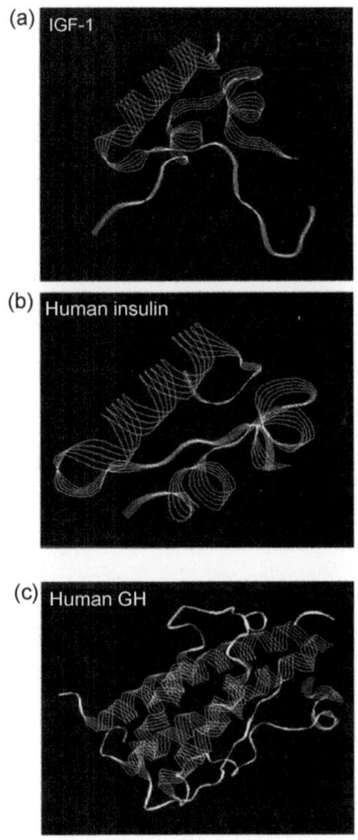

Figure 4: RASMOL generated structures of protein hormones using RCSB Protein Data Bank (PDB) files (http://www.pdb.org/pdb/home/home.do):
(a) Insulin-like growth factor-1 (1 polypeptide chain of 70 residues) PDB reference 1GZR.
(b) Human insulin (2 polypeptide chains A 21 residues & B 30 residues) PDB reference 3I3Z.
(c) Human growth hormone (1 polypeptide chain of 191 amino acid residues,) PDB reference 1HGU.

acute elevation in GH. However, Campos et al. [28] demonstrated that this type of protocol does not result in increased muscular CSA and was the least effective at increasing strength compared to a strength and hypertrophy protocol. These findings suggest that although GH may influence the muscular adaptations to RE, the extent to which GH is acutely elevated is not the ultimate factor determining adaptations. Interestingly, Goto et al. [65] reported that the addition of a single set of high repetitions with 50% 1RM to the end of a strength regimen elicited a much higher GH response than with the strength protocol alone. However, the hypertrophy protocol utilised elicited a higher acute GH response than the strength protocol alone and the strength protocol with the addition of a high-repetitions set. However, the combination of the strength protocol and the high-repetition set did result in increased CSA when compared to the strength protocol without the addition of the high-repetition set (Figure 4).

Conclusion

Traditionally, 1-6RM, 8-12RM and 15+RM loads are recommended to maximize strength, hypertrophy and local muscular endurance, respectively with light loads (~40% 1RM) performed explosively recommended for power training. Most research concerning RE conforms to these ideals however, athletes may experience enhanced adaptations when performing a RE protocol that maximizes hormonal response as this varies inter-individually for the same protocols. To maximize hypertrophy, load needs to be substantial enough to recruit fast twitch muscle fibres but light enough to enable short rest periods and a volume capable of causing metabolic stress. This type of protocol maximizes hormonal response. Approximately 5-6RM appears optimal for increasing maximal dynamic strength. Much smaller loads have increased strength in untrained participants but as individuals become more experienced in RE, a greater load is required to stimulate overload. Commonly, compound exercises (Olympic lifts, dead lifts, squats, bench press) have been prescribed to maximize hypertrophy as they cause a high metabolic stress and stimulate a large hormonal response, thereby increasing protein synthesis. However, hypertrophy has been reported in smaller muscle groups without an anabolic hormone response to the protocol. This suggests that a combination of central and peripheral factors stimulate hypertrophy. Compound exercises are advised for athletes as in the majority of events, large muscle groups are the most utilised (often through locomotion) however, RE should be tailored to the individual athlete's needs. A combination of eccentric and concentric muscle actions is advised for strength and hypertrophy training. Muscle adaptations appear specific to training and isotonic muscle actions are common in most weight lifting events. The exclusion of eccentric muscle actions in a RE protocol has been shown to attenuate muscle growth.

Superior results have been reported for all protocols when incorporating periodization into a training program. A daily-undulating-periodization; characterised by cycling training loads over a short period of time (E.g. 6RM Monday, 10RM Wednesday, 14RM Friday) appears superior to linear periodization and non-periodized training possibly due to more regular overload.

Availability of amino acids is important for protein synthesis associated with hypertrophy and inclusion of CHO may maximize the effect of insulin with creatine also increasing lean body mass. Therefore, a combination of CHO, protein and creatine would be most beneficial to consume pre-, during-, and post-exercise to maximize hypertrophy and recovery. However, creatine is not recommended for athletes who compete in events that require acceleration of one's own body mass. A number of other factors affect the adaptations to RE including age, genetics, gender, time of day trained at, posture and living habits but these are outside the scope of this review.

With regards to previous and future research, it is clear that acute program variables are difficult to examine in isolation and this issue proves problematic in RE research. Therefore, it is difficult to make any certain conclusions about acute RE variables as altering one will normally impact on another. The issue of hypertrophy in the absence of elevated anabolic hormones is an interesting phenomenon that deserves further investigation. Although this phenomenon has been observed, hypertrophy programs have previously been prescribed based on anabolic hormone response and the findings of Cadore et al. [24] suggest that a hypertrophy is superior in increasing muscle growth compared to a strength or muscular endurance protocol. Therefore, another mechanism other than hormone response may determine why a program utilising repetitions of approximately 10 is superior in eliciting hypertrophy. Future investigations could aim to discover this mechanism. With regards to acute program variables, it is still unclear whether a dose response exists; i.e. would utilising 5, 4, 3, 2 and, 1 sets of an exercise result in a stepwise increase in strength or hypertrophy. Then, could this be extrapolated as far as 10 sets and beyond. This hole in the literature is apparent for all program variables, however may be most applicable to volume.

References

1. Kraemer WJ (1983) Exercise Prescription in Weight Training: Manipulating Program Variables. Nat Strength Cond Assoc J 5: 58-59.
2. Chilibeck PD, Calder AW, Sale DG, Webber CE (1998) A comparison of strength and muscle mass increases during resistance training in young women. Eur J Appl Physiol Occup Physiol 77: 170-175.
3. Stone MH, Plisk SS, Stone ME, Schilling BK, O'Bryant HS, et al. (1998) Athletic performance development: Volume load - 1 set vs. Multiple sets, training velocity and training variation. Strength Cond J 20: 22-31.
4. Wilkinson SB, Tarnopolsky MA, Grant EJ, Correia CE, Phillips SM (2006) Hypertrophy with unilateral resistance exercise occurs without increases in endogenous anabolic hormone concentration. Eur J Appl Physiol 98: 546-555.
5. West DWD, Burd NA, Tang JE, Moore DR, Staples AW, et al. (2010) Elevations in ostensibly anabolic hormones with resistance exercise enhance neither training-induced muscle hypertrophy nor strength of the elbow flexors. J Appl Physiol 108: 60-67.
6. Welle S, Totterman S, Thornton C (1996) Effect of age on muscle hypertrophy induced by resistance training. J Gerontol A Biol Sci Med Sci 51: M270-275.
7. Abe T, DeHoyos DV, Pollock ML, Garzarella L (2000) Time course for strength and muscle thickness changes following upper and lower body resistance training in men and women. Eur J Appl Physiol 81: 174-180.
8. Cureton KJ, Collins MA, Hill DW, McElhannon FM Jr (1988) Muscle hypertrophy in men and women. Med Sci Sports Exerc 20: 338-344.
9. Kadi F, Bonnerud P, Eriksson A, Thornell LE (2000) The expression of androgen receptors in human neck and limb muscles: effects of training and self-administration of androgenic-anabolic steroids. Histochem Cell Biol 113: 25-29.
10. Sakamoto A, Sinclair PJ (2006) Effect of movement velocity on the relationship between training load and the number of repetitions of bench press. J Strength Cond Res 20: 523-527.
11. Coburn JW, Housh TJ, Malek MH, Weir JP, Cramer JT, et al. (2006) Neuromuscular responses to three days of velocity-specific isokinetic training. J Strength Cond Res 20: 892-898.
12. Kanehisa H, Miyashita M (1983) Specificity of velocity in strength training. Eur J Appl Physiol Occup Physiol 52: 104-106.
13. Spiering BA, Kraemer WJ, Anderson JM, Armstrong LE, Nindl BC, et al. (2008) Resistance exercise biology: Manipulation of resistance exercise programme variables determines the responses of cellular and molecular signaling pathways. Sports Med 38: 527-540.
14. Eliasson J, Elfegoun T, Nilsson J, Köhnke R, Ekblom B, et al. (2006) Maximal lengthening contractions increase p70 S6 kinase phosphorylation in human skeletal muscle in the absence of nutritional supply. Am J Physiol Endocrinol Metab 291: E1197-1205.
15. Long YC, Widegren U, Zierath JR (2004) Exercise-induced mitogen-activated protein kinase signalling in skeletal muscle. Proc Nutr Soc 63: 227-232.
16. Garma T, Kobayashi C, Haddad F, Adams GR, Bodell PW, et al. (2007) Similar acute molecular responses to equivalent volumes of isometric, lengthening, or shortening mode resistance exercise. J Appl Physiol 102: 135-143.
17. Hather BM, Tesch PA, Buchanan P, Dudley GA (1991) Influence of eccentric actions on skeletal muscle adaptations to resistance training. Acta Physiol Scand 143: 177-185.
18. Spreuwenberg LP, Kraemer WJ, Spiering BA, Volek JS, Hatfield DL, et al. (2006) Influence of exercise order in a resistance-training exercise session. J Strength Cond Res 20: 141-144.
19. Dias I, de Salles BF, Novaes J, Costa PB, Simão R (2010) Influence of exercise order on maximum strength in untrained young men. J Sci Med Sport 13: 65-69.
20. Augustsson J, Thomeé R, Hörnstedt P, Lindblom J, Karlsson J, et al. (2003) Effect of pre-exhaustion exercise on lower-extremity muscle activation during a leg press exercise. J Strength Cond Res 17: 411-416.
21. Baker D, Newton RU (2005) Acute effect on power output of alternating an agonist and antagonist muscle exercise during complex training. J Strength Cond Res 19: 202-205.
22. American College of Sports Medicine (2009) American College of Sports Medicine position stand. Progression models in resistance training for healthy adults. Med Sci Sports Exerc 41: 687-708.
23. Ratamess NA, Falvo MJ, Mangine GT, Hoffman JR, Faigenbaum AD, et al. (2007) The effect of rest interval length on metabolic responses to the bench press exercise. Eur J Appl Physiol 100: 1-17.
24. Lusa Cadore E, Lhullier FL, Arias Brentano M, Marczwski Da Silva E, Bueno Ambrosini M, et al. (2009) Salivary hormonal responses to resistance exercise in trained and untrained middle-aged men. J Sports Med Phys Fitness 49: 301-307.
25. Beaven CM, Gill ND, Cook CJ (2008) Salivary testosterone and cortisol responses in professional rugby players after four resistance exercise protocols. J Strength Cond Res 22: 426-432.
26. Hakkinen K, Alen M, Komi PV (1985) Changes in isometric force-time and relaxation-time, electromyographic and muscle-fiber characteristics of human skeletal-muscle during strength training and detraining. Acta Physiol Scand 125: 573-585.
27. Weiss LW, Coney HD, Clark FC (1999) Differential functional adaptations to short-term low-, moderate-, and high-repetition weight training. J Strength Cond Res 13: 236-241.
28. Campos GE, Luecke TJ, Wendeln HK, Toma K, Hagerman FC, et al. (2002) Muscular adaptations in response to three different resistance-training regimens: specificity of repetition maximum training zones. Eur J Appl Physiol 88: 50-60.
29. Berger RA (1962) Optimum repetitions for the development of strength. Res Q 33: 334-338.
30. O'Shea P (1966) Effects of selected weight training programs on the development of strength and muscle hypertrophy. Res Q 37: 95-102.
31. Wilson GJ, Newton RU, Murphy AJ, Humphries BJ (1993) The optimal training load for the development of dynamic athletic performance. Med Sci Sports Exerc 25: 1279-1286.
32. Staron RS, Karapondo DL, Kraemer WJ, Fry AC, Gordon SE, et al. (1994) Skeletal muscle adaptations during early phase of heavy-resistance training in men and women. J Appl Physiol 76: 1247-1255.
33. Kraemer WJ (1997) A series of studies - The physiological basis for strength training in American football: Fact over philosophy. J Strength Cond ReS 11: 131-142.
34. Nader GA, Esser KA (2001) Intracellular signaling specificity in skeletal muscle in response to different modes of exercise. J Appl Physiol 90: 1936-1942.
35. Atherton PJ, Babraj J, Smith K, Singh J, Rennie MJ, et al. (2005) Selective activation of AMPK-PGC-1alpha or PKB-TSC2-mTOR signaling can explain specific adaptive responses to endurance or resistance training-like electrical muscle stimulation. FASEB J 19: 786-788.
36. Hornberger TA, Chien S (2006) Mechanical stimuli and nutrients regulate rapamycin-sensitive signaling through distinct mechanisms in skeletal muscle. J Cell Biochem 97: 1207-1216.
37. Bodine SC, Stitt TN, Gonzalez M, Kline WO, Stover GL, et al. (2001) Akt/mTOR pathway is a crucial regulator of skeletal muscle hypertrophy and can prevent muscle atrophy in vivo. Nat Cell Biol 3: 1014-1019.
38. Terada N, Patel HR, Takase K, Kohno K, Nairn AC, et al. (1994) Rapamycin selectively inhibits translation of mRNAs encoding elongation factors and ribosomal proteins. Proc Natl Acad Sci U S A 91: 11477-11481.
39. Henneman E, Somjen G, Carpenter DO (1965) Functional Significance of Cell Size in Spinal Motoneurons.
40. McCaulley GO, McBride JM, Cormie P, Hudson MB, Nuzzo JL, et al. (2009) Acute hormonal and neuromuscular responses to hypertrophy, strength and power type resistance exercise. Eur J Appl Physiol 105: 695-704.
41. Linnamo V, Newton RU, Häkkinen K, Komi PV, Davie A, et al. (2000) Neuromuscular responses to explosive and heavy resistance loading. J Electromyogr Kinesiol 10: 417-424.
42. Pincivero DM, Gandhi V, Timmons MK, Coelho AJ (2006) Quadriceps femoris electromyogram during concentric, isometric and eccentric phases of fatiguing dynamic knee extensions. J Biomech 39: 246-254.
43. McCall GE, Byrnes WC, Dickinson A, Pattany PM, Fleck SJ (1996) Muscle fiber hypertrophy, hyperplasia, and capillary density in college men after resistance training. J Appl Physiol 81: 2004-2012.
44. Trappe SW, Trappe TA, Lee GA, Widrick JJ, Costill DL, et al. (2001) Comparison of a space shuttle flight (STS-78) and bed rest on human muscle function. J

Appl Physiol 91: 57-64.

45. Kraemer WJ, Ratamess NA (2004) Fundamentals of resistance training: progression and exercise prescription. Med Sci Sports Exerc 36: 674-688.

46. Peterson MD, Rhea MR, Alvar BA (2005) Applications of the dose-response for muscular strength development: a review of meta-analytic efficacy and reliability for designing training prescription. J Strength Cond Res 19: 950-958.

47. Prestes J, Frollini AB, de Lima C, Donatto FF, Foschini D, et al. (2009) Comparison between linear and daily undulating periodized resistance training to increase strength. J Strength Cond Res 23: 2437-2442.

48. Rhea MR, Ball SD, Phillips WT, Burkett LN (2002) A comparison of linear and daily undulating periodized programs with equated volume and intensity for strength. J Strength Cond Res 16: 250-255.

49. Selye H (1974) Stress without distress. New York: JB Lippincott Company.

50. Tran QT, Docherty D, Behm D (2006) The effects of varying time under tension and volume load on acute neuromuscular responses. Eur J Appl Physiol 98: 402-410.

51. Borst SE, De Hoyos DV, Garzarella L, Vincent K, Pollock BH, et al. (2001) Effects of resistance training on insulin-like growth factor-I and IGF binding proteins. Med Sci Sports Exerc 33: 648-653.

52. Willoughby DS, Chilek DR, Schiller DA, Coast JR (1991) The metabolic effects of 3 different free weight parallel squatting intensities. J Hum Movement Stud 21: 53-67.

53. Dudley GA, Djamil R (1985) Incompatibility of endurance- and strength-training modes of exercise. J Appl Physiol 59: 1446-1451.

54. Hortobágyi T, Barrier J, Beard D, Braspennincx J, Koens P, et al. (1996) Greater initial adaptations to submaximal muscle lengthening than maximal shortening. J Appl Physiol 81: 1677-1682.

55. Housh DJ, Housh TJ, Johnson GO, Chu WK (1992) Hypertrophic response to unilateral concentric isokinetic resistance training. J Appl Physiol 73: 65-70.

56. Ostrowski KJ, Wilson GJ, Weatherby R, Murphy PW, Lyttle AD (1997) The effect of weight training volume on hormonal output and muscular size and function. J Strength Cond Res 11: 148-154.

57. Capen EK (1956) Study of four programs of heavy resistance exercises for development of muscular strength. Res Q 27: 132-142.

58. Krieger JW (2009) Single versus multiple sets of resistance exercise: a meta-regression. J Strength Cond Res 23: 1890-1901.

59. Tang JE, Perco JG, Moore DR, Wilkinson SB, Phillips SM (2008) Resistance training alters the response of fed state mixed muscle protein synthesis in young men. Am J Physiol Regul Integr Comp Physiol 294: R172-178.

60. MacDougall JD, Gibala MJ, Tarnopolsky MA, MacDonald JR, Interisano SA, et al. (1995) The time course for elevated muscle protein synthesis following heavy resistance exercise. Can J Appl Physiol 20: 480-486.

61. Phillips SM (2000) Short-term training: When do repeated bouts of resistance exercise become training? Can J Appl Physiol 25: 185-193.

62. Rhea MR, Alvar BA, Ball SD, Burkett LN (2002) Three sets of weight training superior to 1 set with equal intensity for eliciting strength. J Strength Cond Res 16: 525-529.

63. Moss BM, Refsnes PE, Abildgaard A, Nicolaysen K, Jensen J (1997) Effects of maximal effort strength training with different loads on dynamic strength, cross-sectional area, load-power and load-velocity relationships. Eur J Appl Physiol Occup Physiol 75: 193-199.

64. Marx JO, Ratamess NA, Nindl BC, Gotshalk LA, Volek JS, et al. (2001) Low-volume circuit versus high-volume periodized resistance training in women. Med Sci Sports Exerc 33: 635-643.

65. Goto K, Nagasawa M, Yanagisawa O, Kizuka T, Ishii N, et al. (2004) Muscular adaptations to combinations of high- and low-intensity resistance exercises. J Strength Cond Res 18: 730-737.

66. Creer A, Gallagher P, Slivka D, Jemiolo B, Fink W, et al. (2005) Influence of muscle glycogen availability on ERK1/2 and Akt signaling after resistance exercise in human skeletal muscle. J Appl Physiol 99: 950-956.

67. Kraemer WJ, Gordon SE, Fleck SJ, Marchitelli LJ, Mello R, et al. (1991) Endogenous anabolic hormonal and growth factor responses to heavy resistance exercise in males and females. Int J Sports Med 12: 228-235.

68. Gotshalk LA, Loebel CC, Nindl BC, Putukian M, Sebastianelli WJ, et al. (1997) Hormonal responses of multiset versus single-set heavy-resistance exercise protocols. Can J Appl Physiol 22: 244-255.

69. Kraemer WJ, Noble BJ, Clark MJ, Culver BW (1987) Physiologic responses to heavy-resistance exercise with very short rest periods. Int J Sports Med 8: 247-252.

70. Behm DG, Reardon G, Fitzgerald J, Drinkwater E (2002) The effect of 5, 10, and 20 repetition maximums on the recovery of voluntary and evoked contractile properties. J Strength Cond Res 16: 209-218.

71. Miranda H, Simao R, Moreira LM, de Souza RA, se Souza JAA, et al. (2009) Effect of rest interval length on the volume completed during upper body resistance exercise. J Sport Sci Med 8: 388-392.

72. Robinson JM, Stone MH, Johnson RL, Penland CM, Warren BJ, et al. (1995) Effects of Different Weight Training Exercise/Rest Intervals on Strength, Power, and High Intensity Exercise Endurance. J Strength Cond Res 9: 216-221.

73. Ahtiainen JP, Pakarinen A, Alen M, Kraemer WJ, Häkkinen K (2005) Short vs. long rest period between the sets in hypertrophic resistance training: influence on muscle strength, size, and hormonal adaptations in trained men. J Strength Cond Res 19: 572-582.

74. Crewther BT, Lowe T, Weatherby RP, Gill N, Keogh J (2009) Neuromuscular performance of elite rugby union players and relationships with salivary hormones. J Strength Cond Res 23: 2046-2053.

75. Vermeulen A, Verdonck L, Kaufman JM (1999) A critical evaluation of simple methods for the estimation of free testosterone in serum. J Clin Endocrinol Metab 84: 3666-3672.

76. Florini JR (1987) Hormonal control of muscle growth. Muscle Nerve 10: 577-598.

77. Kraemer WJ, Fleck SJ, Dziados JE, Harman EA, Marchitelli LJ, et al. (1993) Changes in hormonal concentrations after different heavy-resistance exercise protocols in women. J Appl Physiol 75: 594-604.

78. Kvorning T, Andersen M, Brixen K, Madsen K (2006) Suppression of endogenous testosterone production attenuates the response to strength training: a randomized, placebo-controlled, and blinded intervention study. Am J Physiol Endoc Metab 291: 1325-1332.

79. Hansen S, Kvorning T, Kjaer M, Sjøgaard G (2001) The effect of short-term strength training on human skeletal muscle: the importance of physiologically elevated hormone levels. Scand J Med Sci Sports 11: 347-354.

80. Ahtiainen JP, Pakarinen A, Kraemer WJ, Häkkinen K (2003) Acute hormonal and neuromuscular responses and recovery to forced vs maximum repetitions multiple resistance exercises. Int J Sports Med 24: 410-418.

81. Phillips SM, Tipton KD, Aarsland AA, Wolf SE, Wolfe RR (1997) Time course of mixed muscle protein synthesis following resistance exercise in humans. Med Sci Sports Exerc 29: 230.

82. Sinha-Hikim I, Artaza J, Woodhouse L, Gonzalez-Cadavid N, Singh AB, et al. (2002) Testosterone-induced increase in muscle size in healthy young men is associated with muscle fiber hypertrophy. Am J Physiol Endocrinol Metab 283: E154-164.

83. Zitzmann M, Nieschlag E (2003) Effects of androgen replacement on metabolism and physical performances in male hypogonadism. J Endocrinol Invest 26: 886-892.

84. Mauras N, Hayes V, Welch S, Rini A, Helgeson K, et al. (1998) Testosterone deficiency in young men: marked alterations in whole body protein kinetics, strength, and adiposity. J Clin Endocrinol Metab 83: 1886-1892.

85. Beaven CM, Cook CJ, Gill ND (2008) Significant strength gains observed in rugby players after specific resistance exercise protocols based on individual salivary testosterone responses. J Strength Cond Res 22: 419-425.

86. West DW, Kujbida GW, Moore DR, Atherton P, Burd NA, et al. (2009) Resistance exercise-induced increases in putative anabolic hormones do not enhance muscle protein synthesis or intracellular signalling in young men. J Physiol 587: 5239-5247.

87. McCall GE, Byrnes WC, Fleck SJ, Dickinson A, Kraemer WJ (1999) Acute and chronic hormonal responses to resistance training designed to promote muscle hypertrophy. Can J Appl Physiol 24: 96-107.

88. Inoue K, Yamasaki S, Fushiki T, Okada Y, Sugimoto E (1994) Androgen receptor antagonist suppresses exercise-induced hypertrophy of skeletal muscle. Eur J Appl Physiol Occup Physiol 69: 88-91.

89. Lee WJ, McClung J, Hand GA, Carson JA (2003) Overload-induced androgen receptor expression in the aged rat hindlimb receiving nandrolone decanoate. J Appl Physiol 94: 1153-1161.

90. Kraemer WJ, Hatfield DL, Volek JS, Fragala MS, Vingren JL, et al. (2009) Effects of amino acids supplement on physiological adaptations to resistance training. Med Sci Sports Exerc 41: 1111-1121.

91. Kraemer WJ, Patton JF, Gordon SE, Harman EA, Deschenes MR, et al. (1995) Compatibility of high-intensity strength and endurance training on hormonal and skeletal muscle adaptations. J Appl Physiol 78: 976-989.

92. Kraemer WJ, Loebel CC, Volek JS, Ratamess NA, Newton RU, et al. (2001) The effect of heavy resistance exercise on the circadian rhythm of salivary testosterone in men. Eur J Appl Physiol 84: 13-18.

93. Vale RG, de Oliveira RD, Pernambuco CS, de Meneses YP, Novaes Jda S, et al. (2009) Effects of muscle strength and aerobic training on basal serum levels of IGF-1 and cortisol in elderly women. Arch Gerontol Geriatr 49: 343-347.

94. Timon R, Olcina G, Tomas-Carus P, Muñoz D, Toribio F, et al. (2009) Urinary steroid profile after the completion of concentric and concentric/eccentric trials with the same total workload. J Physiol Biochem 65: 105-112.

95. Smilios I, Pilianidis T, Karamouzis M, Tokmakidis SP (2003) Hormonal responses after various resistance exercise protocols. Med Sci Sports Exerc 35: 644-654.

96. Häkkinen K, Pakarinen A (1993) Acute hormonal responses to two different fatiguing heavy-resistance protocols in male athletes. J Appl Physiol 74: 882-887.

97. Duclos M (2008) A critical assessment of hormonal methods used in monitoring training status in athletes. Int Sportmed J 9: 56-66.

98. Duclos M, Gouarne C, Bonnemaison D (2003) Acute and chronic effects of exercise on tissue sensitivity to glucocorticoids. J Appl Physiol 94: 869-875.

99. Pfeffer LA, Brisson BK, Lei H, Barton ER (2009) The insulin-like growth factor (IGF)-I E-peptides modulate cell entry of the mature IGF-I protein. Mol Biol Cell 20: 3810-3817.

100. Adlercreutz H, Härkönen M, Kuoppasalmi K, Näveri H, Huhtaniemi I, et al. (1986) Effect of training on plasma anabolic and catabolic steroid hormones and their response during physical exercise. Int J Sports Med 7 Suppl 1: 27-28.

101. Flynn MG, Pizza FX, Boone JB Jr, Andres FF, Michaud TA, et al. (1994) Indices of training stress during competitive running and swimming seasons. Int J Sports Med 15: 21-26.

102. Fry AC, Kraemer WJ, Ramsey LT (1998) Pituitary-adrenal-gonadal responses to high-intensity resistance exercise overtraining. J Appl Physiol 85: 2352-2359.

103. Adams GR (2002) Invited Review: Autocrine/paracrine IGF-I and skeletal muscle adaptation. J Appl Physiol 93: 1159-1167.

104. Glass DJ (2005) Skeletal muscle hypertrophy and atrophy signaling pathways. Int J Biochem Cell Biol 37: 1974-1984.

105. Barton ER (2006) Viral expression of insulin-like growth factor-I isoforms promotes different responses in skeletal muscle. J Appl Physiol 100: 1778-1784.

106. Fedele MJ, Lang CH, Farrell PA (2001) Immunization against IGF-I prevents increases in protein synthesis in diabetic rats after resistance exercise. Am J Physiol Endocrinol Metab 280: E877-885.

107. Chandler RM, Byrne HK, Patterson JG, Ivy JL (1994) Dietary supplements affect the anabolic hormones after weight-training exercise. J Appl Physiol 76: 839-845.

108. Bamman MM, Shipp JR, Jiang J, Gower BA, Hunter GR, et al. (2001) Mechanical load increases muscle IGF-I and androgen receptor mRNA concentrations in humans. Am J Physiol Endocrinol Metab 280: E383-390.

109. Nindl BC, Kraemer WJ, Hymer WC (2000) Immunofunctional vs immunoreactive growth hormone responses after resistance exercise in men and women. Growth Horm IGF Res 10: 99-103.

110. Hawke TJ (2005) Muscle stem cells and exercise training. Exerc Sport Sci Rev 33: 63-68.

111. Florini JR, Ewton DZ, Coolican SA (1996) Growth hormone and the insulin-like growth factor system in myogenesis. Endocr Rev 17: 481-517.

112. Jurasinski CV, Vary TC (1995) Insulin-like growth factor I accelerates protein synthesis in skeletal muscle during sepsis. Am J Physiol 269: E977-981.

113. Wilborn CD, Taylor LW, Greenwood M, Kreider RB, Willoughby DS (2009) Effects of different intensities of resistance exercise on regulators of myogenesis. J Strength Cond Res 23: 2179-2187.

114. Allen DL, Linderman JK, Roy RR, Grindeland RE, Mukku V, et al. (1997) Growth hormone/IGF-I and/or resistive exercise maintains myonuclear number in hindlimb unweighted muscles. J Appl Physiol 83: 1857-1861.

115. Adams GR, McCue SA (1998) Localized infusion of IGF-I results in skeletal muscle hypertrophy in rats. J Appl Physiol 84: 1716-1722.

116. Wolfe RR (2000) Effects of insulin on muscle tissue. Curr Opin Clin Nutr Metab Care 3: 67-71.

117. Kuo CH, Hunt DG, Ding Z, Ivy JL (1999) Effect of carbohydrate supplementation on postexercise GLUT-4 protein expression in skeletal muscle. J Appl Physiol 87: 2290-2295.

118. Kimball SR, Farrell PA, Jefferson LS (2002) Invited Review: Role of insulin in translational control of protein synthesis in skeletal muscle by amino acids or exercise. J Appl Physiol 93: 1168-1180.

119. Kraemer WJ, Clemson A, Triplett NT, Bush JA, Newton RU, et al. (1996) The effects of plasma cortisol elevation on total and differential leukocyte counts in response to heavy-resistance exercise. Eur J Appl Physiol Occup Physiol 73: 93-97.

120. Nindl BC, Kraemer WJ, Marx JO, Arciero PJ, Dohi K, et al. (2001) Overnight responses of the circulating IGF-I system after acute, heavy-resistance exercise. J Appl Physiol 90: 1319-1326.

121. Bush JA, Kimball SR, O'Connor PM, Suryawan A, Orellana RA, et al. (2003) Translational control of protein synthesis in muscle and liver of growth hormone-treated pigs. Endocrinology 144: 1273-1283.

122. Mulligan SE, Fleck SJ, Gordon SE, Koziris LP, Triplett-McBride NT, et al. (1996) Influence of Resistance Exercise Volume on Serum Growth Hormone and Cortisol Concentrations in Women. J Strength Cond Res 10: 256-262.

123. Hoffman JR, Im J, Rundell KW, Kang J, Nioka S, et al. (2003) Effect of muscle oxygenation during resistance exercise on anabolic hormone response. Med Sci Sports Exerc 35: 1929-1934.

8

Investigation of the Attitudes of Japanese Physical Educational University Students toward Doping in Sports

Masato Takahashi[1]*, Yukitoshi Tatsugi[1] and Tosihiko Kohno[2]

[1]*Faculty of Physical Education, International Budo Univ, Japan*
[2]*Faculty of Nursing, Kameda College of Health Science, Japan*

Abstract

Background: Drug abuse, most notably Anabolic-Androgenic Steroid (AAS) use, in athletes is thought to be widespread. A few drug abusers and persons who express acceptance of drug abuse in sports are known to be present in Japan as well. We investigated the state of drug abuse and attitudes toward drug abuse in sports in a Japanese physical education university from the viewpoint of anti-doping.

Methods: The study sample was comprised of students attending a physical educational university in Japan. An anonymous self-completed questionnaire was given out in two classes at the beginning of the semester from 2008 until 2012, inclusive. Results for the year 2011 are given here. The questionnaire had 5 sections covering responder's drug use, attitudes toward doping, a hypothetical situation on an athlete's drug use, dietary supplements, and what the responder eats or drinks before playing a game.

Results: The response rate for the 2011 questionnaire was 100%. There were 2 admitted drug abusers (0.4%) and 774 (99.6%) non-abusers. The use of diuretics was admitted. In Section II, which included a question on what the responder thought of doping, 144 (19.3%) selected "good" and 592 (79.1%) selected "bad". Section III presented a hypothetical situation whereby the respondent would use a drug undetectable by doping control, win a gold medal and have a lifespan of only 5 years thereafter. In answer to the question of whether the respondent would use the drug under those conditions, 85 (11.4%) answered "yes" and 655 (87.5%) answered "no".

Conclusions: 20% of the students approved of drug use in sports. Furthermore, based on the response to a question in Section III, it can be speculated that 10% of the students might have used drugs in sports.

Keywords: Drug abuse; Doping; Questionnaire; Survey; Stimulant; Anabolic steroid; Dietary supplement

Introduction

A famous track sprinter was ruled out of the 1988 Seoul Korea Olympics for using Anabolic-Androgenic Steroids (AAS), a case that was very shocking. Many athletes were judged positive by doping control measures for using performance enhancing drugs in the 2004 Athens Olympics, too. Drug abuse, most notably AAS use, in athletes is thought to be widespread. Therefore, various surveys on drug abuse among youth have been made in developed countries since that time. Reports of such surveys have been published from Japan also. Takahashi et al. reported on counseling of drug abusers from the viewpoint of anti-doping in Japan [1-2]. Furthermore they surveyed the state of drug abuse through a blog accessed by drug abusers [3]. The drug abusers used the Internet to gain knowledge of information on drug abuse, side effects and the role of the Internet in drug abuse. Furthermore, it was clear that drug abusers exchanged information on doping with each other by blogs.

Meilman et al. performed a cohort study of AAS abusers and nonusers by self-reported data in USA among USA college students in 1990 and 1991 [4]. An official questionnaire survey in Japanese of the state of doping and attitudes toward it was distributed at a National Athletic Meet in Japan. A few drug abusers and persons who accepted the use of such drugs were known to be present. No surveys were performed thereafter in Japan.

We have attempted to investigate the state of drug abuse and attitudes toward drug abuse in sports in a Japanese physical education university. Because physical education university students could easily become connected with drug abuse in sports, we thought that they were an appropriate sample. In addition, it is important to know the state of drug abuse in sports as well as the physical educational college students' attitude toward doping from the viewpoint of anti-doping. From results of this survey, we could clarify the circumstances surrounding permitting drug abuse in Japan and the attitude toward drug abuse in sports.

Materials and Methods

The sample studied was comprised of some of the students who attended a physical educational university, which is located in a rural area. Judo, kendo, naginata, and other Budo event teams from this university are strong in college sports. Field and track events, baseball, volleyball, lifesaving competitions, and power lifting teams are also strong. Some of the participants are candidates for Olympic events.

Participants belonged to one of two "Sports Medicine" classes or a "Health Care Studies" class. An anonymous self-completed questionnaire was given out in each class at the beginning of each semester. Such a questionnaire has been distributed every year since 2006, with the format being changed in 2008 to the one described herein. In this report, we showed the results of the questionnaire distributed in 2011. Almost all of the students who completed the questionnaire were second-year students; however, a few were third- and fourth-year students. In this university, each grade consists of about 500 persons, with 16.7% being female (female's 338/total 2027). In the three classes surveyed, 15.3% were females (female's 131/total 856). To protect the

***Corresponding author:** Dr. Masato Takahashi, Faculty of Phys. Educ, International Budo Univ, Japan, E-mail: t-masato@budo-u.ac.jp

student's anonymity, this questionnaire did not have a question on grade and gender.

We declared that results of this questionnaire would not be given to the university managers, even if someone admitted to using an illegal drug. All of the students answered the questions regarding illegal drug use.

The questionnaire consisted of 5 sections (Table 1). Section I had questions on drug abuse. The first question asked whether or not responders were using a drug and, if so, the second question asked which of the following drugs were used: stimulant, anabolic agent (AAS, β_2 stimulant, and growth hormone), erythropoietin, diuretics, others (please describe). Section II had two questions about attitudes toward doping and the use of medicines in daily life as athletes. Section III presented a hypothetical situation whereby the respondent would use a drug undetectable by doping control, win a gold medal and have a lifespan of only 5 years thereafter; the respondent was asked whether he or she would do this. In Section IV, questions were about dietary supplements. The first question asked whether the responder used dietary supplements and, if the answer was yes, the second question asked which supplements were used. Section V was comprised of a question on eating or drinking before playing a game.

This study was performed according to the Declaration of Helsinki and the guidelines of the ethics board of our university.

Results

The recovery rate of the questionnaire was 100% of those to whom it was distributed.

Responses to Question I-1 showed that there were 2 drug abusers (0.4%) and 744 (99.6%) non-abusers. In Question I-2, 1 drug abuser answered, "Yes" to the use of diuretics and the other gave no answer. There were no responses to Question I-3 to I-7.

In answering Question II-1, 144 (19.3%) selected "good" about doping, 592 (79.1%) selected "bad" and 12 (1.6%) gave "no answer" (Figure 1). In Question II-2 (Figure 2) regarding whether the responder minded taking medicines, 152 (20.3%) said "yes", 573 (74.6%) said "no", and 23 (3.1%) gave "no answer".

In Question III-1 regarding the hypothetical situation regarding drug abuse with the aim of winning a gold medal, 85 (11.4%) answered "yes", 655 (87.5%) "No", and 8 (1.1%) gave "no answer" (Figure 3). As to Question III-2, one of those who answered "yes" said that it was only important to win the gold medal and another stated the desire to win a medal. One of those who answered "no" said that he/she did not want to win a medal if his/her life span would be shortened and another stated that we should win a medal by our own skills without the aid of drugs.

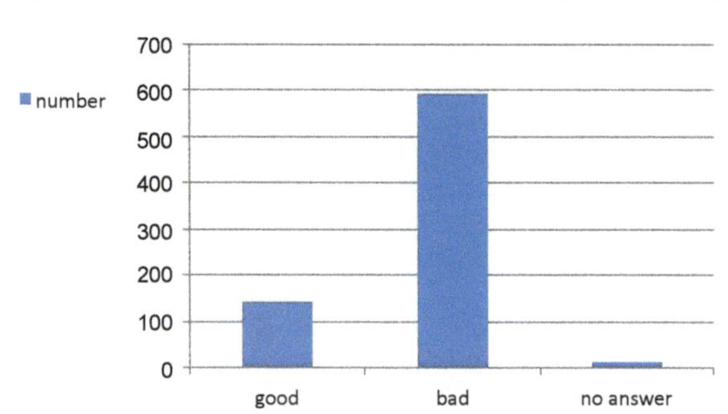

Figure 1: Response to Question II-1 on the self-completed questionnaire (Do you think doping is good or bad?)

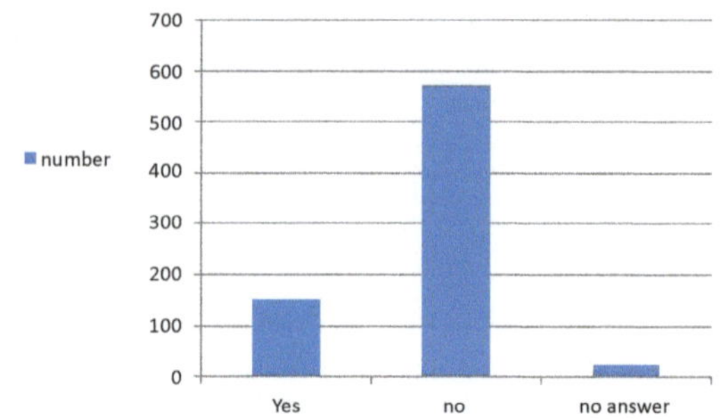

Figure 2: Response to Question II-2 on the self-completed questionnaire (Do you mind using medicines?)

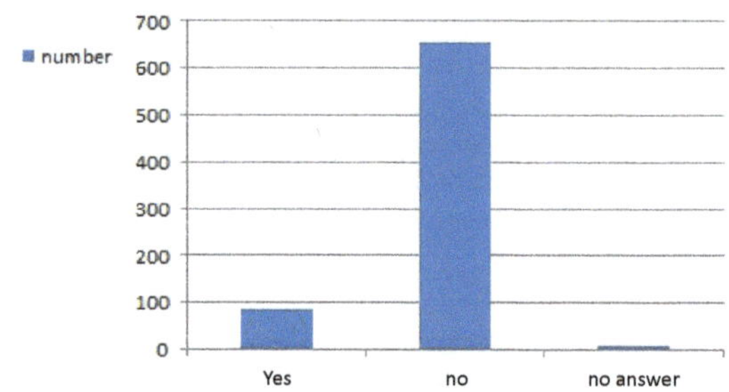

Figure 3: Response to hypothetical situation presented in Section III of the questionnaire whereby the respondent would use a drug undetectable by doping control, win a gold medal a have a lifespan of only 5 years thereafter. Responder was asked to declare whether he would or would not use the agent. Possible responses were "yes," "no" and "no answer".

In Question IV-1, which was on whether the responder used dietary supplements, "yes" was given by 218 (29.1%) responders, "no" by 515 (68.9%), and "no answer" by 15 (2.0%) (Figure 4). Responses to Question IV-2 showed that protein was used by 183 students, amino acids by 66, vitamins by 62, creatine by 42, and iron by 27, and anabolic agent by 6, and a stimulant by 1. As to Question V, which was what the responder might eat or drink before a game, there were no responders.

Discussion

It is important to examine the range and dimensions of the use of AAS. In answer to Question I-1, almost all of the students had not used a performance enhancing drug. Kindlundh et al. reported the results of an anonymous questionnaire on doping among Swedish high school students in 1998 and showed that about 3% of male students used AAS in relation to sports activity [5]. Williamson administered questionnaires on drug abuse in sports, especially AAS in the UK in 1993 [6]. He had the impression that drug abuse was widespread among youths, especially high school students but found that 2.8% of students were using AAS with regard to sports in 1993. In 1996, a survey of the use of AAS by young Canadian students through a self-report questionnaire showed that the rate of anabolic steroid use was 2% in those 16 years of age [7]. In 1997, the report on the state of AAS use in 21 gymnasts in the UK showed that more than 10% of gymnasts of various ages were using AAS [8]. In 1997, the epidemiology of doping in sports was reviewed [9]. In that review, it was stated that the extent of sports doping and its potential health risks indicate that doping in sports should be considered a public health problem. Physicians must consider it as seriously as any other problem, focusing on the wider

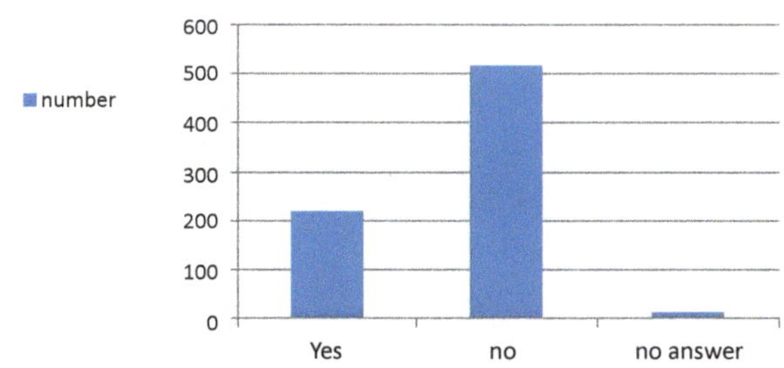

Figure 4: Response to Question IV-1 on the self-completed questionnaire (Are you using dietary supplements?)

issues beyond simply a list of prohibited substances, such as attitudes toward doping. In the US, the use of AAS among high school students is prevalent, and in 2001 1% to 2% of adolescent girls and 4% to 6% of adolescent boys have ever used AAS [10]. In Sweden, the same situation with regard to the use of AAS by adolescents was recognized [11]. In 2007, Laure and Binsinger reported on the state of drug abuse in sports in France [12]. They noted that 1.2% of pupils entering the first year of secondary school in France stated that they had taken doping agents at least once in the preceding 6 months; 4 years later this rate had risen to 3.0%. Of users, 4% reported that they had experienced a health problem related to doping, and 44% reported that they had won at least one sports event as a result of drug use.

Although we did not show the results here, we have distributed the same anonymous questionnaire as described in this report for 5 years. In reality, the rate of use of illegal recreational drugs and performance-enhancing drugs in this physical education university is low. In Japan, the Japan Anti-Doping Agency (http://www.playtruejapan.org/) has announced statistics on the use of performance enhancing agents since 1997. In 2010, 258, 267 samples were examined and 1.08% were positive (http://www.medience.co.jp/doping/03.html). Since 1997, the rate has been below 2%. Therefore it is thought that there may be fewer drug abusers in Japan than in other developed countries. However, in the survey reported here 2 students admitted to the use of drugs, and in the survey in 2010 one student admitted to the use of marijuana. Illegal recreational drugs or AAS might have been used. It was surprising that there were some drug abusers in a physical education college in Japan. It is of interest that no student has answered Questions I-3 to I-7 since the beginning of this investigation.

We asked questions to determine students' attitudes toward doping. In response to Question II-1, which was "What do you think about doping?" 80% of students selected "bad" and 20% selected "good". Over the previous 4 years of the study, that is, from 2008 to 2011, the response of "good" has ranged from 15 to 20%. Although students have attended lectures about illegal drugs, they have not studied the doping control system as a class yet. It is important for elite athletes to become informed about doping.

In addition, we presented a hypothetical situation to elicit the attitude toward doping (Question III-1). About 10% of the responders would use drugs to win a medal even if they would die 5 years later, and about 20% indicated a positive attitude toward doping in sports. Against such a background, the habit of drug abuse in sports will spread if there is a strong motivation.

In 2001, Nilsson et al. reported that AAS abusers use alcohol, growth hormones, and narcotic drugs more than AAS non-users [11]. Laure et al. noted that users of doping agents take cannabis, tranquilizers, hypnotics, and creatine more than non-users [13]. Peterson et al. reported similar results [14]. However, we could not confirm a case of using both AAS and illegal drugs as did these reports. As background, the use of these drugs has not spread among Japanese physical educational students.

German nonathletes, recreational athletes and competitive athletes performed poorly on a knowledge test regarding doping in general with an average below 60% in each case [15]. In our study, each year there were unclear answers to Q I-2 (What drugs are you using if you use performance enhancing drugs?). It is clear that they are not informed about the drugs they are using. It may be the same state from the viewpoint of knowledge of drug abuse. Buckman et al. said that athletes who used performance-enhancing substances compared with nonusers reported more alcohol-related behaviors and alcohol- and drug-use-related problems [16]. Although there were only a few drug users in our study, once such usage spreads, alcohol and various drug problems will spread. In Japan, we will have to warn athletes and others of this possibility. In Germany, the high prevalence of drug abuse in sports was clear. Furthermore the high prevalence of the use of illicit drugs, especially cocaine, was clear [17]. The use of AAS promotes the use of the other drugs [18]. Furthermore, users of performance-enhancing drugs statistically tend to use alcohol [16]. AAS or other performance-enhancing drugs introduce illicit drug use [19-21]. In our study, one case of marijuana abuse was recognized. At present, it is necessary to prevent the growth of the prevalence of illicit or performance enhancing drugs.

AAS abuse in Finnish adolescents was uncommon in a survey [22]. Dietary supplement use is associated with frequent sports participation

I. **Questions about use of performance enhancing drugs**
1. Are you using performance enhancing drugs? Yes / No
2. If you answered "yes", what are you using? Stimulant, anabolic agent (anabolic androgenic steroid, β_2 stimulant, and growth hormone), erythropoietin, diuretics, and others
3. If you are using an anabolic agent, what agent is it?
4. If you are using an anabolic agent, what is your objective?
5. If you are using an anabolic agent, what are its effects?
6. If you are using an anabolic agent, do you have any side effecs?
7. If you used a performance-enhancing drug, what is it?
II. Questions about attitudes toward doping and medicines in daily life as athletes.
1. What do you think about doping? Good / Bad / No answer
2. Do you mind using medicines, for example, when you catch cold?
III. If you could use a drug that would not be detected by doping control and would win a gold medal, would you do so even if your life span would only be 5 years thereafter?
1. Would you use the drug? Yes / No
2. If you have an opinion about this, write it here.
IV. Questions about dietary supplementation.
1. Are you using dietary supplements?
2. If "yes" is it any of the following: protein, amino acids, iron, creatine, and supplement compounded with anabolic agent, supplement with stimulant?
3. If you answered yes, what dietary supplement are you using?
4. If you answered yes, what is the objective?
5. If you answered yes, what are the effects of the supplement?
6. If you answered yes, have you had any side effects?
7. Can you tell us what dietary supplementation you might use?
V. **Can you tell me what you might eat or drink before you play a game?**

Table 1: Questionnaire about doping use, attitudes toward doping, and dietary supplements

and poorer than average health, while AAS use is associated with health-compromising behaviors. This state is similar to Japan. Bahrke et al. reviewed identified risk factors for drug abuse in sports and the rate of AAS use according to geographical regions in the US and South Africa [23]. However, there have been no reports on differences in the rate of AAS use according to country and the cultural background of countries.

In our study, about 30% of the students used dietary supplements. Gardiner et al. reported that herbs and dietary supplements were used by 17% of US young adults [24]. The use of supplements was more prevalent than we expected. However, the motives for the use of dietary supplements were unclear in our study, as in the US.

We think that it is necessary to prevent the spread of drug abuse in sports and of illicit drug use in Japan. Tricker and Connolly reported that drug education could be effective in preventing drug abuse among student athletes [25]. Dawson emphasized the role of the physician in addressing the problem of the use of performance enhancing drugs [26]. Although anti-doping anti-illicit drug measures are taken from official or private viewpoints, still more must be done. We think that it is important provide instruction on these issues at school.

In conclusion, it was ascertained that there were fewer students abusing drugs in Japan than in other developed countries. However, about 20% of the students approved of the use of drugs in sports. Furthermore, about 10% of them indicated that they might use drugs in competition. It is necessary for the government to adopt effective measures to address this issue.

Acknowledgements

We would like to acknowledge all of the students who responded to our questionnaire.

References

1. Takahashi M, Tatsugi Y, Kohno T (2007) Internet-based medical counseling on performance-enhancing drug abuse. J Med Soc Toho 54: 115-119.
2. Takahashi M, Tatsugi T, Kohno Y (2007) Telephone counseling of athletes abusing anabolic-androgenic steroids. J Sports Med Phys Fitness 47: 356-360.
3. Takahashi M, Tatsugi Y, Kohno T (2012) Analysis of communications about drug abuse among players of American football or athletes in Japan. GazzettaMedicaItaliana 171:157-164.
4. Meilman PW, Crace RK, Presley CA, Lyerla R (1995) Beyond performance enhancement: polypharmacy among collegiate users of steroids. J Am Coll Health 44: 98-104.
5. Kindlundh AM, Isacson DG, Berglund L, Nyberg F (1998) Doping among high school students in Uppsala, Sweden: A presentation of the attitudes, distribution, side effects, and extent of use. Scand J Soc Med 26: 71-74.
6. Williamson DJ (1993) Anabolic steroid use among students at a British college of technology. Br J Sports Med 27: 200-201.
7. Melia P, Pipe A, Greenberg L (1996) The use of anabolic-androgenic steroids by Canadian students. Clin J Sport Med 6: 9-14.
8. Korkia P, Stimson GV (1997) Indications of prevalence, practice and effects of anabolic steroid use in Great Britain. Int J Sports Med 18: 557-562.
9. Laure P (1997) Epidemiologic approach of doping in sport. A review. J Sports Med Phys Fitness 37: 218-224.
10. Yesalis CE (2001) Use of steroids for self-enhancement: an epidemiologic/ societal perspective. AIDS Read 11: 157-160.
11. Nilsson S, Baigi A, Marklund B, Fridlund B (2001) The prevalence of the use of androgenic anabolic steroids by adolescents in a county of Sweden. Eur J Public Health 11: 195-197.
12. Laure P, Binsinger C (2007) Doping prevalence among preadolescent athletes: a 4-year follow-up. Br J Sports Med 41: 660-663.
13. Laure P, Lecerf T, Friser A, Binsinger C (2004) Drugs, recreational drug use and attitudes towards doping of high school athletes. Int J Sports Med 25: 133-138.
14. Petersson A, Bengtsson J, Voltaire-Carlsson A, Thiblin I (2010) Substance abusers' motives for using anabolic androgenic steroids. Drug Alcohol Depend 111: 170-172.
15. Wanjek B, Rosendahl J, Strauss B, Gabriel HH (2007) Doping, drugs and drug abuse among adolescents in the State of Thuringia (Germany): prevalence, knowledge and attitudes. Int J Sports Med 28: 346-353.
16. Buckman JF, Yusko DA, White HR, Pandina RJ (2009) Risk profile of male college athletes who use performance-enhancing substances. J Stud Alcohol Drugs 70: 919-923.
17. Simon P, Striegel H, Aust F, Dietz K, Ulrich R (2006) Doping in fitness sports: estimated number of unreported cases and individual probability of doping. Addiction 101: 1640-1644.
18. Skårberg K, Nyberg F, Engström I (2008) The development of multiple drug use among anabolic-androgenic steroid users: six subjective case reports. Subst Abuse Treat Prev Policy 3: 24-34.
19. Nocelli L, Kamber M, François Y, Gmel G, Marti B (1998) Discordant public perception of doping in elite versus recreational sport in Switzerland. Clin J Sport Med 8: 195-200.
20. Black DL, Cawthon B, Robert T, Moser F, Caplan YH, et al. (2009) Multiple drug ingestion by ecstasy abusers in the United States. J Anal Toxicol 33: 143-147.
21. Strano Rossi S, Botrè F (2011) Prevalence of illicit drug use among the Italian athlete population with special attention on drugs of abuse: a 10-year review. J Sports Sci 29: 471-476.
22. Mattila VM, Parkkari J, Laakso L, Pihlajamäki H, Rimpelä A (2010) Use of dietary supplements and anabolic-androgenic steroids among Finnish adolescents in 1991-2005. Eur J Public Health 20: 306-311.
23. Bahrke MS, Yesalis CE, Kopstein AN, Stephens JA (2000) Risk factors associated with anabolic-androgenic steroid use among adolescents. Sports Med 29: 397-405.
24. Gardiner P, Kemper KJ, Legedza A, Phillips RS (2007) Factors associated with herb and dietary supplement use by young adults in the United States. BMC Complement Altern Med 7: 39.
25. Tricker R, Connolly D (1996) Drug education and the college athlete: evaluation of a decision-making model. J Drug Educ 26: 159-181.
26. Dawson RT (2001) Drugs in sport - the role of the physician. J Endocrinol 170: 170: 55-61

Tendon and Ligament Tissue Engineering, Healing and Regenerative Medicine

Ali Moshiri[1] and Ahmad Oryan[2*]

[1]*Veterinary Surgeon, Division of Surgery and Radiology, School of Veterinary Medicine, Shiraz University, Shiraz, Iran*
[2]*Comparative Pathologist, Department of Pathology, School of Veterinary Medicine, Shiraz University, Shiraz, Iran*

Abstract

Tendons transmit forces from muscle to bone and provide the joint function and ligaments transmit forces from bone to bone and provide joint stability. Tendon and ligament injuries have high incidence and management of tendon and ligament injuries is technically demanding because the healing response of these soft connective tissues is low. In addition, number of the available options to be considered as tissue replacement for large defects is low and healing of tendon and ligaments is faced to significant limitations. Among the available options, autografts are still gold standard but all the auto- allo and xenografts have their own limitations. Tissue engineering is a newer option but it is still primitive to be applicable extensively, in clinical setting. Tissue engineering could be divided into four categories including scaffolds, healing promotive factors, stem cells and gene therapy. To be able to have a good judgment regarding the management of tendon and ligament injuries, it is crucial to have a basic knowledge of tendon and ligament healing and regeneration. In this review, we discussed various types of tendon and ligament injuries and their incidence, and introduced the available and future options in managing large and massive tendon and ligament injuries. We specifically discussed the tissue engineering and it's advantageous and disadvantageous. To give a better clarification for the readers, we described different phases and cascades of tendon and ligament healing, modeling and remodeling, host-graft interaction after implantation of the graft and various types of prosthetic implants and finally provided some suggestions for the future investigations.

Keywords: Tendon; Ligament; Tissue engineering; Regenerative medicine; Scaffold; Growth factors; Stem cells; Glycosaminoglycans; Healing; Host-graft interaction; Autograft; Rejection; Repair

Introduction

Tendons transmit forces from muscle to bone and provide the joint function [1,2]. Ligaments transmit forces from bone to bone and provide joint stability [3]. The incidence of tendon and ligament injuries is high and several peoples are presented with these injuries to orthopedic surgery [1-5]. Tendon and ligaments are low vascularized tissues and have low healing capacity and capability; therefore management of tendon and ligament injuries is technically demanding [4-12]. Regardless of the acute or chronic nature of the tendon and ligament injuries, surgical reconstruction of the large and massive tissue defects is a more complicated situation [13-21]. There are some conventional available options in managing such large tissue losses including auto- allo- and xenografts [3,13-15]. Autografts are still gold standard while the allo grafts and xenografts have been introduced as alternative options having lower value than the autografts [3,12-14]. All these available options have their own significant limitations [3]. Tissue engineering is a newer option and is divided into four categories of scaffold, healing promotive factors, stem cells and gene therapy [22-32]. Using each or a combination of them have provided the new insights in orthopedic surgery [12,24,30-32]. To design a proper and well approved tissue engineered based graft to be considered as a substitution of traditional grafts, the knowledge about tendon and ligament healing, modeling and remodeling is important [12,24]. In this review we discussed tendon and ligament injuries, have introduced the available and future options in managing large and massive tendon and ligament defects, specifically focused and discussed about the role of tissue engineering in reconstruction of the tendon and ligament defects and finally, described several important events of tendon and ligament healing, modeling and remodeling. Some important and novel concepts about host-graft interaction after surgical implantation of various grafts and prosthetic implants have also been discussed. In addition, some concepts regarding post-operative management and rehabilitation have been highlighted. Moreover we tried to give some suggestions for future regarding the tendon and ligament tissue engineering researches.

Structure of Tendons and Ligaments

Tendons and ligaments have similar structures with different functions [1,3]. Tendon connects muscle to bone and therefore it provides joint movement but ligament connects bone to bone and produces joint stability [1,3,12]. Although these two structures have different duties but both of them have similar characteristics [1,3]. Both are mainly made up of collagen type I molecules and these molecules are arranged as fibrils, fibers, fiber bundles and fascicles [1,3]. Based on the anatomic position of these structures, extra synovial tendons are covered by paratenon and intrasynovial tendons and ligaments are covered by a synovium or synovial sheath (Figure 1) [1-3,12]. In general tendons and ligaments have low cellularity consisting of mature fibroblast or tenoblasts and fibrocytes or tenocytes [1-11]. Thus, more than 90% of the dry matter of tendons and ligaments are collagenous in nature with a little cellularity and other tissue compositions such as glycosaminoglycans and elastic fibers [3,12]. Normally, the proper body of these structures have low vascularity and they are nourished by peripheral vessels mainly presented in the synovial sheath or paratenon [1,12]. Therefore, the metabolic activity of these structures are low as compared to other orthopedic tissues (e.g. cartilage and bone) [1,3,7]. This unique characteristic of tendon and ligament let the tissue to be more tolerable and resistant when the high energy forces are transmitted through the tissue especially during locomotion and physical activates [1-3]. In such conditions the cellular metabolism is changed from aerobic to anaerobic situation and these tissues are more

***Corresponding author:** Dr. Ahmad Oryan, Department of Pathology, School of Veterinary Medicine, Shiraz University, Shiraz, Iran
E-mail: oryan@shirazu.ac.ir

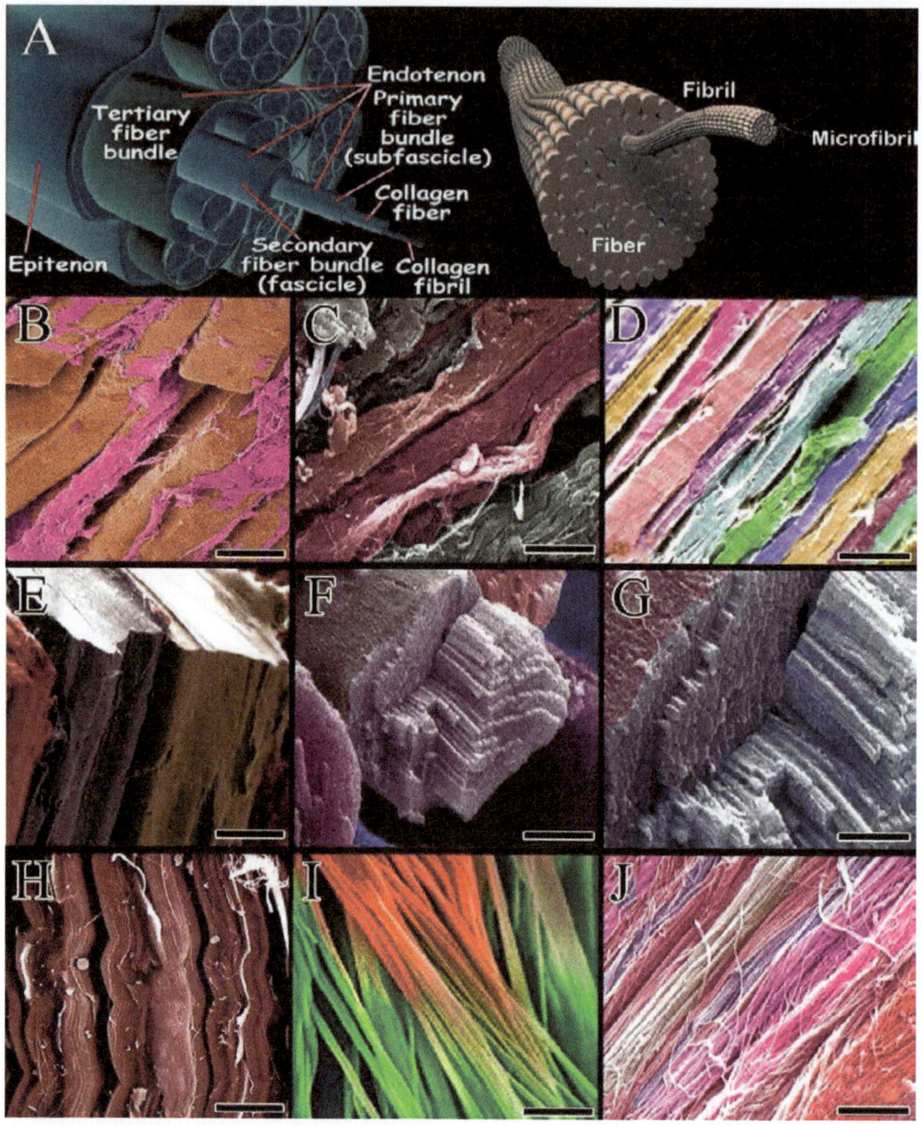

Figure 1: Structure and hierarchical architecture of normal tendon and ligament.
The hierarchical architectures of tendon and ligaments and their tridimensional architectures have significant similarities except that ligaments are denser than tendons and their collagen fibers are twisted. The collagen molecules are polymerized as tropocollagen, micro fibrils, fibrils, fiber bundles and fascicles (A). Endotenon covers the collagen fibers and bundles of collagen fibers internally and epitenon covers the tertiary fiber bundles (the largest bundles of collagen fibers). All these architectures are covered by paratenon in extra-synovial tendons and by tenosynovium or tendon sheath in intra-articular tendons (A). Ligaments (B) are denser than tendons (C, D). (E) is a scanning electron micrograph (SEM) of a normal tendon fascicle. (F) shows a large fiber bundle in which the collagen fibers are densely packed and formed a collagen fiber bundle (F and G). (H) is an ultramicrograph by SEM of the ligament fibers. Normally, these fibers are highly dense and aligned in a unidirectional pattern. (I and G) are the collagen fibrils. The collagen fibrils are aligned in one direction and aggregation of the highly aligned collagen fibrils produces the collagen fibers. B-D and H-J are longitudinal sections while E-G are sagital and cross sections. The ultramicrographs are colored through the structure detection software. Scale bar for B-D: 10 μm, E:100 μm, F:45 μm, G:22 μm, H: 10 μm, I: 700 nm, J: 1.8 μm.

tolerant to anaerobic metabolism compared to other tissues [1]. The low metabolic rate and well-developed anaerobic energy-generation capacity of these structures are essential in carrying loads and maintaining long-standing tensions, and reducing the risk of ischemia and subsequent necrosis [1]. Although this is an excellent tissue characteristic for the normal state of these structures but this could be a negative point in the tendon or ligament injuries and healing [1-3].

Tendon and Ligament Injuries

Tendon and ligament injuries have high incidence in orthopedic surgery and sports medicine [12-21,33,34]. Tendon and ligament injuries are vary in nature and could mainly be divided into acute and chronic injuries [1,12]. In some of the acute tendon or ligament injuries, a simple transection is occurred as a result of sharp traumas or during routine orthopedic surgeries (e.g. bone fixation using plating techniques; tissue dissection, etc.) [4-8]. In addition, these types of injuries have been reported to occur as a result of vehicular trauma [9-11]. In orthopedic surgeries, in order to provide the maximum exposure to bones and joints, it has been suggested to keep the tendons and ligaments free of sharp dissection and it is advised to dissect these structures from their bony insertion [3,12]. This situation is a common condition when exposing joints [3]. Despite of the simple nature of this model of injury, current literature suggests a poor healing response is occurred [7]. Basically, it is a rule to reapposite the transected tendon edges and suture them [4,5]. In the Achilles tendon, simple end-to-end repair is most commonly performed via the Bunnel, Kessler, and Krackow techniques [35]. All these suturing techniques are acceptable for the repair of the Achilles tendon; however, the Krackow method has been shown to be superior in biomechanical and cadaveric studies and has the advantage of allowing 4 threads (and 2 knots) across the rupture site if desired [36].

However, such model of direct suturing is not suggested for the ligaments. It has been stated that direct suturing has low value in torn ligaments because the torn ligaments would not heal in the intra articular space and the inflammatory environment of the joint is degenerative in such condition which do not let an acceptable healing to be processed [3]. Ligament replacement is the best option [3]. The second form of acute tendon or ligament injuries are unsharp or blunt ruptures [12]. This type commonly occurs when high energy forces greater than the ultimate strength of the tissue passes through it [12]. Basically, these high energy forces are produced as a result of high physical activities (e.g. athletics) [3,12]. These sharp tissue ruptures are called strain injuries when a tendon is ruptured or called sprain injuries when a ligament is ruptured [1-3]. Strain and sprain injuries are mainly divided into three degrees [12]. Few collagen fibrils and fibers are microscopically ruptured in degree one but the tissue injury is not obvious at gross morphology [1]. In the second degree, a considerable number of collagen fibrils, fibers and bundles of collagen fibers are ruptured and a partial gap between the ruptured fibers is grossly visible [12,33]. In this condition, the continuity of the tissue in not completely lost [33]. Finally, in the third degree, total collagen fibers and bundles are ruptured and a considerable gap occurs between the edges [25-29]. Treatment of grade one is non-surgical and is limited to supportive strategies; however there is no well accepted method for managing grade two injuries (surgical vs. non-surgical) and in grade three (total rupture), in most instances the ruptured tissue should be surgically repaired [12,29]. Other tendon injuries commonly happen due to traumas, burns, gangrenous and infective ulcers, tumors and several other predisposing factors and mainly result in tissue necrosis [29]. In such conditions it is often necessary to resect the remaining tendon and this results in gap formation [12,29]. The gap should be surgically reconstructed and if it is neglected then joint stiffness occurs which impairs the functionality of the injured limb [26]. Despite of recent advances in orthopedic techniques, however reconstruction of such large and massive tissue defects is technically demanding and variation in surgical techniques in repairing such tissue defects are remarkable and mostly it is hard for surgeons to choose the method of choice [12,26,29]. Many different surgical techniques exist, but only a few of them have been validated in a strict scientific manner [13-21]. The V-Y technique, local tissue augmentation, turn-down flaps, tissue transfer, free tissue transfer, and use of synthetic materials are some of the examples [13-15,29]. Each has its own significant limitations [14-19]. Here we described some surgical techniques useful in Achilles tendon reconstruction.

End-to-end repair with augmentation can be performed with additional autografts, allografts, and synthetic grafts. Graft options have been discussed separately in the following sections of this review. The most common and easiest autograft to harvest is with the plantaris tendon, which is usually intact after a rupture and easily available through the same surgical wound. The tendon is cut from its insertion on the calcaneus and stretched or "fanned out" and can be placed over the rupture site with absorbable sutures [37-39].

Fascial turn down flaps of the proximal gastrocnemius fascia have also been advocated. The most common being the single strip or Silfverskio¨ ld procedure and the double strip or Lindholm procedure, and these fascial slips are made approximately 3 cm proximal to the rupture site and rotated 180° and flapped down to cover and reinforce the rupture site. It should be noted that doing a turndown flap requires a longer proximal skin incision with more dissection that increases the potential for wound healing issues and sural nerve injury [40].

Minimal incisional and percutaneous techniques were introduced and advocated to decrease potential wound complications, scar adhesions, and sural nerve injuries [41-43]. Ma and Griffith first described a percutaneous technique using multiple stab incision of 18 acute Achilles tendon ruptures to minimize postoperative complications and reported no complications of sural nerve injury [41]. It should be noted that percutaneous repairs are not completely benign and every surgeon should appreciate this and use caution when placing a proximal and especially proximal lateral incision even with this technique. Martinelli described percutaneous repair on 50 acutely ruptured Achilles tendon [42]. In this study, 30 patients practiced amateur or professional sports and were able to return to preinjury sporting levels after 120 to 150 days. Favorable arguments for mini-open technique are allowing for early postoperative ROM and rehabilitation to assist proper tendon healing with the reduction of scar adhesions and allowing athletes an earlier return to sporting activities.

Among all chronic tendon injuries, tendinopathy has the highest incidence and importance [1]. Excessive loading on tendons during vigorous physical training is regarded as the main pathological stimulus for degeneration, and there may be a greater risk of excessive loading inducing tendinopathy in the presence of intrinsic risk factors [12]. Tendons respond to repetitive overload beyond the physiological threshold with either inflammation of their sheath or degeneration of their body, or both [1,2]. Different stresses induce different responses [19]. Unless fatigue damage is actively repaired, tendons will weaken and eventually rupture. The repair mechanism is probably mediated by resident tenocytes, which maintain a fine balance between extracellular matrix network production and degradation [4]. Tendon damage may even occur from stresses within the physiological limits, as frequent cumulative microtrauma may not allow enough time for repair [12]. Microtrauma can also result from nonuniform stress within tendons, producing abnormal load concentrations and frictional forces between the fibrils and causing localized fiber damage [1]. The etiology and importance of tedinopathy has been extensively discussed [1].

Epidemiologic Aspects of Tendon and Ligament Injuries

Of the 33 million musculoskeletal injuries reported in the United States per year, roughly 50% involve injuries to the soft tissue including tendon and ligament [1,13,44,45,47-50]. As larger portions of the general population participate in physical and recreational activities every year, the frequency of tendon and ligament injuries is likely to increase as well, resulting in increasing health care costs and patient morbidity [1-5,46,48]. Twenty-five percent of all athletic injuries, irrespective of the specific sport or level of play, involve the foot and ankle [14,15,44]. Here, some epidemiologic aspects of tendon and ligament injuries have been shortly discussed.

Achilles tendon ruptures were apparently rare before the year 1950, but the incidence has recently increased in developed countries [15,51]. A bimodal age distribution (peak in the fourth decade of life followed by a second, but lower, peak in the sixth to eighth decade of life) among patients with a rupture has been noted in most of the studies, and this probably represents two different etiologies of Achilles tendon rupture [16-19,51]. Especially in the younger age group, the majority of Achilles tendon ruptures are related to sports that require sudden acceleration and jumping [19]. It has been shown that 755 of nearly 4000 ruptures of the Achilles tendon were related to sports activities [21,44]. The incidence of Achilles tendon rupture in men is about 1.7 to 7 times greater than in women [15,16]. The first peak in incidence of Achilles tendon rupture, is between 30 and 40 years of age, lower than the age in patients with other spontaneous tendon ruptures [1,15,44,51]. In some studies, the second peak has been suggested to be between 50 and 60 years and in some others between 70 and 80 years, closer to the mean age of patients with other types of tendon ruptures [19,20,45,47].

The distribution of Achilles tendon rupture by different sports varies considerably from country to country [15,44]. For example, in northern and middle Europe, soccer, tennis, track and field, indoor ball games and downhill skiing and in North America, football, basketball, baseball, tennis and downhill skiing dominate the statistics [15-17,44,51,52]. However, during the last decade, it has been suggested that ball games covered about 90% of all sports related Achilles tendon ruptures and the incidence of badminton induced ruptures is increasing yearly, so that this sport is now placed in the first cause of Achilles tendon rupture in Finland and Sweden [15-17,51,52]. In some other countries, downhill skiing has been shown to be the most common cause of Achilles tendon rupture. Although people's general lifestyle has become more sedentary and physically less demanding during recent decades, increasing leisure time, and especially increased recreational and competitive sport activities, has resulted in a greater incidence of acute and overuse sports injuries [53,54].

Chronic problems caused by overuse of tendons probably account for 30% of all running-related injuries, and as an example, the prevalence of elbow tendinopathy in tennis players can be as high as 40% [1,50]. The occurrence of Achilles tendon overuse injuries is the highest in middle- and long distance running, orienteering, track and field, tennis and other ball games [53,55]. An annual incidence of Achilles tendon overuse injuries in top level runners has been shown to be of 7 to 9% [55]. The most common clinical diagnosis of Achilles overuse injuries is tendinopathy of the main body of the tendon (55 to 65%), followed by insertional problems such as retrocalcaneal bursitis and insertion tendinopathy (20 to 25%) [55]. The etiology of Achilles tendon overuse injuries is multifactorial [1]. Training errors have been reported in 60 to 70% of the running injuries [55]. The most common training errors associated with Achilles tendinopathy as for many other overuse injuries are a rapid increase in mileage, increased intensity of training, and running on sloping and slippery roads [53,56]. The symptoms of Achilles tendon overuse injuries are usually initially unilateral however it has been suggested that the patients with unilateral tendinopathy seem to have a relatively high risk (reported to be about 41%) to get the symptoms of overuse (exertional pain with or without swelling and stiffness) to the initially uninvolved contralateral Achilles tendon, too [52].

About one-third of sport injuries that are treated at outpatient sports clinics involve the knees [57]. Patellar tendinopathy has high incidence in knee disorders that are yearly presented in the clinics [58]. It has been shown that the highest incidence is in soccer (21%), long distance running (13%), volleyball (12%), orienteering (8%) and ice hockey (7%) [58]. Men are affected about 4 to 6 times more than women [57]. Overuse injuries of the patellar tendon are most common in athletes involved in some types of repetitive activities, such as jumping (volleyball, basketball, high jump, and triple jump), kicking (soccer, football), quick stops and starts (tennis, squash, badminton), running (sprinters, endurance runners), weightlifting and powerlifting, and bicycling [58]. It has been shown that increased laxity of the knee joint correlated with patellar tendinopathy [58]. The pathologic changes are most often located at the insertional areas, where micro- or macroruptures and tissue degeneration are often found. In volleyball, landing from jump (eccentric loading) and repeated direct striking of the knees on the floor may play a role in the etiology of the patellar tendinopathy [57,58].

A rotator cuff tendon injury involves any type of irritation or damage to the rotator cuff tendons [59]. This can be caused from traumatic injuries (falling on an outreached arm), lifting, or repetitive arm activities done overhead, such as throwing a baseball or placing an item on a shelf [60]. These injuries can be as simple as a strain or tendonitis, and as severe as partial or complete tear of the tendon [59]. The incidence of rotator cuff tendon damage increases with age and is most frequently due to degeneration of the tendon, rather than injury from sports or trauma [59-61]. Though found to be more common in older populations, rotator cuff injuries do not discriminate and occur in males and females of all ages [61,62]. Due to the aging process, the rotator cuff tendon tissue loses its elasticity, become more susceptible to injury, and is more frequently damaged while performing everyday activities [63]. In younger patients, these injuries are typically due to unusually high demand of the shoulders or traumatic injuries [59]. In addition to primary causes of injuries, the risks of developing weakness or injury to the rotator cuff include: being an athlete (using repetitive motions, such as baseball pitchers, swimmers, archers and tennis players), working in the construction trades (carpenters and painters), poor posture, and weak shoulder muscles [60-63].

Flexor tendon injuries are common events as the tendons lie close to the skin and so are usually the result of either lacerations such as those from knives or glass, from crush injuries and occasionally they can rupture from where they are joined to bone during contact sports such as football, rugby and wrestling [2,64,65]. Flexor tendon injuries are challenging problems for orthopedic surgeons due to three main reasons [2,4,64]. Firstly, flexor tendon injury in hand is a clinical problem because it cannot heal without surgical treatment, as the two ends need to be surgically brought together for the healing to occur unlike other tendons including the Achilles tendon where it could be placed into plantar flexion to heal [8-11,64]. Secondly postoperative management needs to be carefully planned as mobilization has shown to be essential to prevent adhesions and improve gliding but this can risk rupture. Lastly due to the unique anatomy of the tendons running through flexor tendon sheaths to function, surgeons need to plan preventing increasing the bulkiness of the tendon through its sheath, which is not always possible from scarring as this affects the functional outcome of the tendon [2,5-7,64]. Unfortunately there is no well-known incidence of flexor tendon injury but to the authors experience it seems to be high both in humans and animals.

Among all the ligament injuries which are yearly presented in the orthopedic practice, ACL has been shown to have the highest incidence [66]. Ligament injuries are most often a result of low-velocity, noncontact, deceleration injuries and contact injuries with a rotational component [67]. Contact sports also may produce injury to the anterior cruciate ligament secondary to twisting, valgus stress, or hyperextension all directly related to contact or collision. When matched for activities, a greater prevalence for ACL injury is found in females compared with males. In one meta-analysis study by Prodromos et al. [34], it has been shown that female subjects have a roughly 3 times greater incidence of ACL tears in soccer and basketball versus male subjects. They showed that recreational Alpine skiers had the highest incidences of ACL tear, whereas expert Alpine skiers had the lowest incidences. Volleyball may in fact be a low-risk sport rather than a high-risk sport. Alpine skiers and lacrosse players had no gender difference for ACL tear rate. Year-round female athletes who play soccer and basketball have an ACL tear rate of approximately 5% [34].

Approximately 50% of patients with ACL injuries have meniscal tears too. In acute ACL injuries, the lateral meniscus is more commonly torn; in chronic ACL tears, the medial meniscus is more commonly torn [3]. The incidence of ACL tears has been estimated as 1 case in 3,500 people, resulting in 95,000 new ACL ruptures per year [66]. The importance of the ACL has been emphasized in athletes who require stability in running, cutting, and kicking. The ACL-deficient knee has also been linked to an increased rate of degenerative changes and meniscal injuries. For these reasons, approximately 60,000-75,000 ACL reconstructions are performed annually in the United States [66]. For restoration of activity and stability, the expected long-term success rate of ACL reconstruction is between 75-95%. The current failure rate is 8%, which may be attributed to recurrent instability, graft failure, or arthrofibrosis [3,34].

Managing Mild Tendon Injuries with Least Tissue Defect

In order to manage mild tendon injuries, several factors have a role on the final decision [44]. Physical therapy, rest, and gradual return to the activity in which tendinosis was experienced is a common therapy [1,46,47]. There is evidence to suggest that tendinosis is not an inflammatory disorder; anti-inflammatory drugs are not an effective treatment, and inflammation is not the cause of this type of tendon dysfunction [48]. There is a variety of treatment options, but more research is necessary to determine their effectiveness [48,49]. Initial recovery is usually within 2 to 3 months, and full recovery usually within 3 to 6 months. About 80% of the patients will fully recover within 12 months. If the conservative therapy doesn't work, then surgery can be an option [50]. This surgery consists of the excision of abnormal tissue and reconstruction of the defect area [13-20]. Time required to recover from surgery is about 4 to 6 months [15].

Controversy regarding operative versus non-operative treatment exist in the treatment of tendon ruptures that focuses on re-rupture rates and wound complications related to surgery [15,35-38,54]. Re-rupture rate of 3.5% in the operatively treated patients and 12.6% in the non-operative patients has been reported previously [38]. Complications such as adhesions, altered sensation, and wound infection, however, were more common in operatively treated patients with 34.1% in the operative patients versus 2.1% in the non-operative patients [39]. Due to the similar percentage of re-rupture between most studies advocating surgery and their promising results with non-operative management, the necessity for surgical repair of Achilles tendons, with all of its risks and high cost is questionable [38]. Therefore, for mild tendon ruptures with the least tissue loss, conservative or non-surgical or non-invasive treatment may be a first line approach [15-17,54]. Patients with pain, whose function is reasonably maintained, are suitable candidates for non-operative management [38]. A conservative physical therapy program begins with preliminary rest and restriction from engaging in the event which gave rise to the symptoms [44,48,50]. Oral medications that provide pain relief such as anti-inflammatory agents, topical pain relievers such as cold packs and, if warranted, local anesthetic injection may be used [50,54]. A sling may be offered for short-term comfort, with the understanding that undesirable joint stiffness can develop with prolonged immobilization. Early physical therapy may afford pain relief and help to maintain motion. As pain decreases, strength deficiencies and biomechanical errors can be corrected [54,55]. A gentle, passive range-of-motion program should be started to normalize the stiffness and maintain range of motion during this resting period [55,58]. Exercises should be a part of this program [54]. After a full, painless range of motion has been achieved, the patient may advance to a gentle strengthening program [51].

There are several instances in which non-operative treatment would not be suggested [15,34,52,54]. The first is the 20 to 30-year-old active patients with an acute tear and severe functional deficit from a specific event [54,59]. The second is the 30 to 50-year-old patients with acute tendon tear secondary to a specific event [61,63]. The third instance is the highly competitive athlete who is primarily involved in overhead or throwing sports [51,54]. These patients need to be treated operatively because tendon repair is necessary for restoration of the normal strength required to return these athletes to the same competitive preoperative level of function [51]. Patients who do not respond or are unsatisfied with conservative treatment should seek an opinion concerning surgery [54]. Patients associated with significant tendon defect should be surgically treated and the defect area should be surgically reconstructed by grafts [29].

Managing Large Tendon and Ligament Injuries

Patients associated with significant tendon defect should be surgically treated and the defect area should be surgically reconstructed by grafts [15-18]. Also most of the torn ligaments especially the intrasynovial ones such as ACL should be surgically replaced by a graft and therefore no medical or conservative treatment option is warranted for these patients [3,23,34,35].

Graft Options In Managing Large and Massive Tendon and Ligament Injuries

Using autografts is currently the only gold standard method for managing large tendon and ligament deficits [26,29]. However, reconstruction of such large defects requires massive tissue harvesting from the donor site and therefore the donor site morbidity and pain is a considerable challenge to autografts [3,12-14]. In addition there may not be enough autografts in the patient's body at the time of reconstruction and cosmetically this method is not pleasant [3,13]. Another limitation of this treatment strategy is that it is commonly necessary to make a second surgery in the patient which increases the surgical time and cost [15]. In contrast to autografts are allo- and xenografts [13,16]. Allografts have lower immunogenicity than xenografts but both of them have this chance to be acutely or chronically rejected by the host [12]. Thus rejection is one of their limitations [68-71]. In addition, it has been stated that using allo- or xenografts increases the chance of disease transmission of several hazardous and dangerous viruses and prions such as human immune deficiency virus, hepatitis type B and more importantly type C and bovine spongiform encephalitis [3,12,26,29]. Disease transmission in xenografts is a more serious concern than allografts because there are well known human diseases that could be detected in the allografts using the standard screening technologies but in xenografts there are several unknown zoonotic diseases that are more hazardous for the humane body than those of the well-known humane diseases [3,12,29]. In addition to these disadvantageous there are also several ethical concerns regarding usage of allo- and xenografts in the human body [13-16].

Comparing auto- to allo- and xenografts options, autografts have better incorporative properties than the other grafts because basically the autografts are viable tissues and their cells can collaborate at different stages of healing [3,71-73]. In addition the resorption rate of autografts are lower than other grafts; therefore the healing in autografts would be faster [3,72]. In contrast to autografts, the most important positive and beneficial issue regarding allo- and xenografts is their availability [13-15]. However, to reduce the immunogenicity of the allo- and xenografts, several processes have been made (e.g. sterilization, cell rinsing, freeze drying, etc.); therefore these types of grafts are not viable in nature because their cellular structures are commonly destroyed during sterilization and other important tissue processing [72-85]. Therefore, it is a fact that the allo- and xenografts have significantly lower incorporative properties with the healing tissue and this is another major limitation which results in rapid absorption of the graft during tendon or ligament healing [69,72].

Tissue Engineering

Tissue engineering is another option which has been introduced in the last decade and currently it is the final option in managing large and massive tendon and ligament injuries [22-32]. Tissue engineering is defined as "a process that affects the structure and architecture of any viable and nonviable tissue with the aim to increase the effectiveness of the construct in biologic environments" [12]. Therefore, all of the non-fresh grafts which are processed for acellularization belong to the tissue engineering category [68-72]. In fact, acellularization is the basic tissue engineering technology as described for the allo- and xenografts [68,70,72]. This method of tissue engineering has been used for many years to decrease the antigenicity of the viable grafts [68-72]. Newer approaches have been developed by many and newer tissue engineered products are introduced in the recent years [73-85]. Basically, tissue engineering could be divided into four major categories including tissue scaffolds, healing promotive factors, stem cells and gene therapy [12]. The fourth category "Gene Therapy" has been recently included in tissue engineering [12,24].

Scaffolds

Scaffolds are the most important part of tissue engineering because they have many applications and without them application of promotive factors and stem cells have low clinical value because their long term availability without attachment to the scaffolds is questionable [12,22-32]. Tissue scaffolds have several duties but their major role is to provide a suitable environment for cell attachment, migration, proliferation and matrix remodeling and regeneration [12]. In addition, tissue scaffolds have been used in drug delivery, vehicle for healing promotive factors and stem cells and also as tissue filler [24-32]. Based on their stiffness, scaffolds could be divided into three major categories including hard, soft and hybrid scaffolds [12,24]. Based on the source, tissue scaffolds could be divided into three major categories including biologic, synthetic and hybrid scaffolds [22-24]. The acellularized cadaveric tissues or grafts are the most well-known biologic scaffolds [24,68-73,75-81]. However, the newer ones are those constructed by the biologic based molecules such as collagen, elastin, chitosan, demineralized bone matrix, fibrin, gelatin, hyaluronic acid, chondroitin sulphate, silk, etc [12,25-28]. In contrast to biologic scaffolds, the synthetic scaffolds are produced by polymerization of the synthetic materials [12,28,29]. The major category of synthetic based scaffolds are the oil based polymers such as those constructed by polypropylene, polycaprolacton, polydioxanone, polygalactin 910, nylon, etc [12,29]. Other synthethic based materials used to construct synthetic tissue scaffolds are carbon fiber, hydroxyapatite, several forms of calcium phosphate (e.g. mono, bi, tri and octa calcium phosphate), ceramics, etc [12].

Both the biologic and synthetic based scaffolds could be divided into two major categories based on their absorbability [12,24,26]. As a general rule, materials such as collagen, gelatin, elastin, fibrin, hyaluronic acid, chondroitin sulphate, polydioxanone, polygalactin 910, polyglycolic acid, and several forms of hydroxyapatite and calcium phosphates are absorbable materials and the other materials such as silk and nylon are none absorbable materials in the host environment [12,24]. Among the above mentioned absorbable materials the synthetic polymers such as polydioxanone have higher biocompatibility than collagen, elastin, fibrin, etc [86]. This is because the polymer based biodegradable materials are absorbed through a hydrolysis mechanism [12,24,86]. In this mechanism the polymers are degraded to Carbone dioxide and water and therefore this polymer based scaffolds have least tissue reaction after their surgical implantation in the host [12]. In contrast to synthetic polymer based scaffolds, the biologic based polymers such as collagen and elastin are absorbed through a different mechanism which is named, phagocytosis [87,88]. In fact, the exogenous biologic based absorbable scaffolds such as those constructed by collagen Type I, accelerate the inflammation because their surface antigens chemotactically attract the neutrophils and macrophages and this lead to neutrophil and macrophage accumulation in the tissue scaffold [76,77,87]. Therefore, the absorption rate of the biologic based scaffolds are much faster than those of the synthetic based biodegradable scaffolds [28,29]. Similar behavior has been suggested for the none absorbable materials in which the silk has been shown to be more immunogenic than nylon after surgical implantation in the host [12,24]. Despite these explanations, it should be highlighted that the biologic based biodegradable scaffolds such as those constructed by collagen have an acceptable biocompatibility but also they have much better healing incorporative capacity and biodegradability [12,24,29,69,72]. One of the most important goals in tendon and ligament tissue engineering is that the scaffolds should simulate native tendon characteristics in short term but should be gradually degraded and replaced by the new tissue [29]. This newly developed tissue should be comparable to the normal tissue in the least possible time in order to be able to carry out its duty [12].

Synthetic scaffolds have another superiority over the biologic scaffolds and the synthetic based scaffolds have higher biomechanical characteristics than the biologic based scaffolds; therefore application of the synthetic scaffolds has superior outcome at short term while the biologic based scaffolds have better outcome at long term [25-29]. This is a very important concept in reconstructing large and massive tissue defects with tissue engineered based scaffolds [12]. After implantation of a tissue engineered graft, the graft should have an optimum biomechanical property in order to be able to resist against functional weight bearing forces and physical activities of the patient [12,24,29]. The higher biomechanical properties of a scaffold, the lower incidence of dehiscence and gap formation at short term [27,29]. However, as mentioned, those scaffolds with the higher biomechanical properties have lower degradation rate and healing incorporative properties which leads to dehiscence and rupture of the healing tissue at long term [12,24]. This is because the biomechanical properties of the biodegradable scaffolds decreases by time and if a newly developed tissue would not be able to completely substitute the graft, then the rupture could occur [27]. To overcome these limitations regarding the outcome of biologic materials at short term and long lasting synthetic materials at long term, scientists have invented the hybrid scaffolds in which they combined the synthetic materials with biologic materials to increase the biodegradability, biocompatibility, biomechanical properties and healing incorporative characteristics of the implant in order to overcome the above mentioned limitations [22,23,29,75].

In addition, technically it is possible to increase the biomechanical properties of the natural based scaffolds such as collagen [28,75,80,82].

Cross linking of the scaffold fibers is one of these technologies (Figure 2) [80,82]. It is possible to crosslink the scaffold fibers, using various techniques including dehydrothermal, chemical, ultraviolet, etc. [26-29]. Among these well-known technologies, chemical crosslinking has been suggested as the most effective method but crosslinking in chemical solutions such as glutaraldehyde and formalin has been reported to be hazardous for the host because the remaining solvent in the scaffold may be preserved even after several washings [26-29]. Dehydrothermal crosslinking has a low value because it has least effectiveness on the biomechanical properties of the graft but it can decrease the biodegradability of the implant so that by dehydrothermal crosslinking it is possible to increase the persistence time of the implant in the host [27]. The newer approach in cross linking is UV method which is a safe and effective method in both sterilization and crosslinking of the implant with no deleterious effects in the host [25-28,82]. As a general rule it is important to make some degrees of cross linking in the scaffolds in order to increase the persistence time of implant in the host with the aiming to increase the effectiveness of the implant at various stages of healing [12,24,27]. Without cross linking the biologic scaffolds are soluble in water and therefore they are acutely absorbed by the host immune response [28,29].

By combining the biologic based materials with the synthetic materials it is therefore possible to decrease the crosslinking degree but also increase the biomechanical properties of the scaffold [12,29]. Well comprehensive detailed studies have shown that it is better to construct the main part of the scaffold with biologic based materials such as collagen and cover it with a synthetic based scaffold such as polydioxanone [24-29]. This strategy has been shown to be as effective as the natural autografts *in vivo* [24,29]. For example, to simulate tendon proper, a novel tridimensional collagen scaffold has been made and covered with polydioxanone sheath to simulate paratenon [28,29]. It has been suggested that the new tendon have formed through the polydioxanone sheath and at long term no part of collagen implant existed in the defect area and has totally been replaced by the new tendon that had optimum biomechanical properties at long term [28,29]. It has been shown that polydioxanone sheath can provide the initial biomechanical characteristics required for the short term weight bearing which is substituted by the long term biomechanical performance due to the newly regenerated tendon [29]. Another possible strategy is to reduce the weight bearing forces from the tissue scaffold and transfer it on a suture material [27]. This has been shown to be effective in short term, *in vivo* [27]. It is also possible to reduce the weight bearing by casting the injured limb [4-11]. However, the first and second strategies are more advantageous than the latter one because casting the injured limb increases the development of peritendinous adhesion, muscle fibrosis and atrophy [2]. As a new strategy it is possible to chemically combine the synthetic and biologic based materials and produce a new scaffold with hybrid polymeric fibers [12,24]. This is a new area of research and its effectiveness on the biomechanical properties and the healing incorporative capacity of the graft is not clear as yet [12].

In designing a tissue engineered scaffold for tendon and ligaments it is important to consider the above important issues [12,22,23,26]. As suggested, the implant should have some degree of crosslinking to have optimum biomechanical properties at short term but also it should be cytocompatible *in vitro*, biocompatible, biodegradable and healing incorporative *in vivo* [12,24,26-29]. These are general guidelines [12]. In addition to the above features, the architecture of the scaffold is also important (Figure 2) [1,25]. Tendon and ligaments are highly aligned tissues (Figure 1) and the collagen fibrils and fibers are unidirectionally arranged and are densely packed [4-11]. In addition, these tissues consist of nano and micro collagen fibrils and fibers [12]. In designing a scaffold for tendon and ligament replacement it is important to produce an aligned scaffold and the scaffold should have both micro and nano scaled fibers in its architecture (Figure 2) [12,89].

As another issue, tendon and ligaments are tridimensional structures but their sheath is a bidimensional structure [25-29]. This should be considered that the healing cells have better migration, proliferation and production properties in tridimensional environments [29]. As another factor, the scaffolds should have porosity in their internal architecture and regarding current literature the pore size could be lower than those used for bone and cartilage tissue engineering [12,24]. Therefore the pore size could vary but should consists of pore diameters between 10 to 100 micrometer [12,24,25-29]. In addition the internal pores should

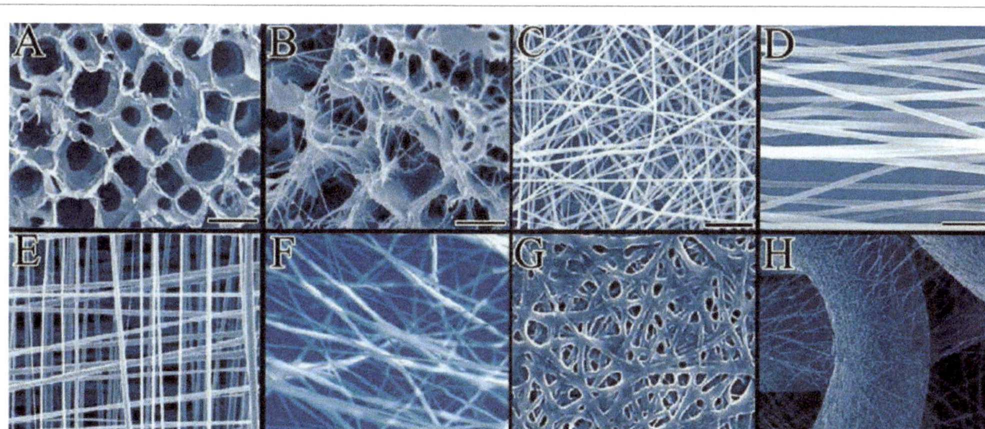

Figure 2: Ultramicrographs by SEM of different tissue engineered based scaffolds.
(A and B) are porous scaffolds. These types of scaffolds are porous in nature and their porosity is high. The pore size is usually between 10 to 100 μm but it may be larger. No fiber structure is visible in these scaffolds and the molecules are not arranged as fibers. The density of the pores is more than 50% in these types of scaffolds. (C to F) are fibrous or fiber based scaffolds. (C) is an amorphous scaffold which has some porosity between its fibers while (D) is a highly aligned scaffold which has lower porosity than (C). (E) is a unique highly aligned scaffold but the fibers have been polymerized and aligned in two different directions so that some of the fibers are perpendicular to others. This unique configuration of the fibers has produced large pores between the fibers. (F) is a moderately aligned scaffold in which the collagen fibers are mostly aligned but an acceptable porosity exists between the fibers. (G) is a fibrous scaffold which have been cross-linked so that the fibers have been fused together but some porosity is still preserved in the scaffold. (H) is a hybrid scaffold in which both the micro and nano structured fibers are present in the scaffold. Scale bar for A: 1 μm, B: 500 nm, C to F: 1 μm, G: 2 μm, H: 2.4 μm.

be connected with the external pores at only two sides of the scaffold [12]. These are those sides that are laid between the tendon or ligament edges after graft implantation *in vivo* [89]. The surface of other sides of the scaffold should be none porous because porosity at other sides could accelerate peri-tissue adhesion formation [12,89].

Careful attention should be paid on the sterility and endotoxin content of the scaffolds [84]. Several hazardous solvents and microorganisms could contaminate the implant during production and therefore quality control tests regarding the sterility and endotoxin content should be performed before surgical implantation [12,27]. As a general rule the scaffolds could be sterilized with ethanol 70% for 1 hr [29]. However ethanol has some effect on tissue architecture and it may not be sufficient to kill all the microorganisms such as bacterial spores [12]. Newer technologies have been introduced and among them UV and gamma irradiation have been found much effective in eliminating all the contaminations [12,24,83,84].

Healing Promotive Factors

"Healing Promotive Factors" is another category of tissue engineering [12,30,31]. These are basically divided into four categories including glycosaminoglycans, growth factors, pro-inflammatory mediators and healing agents [12,30,31]. Glycosaminoglycans are present in the tissue matrix of all the connective tissues [4,9,31,90]. Hyaluronic acid, chondroitin sulphate, dermatan sulphate, keratin sulphate and glucosamine are some examples of this category [1]. Glycosaminoglycans have several important characteristics in tissue healing and remodeling [4,9]. For example, hyaluronic acid has been shown to modulate the inflammation at short term but also has a role in collagen fibril aggregation and development in later stages of tendon or ligament healing [4,9]. It can reduce cell proliferation over the tendon and ligament surface thus has a role in decreasing peritendinous adhesion and it also increase cell migration and proliferation in the internal parts of the injured tendon and ligaments and therefore it can increase the healing quality of the injured tissues [9,31]. Poly-sulphated glycosaminoglycans such as chondroitin sulphate has been shown to increase the collagen fibrils' diameter and aggregation and have a role in matrix remodeling at later stages of healing [4]. Although the major role of glycosaminoglycans is to increase the healing quality of the regenerated tissue but they have been used as architectural polymers in combination with other materials such as collagen and elastin [12,24,31]. Therefore, this category has an important role in tissue engineering [31].

During tissue repair growth factors play an important role in regulating several events [30]. To date, several growth factors have been characterized and introduced [91-99]. The main important well-known growth factors are basic and acidic Fibroblast Growth Factor (FGF), Vasculoendothelial Growth Factor (VEGF), Transforming Growth Factor beta (TGF-β), Platelet Derived Growth Factor (PDGF), bone morphogenic protein (BMP), etc. [3,5,6,10,30]. The role of basic fibroblast growth factor has been well shown previously [5,6,10]. FGF increases migration, proliferation, and collagen production of fibroblasts and regulate inflammation, fibroplasia and remodeling, thus can increase the collagen fibrillogenesis and density during different stages of tendon healing [5,6]. It has a role in migration and proliferation of endothelial cells and therefore can accelerate angiogenesis, short term after injury [94,96,97]. VEFG regulates and increases the migration and proliferation of endothelial cells and both the FGF and VEGF have a strong role in cell differentiation shortly after injury induction and during the initial stages of wound healing [30,95-99]. PDGF is released from the alpha granules of the aggregated and activated platelets after injury and have crucial roles in regulating different stages of healing [30,91,100]. They also enhance activation of macrophages and facilitate the fibroplasia and remodeling at long term [30]. TGF-β has a role in matrix remodeling and increase tissue alignment and density of the collagen fibers during healing process [93]. It also has a role in reducing the tissue metabolism at long term and regulates cell behavior and production at different stages of healing [1,93]. Therefore the role of growth factors in tissue healing and regeneration should not be neglected [30]. Platelet Rich Plasma (PRP) has been shown to have some of these growth factors and has effective value in healing and regeneration [30]. PRP is prepared via the circulating blood using one or two step centrifugation. There are several types of PRP tested in the literature with variable results [30,100]. Several important issues exist with PRP that should be addressed in future investigations. Perhaps, preparation method of PRP, its concentration, source (e.g. auto- allo- and xenogenic base) and its constitutions (platelet or platelet with buffy coat) are suggested to be different between several studies [30,101-103]. As a general rule, effective PRP is prepared via two steps centrifugation with the combination of platelets and buffy coats (inflammatory cells) and has a 6 to 7 times more platelets than the circulating blood [30]. PRP could also be activated to form a gel. It has been suggested that PRP-gel has a higher efficacy in biologic environments because the gel form releases more growth factors during wound healing [30].

In vivo animal based investigations have showed beneficial effects of PRP in tendon and ligament healing while its value in clinical trial studies is questionable [103-106]. This substantial differences has been suggested to be related to the source of PRP [30]. In the animal experiments allogenous PRP have been used while in the clinical studies the autogenous form has been used [30]. Therefore it has been suggested that the effect of PRP may be related to its effectiveness on inflammation in which the allogenous PRP results in more inflammatory reaction than the autogenous PRP [30].

Pro-inflammatory mediators such as Matrix Metalloproteinases (MMPs), Interleukins (IL) and Tumor necrosis factor-α (TNF- α), are important factors which regulate the inflammation phase of healing directly and fibroplasia and remodeling indirectly [1]. These mediators activate different cells and regulate their behavior during healing process and have a role in graft acceptance or rejection [68,70,71]. Th1 lymphocytes produce pro-inflammatory cytokines such as Interleukin-2 (IL-2), Interferon-γ (IFN-γ), and Tumor Necrosis Factor-β (TNF-β) leading to macrophage activation, and can be associated with poor tissue remodeling outcome as well as rejection of both allogenic and xenogenic transplants. On the other hand, Th2 lymphocytes produce IL-4, IL-5, IL-6, and IL-10, cytokines that do not activate macrophages and are probably associated with transplant acceptance [68].

Macrophages are characterized as M1 or M2 phenotypes based on receptor expression, function and production of cytokines. M1 macrophages produce large amounts of pro-inflammatory cytokines such as IL-12 and TNF-α which promote inflammation and express CD68 and CD80 surface markers in rats. On the other hand, M2 macrophages produce large amounts of IL-10 and TGF-β, inhibit release of pro-inflammatory cytokines, promote constructive tissue remodeling and express CD163 surface markers in rats [70]. M2 macrophages induce the Th2 response which is beneficial for the constructive tissue remodeling [70]. The presence of cellular material within an Extracellular Matrix (ECM) scaffold modulates the phenotype of the macrophages and lymphocytes involved in the recipient immunity response after implantation; this can be related to tissue remodeling outcome, acceptance or rejection [29]. Indeed, a cellular graft elicits M1 macrophage and Th1 lymphocyte response, and can result in the deposition of connective tissue and rejection of the graft [29]. An acellular graft elicits M2 macrophage and Th2 lymphocyte response, leading to more constructive tissue remodeling outcome and acceptance of the graft [68,70,71]. It may be possible that the exogenous pro-inflammatory mediators affect the graft acceptance and rejection *in vivo* [1,12].

Large numbers of healing agents have been extensively tested in the literature with beneficial outcomes [3-11,107-115]. Honey and aloe Vera have been used for skin wound healing and have shown that they can modulate inflammation and increase collagen production and aggregation [110,114]. Tarantula cubensis is a novel therapeutic agent which is commercially available in market as theranekron and has been shown to lyse the necrotic tissues formed after tendon injury thus increases the healing rate [8,11]. Tarantula cubensis has also been shown to regulate different stages of inflammation in order to increase the healing response at further stages of tendon healing [8,11]. Garlic and sylimarin has been shown to be anti-inflammatory and anti-oxidant agents who their effectiveness on wound healing have been extensively described [115,116]. Several other agents such as vitamin C, non-steroidal anti-inflammatory agents such as indomethacin and celecoxib have been shown to regulate the inflammation and are effective in the healing quality [1,117,118]. Piascledine is a novel therapeutic supplement which is produced by a combination of soybean and avocado with a unique proportion and have been shown to increase the collagen production and matrix remodeling [119]. All these agents together with others that have not been listed here could be used in combination with scaffolds, glycosaminoglycans, growth factors and pro inflammatory mediators in order to increase the efficacy of each well designed treatment strategy.

Stem Cells

Stem cells are another category of tissue engineering [32]. Large varieties of stem cells have been differentiated and tested both *in vitro* and *in vivo* [32]. The most well-known stem cells are the mesenchymal types which are differentiated from bone marrow, adipose tissue and blood [120-123]. The bone marrow types have been extensively used in clinical practice but its efficacy is not well described both in clinical trials and animal studies [32,120-123]. Other types of stem cells including pluripotent embryonic stem cells, cord blood stem cells and fetal stem cells are currently under investigation [32]. Cells are the most important factor in wound healing [124-126]. It is a fact that without cells there is no healing response [1]. Endogenous healing cells migrate, proliferate, differentiate and produce matrix during healing process, but the role of exogenous stem cells is in doubt [120-126]. It has been suggested that the effectiveness of stem cells is related to their differentiation state [32]. The higher the differentiated state, the more effective in the healing [32,126]. Based on this statement it has been suggested that the more undifferentiated stem cells have the more capacity to produce tumor or undesirable tissue in the wound [32]. There is also another challenge. The higher differentiated cells generally have lower telomere length and aged during wound healing thus they may not be able to present at later stages of healing in order to be able to produce useful matrix [126]. The most important concern regarding stem cells usage is their viability during the inflammatory phase of tendon and ligament healing [32]. By inflammatory phase, several cytokines and cytotoxic proteins and inflammatory factors are released by the necrotized tissues and inflammatory cells which reduce the viability chance of the stem cells in the host [1,12]. There is no well approved and comprehensive study to answer this question [12]. The results of various investigations are also contraindicated [120-127]. Some studies suggested the effectiveness of various stem cell types including differentiated and undifferentiated ones while others suggest no effectiveness [126-128]. Therefore use of stem cells is only primitive, limited to *in vitro* and animal experimental studies, and thus it could not be suggested as a first line of treatment [30]. If the above concerns are going to be solved one day then the stem cell option could be a new insight in tissue engineering and regenerative medicine [32]. Cell seeding is one of the interesting area in tissue engineering research, it is possible to seed each scaffold with stem cells in order to produce a viable graft similar to autograft [27-29]. This increases the healing incorporative characteristics of the graft and increases the tendon and ligament regeneration capacity [12,32]. Healing promotive factors could be used as a culture medium for stem cells which seeded in the scaffolds [30-32]. Therefore combination of stem cells, healing promotive factors and scaffolds is the newest strategy with the aiming to produce a viable and effective tissue graft [12]. However, despite many advances in the recent years, more investigations are required to confirm this strategy [3].

Gene Therapy

Gene therapy is the final category in tissue engineering and it involves in the transfer of genetic information to target cells, and may introduce safe and effective strategies to induce tissue healing [129-131]. Gene therapy can be used for delivery of growth factors in tissue engineering [130]. The vehicle for gene delivery can be either viral (adenovirus, retrovirus, adeno-associated viruses) or non-viral (liposomes). However, this approach, as others, has a series of limitations, including trans-infection of the target cells with the foreign genes [129]. Furthermore, an unsolved issue of gene therapy is to target the right gene at the right location in the right cells, and express it sufficiently at the right time while minimizing adverse reactions [129,131]. A short controlled expression is desirable and often sufficient to accelerate bone healing, while achieving permanent or long-term expression of a therapeutic gene is more difficult [129]. Therefore, providing controlled and sufficient expression by adaptation of gene therapy to tissue engineering is a key and critical aspect in this field [130].

Tendon and Ligament Healing

Tendons have three different areas including tendon proper which is completely tendinous in nature, musculo-tendinous junction and finally the tendon to bone junction which has three areas of bone, cartilage and tendon [1,12]. Ligaments have two different areas including the ligament part, and bony attachments [3]. In the bony attachment site there are different parts including ligament fibers, sharpey's fibers, cartilage and bone [3,132,133]. Therefore healing of tendons and ligaments are different based on the above mentioned areas [133]. In the tendinous and ligamentous part which are mostly consist of collagen fibers, there are three overlapping healing phases following injury induction [1-3]. These phases are inflammatory, fibroplasia and remodeling [12]. After tendon and ligament injuries, a lag phase is started [1]. In this healing phase, the vessels are disrupted due to injury and the blood enters the injured area [12]. By exposing the circulating blood to the injured collagen fibers, the platelets aggregate and by regulating several mechanisms a blood clot is formed in the wound area [30]. This clot have several roles in the healing process [1,30]. It acts as a scaffold for the inflammatory and mesenchymal cells, thus it creates a tridimensional environment which enables the cells to migrate, attach, proliferate and do their pathophysiological duties [12]. During this phase the platelets release their growth factors and pro inflammatory mediators consisting of mainly PDGF, IGF, FGF and VEGF from their α-granules and the injured cells release pro inflammatory cytokines which regulate migration and activation of inflammatory cells [1-3,12,24,30]. Neutrophils and macrophages are the first line inflammatory cells which enter and release several growth factors and cytokins in the wound area which accelerate the inflammation and absorb more inflammatory cells in the wound area [132,133].

Transforming growth factor-β (TGF-β) is a product of most cells that are involved in the healing process; its 3 isoforms give rise to distinct spatial responses leading to its diverse effects that regulate several events [93]. During the initial inflammatory phase after trauma, TGF-β expression is elevated and stimulates cellular migration and proliferation, as well as interactions within the repair zone [1]. Synthesis of collagen type I and collagen type III is greatly increased during the later phases [4]. One of the isoforms of the growth factors, TGF-β1, is responsible for the initial scar tissue formation which establishes tissue continuity at the wound site [91]. In the later phases of wound healing, enhanced expression of TGF-β1 leads to scar proliferation and reduced functionality [96]. Transforming growth factor-β3 acts as a negative regulator of scarring at the wound site. Transforming growth factor-β also serves to mechanically regulate the synthesis of collagen in tendon during physical exercise [97].

During the initial repair process and the inflammatory phase, upregulation of growth factors and cytokines such as Insulin-like Growth Factor-1 (IGF-1) stimulate the migration and proliferation of fibroblasts and inflammatory cells to the wound site [91]. Insulin-like growth factor-1 may be stored as an inactive precursor protein in normal tendon and, upon injury, enzymes release the growth factor to exert its biological activity [12]. During the later phases such as remodeling, IGF-1 stimulates synthesis of collagen and other extracellular matrix components. The effects of IGF-1 on matrix metabolism are dose dependent [1]. Cell proliferation and collagen content increase on treatment with IGF-1 [30]. These changes are accompanied by increased stiffness in the treated tendons. Platelet Derived Growth Factor (PDGF) induces the expression of other growth factors such as IGF-1 during the initial repair phase [30]. In addition, the delivery of PDGF to tendon injuries in animal models increases cell proliferation and stimulates the synthesis of collagen and other ECM components in a dose dependent manner during the remodeling phase [30]. Some studies have shown that a phased delivery of PDGF over a longer duration may be desirable to obtain repair that leads to regeneration of a tissue that is functionally closer to normal tendon [95]. Experiments conducted *in vivo* and *in vitro* attest to the mitogenic activity of basic Fibroblast Growth Factor (bFGF), a potent factor that is involved in cell migration and angiogenesis in addition to cell proliferation. Basic fibroblast growth factor has been immunolocalized during tendon repair and is expressed by fibroblasts and inflammatory cells [1,12]. Wound healing models has shown distinctly faster wound closure on treatment with increasing doses of bFGF [5].

Vascular Endothelial Growth Factor (VEGF) is critical for neovascularization, and in the later phases, VEGF is essential in establishment and maintenance of the vasculature present in the endotenon and epitenon [98]. Postoperatively, VEGF expression in healing tendons shows a biphasic expression by majority of the cells within the repair site [30]. Delivery of the bone morphogenetic proteins (BMP) -12, -13, and -14 (also known as Growth/Differentiation Factor [GDF] -7, -6, and -5 or Cartilage Derived Morphogenetic Protein [CDMP] -3, -2, and -1, respectively) to ectopic sites leads to the formation of tendon-like connective tissue [1]. GDFs also increases tendon's callus [30]. Growth/differentiation factors regulate synthesis of the ECM components and expression of collagen type I and collagen type III [1]. These polypeptide factors regulate the expression of specific genes that are found in common among tendons and ligaments, and the expression of these genes serve as markers of tendinogenesis [91-93].

MMPs are important regulators of extracellular matrix network remodeling, and their levels are altered during tendon healing [1]. Expression of the MMP-9 and MMP-13 (collagenase-3) peaks between the first two weeks of injury [12]. MMP-2, MMP-3, and MMP-14 (MT1-MMP) levels increase after the injury and remain high until one month after injury [12]. MMP-9 and MMP-13 participate only in collagen degradation, whereas MMP-2, MMP- 3, and MMP-14 participate both in collagen degradation and in collagen remodeling [1].

The main role of neutrophils is in the acute inflammation is phagocytosis [29]. Macrophages are blood monocytes which migrated from circulating blood through a process called *diapedesis* [12]. Macrophages have more role than phagocytosis and they are the main cells responsible for growth factor and MMPs delivery at the wound site [27-29]. Neutrophils and macrophages phagocytize the necrotic tissues and macrophages regulate important events in the inflammation which is responsible for the transition to fibroplasia of healing as the second stage [25,26]. Macrophages activate the mesenchymal cells' migration, attachment and proliferation in the wound site [4]. At later stages of inflammation the neutrophils decrease in number and the lymphocytes migrate in the wound area thus regulate the macrophage behavior [5]. As suggested Th lymphocytes regulate macrophage response and can determine whether the graft should be accepted or rejected and this completely depends on several important characteristics of the graft which is mainly due to the immunogenicity of the graft [68-72]. When the mesenchymal cells infiltrated in the injured area, the growth factors regulate their behavior thus those cells are in the exposure of bFGF and some other growth factors, are differentiated to fibroblasts and those are mainly exposed to VEGF are differentiated to endothelial cells [5,6,10,12]. Fibroblasts are the main cell types responsible in collagen production while the endothelial cells are responsible for angiogenesis and vessel production [1]. When these cells are differentiated large amounts of glycosaminoglycans (primarily hyaluronic acid), collagen and immature blood vessels are produced in the wound area and at this time the fibroplasia is in progress [7]. Gradually the fibroblasts produce more collagen than glycosaminoglycans and also they produce more polysulphated glycosaminoglycans than hyaluronic acid [12]. As stated, hyaluronic acid is produced at earlier stages of fibroplasia while the polysulphated glycosaminoglycans are produced at later stages of fibroplasia and in the earlier stages of remodeling phase of the healing process [3]. Hyaluronic acid plays an important role in formation of the initial extra cellular matrix thus providing an optimum environment for collagen deposition and cell activity while the polysulphated glycosaminoglycans play important role in collagen aggregation and maturation and regulate collagen fibril diameter and density [12].

The quality of fibroplasia is well correlated with the higher number of fibroblasts and blood vessels [28]. At this moment the immature blood vessels connect to each other and several unconnected immature blood vessels lyse and removed from the healing matrix [29]. The connected blood vessels establish the tissue circulation and nourish the healing fibroblasts to produce more collagenous matrix [12]. In the early fibroplasia the collagen fibers mainly consist of type III which is an immature collagen type while at later stages the matrix consists of mainly of collagen type I which is a mature collagen type [9]. Ultrastructural investigations suggest that the collagen fibrils of type III are disconnected from each other, have low longitudinal and transverse diameter while gradually these collagen fibrils connect each other to produce larger diameter collagen type I fibrils [4-11]. These fibrils are longer and also have larger transverse diameter at the end of fibroplasia and at remodeling phase of tendon and ligament healing and can transfer the weight bearing forces thus have biomechanical characteristics [7]. By time, the weight bearing forces gradually increase and therefore, the collagen fibers became more aligned along the direction of the stress line that is transmitted between muscle to bone in tendons and between bone to bone in ligaments [12]. By increasing in the exogenous forces and aligning the collagen fibers, the cellularity gradually decreases and tendon metabolism decreases [7-10,134,135]. At this time the remodeling phase of tendon healing which has started by collagen fiber alignment and cell reduction is in progress and gradually moves to maturation and consolidation stages [1]. During the maturation stage of remodeling phase the vascularity gradually decreases, the alignment increases and the metabolism of fibroblasts' decreases and these cells shift from mature fibroblast to highly matured fibrocytes [12]. The fibrocytes have least transverse diameter and the nucleus/cytoplasm ratio is maximum as compared to immature and mature fibroblasts [4,29]. At this stage the collagen fibrils aggregate laterally and pack to form the bundles of collagen fibers [27]. Collagen fibers could be detected under light microscopy and are well responsible for the higher biomechanical properties of the healing tissue [1]. Collagen fibrils have diameter ranging from 30 to 300 nm while the collagen fibers' diameter starts from few to several micrometers [12]. At consolidation stage the endotenon is well developed between the packs of collagen fibers and produce the secondary collagen fiber bundles and fascicles [12]. Collagen differentiation may be terminated at fiber level or may be progressed to produce large fascicles and bundles of collagen fibers [25,134,135]. Consolidation stage of tendon and ligament healing takes several months to years to be terminated and despite of these improvements the biomechanical properties of the healing tendon would never be achieved [1].

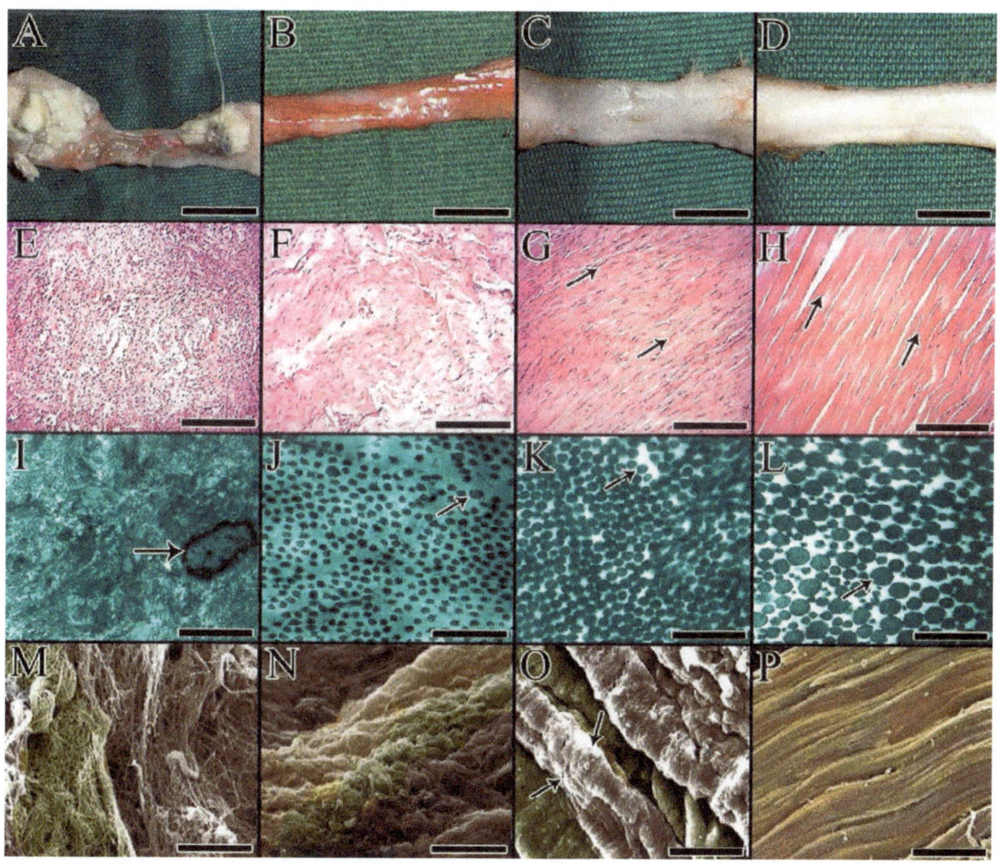

Figure 3: Three different stages of tendon healing under gross morphology, transmission electron-, and scanning electron microscopies.
(A to D) are gross morphologic Figures, (E to H) are light microscopic micrographs, (I to L) are transmission electron ultramicrographs and (M to P) are scanning electron micrographs. (A, E, I and M) show an injured healing tendon in the inflammatory phase of tendon healing. (B, F, J and N) show an injured healing tendon in the fibroplasia phase of tendon healing. (C, G, K and O) show an injured healing tendon in the early remodeling phase of tendon healing. (D, H, I and P) show an injured healing tendon in the late remodeling phase of tendon healing. In the inflammatory phase of tendon healing the injured tendon is inflamed and the tendon edges are necrotized (A). The inflammatory cells consisting of neutrophils, lymphocytes and macrophages are infiltrated in the defect area and start to lyse the necrotic tissues (E). By transmission electron microscopy (I), a macrophage (arrow) could be seen in the injured area and the ultrastructure of the injured area is highly amorphous and no fibrillar pattern could be detected because most of the collagen fibrils of the scaffold have been lysed and no characteristic fibrillogenesis has still occurred. Under scanning electron microscopy the density of the collagen fibrils is much low and most of the tissue spaces between the collagen fibrils are free of collagen fibrils. In fibroplasia, the vascularity of the tissue is high and the injured area of the tendon is hyperemic (B), the collagenous matrix is formed but it is immature in nature because the collagen fibers are not still formed but the number of collagen fibrils is gradually increasing (F). Generally the tissue is hypercellular and the density of the collagenous mass is low (F). At ultrastructural level, the immature collagen fibrils have newly developed (arrow) but their density is low (J). Under scanning electron microscopy (N) the collagen fibrils have developed but they have not still developed to collagen fibers. At early remodeling phase, the hyperemia have reduced and the density of the new tissue has increased but still is not comparable to normal (C). The collagen fibers are recently formed and are unidirectionally aligned (G, arrows). At ultrastructural level, the density and diameter of the collagen fibrils have increased (K) so that the collagen fibers are formed which could be well detected under scanning electron microscopy (O, arrows). In the late remodeling phase, the density of the new tendon have greatly increased (D), and the bundles of collagen fibers are clearly detectable (H) and are highly aligned (H). Under transmission electron microscopy (I) the collagen fibrils are distributed in multimodal pattern so that more than three different categories of collagen fibrils could be detected based on their transverse diameter (I). Under scanning electron microscopy, the collagen fibers that have well differentiated and are densely packed could be seen. Scale bar: A to D: 1 cm, E to H: 50 μm, I to L: 900 nm, M to P: 2 μm.

Two distinct models have been proposed to explain the mechanism of tendon healing including extrinsic and intrinsic mechanisms [1,2,12,29]. In the extrinsic mechanism, tenoblasts and inflammatory cells move from the periphery or external tissue sources to invade the healing site and initiate, and later promote, repair and regeneration [12]. This process includes the initial formation of adhesions and requires a well-established vascular network for the tissue to heal effectively [12]. Intrinsic healing occurs through a mechanism that entails the migration and proliferation of cells from the tendon proper including edges of tendon defect into the injury site; these cells establish an extracellular matrix and an internal neovascular network [1]. In most cases, both mechanisms are involved in the healing phenomenon that is dependent on several factors, including tendon location, extent of trauma, and postoperative motion [7,12]. The extrinsic mechanism, activated earlier than the intrinsic mechanism, is responsible for the formation of adhesions that occur initially, the disorganized collagen matrix with high cellularity, and high water content in the injury site [1,2]. By contrast, the intrinsic mechanism is responsible for the reorganization of the collagen fibers and maintenance of the fibrillar continuity [4,5,12]. It has been suggested that the intrinsic mechanism is the sole responsible for most of the beneficial events that regulates the structure and strength of the new tendon (Figure 3) [12].

Tendon to Bone Healing

As stated tendon and ligaments have bony attachments [3]. Tendon-bone incorporation of a tendon graft within the bone tunnel is a major concern when using a tendon graft for ligament reconstruction [132]. Successful ligament reconstruction with a tendon graft requires solid healing of the tendon graft in the bone tunnels [3]. Improvement of graft healing to bone is crucial to facilitate early and aggressive rehabilitation and a rapid return to full activity [133]. Healing of a tendon graft in a bone tunnel requires bone ingrowth into the tendon [132]. Indirect Sharpey's fibers and direct fibrocartilage fixation of the tendon-bone interface provide different anchorage strength and interface properties [133]. The insertion of the native ligament is characterized in four layers: ligament, fibrocartilage, mineralized fibrocartilage, and bone (Figure 4) [1]. The collagen fibers of the ligament extend into both the fibrocartilage and the mineralized layer [3]. This structure usually is destroyed when the ligament is removed and the bone tunnel is drilled [3]. A replication of this direct type of insertion may be considered desirable when assessing bone tunnel healing for ligament grafts [132]. Based on normal ligament structure and function of the insertion site, the ideal tendon graft would attach broadly to the surface of the bone at the origin and insertion attachment sites by an intermediate zone of fibrocartilage (Figure 4) [3]. The bone-tendon-bone graft undergoes a process of ligamentization [3]. The graft undergoes initial processes of necrosis, revascularization, cellular proliferation, and then remodeling [132,133]. The remodeling phase could be divided into consolidation and maturation phases [1]. The biochemical and morphological changes occur in the graft as it assumes a histologic pattern similar to native ligament, but it is not identical to either native ligament or tendon [3]. The most rapid healing time at the insertion sites is in bone-tendon-bone autograft (e.g. patellar tendon bone autograft) or allograft with bone-to-bone healing times of 4-6 weeks [136]. This graft has the additional benefit of having the natural insertion site of tendon preserved on the bone plug as previously described [3].

The mechanism by which graft-bone healing occurs depends on the type of the graft used. For bone-tendon-bone grafts, healing in the tunnel resembles normal fracture healing but may be a more complex process [3]. Incorporation of the bone block in the tunnel has been observed as early as 16 weeks after surgery [133]. Bone-tendon-bone grafts (e.g. bone- patellar tendon- bone grafts) have the advantage of allowing rigid fixation of the graft in the bone tunnel [133]. The tendon-bone healing process occurs through a different mechanism after implantation of a soft-tissue graft without bone plugs [3]. First, fibrovascular interface tissue forms between graft and bone, and progressive mineralization of the interface tissue occurs with subsequent bone ingrowth into the outer tendon and incorporation of the tendon graft into the surrounding

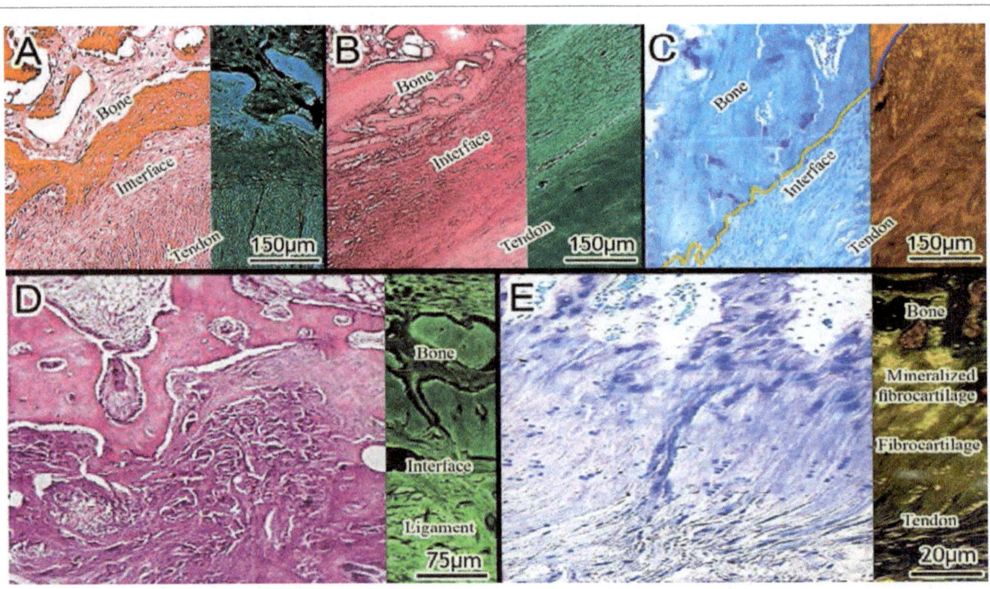

Figure 4: Tendon to bone junction.
The insertion of the native tendon is characterized in four layers: tendon, fibrocartilage, mineralized fibrocartilage, and bone (A to E). The collagen fibers of the tendon extend into both the fibrocartilage and the mineralized layer (E). The tendon-bone healing process occurs as follows: First, fibrovascular interface tissue forms between the graft and bone, and progressive mineralization of the interface tissue occurs with subsequent bone in growth into the outer tendon and incorporation of the tendon graft into the surrounding bone. Sharpey's fibers are made up of type I collagen and connect the periosteum to the bone. Progressive reestablishment of the continuity of collagen fibers between the tendon and the bone results in re-establishment of a tendoosseous junction. Tendoosseous junction is the interface zone (A to D). A and B stained with H and E. C to E stained with toluidine blue.

bone [132,133]. Sharpey's fibers are made up of type I collagen and connect the periosteum to the bone. Progressive re-establishment of the continuity of collagen fibers between the tendon and the bone results in re-establishment of a tendoosseous junction [133]. Formations of the Sharpey-like fibers within the bone tunnel often are identified as a marker of indirect healing between the tendon and bone. Formation of these collagenous fibers may start from 6 weeks after surgery [132]. However, complete bone tunnel healing of a ligament graft may occur as late as 6 to12 months after surgery [136]. It has been postulated that tendon graft incorporation occurs more slowly than bone-tendon-bone healing [3]. In addition to the choice of graft, surgical fixation, graft position, and interfacial motion within the bone tunnel may affect healing [3]. Graft motion within the bone tunnel has been shown to be inversely proportional to healing in animal models [132]. Histology taken at revision surgery for mid-substance tears, shows that free tendon autograft has adequate osteointegration between 6-15 weeks [3]. If soft tissue-to-bone integration occurs at this time, a tendon graft may allow for earlier recovery and return to activity because of less donor site morbidity [12]. A number of studies have shown no significant difference in clinical outcomes between bone-tendon-bone graft and tendon graft for ligament reconstruction [3,132,133]. The healing potential of a ruptured ligament as described before is considered to be extremely poor [12]. It is suggested that the intra-articular environment that inhibits ligament healing also may interfere with bony healing in the proximal parts of the osseous tunnels [3].

Limitations of tendon and ligament healing

Adhesion formation after intrasynovial tendon injury poses a major clinical problem. Disruption of the synovial sheath at the time of the injury or surgery allows granulation tissue and tenocytes from around the tissue to invade the repair site [1,12]. Exogenous cells predominate over endogenous tenocytes, allowing the surrounding tissue to attach to the repair site and resulting in adhesion formation [12]. We showed such limitation happens in the extra synovial flexor tendons healing too [25-29].

As another limitation, despite remodeling the biochemical and mechanical properties of healed tendon never match those of the intact tendon [28]. Finally, healing of large tissue deficits is a complicated process and the healing response and rate is low, resulting in formation of non-functional scar tissue. In tendon to bone junction, dehiscence at the attachment site is one of the most important limitations especially in ligament reconstruction [3].

Host-graft interaction

At least five possible biologic responses have been suggested after implantation of extracellular matrixes including: extracellular matrix nonincorporating responses (ie, encapsulation and rejection) and extracellular matrix incorporating responses (i.e., resorption, integration with progressive degradation, adoption, and adaptation) [29,69]. These responses are dependent to several factors [69]. The best results have been suggested for autografts because their cellular structures are the same as host and also they have least post-implantation immunological reaction [72]. In such condition the inflammation is not triggered by the graft thus there is no rapid absorption [72]. The cellular structures of autografts could well collaborate in the healing process and can produce matrix as the healing fibroblasts do [69-72]. The collagen fibers of autograft are also participate in regeneration mechanism [87,89]. In the other meaning, the host uses most portions of the autograft matrix and therefore there is no need for the host to produce large amounts of collagenous materials and therefore the risk of adhesion formation reduces [87]. Investigations have shown that following autograft implantation the inflammatory cells infiltrate through the graft but they do not accumulate [69-72]. The matrix is partially degraded by phagocytosis and MMPs but most of the matrix is preserved [72]. At fibroplasia the fibroblasts infiltrate the healing graft and the graft is accepted as a part of the new tendon or ligament [12,72]. In this case, the inflammation is minimum and the healing rate is maximum [12]. The autografts have excellent tendoinductivity, tenoconductivity and tenogenisity thus the host behavior following autograft implantation is a combination of integration with progressive degradation, adoption, and adaptation [3]. However the host behavior is different between individuals and species [3,12,29].

Allografts have lower healing capability because most of their cells are not alive; therefore their tendinogenesis properties is lower than the autografts and this leads to inferior healing response to allografts as compared to autografts [3,12,29]. Allografts have two forms including fresh and processed tissues [25-28]. After implantation of a fresh allograft most of its cellular structures are degraded by the apoptosis mechanism and or died and lysed by phagocytosis by the inflammatory cells in the inflammatory phase of healing [69]. As a general rule, the allografts accelerate the inflammatory reaction; therefore more inflammatory cells enter the graft following implantation [12,68]. These cells may accumulate in some areas of the graft to completely lyse the implanted tissue. In the case of fresh allografts the phagocytosis activity of the immune response is much high thus it leads to rapid absorption of the graft [3]. In fresh allograft there is a risk of rejection and the model of rejection is likely to be a rapid absorption [3]. In human and animals models, rejection may occur by different mechanisms [29]. If the graft would be biodegradable such as fresh allografts, then the rejection is activated through the rapid absorption mechanism [69]. If the graft was not biodegradable then the rejection occurs through encapsulation [12]. Therefore application of fresh allograft have not been selected by many surgeons and the processed allograft that have lower antigenicity have been used widely [12,24]. Following implantation of the processed allografts the degree of host inflammatory response is completely dependent on the immunogenicity of the graft and the method of processing [12]. If the antigenicity of the graft was low, then a better outcome could be expected [72]. In that case, the inflammatory is milder and some parts of the graft is persevered and partial matrix replacement occurs by the new tissue [12]. In such situation the processed allograft tissue has no teno- or ligamentoinductivity but has teno- or ligamentoconductivity; it means the graft can act as a scaffold for tissue regeneration and therefore satisfactory results could be expected; however the results are inferior to autografts even with the best outcome [3]. Xenografts are acutely rejected [12,29]. It has been postulated that following xenograft implantation in the tendon defect, the inflammatory cells immediately accumulate in the graft and completely degrade the graft thus only a loose areolar and amorphous tissue replaces the matrix [68-72]. In this case, neutrophils, macrophages and giant cells infiltrate and accumulate in most parts of the graft and degrade it [72]. No acceptable outcome has been reported for the xenografts [72].

As stated, the tissue engineered grafts could be divided into absorbable and non-absorbable ones [25]. Both of the absorbable and non-absorbable materials could be immunogenic i.e. they must be free of immunological characteristics [26]. The host behavior is completely dependent on the above factors [27-29]. If the tissue engineered graft has low immunogenicity and is biodegradable when it is seeded with autogenous stem cells, then it is possible to be accepted as a part of new tendon or ligament similar to the mechanism that was described for autografts [12]. In this case the severity of the inflammation may be higher than that of the autografts but the duration would not be longer [68,70,71]. These types of tissue engineered cell seeded scaffolds have all the autografts characteristics including tissue inductivity, genesis and conductivity [26]. If the allologous or xenologous cells were seeded in the biodegradable low immunogenic scaffolds, then similar results could be expected as we have described for the fresh allografts and xenografts in which the duration and severity of the inflammation may be prolonged, the graft is acutely absorbed and an amorphous tissue fills the defect [68-72]. Another option is application of scaffolds without stem cells [25-29]. In that case if the scaffold has high immunogenicity and is none resorbable then the scaffold is expected to be rejected by the host through encapsulation mechanism [69]. In fact, fibrous connective tissue covers the scaffold in order to reduce the immunogenic signals and by this mechanism it decreases the duration of the inflammation [12]. In this case the scaffold is preserved in the body but has no function after the healing process [87-89]. If the scaffold was not immunogenic, then it is expected to be preserved and be accepted as a part of the newly developed tissue [25-29]. In that case, the new tissue regenerates through the free spaces of the inner parts of the non-absorbable scaffold but the newly regenerated tissue cannot replace the graft [25]. If the scaffold was not immunogenic but was also biodegradable, an acceptable outcome would be expected and achieved [76,77,85]. Studies suggest that these types of scaffolds would not be completely rejected by the host and some portion of the scaffold may be preserved [28]. In this case some areas of the scaffold may be rapidly infiltrated by the host immune cells and are phagocytized and some remnants parts of the scaffold may be covered by fibrous connective tissue and are encapsulated [27]. It is well shown that following implantation of such bio-absorbable grafts the inflammatory reaction is accelerated but does not last for a long period [25-29]. Therefore, the inflammatory cells consisting of neutrophils and macrophages infiltrate in the scaffold and degrade some parts but rapidly these free spaces are filled with new connective tissue [29].

The portion to be deleted by the host immune response is depended to two factors including the cross linking degree and the immunogenicity of the implant [12]. If the cross linking degree is moderate and the immunogenicity is acceptable, then approximately more than 50% percent of the scaffold is preserved in the fibroplasia stage and numerous small pieces of the implant could be seen as islands of the scaffold. It has been shown that such remnant have major roles in further alignment of the newly developed connective tissue [12,24]. From fibroplasia to the end of healing such remnants could participate in tendon healing and the healing is continued by three major mechanisms [28,29]. In the first mechanism the volume of some of the preserved remnant of the scaffolds gradually decrease but they still act as micro scaffolds and align the new tissue along their longitudinal orientation [28]. In this mechanism the graft remnants are not infiltrated by the fibroblasts and fibrocytes [28]. In the second mechanism the preserved remnants are absorbed faster than the first mechanism [29]. In this mechanism, those free spaces of the implant that were filled with new connective tissue sooner, act as microscaffolds for the newly developed connective tissues that filled the free spaces of the graft later [25]. Therefore, under light microscopy two distinct areas could be seen in the injured area consisting of mature and immature collagen fibers. In the third mechanism the preserved remnant parts are infiltrated by the host fibroblasts and are accepted as parts of the new tendon or ligament [28]. At the remodeling phase most of the implant should be degraded and most of the defect area should be filled with the new but highly aligned tissue (Figure 5) [29].

Postoperative management

The aim of rehabilitation after surgically repaired or reconstructed tendon is to achieve function and gliding but avoiding rupture of the tendon. Although several protocols have been introduced to date, however, the ideal protocol, which gives the best functional outcome, is still under debate.

Historically, patients with Achilles or patellar tendon or ACL rupture are immobilized in a rigid cast for at least 4-6 weeks to allow the presumed tendon healing [137]. Current trends, however, favor minimizing postoperative immobilization and focus on early weight

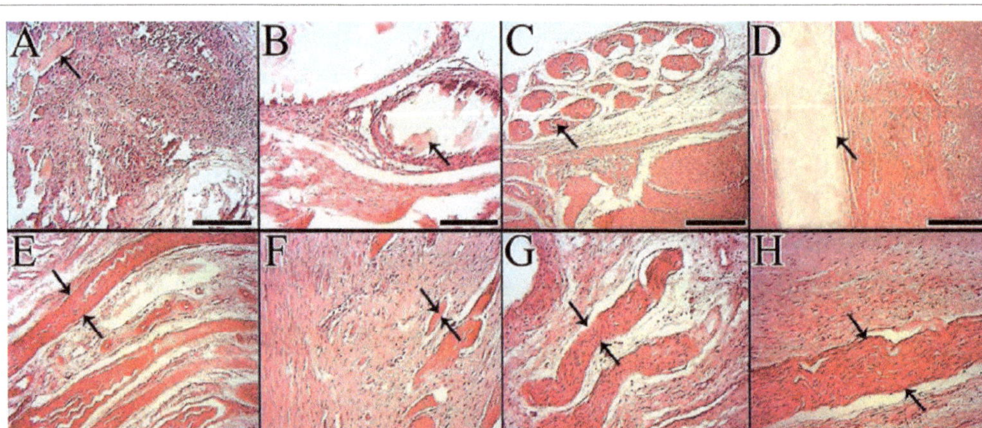

Figure 5: Mechanisms of host graft interactions.
Implantation of various prosthetic implants causes different host behavior based on the nature of the implant. Implantation of the highly antigenic implants cause rapid absorption (A and B) which is described as one of the host rejection mechanisms. Vigorous inflammatory reaction occurs after implantation of the antigenic graft (A) and the inflammatory cells surround the scaffold remnants to completely lyse them at a short period of time. Arrows in A and B show the scaffold remnants. The host can reject the implanted graft by another mechanism which is called encapsulation (C). In fact, the body fails to lyse all parts of the graft, thus the fibrous connective tissue surrounds the graft (C, arrow). If the implant would not be rejected by the host then it can collaborate at different stages of tendon and ligament healing and regeneration by different mechanisms (D to H). D to F is progressive degradation mechanism in which some part of the implant have been absorbed and the new tissue filled the free spaces in the graft and the remnant parts (arrow) are not surrounded by the inflammation and are not encapsulated. The remnant parts are progressively degraded at later stages and the new tissue fills their free spaces (D). The absorption rate in this mechanism is high but is lower than the acute degradation mechanism which we showed in A and B. The final mechanism is adoption and adaptation of the graft (G and H). Some remnants of the graft (arrows) are not rejected by the host, also are not slowly degraded but also infiltrated by the host fibroblasts and accepted as part of the new tendon or ligament. Color staining: H & E. Scale bar for A, C, D, and E: 125 μm and for B, F, G and H: 50 μm.

bearing with excellent results. In a rat model of tendon rupture, using wheel running for early tendon motion, Bring et al. [137] were able to show that physical activity speeds up tendon healing as compared to plaster immobilization. This suggests that there may be some stimulatory effect of mechanical loading on tendon healing. In a clinical prospective study with full postoperative weight bearing in a controlled ankle motion walker accompanied by active stretching, Jacob and Paterson [138] showed few minor complications, high patient satisfaction, and no re-ruptures. Patients with both acute and chronic tears repaired with an open technique did equally well under this treatment protocol. In their meta-analysis of randomized trials comparing early postoperative weight bearing with cast immobilization, Suchak et al. [139] found no difference in re-rupture rates and more excellent rated subjective patient responses. Patients preferred the early function protocol with a mobile cast for multiple reasons including a decrease in leg edema, the ability to bear weight, and easier and faster ability to obtain normal gait after removal of the cast [140].

Here we discussed the rehabilitative protocols of those patients that their hand flexor tendons have been surgically repaired which could be a good example for post-operative rehabilitation program. For hand flexor tendons, there are 3 main methods. Firstly, there is active extension with rubber band flexion, also called the active extension-passive flexion method [141]. Secondly there is passive motion method, which uses a range of 3-5mm of passive motion in the involved tendon and then lastly there is controlled passive motion with the patient actively flexing the digit rather than someone else [141]. There are variations of these methods in clinical practice today. The once popular rubber band technique made known by Kleinert et al., has now been favoured against by passive and active motion protocols [142]. The mobilized tendons have shown to heal quicker and are stronger with lesser adhesions than the immobilized tendons [143]. Programs involve a step-wise progression of passive movement to reduce adhesion but preventing excessive loading and the active motion to overcome stiffness and swelling of the joints. It has been shown that early active protocols and combined Kleinert (passive flexion and active extension) and Durran (controlled passive motion) protocols resulted in low rates of tendon ruptures and acceptable range of motion following flexor tendon repair in zone 2 [144]. Patient compliance is vitally important for success of flexor tendon repairs as patients who negatively ignore the rehabilitation protocols can impact on their results. The trend to more active mobilization seems to be favored but further studies in this area are needed.

The Future

Management of tendon and ligament injuries is technically demanding and the acceptable options are limited [3,12,29]. In addition, tendon and ligament healing and regeneration are complicated processes and have significant limitations including development of post-operative adhesion, low healing response and rejection of the graft [1,12,25]. Autografts are still the gold method; however tissue engineering produced new insights but is still a primitive choice [13-18]. Despite of several achievements in tendon and ligament tissue engineering, the outcome is unclear because the investigations are not organized in order to solve the problems [23,24]. The necessity of animal based studies is felt and it is expected to be done in future in order to better clarify the possible mechanisms and solutions [29]. There are few studies that compared the differences between auto- allo- xeno- and tissue engineered grafts with or without cell seeding methods and other tissue processizations [12,24]. Tissue engineering should answer this question whether is it possible to produce a viable graft alternative to autografts with the same desirable outcome after *in vivo* application. The role of inflammation in tissue healing and regeneration should not be neglected and the possible mechanisms after implantation of various grafts should be better clarified and described [25-29,30-32]. One major problem is that different studies used different methodologies and viable species, thus possible comparison is not logic. It is suggested that the researchers use more standard methods in their investigations and systematic reviews and meta-analyses studies, and comparing the results and concluding their outcomes are highly recommended in future. The role of scaffolds, healing promotive factors including growth factors, glycosaminoglycans, and healing agents, together with stem cells and gene therapy has been discussed in this review. Future investigations should focus on the effectiveness of the combinations of these materials and factors. In designing such novel but interesting tissue engineered based viable bioactive grafts, it is important that the grafts have optimum biomechanical properties at short term and high healing incorporative properties in order to be tissue inductive, -conductive and –genesis at long term. Tissue engineering could open new insights and present a significant achievement in near future and this could be a revolution in healing and regeneration.

Author Contribution

Dr Ali Moshiri and Professor Ahmad Oryan had equal contribution in all parts of the study.

References

1. Sharma P, Maffulli N (2005) Tendon injury and tendinopathy: healing and repair. J Bone Joint Surg Am 87: 187-202.
2. Khanna A, Friel M, Gougoulias N, Longo UG, Maffulli N (2009) Prevention of adhesions in surgery of the flexor tendons of the hand: what is the evidence? Br Med Bull 90: 85-109.
3. Oryan A, Moshiri A, Meimandi-Parizi AH (2013) Graft selection in ACL reconstructive surgery: Past, Present and Future. Current Orthopaedic Practice. Curr Orthop Pract 24: 321-333.
4. Oryan A, Moshiri A, Meimandiparizi AH (2011) Effects of sodium-hyaluronate and glucosamine-chondroitin sulphate on remodeling stage of tenotomized superficial digital flexor tendon in rabbits: a clinical, histopathological, ultrastructural, and biomechanical study. Connect Tissue Res 52: 329-339.
5. Moshiri A, Oryan A (2011) Structural and functional modulation of early healing of full-thickness superficial digital flexor tendon rupture in rabbits by repeated subcutaneous administration of exogenous human recombinant basic fibroblast growth factor. J Foot Ankle Surg 50: 654-662.
6. Oryan A, Moshiri A (2011) A long term study on the role of exogenous human recombinant basic fibroblast growth factor on the superficial digital flexor tendon healing in rabbits. J Musculoskelet Neuronal Interact 11: 185-195.
7. Oryan A, Moshiri A, Meimandi-Parizi AH (2012) Short and long terms healing of the experimentally transverse sectioned tendon in rabbits. Sports Med Arthrosc Rehabil Ther Technol 4: 14.
8. Oryan A, Moshiri A, Raayat AR (2012) Novel application of Theranekron® enhanced the structural and functional performance of the tenotomized tendon in rabbits. Cells Tissues Organs 196: 442-455.
9. Oryan A, Moshiri A, Meimandi Parizi AH, Raayat Jahromi A (2012) Repeated administration of exogenous Sodium-hyaluronate improved tendon healing in an in vivo transection model. J Tissue Viability 21: 88-102.
10. Oryan A, Moshiri A (2012) Recombinant fibroblast growth protein enhances healing ability of experimentally induced tendon injury in vivo. J Tissue Eng Regen Med.
11. Oryan A, Moshiri A, Meimandi Parizi A (2012) Alcoholic extract of tarantula cubensis improves sharp ruptured tendon healing after primary repair in rabbits. Am J Orthop (Belle Mead NJ) 41: 554-560.
12. Moshiri A, Oryan A (2012) Role of tissue engineering in tendon reconstructive surgery and regenerative medicine: current concepts, approaches and concerns. Hard Tissue 1: 11.
13. Beals TC, Severson EP, Kinikini D, Aoki S (2010) Complex Achilles reconstruction for massive soft tissue loss: allograft, autograft, and use of a temporary cement spacer. J Orthop Trauma 24: e78-80.

14. Park YS, Sung KS (2012) Surgical reconstruction of chronic achilles tendon ruptures using various methods. Orthopedics 35: e213-218.

15. Maffulli N, Spiezia F, Testa V, Capasso G, Longo UG, et al. (2012) Free gracilis tendon graft for reconstruction of chronic tears of the Achilles tendon. J Bone Joint Surg Am 94: 906-910.

16. Ronel DN, Newman MI, Gayle LB, Hoffman LA (2004) Recent advances in the reconstruction of complex Achilles tendon defects. Microsurgery 24: 18-23.

17. Bullocks JM, Hickey RM, Basu CB, Hollier LH, Kim JY (2008) Single-stage reconstruction of Achilles tendon injuries and distal lower extremity soft tissue defects with the reverse sural fasciocutaneous flap. J Plast Reconstr Aesthet Surg 61: 566-572.

18. Longo UG, Lamberti A, Maffulli N, Denaro V (2010) Tendon augmentation grafts: a systematic review. Br Med Bull 94: 165-188.

19. Duthon VB, Lübbeke A, Duc SR, Stern R, Assal M (2011) Noninsertional Achilles tendinopathy treated with gastrocnemius lengthening. Foot Ankle Int 32: 375-379.

20. Maheshwari AV, Walters JA, Henshaw RM (2012) Extensile posterior approach to the ankle with detachment of the achilles tendon for oncologic indications. Foot Ankle Int 33: 430-435.

21. Yang M, Wang Z, Li Y, Guo B (2013) Bilateral cadaveric Achilles tendon graft in reconstruction after Achilles tendon tumor resection. J Foot Ankle Surg 52: 103-106.

22. Shearn JT, Kinneberg KR, Dyment NA, Galloway MT, Kenter K, et al. (2011) Tendon tissue engineering: progress, challenges, and translation to the clinic. J Musculoskelet Neuronal Interact 11: 163-173.

23. Chen J, Xu J, Wang A, Zheng M (2009) Scaffolds for tendon and ligament repair: review of the efficacy of commercial products. Expert Rev Med Devices 6: 61-73.

24. Oryan A, Moshiri A, Sharifi P (2012) Advances in injured tendon engineering with emphasis on the role of collagen implants. Hard Tissue 1: 12.

25. Moshiri A, Oryan A, Meimandi Parizi AH, Silver IA, Tanideh N, et al. (2013) Effectiveness of hybridized nano and micro-structure biodegradable and biocompatible collagen-based, three-dimensional bioimplants, in repair of a large tendon-defect model in rabbits. J Tissue Eng Regen Med.

26. Meimandi-Parizi A, Oryan A, Moshiri A (2013) Role of tissue engineered collagen based tridimensional implant on the healing response of the experimentally induced large Achilles tendon defect model in rabbits: a long term study with high clinical relevance. J Biomed Sci 20: 28.

27. Meimandi-Parizi A, Oryan A, Moshiri A, Silver IA (2013) Novel application of a tissue-engineered collagen-based three-dimensional bio-implant in a large tendon defect model: A broad-based study with high value in translational medicine. Tissue Cell 45: 282-294.

28. Moshiri A, Oryan A, MeimandiParizi A (2013) A novel application of biosynthetic tissue-engineered tridimensional implant on large tendon defects: a comprehensive, detailed, in vivo investigation with significant clinical value. Connect Tissue Res 54: 227-243.

29. Moshiri A, Oryan A, Meimandi-Parizi A (2013) Role of tissue-engineered artificial tendon in healing of a large achilles tendon defect model in rabbits. J Am Coll Surg 217: 421-441.

30. Moshiri A, Oryan A (2013) Role of platelet rich plasma in soft and hard connective tissue healing: an evidence based review from basic to clinical application. Hard Tissue 2: 6.

31. Oryan A, Moshiri A (2013) Exogenous acellular synovial fluid as a new therapeutic option in tissue engineering and regenerative medicine. Hard Tissue 2: 21.

32. Moshiri A, Oryan A, Meimandi-Parizi A (2013) Role of stem cell therapy in orthopaedic tissue engineering and regenerative medicine: a comprehensive review of the literature from basic to clinical application. Hard Tissue 2: 31.

33. Sarrafzadehrezaei F, Oryan A, Dehghani S (1999) Effects of electrical stimulation on biomechanics of partial and completed ruptured tendon. Res Med 23: 169-175.

34. Prodromos CC, Han Y, Rogowski J, Joyce B, Shi K (2007) A meta-analysis of the incidence of anterior cruciate ligament tears as a function of gender, sport, and a knee injury-reduction regimen. Arthroscopy 23: 1320-1325.

35. Krackow KA, Thomas SC, Jones LC (1986) A new stitch for ligament-tendon fixation. Brief note. J Bone Joint Surg Am 68: 764-766.

36. Watson TW, Jurist KA, Yang KH, Shen KL (1995) The strength of Achilles tendon repair: an in vitro study of the biomechanical behavior in human cadaver tendons. Foot Ankle Int 16: 191-195.

37. Akgün U, Erol B, Karahan M (2006) [Primary surgical repair with the Krackow technique combined with plantaris tendon augmentation in the treatment of acute Achilles tendon ruptures]. Acta Orthop Traumatol Turc 40: 228-233.

38. Beskin JL, Sanders RA, Hunter SC, Hughston JC (1987) Surgical repair of Achilles tendon ruptures. Am J Sports Med 15: 1-8.

39. Rosenzweig S, Azar FM (2009) Open repair of acute Achilles tendon ruptures. Foot Ankle Clin 14: 699-709.

40. Lindholm A (1959) A new method of operation in subcutaneous rupture of the Achilles tendon. Acta Chir Scand 117: 261-270.

41. Ma GW, Griffith TG (1977) Percutaneous repair of acute closed ruptured achilles tendon: a new technique. Clin Orthop Relat Res: 247-255.

42. Martinelli B (2000) Percutaneous repair of the Achilles tendon in athletes. Bull Hosp Jt Dis 59: 149-152.

43. Davies MS, Solan M (2009) Minimal incision techniques for acute Achilles repair. Foot Ankle Clin 14: 685-697.

44. Thompson J, Baravarian B (2011) Acute and chronic Achilles tendon ruptures in athletes. Clin Podiatr Med Surg 28: 117-135.

45. Winwood PW, Hume PA, Keogh JW, Cronin JB (2013) Retrospective Injury Epidemiology of Strongman Competitors. J Strength Cond Res.

46. Lam KK (2013) Comparative epidemiology of tendon injuries in different racing disciplines. Vet J 195: 265-266.

47. Lopes AD, Hespanhol Júnior LC, Yeung SS, Costa LO (2012) What are the main running-related musculoskeletal injuries? A Systematic Review. Sports Med 42: 891-905.

48. Clegg PD (2012) Musculoskeletal disease and injury, now and in the future. Part 2: Tendon and ligament injuries. Equine Vet J 44: 371-375.

49. Patillo D, Rayan GM (2012) Open extensor tendon injuries: an epidemiologic study. Hand Surg 17: 37-42.

50. Taylor SA, Hannafin JA (2012) Evaluation and management of elbow tendinopathy. Sports Health 4: 384-393.

51. Gajhede-Knudsen M, Ekstrand J, Magnusson H, Maffulli N (2013) Recurrence of Achilles tendon injuries in elite male football players is more common after early return to play: an 11-year follow-up of the UEFA Champions League injury study. Br J Sports Med 47: 763-768.

52. Vosseller JT, Ellis SJ, Levine DS, Kennedy JG, Elliott AJ, et al. (2013) Achilles tendon rupture in women. Foot Ankle Int 34: 49-53.

53. Raikin SM, Garras DN, Krapchev PV (2013) Achilles tendon injuries in a United States population. Foot Ankle Int 34: 475-480.

54. Wilkins R, Bisson LJ (2012) Operative versus nonoperative management of acute Achilles tendon ruptures: a quantitative systematic review of randomized controlled trials. Am J Sports Med 40: 2154-2160.

55. Ackermann PW, Renström P (2012) Tendinopathy in sport. Sports Health 4: 193-201.

56. Joseph MF, Crowley J, Dilieto L, O'Neil B, Denegar CR (2012) Incidence of morphologic changes in asymptomatic Achilles tendons in an active young adult population. J Sport Rehabil 21: 249-252.

57. Swenson DM, Collins CL, Best TM, Flanigan DC, Fields SK, et al. (2013) Epidemiology of knee injuries among U.S. high school athletes, 2005/2006-2010/2011. Med Sci Sports Exerc 45: 462-469.

58. Benner RW, Shelbourne KD, Urch SE, Lazarus D (2012) Tear patterns, surgical repair, and clinical outcomes of patellar tendon ruptures after anterior cruciate ligament reconstruction with a bone-patellar tendon-bone autograft. Am J Sports Med 40: 1834-1841.

59. Weiss JM, Arkader A, Wells LM, Ganley TJ (2013) Rotator cuff injuries in adolescent athletes. J Pediatr Orthop B 22: 133-137.

60. Horsley IG, Fowler EM, Rolf CG (2013) Shoulder injuries in professional rugby: a retrospective analysis. J Orthop Surg Res 8: 9.

61. Mall NA, Lee AS, Chahal J, Sherman SL, Romeo AA, et al. (2013) An evidenced-based examination of the epidemiology and outcomes of traumatic rotator cuff tears. Arthroscopy 29: 366-376.

62. Tekavec E, Jöud A, Rittner R, Mikoczy Z, Nordander C, et al. (2012) Population-based consultation patterns in patients with shoulder pain diagnoses. BMC Musculoskelet Disord 13: 238.

63. Tashjian RZ (2012) Epidemiology, natural history, and indications for treatment of rotator cuff tears. Clin Sports Med 31: 589-604.

64. Starr HM, Snoddy M, Hammond KE, Seiler JG 3rd (2013) Flexor tendon repair rehabilitation protocols: a systematic review. J Hand Surg Am 38: 1712-1717.

65. McCarthy MM, Voos JE, Nguyen JT, Callahan L, Hannafin JA (2013) Injury profile in elite female basketball athletes at the Women's National Basketball Association combine. Am J Sports Med 41: 645-651.

66. Sri-Ram K, Salmon LJ, Pinczewski LA, Roe JP (2013) The incidence of secondary pathology after anterior cruciate ligament rupture in 5086 patients requiring ligament reconstruction. Bone Joint J 95-95B: 59-64.

67. Goddard M, Bowman N, Salmon LJ, Waller A, Roe JP, et al. (2013) Endoscopic anterior cruciate ligament reconstruction in children using living donor hamstring tendon allografts. Am J Sports Med 41: 567-574.

68. Badylak SF, Valentin JE, Ravindra AK, McCabe GP, Stewart-Akers AM (2008) Macrophage phenotype as a determinant of biologic scaffold remodeling. Tissue Eng Part A 14: 1835-1842.

69. Cornwell KG, Landsman A, James KS (2009) Extracellular matrix biomaterials for soft tissue repair. Clin Podiatr Med Surg 26: 507-523.

70. Allman AJ, McPherson TB, Badylak SF, Merrill LC, Kallakury B, et al. (2001) Xenogeneic extracellular matrix grafts elicit a TH2-restricted immune response. Transplantation 71: 1631-1640.

71. Palmer EM, Beilfuss BA, Nagai T, Semnani RT, Badylak SF, et al. (2002) Human helper T cell activation and differentiation is suppressed by porcine small intestinal submucosa. Tissue Eng 8: 893-900.

72. Veillette CJ, Cunningham KD, Hart DA, Fritzler MJ, Frank CB (1998) Localization and characterization of porcine patellar tendon xenograft antigens in a rabbit model of medial collateral ligament replacement. Transplantation 65: 486-493.

73. Pridgen BC, Woon CY, Kim M, Thorfinn J, Lindsey D, et al. (2011) Flexor tendon tissue engineering: acellularization of human flexor tendons with preservation of biomechanical properties and biocompatibility. Tissue Eng Part C Methods 17: 819-828.

74. Fini M, Torricelli P, Giavaresi G, Rotini R, Castagna A, et al. (2007) In vitro study comparing two collageneous membranes in view of their clinical application for rotator cuff tendon regeneration. J Orthop Res 25: 98-107.

75. T Shu-Hua Teng, Eun-Jung Lee, Peng Wang, Hyoun-Ee Kim (2008) Collagen/hydroxyapatite composite nanofibers by electrospinning. Mat Let 62: 3055-3058.

76. Postlethwaite AE, Seyer JM, Kang AH (1978) Chemotactic attraction of human fibroblasts to type I, II, and III collagens and collagen-derived peptides. Proc Natl Acad Sci U S A 75: 871-875.

77. Ghanaati S, Schlee M, Webber MJ, Willershausen I, Barbeck M, et al. (2011) Evaluation of the tissue reaction to a new bilayered collagen matrix in vivo and its translation to the clinic. Biomed Mater 6: 015010.

78. Tsai S, Hsieh C, Hsieh C, Wang D, Huang LL, et al. (2007) Preparation and Cell Compatibility Evaluation of Chitosan/Collagen Composite Scaffolds Using Amino Acids as Crosslinking Bridges. J Appl Polym Sci 105: 1774-1785.

79. Foltran I, Foresti E, Parma B, Sabatino P, Norberto R (2008) Novel Biologically Inspired Collagen Nanofibers Reconstituted By Electrospinning Method. Macromol Symp 269: 111-118.

80. Wray LS, Orwin EJ (2009) Recreating the microenvironment of the native cornea for tissue engineering applications. Tissue Eng Part A 15: 1463-1472.

81. Dubey N, Letourneau PC, Tranquillo RT (2001) Neuronal contact guidance in magnetically aligned fibrin gels: effect of variation in gel mechano-structural properties. Biomaterials 22: 1065-1075.

82. McCall AS, Kraft S, Edelhauser HF, Kidder GW, Lundquist RR, et al. (2010) Mechanisms of corneal tissue cross-linking in response to treatment with topical riboflavin and long-wavelength ultraviolet radiation (UVA). Invest Ophthalmol Vis Sci 51: 129-138.

83. Stillaert FB, Di Bartolo C, Hunt JA, Rhodes NP, Tognana E, et al. (2008) Human clinical experience with adipose precursor cells seeded on hyaluronic acid-based spongy scaffolds. Biomaterials 29: 3953-3959.

84. Siritientong T, Srichana T, Aramwit P (2011) The effect of sterilization methods on the physical properties of silk sericin scaffolds. AAPS PharmSciTech 12: 771-781.

85. Gigante A, Cesari E, Busilacchi A, Manzotti S, Kyriakidou K, et al. (2009) Collagen I membranes for tendon repair: effect of collagen fiber orientation on cell behavior. J Orthop Res 27: 826-832.

86. Ping Ooi C, Cameron RE (2002) The hydrolytic degradation of polydioxanone (PDSII) sutures. Part II: Micromechanisms of deformation. J Biomed Mater Res 63: 291-298.

87. Oryan A (1995) Role of collagen in soft connective tissue wound healing. Transplant Proc 27: 2759-2761.

88. Oryan A (1995) Induction of soft connective tissue formation by various prosthetic implants. Transplant Proc 27: 2754-2755.

89. Oryan A, Moshiri A (2013) Tissue Engineering: Alternative Option in Managing Large and Massive Tissue Deficits. Tropical Medicine & Surgery 1:e101.

90. Oryan A, Goodship AE, Silver IA (2008) Response of a collagenase-induced tendon injury to treatment with a polysulphated glycosaminoglycan (Adequan). Connect Tissue Res 49: 351-360.

91. Barnes GL, Kostenuik PJ, Gerstenfeld LC, Einhorn TA (1999) Growth factor regulation of fracture repair. J Bone Miner Res 14: 1805-1815.

92. Wang JS (1996) Basic fibroblast growth factor for stimulation of bone formation in osteoinductive or conductive implants. Acta Orthop Scand Suppl 269: 1-33.

93. Rosier RN, O'Keefe RJ, Hicks DG (1998) The potential role of transforming growth factor beta in fracture healing. Clin Orthop Relat Res: S294-300.

94. Friesel RE, Maciag T (1995) Molecular mechanisms of angiogenesis: fibroblast growth factor signal transduction. FASEB J 9: 919-925.

95. Canalis E, McCarthy TL, Centrella M (1989) Effects of platelet-derived growth factor on bone formation in vitro. J Cell Physiol 140: 530-537.

96. Steenfos HH (1994) Growth factors and wound healing. Scand J Plast Reconstr Surg Hand Surg 28: 95-105.

97. Lieberman JR, Daluiski A, Einhorn TA (2002) The role of growth factors in the repair of bone. Biology and clinical applications. J Bone Joint Surg Am 84-84A: 1032-44.

98. Peng H, Wright V, Usas A, Gearhart B, Shen HC, et al. (2002) Synergistic enhancement of bone formation and healing by stem cell-expressed VEGF and bone morphogenetic protein-4. J Clin Invest 110: 751-759.

99. Hom DB, Maisel RH (1992) Angiogenic growth factors: their effects and potential in soft tissue wound healing. Ann Otol Rhinol Laryngol 101: 349-354.

100. Tohidnezhad M, Varoga D, Wruck CJ, Brandenburg LO, Seekamp A, et al. (2011) Platelet-released growth factors can accelerate tenocyte proliferation and activate the anti-oxidant response element. Histochem Cell Biol 135: 453-460.

101. Muto T, Kokubu T, Mifune Y, Sakata R, Nagura I, et al. (2013) Platelet-rich plasma protects rotator cuff-derived cells from the deleterious effects of triamcinolone acetonide. J Orthop Res 31: 976-982.

102. de Jonge S, de Vos RJ, Weir A, van Schie HT, Bierma-Zeinstra SM, et al. (2011) One-year follow-up of platelet-rich plasma treatment in chronic Achilles tendinopathy: a double-blind randomized placebo-controlled trial. Am J Sports Med 39: 1623-1629.

103. Oryan A, Meimandi-Parizi AH, Shafiei-Sarvestani Z, Bigham AS (2011) Effects of combined hydroxyapatite and human platelet rich plasma on bone healing in rabbit model: radiological, macroscopical, histopathological, ultrastructural and biomechanical studies. Cell Tissue Bank 13: 639-651.

104. Aspenberg P, Virchenko O (2004) Platelet concentrate injection improves Achilles tendon repair in rats. Acta Orthop Scand 75: 93-99.

105. Wnuk T, Blacha J, Mazurkiewicz T, Olchowik G, Chyżyńska M (2012) The mechanical and histological estimation of calcaneal tendon callus in rats after PRP injection. Pol Orthop Traumatol 77: 5-9.

106. Kaux JF, Drion PV, Colige A, Pascon F, Libertiaux V, et al. (2012) Effects of platelet-rich plasma (PRP) on the healing of Achilles tendons of rats. Wound Repair Regen 20: 748-756.

107. Oryan A, Silver IA, Goodship AE (2010) Metrenperone enhances collagen turnover and remodeling in the early stages of healing of tendon injury in rabbit. Arch Orthop Trauma Surg 130: 1451-1457.

108. Oryan A, Silver IA, Goodship AE (2009) Effects of a serotonin S2-receptor blocker on healing of acute and chronic tendon injuries. J Invest Surg 22: 246-255.

109. Naeini AT, Oryan A, Nikahval B, Toosinezhad M (2012) Evaluation of Glycyrrhiza glabra (Licorice) on wound healing in rats. Online J Vet Res 16: 138-146.

110. Oryan A, Tabatabaeinaeini A, Nikahval B, Gorgian E (2010) Effects of aqueous extract of Aloe vera on experimental cutaneous wound healing in rat. Vet Arhiv 80: 509-522.

111. Tabatabaei AT, Oryan A, Dehghaninazhvani S, Nikahval B (2008) Effects of topical and parentral application of Phenytoin on cutaneous wound healing in rabbit. J Ani Vet Adv 7: 1537-1545.

112. Tabatabaei AT, Oryan A, Dehghani S, Nikahval B (2008) Experimental cutaneous wound healing in rabbits: Using continuous microamperage low voltage electrical stimulation. Comp Clin Pathol 17: 203-210.

113. Oryan A, Khalafi-Nezhad A, Toloo N, Soltani Rad MN (2007) Effects of 4-chloro-2,6-bis-(2-hydroxyl-benzyl)-phenol on healing of skin wounds and growth of bacteria. J Vet Med A Physiol Pathol Clin Med 54: 585-591.

114. Oryan A, Zaker SR (1998) Effects of topical application of honey on cutaneous wound healing in rabbits. Zentralbl Veterinarmed A 45: 181-188.

115. Oryan A, Tabatabaei Naeini A, Moshiri A, Mohammadalipour A, Tabandeh MR (2012) Modulation of cutaneous wound healing by silymarin in rats. J Wound Care 21: 457-464.

116. Nidadavolu P, Amor W, Tran PL, Dertien J, Colmer-Hamood JA, et al. (2012) Garlic ointment inhibits biofilm formation by bacterial pathogens from burn wounds. J Med Microbiol 61: 662-671.

117. Hung LK, Fu SC, Lee YW, Mok TY, Chan KM (2013) Local vitamin-C injection reduced tendon adhesion in a chicken model of flexor digitorum profundus tendon injury. J Bone Joint Surg Am 95: e41.

118. Pavelka K, Coste P, Géher P, Krejci G (2010) Efficacy and safety of piascledine 300 versus chondroitin sulfate in a 6 months treatment plus 2 months observation in patients with osteoarthritis of the knee. Clin Rheumatol 29: 659-670.

119. Ai J, Ebrahimi S, Khoshzaban A, Jafarzadeh Kashi TS, Mehrabani D (2012) Tissue engineering using human mineralized bone xenograft and bone marrow mesenchymal stem cells allograft in healing of tibial fracture of experimental rabbit model. Iran Red Crescent Med J 14: 96-103.

120. Al Faqeh H, Nor Hamdan BM, Chen HC, Aminuddin BS, Ruszymah BH (2012) The potential of intra-articular injection of chondrogenic-induced bone marrow stem cells to retard the progression of osteoarthritis in a sheep model. Exp Gerontol 47: 458-464.

121. Behfar M, Sarrafzadeh-Rezaei F, Hobbenaghi R, Delirezh N, Dalir-Naghadeh B (2012) Enhanced mechanical properties of rabbit flexor tendons in response to intratendinous injection of adipose derived stromal vascular fraction. Curr Stem Cell Res Ther 7: 173-178.

122. Behnia H, Khojasteh A, Soleimani M, Tehranchi A, Atashi A (2012) Repair of alveolar cleft defect with mesenchymal stem cells and platelet derived growth factors: a preliminary report. J Craniomaxillofac Surg 40: 2-7.

123. Cheung WH, Chin WC, Wei FY, Li G, Leung KS (2013) Applications of exogenous mesenchymal stem cells and low intensity pulsed ultrasound enhance fracture healing in rat model. Ultrasound Med Biol 39: 117-125.

124. Chong AK, Ang AD, Goh JC, Hui JH, Lim AY, et al. (2007) Bone marrow-derived mesenchymal stem cells influence early tendon-healing in a rabbit achilles tendon model. J Bone Joint Surg Am 89: 74-81.

125. Clarke AW, Alyas F, Morris T, Robertson CJ, Bell J, et al. (2011) Skin-derived tenocyte-like cells for the treatment of patellar tendinopathy. Am J Sports Med 39: 614-623.

126. Pascual-Garrido C, Rolón A, Makino A (2012) Treatment of chronic patellar tendinopathy with autologous bone marrow stem cells: a 5-year-followup. Stem Cells Int 2012: 953510.

127. Silva A, Sampaio R, Fernandes R, Pinto E (2012) Is there a role for adult non-cultivated bone marrow stem cells in ACL reconstruction? Knee Surg Sports Traumatol Arthrosc.

128. Egermann M, Lill CA, Griesbeck K, Evans CH, Robbins PD, et al. (2006) Effect of BMP-2 gene transfer on bone healing in sheep. Gene Ther 13: 1290-1299.

129. Schwabe P, Greiner S, Ganzert R, Eberhart J, Dähn K, et al. (2012) Effect of a novel nonviral gene delivery of BMP-2 on bone healing. ScientificWorldJournal 2012: 560142.

130. Heyde M, Partridge KA, Oreffo RO, Howdle SM, Shakesheff KM, et al. (2007) Gene therapy used for tissue engineering applications. J Pharm Pharmacol 59: 329-350.

131. Lui P, Zhang P, Chan K, Qin L (2010) Biology and augmentation of tendon-bone insertion repair. J Orthop Surg Res 5: 59.

132. James R, Kesturu G, Balian G, Chhabra AB (2008) Tendon: biology, biomechanics, repair, growth factors, and evolving treatment options. J Hand Surg Am 33: 102-112.

133. Oryan A, Shoushtari AH (2008) Histology and ultrastructure of the developing superficial digital flexor tendon in rabbits. Anat Histol Embryol 37: 134-140.

134. Oryan A, Shoushtari AH (2009) Biomechanical properties and dry weight content of the developing superficial digitalflexor tendon in rabbits. Comp Clin Pathol 18: 131-137.

135. Oryan A, Alidadi S, Moshiri A (2013) Current concerns regarding healing of bone defects. Hard Tissue 2: 13.

136. Metzl JA, Ahmad CS, Levine WN (2008) The ruptured Achilles tendon: operative and non-operative treatment options. Curr Rev Musculoskelet Med 1: 161-164.

137. Bring DK, Kreicbergs A, Renstrom PA, Ackermann PW (2007) Physical activity modulates nerve plasticity and stimulates repair after Achilles tendon rupture. J Orthop Res 25: 164-172.

138. Jacob KM, Paterson R (2007) Surgical repair followed by functional rehabilitation for acute and chronic achilles tendon injuries: excellent functional results, patient satisfaction and no reruptures. ANZ J Surg 77: 287-291.

139. Suchak AA, Spooner C, Reid DC, Jomha NM (2006) Postoperative rehabilitation protocols for Achilles tendon ruptures: a meta-analysis. Clin Orthop Relat Res 445: 216-221.

140. Boyer MI, Strickland JW, Engles DR, Sachar K, Leversedge FJ (2002) Flexor tendon repair and rehabilitation, state of the art in 2002. J Bone Joint Surg Am 84: 1684-1706.

141. Small JO, Brennen MD, Colville J (1989) Early active mobilisation following flexor tendon repair in zone 2. J Hand Surg Br 14: 383-391.

142. Kleinert HE, Kutz JE, Atasoy E, Stormo A (1973) Primary repair of flexor tendons. Orthop Clin North Am 4: 865-876.

143. Tang JB (2007) Indications, methods, postoperative motion and outcome evaluation of primary flexor tendon repairs in Zone 2. J Hand Surg Eur Vol 32: 118-129.

144. Chesney A, Chauhan A, Kattan A, Farrokhyar F, Thoma A (2011) Systematic review of flexor tendon rehabilitation protocols in zone II of the hand. Plast Reconstr Surg 127: 1583-1592.

Football Scores on the Big Five Personality Factors across 50 States in the U.S.

Xuan Tran*
University of West Florida, USA

Abstract

Despite the growing evidence of role personality plays on sport and exercise related behavior, little is known about the influence of personality traits on football players in the U.S. The purpose of this study was to explore the effects of the big five personality traits on football achievements. Extraversion (E), Agreeableness (A), Conscientiousness (C), Neuroticism (N), and Openness (O) traits obtained from 619,397 U.S. respondents in a previous study were used as predictors to state-level football scores in this study. Across 50 states in the U.S., football ranks were positively correlated with state scores on the Big Five personality factors of conscientiousness and agreeableness. However, when applying multiple regression analyses to the prediction model for football ranks based on five independent variables of the Big Five personality factors, only conscientiousness and neuroticism would significantly predict football ranks. Agreeableness correlates with football ranks but does not contribute to the prediction model since agreeableness is collinear with conscientiousness, extraversion, and openness. Neuroticism insignificantly correlates with football ranks but contributes to the prediction because the suppressor effect of conscientiousness by neuroticism has improved its predictor of football ranks. The findings implied that in order to increase high ranks in football practice, selection for athletics would focus on persons with high conscientiousness and neuroticism.

Keywords: Conscientiousness; Neuroticism; Extroversion; Agreeableness; Openness; Football

Introduction

Personality can be defined as the intrinsic organization of an individual's mental world that is stable over time and consistent over situations [1]. The importance of personality as a predictor for behavior performance has been recognized in psychology [2]. Researchers have recently reported the significant effects of personality on sports [3].

What personality type of person is the successful athlete playing football? Are the athletes' personality traits related to their performance on the football field? Using the Profile of Mood States [4-6] had different answers to these questions. It has been reported that no unifying theory of personality and no consensus about which personality dimensions to measure or how to measure them, comparisons of personality were difficult to interpret and, arguably, unreliable [7].

Contemporary research uses the Big Five personality factor model (Extraversion (E), Agreeableness (A), Conscientiousness (C), Neuroticism (N), and Openness (O)) as a reliable and valid measurement for psychological characteristics [8] based on the three main reasons. First, the five dimensions are rooted in biology [9]. Second, the dimensions are relatively stable throughout life [10], and third, the dimensions are found in several cultures [11].

Most research has focused on the effects of the five personality traits on human behavior. Agreeableness reflects warmth, compassion, cooperativeness, and friendliness. Agreeableness was negatively related to rates of robbery, murder, and property crime [12]. Extraversion is associated with sociability, energy, and health. Different from agreeableness, extraversion reflects sociability and outgoingness more than friendliness and warmth [13]. Conscientiousness reflects dutifulness, responsibility, and self-discipline. Low-conscientiousness individuals are more likely to commit acts of violence and deviance than are high-conscientiousness individuals [12]. Neuroticism reflects anxiety, stress, impulsivity, and emotional instability and is related to antisocial behavior, poor coping, and poor health [12]. Openness reflects curiosity, intellect, and creativity. Open individuals prefer jobs that involve a high degree of abstract and creative thought [12].

Little contemporary research has explored the effects of the five personality traits on football although football is one of the key sports in the United States. This research attempted to explore the influence of football players' personality traits on their achievements. The purpose of this study was thus to examine the effects of neuroticism, extraversion, openness, conscientiousness, and agreeableness on football ranks across 50 states to propose the most effective way to develop a successful football team based on personality traits.

Literature

Some studies have specifically examined the role of the Big Five in predicting academic performance [14]. Studies have also indicated a positive relationship between conscientiousness and job performance [15]. Piedmont et al. [16] examined the coaches' ratings on their games and found that there were significant correlations between athletic ability and personality. Kovacs [17] reported that conscientiousness and neuroticism have a direct correlation to athletic performance. Extraversion has been found to predict sport performance, particularly in team athletes [18]. Aidman and Schofield [3] reported that Agreeableness and Openness are not correlated with sport performance.

The present study has focused on the five personality traits at state level based on the assumption that psychological characteristics are geographically clustered across the country. There are at least three main reasons for geographic variations on personality across 50 states in the United States. First, the early child rearing practices form psychological characteristics and these practices are shaped by larger societal institutions in which individual lives [19]. Secondly, in the United States the groups of immigrants who chose to leave their homeland possess

***Corresponding author:** Xuan Tran, University of West Florida, USA, E-mail: xtran@uwf.edu

restricted gene pools of nonrandom samples of personality traits [20]. Finally, there appear geographic variations on personality because the specific personality of social founders may influence regional people's personality traits [21]. Rentfrow et al. [20] examined big five personality traits from over half a million U.S. residents and found that (1) North Dakota was ranked as the state with highest extroversion but Maryland as the state with lowest extroversion; (2) North Dakota was again ranked as the state with the highest agreeableness but Alaska as the state with lowest agreeableness; (3) New Mexico was ranked as the state with the highest conscientiousness but Alaska as the state with the lowest conscientiousness; (4) West Virginia was ranked as the state with the highest neuroticism but Utah as the state with the lowest neuroticism; (5) Washington, D.C. as the district with highest openness but North Dakota as the state with the lowest openness. As a result, fifty U.S. states possessed different levels of big five personality traits [20].

When 50 states are differentiated by their own personality, they will influence athletic performance since the five personality factors (neuroticism, extraversion, openness, conscientiousness, and agreeableness) reflect the core aspects of humans in the sport domain. Therefore, this study hypothesized that there would be significant relationship between football ranks and the big five personality factors across 50 states.

Methods

Ethical clearance

According to Rentfrow et al. [20], the personality data were collected as part of an ongoing study of personality involving volunteers assessed over the World Wide Web. The website is a noncommercial, advertisement-free website containing a variety of personality measures. Potential respondents could find out about the site through several channels, including search engines, or unsolicited links on other websites. The data reported in the present research were collected between December 1999 and January 2005. Respondents volunteered to participate in the study by clicking on the personality test icon; they were then presented with a series of questions about their personalities, demographic characteristics, and state of residence. After responding to each item and submitting their responses, participants were presented with a customized personality evaluation based on their responses to all the items [20].

Study design

The present study explored a model of the relationships between the state-level five personality factors and the state-level football scores. The independent variables are state ranks for each personality dimension, adapted from Rentfrow et al. [20]. The dependent variable is the state ranks for football scores, adapted from Bleacher report [22].

Sampling

Table 1 provides 51 state ranks for each personality dimension and football score, which were adapted from Rentfrow et al. [20] and the Bleacher report [22].

According to Rentfrow et al. [20], in order to avoid the possibility that respondents may complete a survey multiple times resulting in unreliable and misleading results, the researchers used several criteria to eliminate repeat responders. "First, one question included in the survey asked: "Have you ever previously filled out this particular questionnaire on this site?" If respondents reported completing the questionnaire before, their data were excluded. Second, IP addresses were used to identify repeat responders. If an IP address appeared two or more times within a 1-hr period, all responses were deleted. Third, if an IP address appeared more than once in a time span of more than 1 hour, consecutive responses from the same IP address were matched on several demographic characteristics (gender, age, ethnicity etc.) and eliminated if there was a match. Finally, only respondents who indicated that they lived in the 50 U.S. states or in Washington D.C. were included." [20].

The sample size was 619,397 respondents (55% female). The median age of respondents was 24 years (SD 59.8 years). The sample was comprised of White (80.2%), African American (4%), Asian (6.6%), Latino (4.6%), and other (4.6%). The respondents included social class (13.5%), working class (15.6%), middle class (42.8%), and upper-middle class (25.7%) and upper class (2.4%). Overall, these analyses indicate that our Internet-based sample was generally representative of the population at large [23].

Procedure-data collection and data analysis

Independent variables were extraversion, agreeableness, conscientiousness, neuroticism, and openness. The five personality traits were obtained from The Big Five Inventory [13]. The Big Five Inventory consists of 44 short statements designed to assess the prototypical traits defining each of the five factor model dimensions based on a 5-point Likert-type rating scale ranging from 1 (disagree strongly) to 5 (agree strongly). The Big Five Inventory scales have shown reliability and validity compared with other five factor model measures at the individual level [24].

Dependent variable was state-level football scores ranked in order for 50 states, which were available online from the Bleacher report [22].

Multiple regression analyses were conducted to find the causative relationship between football scores and five personality traits.

Results

The means and standard deviations of the data were summarized in table 2 as follows

Table 3 indicates that football ranks were positively associated with scores on the Big Five Inventory factors of Agreeableness (r=.40, two-tailed p=.003) and conscientiousness (r=.42, two-tailed p=.002) but were not significantly correlated to extraversion, neuroticism, and openness (rs=.21, .11, and -.02, respectively). Using the Spearman rank-order correlation coefficient yielded similar results. Football ranks were positively correlated with Agreeableness and Conscientiousness (rs=.40 and .43, two tailed ps<.001), but were not significantly correlated to Extraversion, Neuroticism, and Openness (rs=.20, .10, and -.01, respectively).

Multiple regression analyses were used to test the causative relationships between football ranks and five personality traits (Extroversion, Agreeableness, Conscientiousness, Neuroticism, and Openness) as illustrated in table 4 as follows:

The result of the regression for football ranks indicated conscientiousness and neuroticism explained 27% of the variance ($R2$=.27, F(5, 44)=3.29, p<.05). It was found that conscientiousness and neuroticism predicted football rank (βs=.37 and .28, respectively, ps<.05).

Discussions

Agreeableness correlates football rankings but does not contribute to the prediction model since Agreeableness is collinear with Conscientiousness, Extraversion, and Openness. Neuroticism does not

State	Football	Extraversion	Agreeableness	Conscientiousness	Neuroticism	Openness
Alabama	1	20	36	36	30	48
Alaska	42	49	51	51	47	49
Arizona	29	24	31	9	45	31
Arkansas	15	31	41	37	10	27
California	4	38	28	27	37	6
Colorado	32	28	29	15	50	8
Connecticut	38	33	43	46	15	12
Delaware	42	21	37	34	19	42
District of Columbia	42	3	50	40	31	1
Florida	2	10	14	8	36	13
Georgia	10	6	8	3	33	20
Hawaii	37	39	24	49	40	46
Idaho	22	46	39	26	32	30
Illinois	17	9	26	11	20	21
Indiana	8	34	19	14	13	34
Iowa	26	15	15	33	22	43
Kansas	31	13	17	5	34	38
Kentucky	27	36	21	19	7	45
Louisiana	9	30	13	30	8	29
Maine	42	11	46	50	12	35
Maryland	33	51	38	35	17	10
Massachusetts	34	42	40	43	11	4
Michigan	5	17	11	21	26	36
Minnesota	35	5	2	22	41	40
Mississippi	13	19	3	12	4	41
Missouri	25	18	16	10	25	32
Montana	42	43	42	29	39	16
Nebraska	11	4	10	7	44	44
Nevada	39	37	48	24	42	9
New Hampshire	42	50	30	44	14	14
New Jersey	36	14	34	45	5	15
New Mexico	41	22	33	1	29	23
New York	30	32	47	42	3	2
North Carolina	23	35	7	2	24	33
North Dakota	42	1	1	23	43	51
Ohio	6	25	27	38	9	24
Oklahoma	7	27	9	6	27	37
Oregon	21	44	18	31	48	3
Pennsylvania	14	12	35	28	6	25
Rhode Island	42	40	45	48	2	28
South Carolina	12	26	20	16	16	26
South Dakota	42	7	23	17	49	39
Tennessee	24	29	6	13	23	19
Texas	3	16	25	18	28	17
Utah	18	8	4	4	51	18
Vermont	42	47	12	41	18	7
Virginia	16	45	44	39	21	11
Washington	28	48	22	25	46	5
West Virginia	20	23	32	32	1	22
Wisconsin	19	2	5	20	35	47
Wyoming	40	41	49	47	38	50

Table 1: State Rankings for Each Five Factor Personality Dimension and Football Score. (Rentfrow et al. [20] and the Bleacher Report [22])

correlate football rankings but contribute to the prediction because the suppressor effect of Conscientiousness by Neuroticism has improved its predictor of football rankings [25].

Like Kovacs' [17] finding, there is an association between conscientiousness and sport ranking. Conscientiousness is significantly positively correlated with football ranking. Moreover, the present analysis indicated that conscientiousness would predict football rankings. In addition, the study found the football rankings were significantly associated with neuroticism. A state with higher neuroticism would get higher football rankings because neuroticism is a strong predictor for football rankings. In sum, the significance of these relationships may contribute to selection and management of football teams. It also helps forecasting the results of football competition based on the profile of big five personality traits. In order to increase high ranks in football practice, selection for athletics would focus on

Average of 50-state data	Mean	Std.Deviation
Football rank	24.78	13.54
Extroversion rank	26.10	14.99
Agreeableness rank	25.78	14.93
Conscientiousness rank	25.84	14.92
Neuroticism rank	26.14	14.98
Openness rank	25.68	14.83

Table 2: Descriptive Statistics of Football and the Big Five Personality Traits Enrollment in local colleges.

	(1)	(2)	(3)	(4)	(5)	(6)
1. Football rank		.22	.39**	.41**	.12	-.05
2. Extroversion rank			.43**	.44**	-.12	-.31*
3. Agreeableness rank				.65**	-.18	-.30*
4. Conscientiousness rank					-.32*	-.12
5. Neuroticism rank						.10
6. Openness rank						

(**) Correlation is significant at 0.01 levels (1-tailed)

(*) Correlation is significant at 0.05 levels (1-tailed)

Table 3: Pearson Correlations of Football Rank, Extroversion Rank, Agreeableness Rank, Conscientiousness Rank, Neuroticism Rank, and Openness Rank.

persons with high Conscientiousness and Neuroticism. Future research might also find the model of these relationships useful when expanding athletic departments.

Since low-Conscientiousness individuals are more likely to commit acts of violence and deviance than are high-Conscientiousness individuals [12], football players with low conscientiousness may be likely to commit doping or other deviant behavior. Conscientiousness reflects the degree to which football players prefer systematic and focused tasks and clearly defined rules and regulations so conscientious individuals tend to engage in health promoting behavior and live long healthy lives, which is consistent with previous research [26]. Conscientiousness was negatively related to spending time in a bar and entertaining guests at home [20] so conscientious football players were not related to social involvement. Rentfrow et al. [20] also reported that large proportions of computer scientists and mathematicians in high Conscientiousness states and more artists and entertainers are in low Conscientiousness states.

Neuroticism reflects anxiety, stress, impulsivity, and emotional instability. Table 4 indicates that Neuroticism is a significant predictor in the model although the correlation between Neuroticism and Football scores is not significant. The reason for this is Neuroticism is a suppressor. According to Cohen et al. [25], a suppressor that is uncorrelated with Y may be significant in a multiple regression model. The suppressor effect of Conscientiousness by Neuroticism has improved its predictor of football rankings. A football player with high Neuroticism may take a risk to attain the goal by doping or anti-social behavior; however, the direction of these relationships changed when controlling for urbanization and income [20]. The research showing inverse relationships between Neuroticism and longevity and Neuroticism is negatively related social involvement [12,27].

Agreeableness reflects warmth, compassion, cooperativeness, and friendliness at the individual level. Agreeableness was correlated with football scores but it did not predict football scores since football players with high agreeableness were positively associated with activities that promote tight social relations so it correlates with the football scores when the players help others in their team but in order to attain the goal, the cooperativeness should be replaced by competition.

An increase in conscientiousness is associated with an increase

*Predictor	C	E	A	O	N
r (p)	.43(.00)	.20(.15)	.40(.00)	-.01(.91)	.10(.44)
β (p)	.36(.05)	.00(.96)	.22(.20)	.05(.68)	.27(.05)

Predictors: C: Conscientiousness; E: Extraversion; A: Agreeableness; O: Openness; N: Neuroticism

Dependent Variable: Football rank

Table 4: Spearman's rho Bivariate and Multivariate Contributions–DV=Football ranks.

in football ranking. Moreover, the present analysis indicated that conscientiousness would predict football ranks. In addition, the study found the football ranks were significantly associated with neuroticism. A state with higher neuroticism would get higher football ranks and neuroticism is a strong predictor for football ranking. In sum, the significance of these relationships may contribute to selection and management of football teams. It also helps forecasting the results of football competition based on the profile of big five personality traits. In order to increase high ranks in football practice, selection for athletics would focus on persons with high conscientiousness and neuroticism. Future research might also find the model of these relationships useful when expanding athletic departments.

References

1. Piedmont RL (1998) The Revised NEO Personality Inventory: Clinical and Research Applications. Springer, New York.
2. Sternberg RJ (2000) Handbook of intelligence. New York: Cambridge University Press.
3. Aidman E, Schofield G (2004) Personality and Individual Differences in Sport. (2ndedn), Sport psychology: theory, applications and issues Wiley, Milton, Australia.
4. McNair DM, Lorr M, Droppleman LF (1981) Profile of Mood States manual. Educational and Industrial Testing Service, San Diego, CA.
5. Newby RW, Simpson S (1991) Personality profile of nonscholarship college football players. Percept Mot Skills 73: 1083-1089.
6. Leunes A, Nation JR (1982) Saturday's heroes: a psychological portrait of college Football players. Journal of Sport Behavior 5: 139-149.
7. Levine RA (2001) Culture and personality studies, 1918-1960: myth and history. J Pers 69: 803-818.
8. Costa PT, McCrae RR (1992) The Revised NEO Personality Inventory (NEO-PI-R). Odessa, FL: Psychological Assessment Resources.
9. Jang KL, McCrae RR, Angleitner A, Riemann R, Livesley WJ (1998) Heritability of facet-level traits in a cross-cultural twin sample: support for a hierarchical model of personality. J Pers Soc Psychol 74: 1556-1565.
10. McCrae RR, Costa PT Jr (2003) Personality in Adulthood: A Five-Factor Theory perspective. (2ndedn), Guilford Press, New York, USA.
11. Benet-Martinez V, John OP (2000) Toward the Development of Quasi-Indigenous Personality Constructs. American Behavioral Scientist 44: 141-157.
12. Ozer DJ, Benet-Martínez V (2006) Personality and the prediction of consequential outcomes. Annu Rev Psychol 57: 401-421.
13. John OP, Srivastava S (1999) The Big Five Trait taxonomy: History, measurement, and theoretical perspectives. In LA Pervin, OP John (Eds.), Handbook of personality: Theory and research (2nd ed., pp. 102–139). New York: Guilford.
14. Busato VV, Prins FJ, Elshout JJ, Hamaker C (2000) Intellectual ability, learning style, personality, achievement motivation and academic success of psychology students in higher education. Pers Indiv Differ 29: 1057-1068.
15. Salgado JF (1997) The Five Factor Model of personality and job performance in the European Community. J Appl Psychol 82: 30-43.
16. Piedmont RL, Hill DC, Blanco S (1999) Predicting athletic performance using the five-factor model of personality. Pers Indiv Differ 27: 769-777.
17. Kovacs M (2008) Relationship between personality and collegiate tennis rankings. Medicine and Science in Sports and Exercise 40: 209-210.

18. Taylor DM, Doria JR (1981) Self-serving and group-serving biases in attribution. J Soc Psychol 113: 201-211.

19. Peabody D (1988) National characteristics. Cambridge, United Kingdom: Cambridge University Press and Maison des Sciences de l'Homme.

20. Rentfrow P, Gosling S, Potter J (2008) A theory of the emergence, persistence, and expression of geographic variation in psychological characteristics. Perspective on Psychological Science 3: 339-369.

21. Kitayama S, Ishii K, Imada T, Takemura K, Ramaswamy J (2006) Voluntary settlement and the spirit of independence: evidence from Japan's "Northern frontier". J Pers Soc Psychol 91: 369-384.

22. Vasta D (2012) Power Ranking All 50 States by Their College Football Teams.

23. Gosling SD, Vazire S, Srivastava S, John OP (2004) Should we trust web-based studies? A comparative analysis of six preconceptions about internet questionnaires. Am Psychol 59: 93-104.

24. Benet-Martínez V, John OP (1998) Los Cinco Grandes across cultures and ethnic groups: multitrait multimethod analyses of the Big Five in Spanish and English. J Pers Soc Psychol 75: 729-750.

25. Cohen J, West SG, Aiken L, Cohen P (2003) Applied multiple regression/correlation analysis for the behavioral sciences, (3rdedn). Mahwah, NJ.: Erlbaum Associates.

26. Bogg T, Roberts BW (2004) Conscientiousness and health-related behaviors: a meta-analysis of the leading behavioral contributors to mortality. Psychol Bull 130: 887-919.

27. Roberts BW, Kuncel NR, Shiner R, Caspi A, Goldberg LR (2007) The Power of personality: The comparative validity of personality traits, socioeconomic status, and cognitive ability for predicting important life outcomes. Perspective Psych Sci 2: 313-345.

11

Posterior Talar Intraosseous Ganglion Treated with Arthroscopic Debridement, Microfracture and Injectable Bone Graft Substitute

Roland Walker*, William J Nash, Rajiv S Patel and Sam Singh

Orthopaedic Department, Guy's Hospital, Great Maze Pond, London, UK

Abstract

We report the case of a 57 year old female patient presenting with longstanding diffuse ankle pain. SPECT-CT was useful in making the diagnosis of an intraosseous ganglion of the posterior talus. The patient was treated with posterior arthroscopic debridement of the cyst via a two portal approach and grafting with an injectable synthetic bone graft substitute (PRO-DENSE®). The patient experienced rapid relief of pain and made a quick recovery. The surgical technique is discussed as well as a review of the current literature.

Keywords: Intraosseous ganglion; Talus; Arthroscopy; Bone graft

Introduction

Simple, benign cystic lesions of the talus are relatively rare and must be differentiated from degenerative cystic lesions associated with osteochondral injury or established osteoarthritis. The diagnoses include unicameral bone cyst, more commonly seen in children, and intraosseous ganglion seen more commonly in middle-aged adults and first described by Hicks in 1956 [1]. Patients may often attribute the associated ankle pain to a previous minor injury and this may erroneously lead the clinician toward treating a ligamentous injury.

The gold standard surgical management of a talarintraosseous ganglion has been open debridement, curettage and bone grafting with good result [2-4]. More recently, arthroscopic treatment of a variety of ankle conditions has gained popularity and widespread acceptance due to the reduced morbidity and more rapid recovery associated with the technique. The method of hind foot arthroscopy popularized by van Dijk gives good access to the posterior talus and offers an attractive surgical approach to cysts of the posterior talus [5]. Three authors have so far reported their experience treating posterior talarintraosseous ganglions with posterior arthroscopy [6-8]. This is the first case report combining this technique with an injectable synthetic bone graft substitute containing a combination of calcium sulphate and calcium phosphate, designed specifically for the treatment of these types of defects.

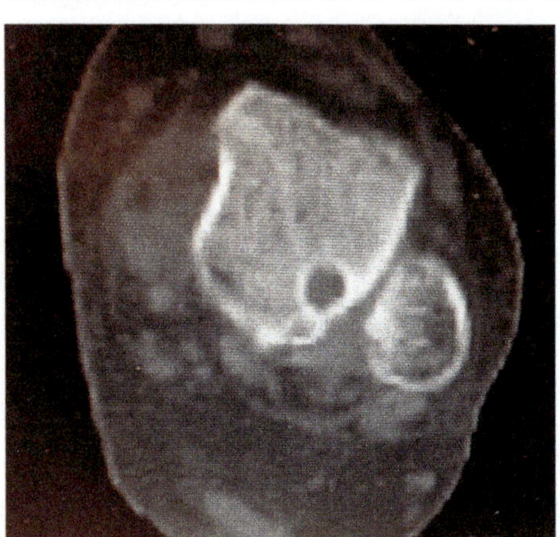

Figure 1: Axial CT showing cyst in posterior talar dome.

Case Report

A 57 year old female patient presented with longstanding ankle pain, after a mild ankle sprain some years previously. She had failed conservative treatment options with NSAIDs, physiotherapy and bracing and had been recommended a range of surgical options before presenting to the senior author for a second opinion.

Clinical examination revealed some swelling of the ankle, quite generalized tenderness both anteriorly and posteriorly. Anterior draw test was negative and there was clinical evidence of posterior impingement with pain on forced plantar flexion of the ankle. Previous CT and MRI scans revealed a large posterior talar cyst (Figure 1), likely to be an intraosseous ganglion; a small ostrigonum and thickening of the posterior tibiofibular ligament with partial tear and a small avulsion fragment. The ankle joint space was preserved, with no radiological evidence of a chondral or osteochondral lesion. Given she reported pain in 3 different areas of the ankle, to help clarify which pathology was the main pain generator, a SPECT CT scan was requested. This revealed high signal around the talarintraosseous ganglion only (Figure 2) and

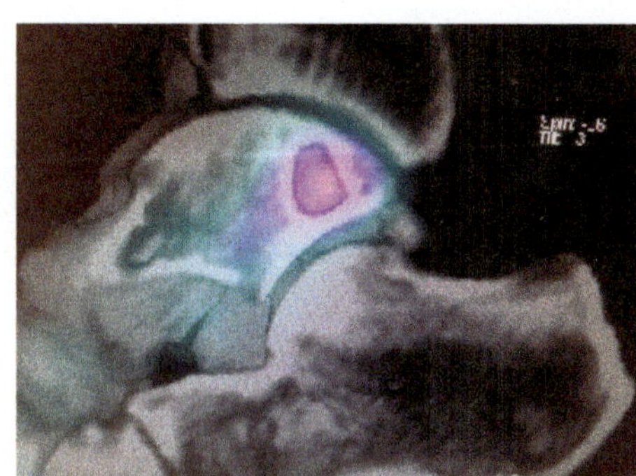

Figure 2: Sagittal SPECT CT showing metabolic activity in cyst.

***Corresponding author:** Roland Walker, FRCS (Tr&Orth), Foot & Ankle Fellow, Orthopaedic Department, Guy's Hospital, Great Maze Pond, London, SE1 9RT, UK, E-mail: rsrpatel@doctors.org.uk

confirmed the clinical suspicion that the cyst was the most likely cause of the patient's ongoing ankle pain. She was advised that arthroscopic surgery to decompress, microfracture and bone graft the cyst would be most likely to address her pain given other simpler non-surgical modalities had been exhausted.

In theatre a tourniquet was placed around the thigh. The patient was positioned in the recovery position with the affected side lowermost and the foot just off the end of the operating table. This position gives excellent access to the posterior ankle and is used by the senior author for posterior ankle arthroscopy as well as Achilles tendon surgery. The limb was exsanguinated and the tourniquet inflated. Two arthroscopy portals were made either side of the Achilles tendon, to access the ankle and subtalar joint, following the principles described van Dijk [5]. The retrocalcaneal fat pad was carefully incised to create a working space and the FHL tendon and the small ostrigonum were then identified as key landmarks. Cross sectional imaging had shown that the posterior talarintraosseous ganglion lay just deep to the small ostrigonum. The small ostrigonum was therefore resected, exposing the posterior ankle joint and the subtalar joint. The cyst revealed itself as a pinhole opening in the posterior talus (Figure 3) and the opening was dilated revealing a fibrous tissue membrane lining the cyst (Figure 4). This was easily and completely excised with arthroscopic curettes. Once the floor of the cyst had been exposed a 1.2 mm kirschner wire was used to create a series of holes into the cancellous bone beneath (Figure 5) in order to release osteoprogenitor cells into the cyst cavity. The cavity was then filled with

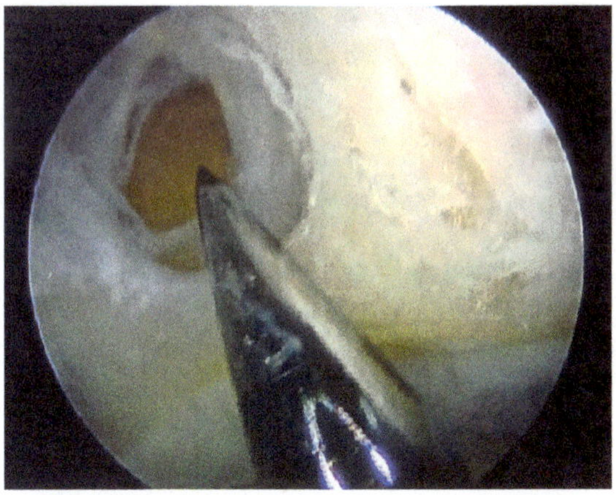

Figure 3: Cyst neck exposed after resection of ostrigonum.

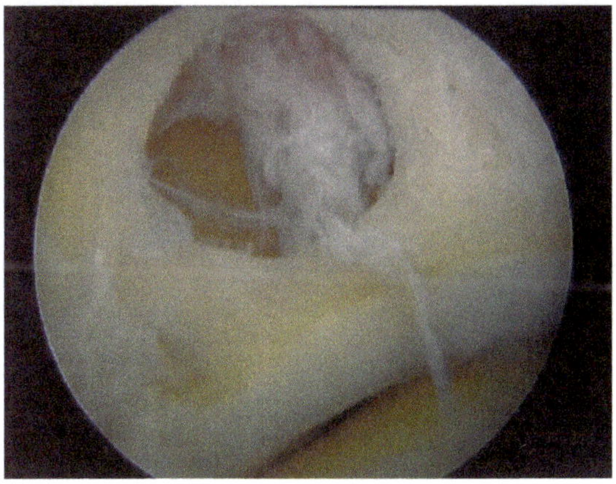

Figure 4: Fibrous tissue within the cyst.

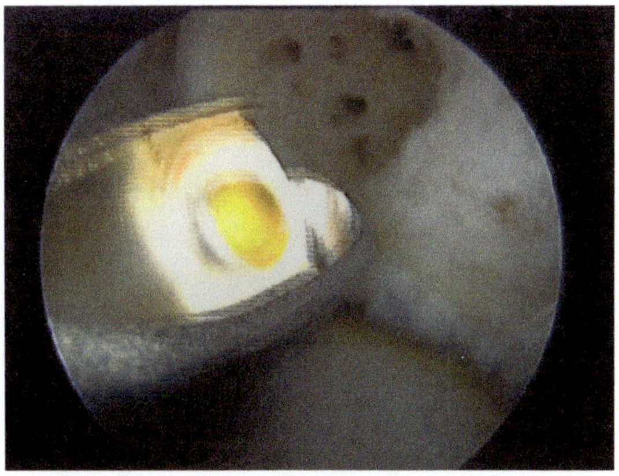

Figure 5: Base of the cysts following microfracture.

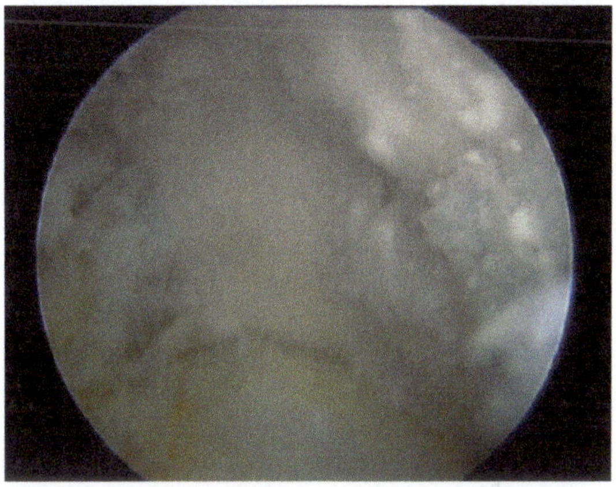

Figure 6: Cyst following grafting with an injectable bone graft substitute.

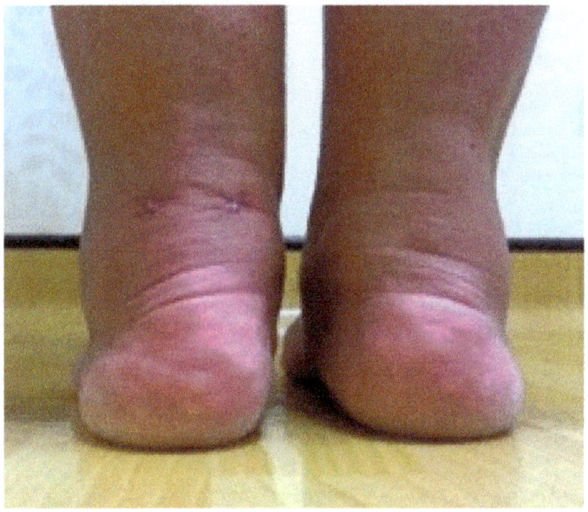

Figure 7: Hindfoot at 6 weeks post op (left side operated).

an injectable bone graft substitute (PRO-DENSE®, Wright Medical) (Figure 6). The portals were closed and the patient was immobilized in a back slab, non-weight bearing for 2 weeks. She then went into a boot, fully weight bearing for a further 2 weeks. By 6 weeks the patient was already making excellent progress, with good portal healing and only a small amount of residual swelling (Figure 7). She was able to stand on tiptoes without pain (Figure 8) and was able to walk 45 minutes without needing to rest. Even at this early stage she reported an improvement in her pain. Her 8 week post-operative X-ray showed some in-fill on the cyst (Figure 9) and the patient is doing very well and is able to walk a few hours a day without experiencing pain. She occasionally gets swelling but only for short periods of time.

Discussion

In 1972 Ogden and Griswold reported the first surgically managed case involving a unicameral bone cyst located in the anterior talar dome of a 15 year old [2]. This was successfully treated with curettage and autologous iliac crest bone grafting via an open antero-medial approach to the ankle. A year later Paaby reported two cases of talar intraosseous ganglions in adult patients, both successfully treated by open curettage and bone grafting with cancellous chips [3]. The first two cases of entirely arthroscopic treatment of a talar ganglion cyst were reported by van Dijk's group in 2003 and both cases utilized posterior ankle arthroscopy to debride and graft the ganglion cysts [8]. Subsequently two other authors have reported the technique. In 2011 Ogut et al. reported a small case series of 6 ankles in 5 patients, where posterior ankle arthroscopy was used to access and treat the posteriorly located talar cyst in a minimally invasive manner [7]. In these cases autologous bone was used to graft the defects in five ankles and hydroxyapatite in one. Good results were reported. In 2014 Dawe reported a single case study of posterior talar cyst treated with posterior ankle arthroscopy and injection of demineralized bone allograft in a gel, with good results at 3 years [6]. Due to the rarity of talarintraosseous ganglion cysts there are no studies in the literature comparing open versus arthroscopic methods of treatment or comparing the treatment methods of dealing with the cyst itself.

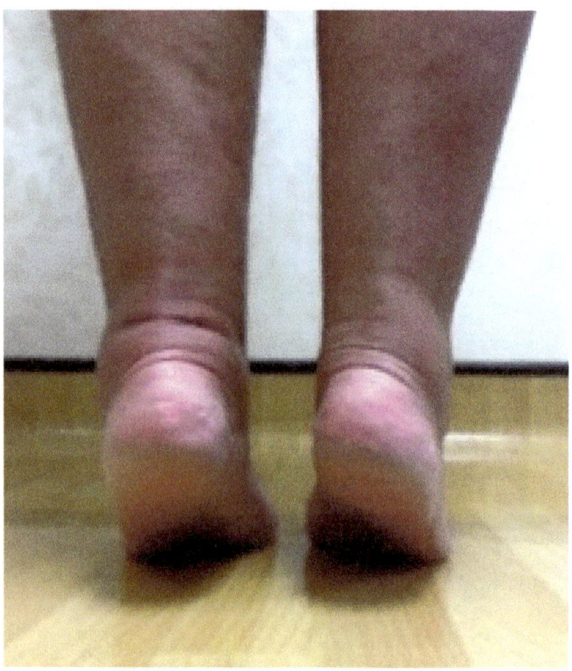

Figure 8: Full tiptoe possible at 6 weeks.

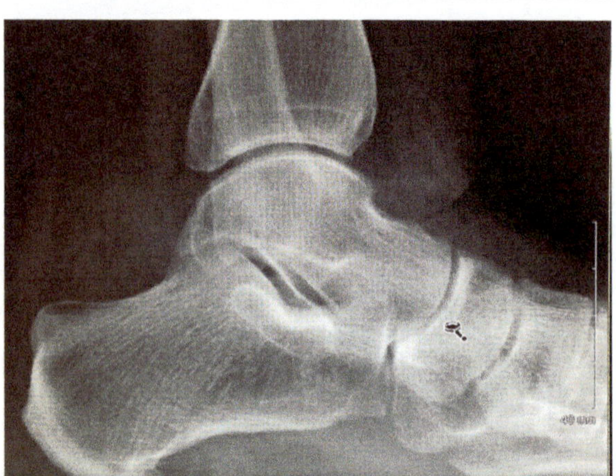

Figure 9: 8 week post-op X-ray showing some in-fill on the cyst.

Another important feature in this case report was the utility of SPECT CT in the pre-operative assessment. There is increasing evidence supporting the use of SPECT CT for the diagnosis of non-specific or poorly localized musculoskeletal pain. This is particularly useful in the hands and feet where the number of small bones and proximity of joints can make the diagnosis of the true pain generator challenging [9]. In our practice we have found SPECT CT very useful and in this case study we believe that the SPECT scan correctly identified the talar cyst as the patient's main problem and allowed us to target treatment appropriately.

Compared with previously published cases, the technique presented here avoids the need for autologous bone graft to be taken, therefore reducing donor site morbidity by using an injectable bone graft substitute. This consisted of 75% calcium sulphate and 25% calcium phosphate. This bone graft substitute has been developed to treat benign bone cysts in areas where structural integrity is maintained by the surrounding bone. It acts as an osteo-conductive filler, curing in around 2 hours, and gradually resorbing over time. The calcium sulphate component resorbs more quickly, in theory leaving voids for vascular ingrowth. The other main advantage was the delivery method, as the bone graft substitute comes as a putty in a pre-filled syringe with an introducer, and will set hard even in a wet environment. These features make it very user friendly in the arthroscopic setting. Compared with demineralized bone matrix gel, PRO-DENSE® cures hard in situ, which may facilitate earlier mobilization of the patient. There is little clinical data in publication regarding PRO-DENSE® however one initial study of 24 patients being treated with the bone graft substitute after resection of benign bone tumours showed rapid biological integration with few complications [10].

In summary we feel that our technique builds on the principles pioneered by other authors. An arthroscopic approach to the cyst and the use of an injectable bone graft substitute which can cure in a wet environment is advantageous to both the surgeon and patient. Long-term follow up is now needed to establish whether the clinical improvement is sustained and that there is resorption of the bone graft substitute and subsequent bony infill of the cyst.

Conclusion

We present a case study which demonstrates the successful treatment of a posterior talarintraosseous ganglion using a posterior ankle arthroscopic approach and injectable bone graft substitute.

References

1. Hicks J (1956) Synovial Cysts in Bone. Aust N Z J Surg 26: 138-143.
2. Ogden J, Griswold D (1972) Solitary Cyst of the Talus a case report. J Bone Joint Surg Am 54: 1309-1310.

3. Paaby H (1973) Solitary Cysts of the Talus. Report of Two Operated Cases. Acta Orthop Scand 44: 560-563.

4. Barth E, Hagen R (1982) Juxta-Articular Bone Cyst. ActaOrthopScand 53: 215-217.

5. Van Dijk CN (2004) Hindfoot Endoscopy for Posterior Ankle Pain. Springer-Verlag New York, Inc. Foot and Ankle Arthroscopy : 219-234.

6. Dawe EJ, Jukes C, Gougoulias N, Wee A (2014) Successful Arthroscopic Decompression and Synthetic Grafting of a Posterior Talar Cyst: A Case Report. J Foot Ankle Surg 20:35-36.

7. Ogut T, Seker A, Ustunkan F (2011) Endoscopic Treatment of Posteriorly Localized Talar Cysts. Knee Surg Sports TraumatolArthrosc 19: 1394-1398.

8. Scholten P, Altena M, Krips R, Niek van Dijk C (2003) Treatment of a Large IntraosseousTalar Ganglion by Means of Hindfoot Endoscopy. Arthroscopy 19: 96-100.

9. Huellner M, Strobel K (2014) Clinical Applications of SPECT/CT in Imaging the Extremities. Eur. J.Nucl. Med. Mol. Imaging 41: 50-58.

10. Evaniew N, Tan V, Parasu N, Jurriaans E, Finlay K et al. (2013) Use of a Calcium Sulfate-Calcium Phosphate Synthetic Bone Graft Composite in the Surgical Management of Primary Bone Tumors. Orthopedics 36: 216-222.

12

Effectiveness of Whey Protein Supplement in Resistance Trained Individuals

Fernando Naclerio[1,3]* Ahmad Alkhatib[1] and Alfonso Jimenez[2]

[1]*Centre of Sport Science and Human Performance, School of Science, University of Greenwich, UK*
[2]*School of Sports Science, European University of Madrid, Spain*
[3]*Institute of Sport, Exercise and Active Living (ISEAL), Victoria University, Melbourne, Australia*

Abstract

Athletes and recreationally resistance-trained individuals often use protein supplements in an attempt to maximize their training gains and performance. Because of the high bioavailability and solubility and its higher proportion of essential amino acids including Leucine, whey protein extract has been proposed as the best optimal form of protein for strength and power athletes. The objective of this review is to examine the current evidence for the efficacy of whey protein containing supplements to optimize strength training adaptation and outcomes for regular resistance training practitioners.

A limited numbers of studies have reported positive effects of whey protein containing supplements (including those with carbohydrate and creatine) for optimizing the anabolic responses and adaptations process in resistance-trained individuals.

In order to promote a more anabolic environment and maximize muscle protein synthesis along the day, an eating pattern behavior involving frequents meals (every 3 to 5 h) containing 17 to 20 g of high quality protein (200 to 250 mg/kg) providing 8 to 10 g of EAA (90 to 110 mg/kg) and about 2 g of Leucine (20 to 25 mg/kg) have been recommended. Special attention should be given to the periworkout hours where the ingestion of whey proteins combined with carbohydrates, creatine monohydrate (0.1 g/kg/d) and other proteins sources such as casein before, during and after workout have been shown to improve training adaptations and enhance the recovery process. However, when considering that the training conditions (workout volume, organization, number of exercises) used in the available studies are substantially different than what athletes actually perform. Optimal whey protein supplementation protocols need to specifically be based on the regular resistance training workout organization and would probably need to consider other doses and timing strategies than what is currently recommended.

Keywords: Multinutrient; Supplementation; Strength and power athletes; Amino acid; Leucine; casein; Sport-nutrition

Abbreviations: LBM: Lean Body Mass; AA: Amino Acid; PDCAAS: Protein Digestibility Corrected Amino Acid Score; DIAAS: Digestible Indispensable Amino Acid Score; EAA: Essential Amino Acid; BCAA: Branched Chain Amino Acid

Introduction

The protein requirements for athletic populations have been the subject of extensive scientific debate. During the last decade the notion that athletes as well generally active population require greater protein intake than the currently RDA recommendation of 0.8 g/kg of body weight per day in healthy adults has become well accepted [1,2]. In addition, high protein diets have also become quite popular in general population as part of many weight reduction programs [3,4]. Differences in protein requirements for different types of athletes (i.e., endurance, strength/power) and non-athletes are well documented [5-8]. Many studies have investigated the effects of protein obtained from different sources such as milk eggs soy rice or bovine colostrum as well as the technique used to manufacture the protein supplements or the methodology recommended for their ingestion [9-15]. In fact, these factors can be very relevant when the protein supplements are ingested with the scope to optimize training adaptations [16].

Although some studies have shown greater strength, muscular hypertrophy and/or Lean Body Mass (LBM) gains when resistance training is combined with whey protein alone or in conjunction with carbohydrates other protein sources enriched with amino acids or creatine; there are still some inconsistencies regarding the most appropriate effective doses and ingestion-timing strategy for optimizing resistance training induced adaptations and outcomes (strength gain or muscle mass accretion) [17-21].

As the focus of this review is on the effects of whey protein supplementation on both resistance training performances and their outcomes in trained individuals, we have focused on reviewing the evidence that have used whey protein preparation alone or combined with other protein sources or amino acid derivatives for optimizing resistance training responses for regular athletes and recreationally resistance training individuals. Thus, after describing the main characteristics of whey protein supplements, manufacture process, quality and Amino Acid (AA) profile; we will analyze the documented effects of whey protein containing supplements for resistance-trained individuals. In addition some practical recommendations about the most appropriate serving sizes and feeding distribution strategies will be provided based on current level of evidences.

Protein Supplements

Most of protein extract are obtained from milk, eggs, bovine colostrums, soy and to less extend from bean, wheat or rice. The quality of these extracts may vary depending on the type and quality

***Corresponding author:** Fernando Naclerio, Centre of Sport Science and Human Performance, School of Science, University of Greenwich, Medway Campus, Central Avenue, Chatham Maritime, Kent ME4 4TB, UK
E-mail: f.j.naclerio@gre.ac.uk

of the manufacturing process. A range of processed milk proteins (concentrates, isolates, hydrolyzate or peptides) has been used for different purposes including change in metabolic health in young or elderly people or training optimization outcomes in untrained recreationally active or well trained athletes [19,22-26].

Milk composition: Protein sub-fractions manufacturing and main differences

Whole milk is approximately 87% water, with the remaining 13% as solids. The 13% solids are composed of 30% fat, 37% lactose, 27% protein, and 6% minerals. Of the 27% of milk that is protein, 20% is whey protein and 80% is casein protein [27]. During the process of making cheese, whey protein is separated out into a transparent liquid fraction that has shown to be a good source of high quality protein currently used to produce protein powders and many other products.

Milk protein concentrate, produced by ultrafiltration of skimmed milk, contains both casein and whey proteins in similar proportions to whole milk, but the total amount of protein, lactose and mineral content may vary between different formulations [14].

The casein fraction comprises α-casein, β-casein, and κ-casein whilst whey contain multiple globular proteins including β-lactoglobulin (50 to 55%), α-lactalbumin (20 to 25%) bovine serum albumin (5 to 10%) lactoferrin (1 to 2%) immunoglobulins (10 to 15%) lactoperoxidase enzymes (~0.5%) and glycomacropeptides (10 to 15%), enzymes and growth factors. All of these components have been associated with the potential to improve general health outcomes and disease prevention reduce immunosuppression attenuate muscular inflammatory related damage optimize recovery process and resistance training outcomes in athletes and enhance metabolic health in general population [19-22,28-30].

Whey fraction of the milk is particularly rich in essential amino acid, vitamins and mineral [14]. Protein concentrates obtained from whey are produced by coagulation of milk with the enzyme rennet or acid, resulting in separation of curds and whey, further ultrafiltration and drying produces whey protein concentrates containing ≈25-80% protein [31]. Additional processing can produce whey protein isolates containing >90% protein with very low amounts of lactose and lipids [28]. Selective elution, also known as ion exchange chromatography, is the process most often used to produce whey protein isolates [14]. Additional hydrolysis with enzymes or acids provides a way to breakdown the structure of protein containing in whey [22]. As the acids hydrolysis process would also lower the quality and biological value of protein, the addition of proteolytic enzymes, followed by purification procedures is greatly preferred [32]. The main advantage of high quality whey protein ion exchanges hydrolyzates preparations would be the rapid uptake and availability of AA and a possible strong insulinotropic effect that would elicited a fast and powerful stimulus on muscle protein synthesis during the 3 h postprandial period [33,34]. This advantageous postprandial effect of whey protein contributes to numerous anabolic responses following resistance training and its supplementation has been recently shown to have superior cardio-protective effects on postprandial lipemia compared with other common dietary protein supplementations such as cod or gluten [25,35].

With high quality of manufacturing the native structures of whey protein can be retained. However, some minor peptides such as lactoferrin may have a decreased concentration, while the β-lactoglobulin protein fraction tends to increase in whey protein isolates [27]. Thus, protein isolates tend to be low in glycomacropeptides, lactoferrin, lactoperoxidase and some bioactive peptides. However, a high quality process of microfiltration/ultrafiltration would produce whey protein isolates with higher amounts of glycomacropeptides, lactoferrin, lactoperoxidase and the bioactive peptides, and lower in bovine serum albumin. Cross-flow microfiltration gives a whey protein isolate which is greater than 90% in protein that is under-natured and that retains all important sub-fractions in natural ratios, with no fat or lactose [14].

There is indication that lactoferrin and some of the immunoglobulins in whey proteins may be more resistant to proteolytic degradation than are other types of proteins. Some proteins e.g. bovine serum albumin or beta-lactoglobulin may yield glutamylcysteine during their digestion, which may be absorbed and serve as a precursor to glutathione (potent antioxidant precursor) in some tissues [36].

In summary, when whey proteins preparation are processed with high quality process using low temperatures and not exposed to fluctuating pH changes the undesirable denaturing of native structures would be avoided.

Casein is the protein source of cheese and forms curds during processing because it exists as a micelle in milk [27]. As nutritional supplements casein is made of to rennet casein or caseinates; which is an acid form usually combined with sodium, calcium, or potassium. The low pH conditions in the stomach cause casein to clot, forms clumps or curds and delay gastric emptying [37]. Different from whey protein that remain soluble in the stomach, and thus are emptied rapidly, casein is converted into a solid clot, and emptied more slowly from the stomach [38]. These differences in digestive properties are likely to contribute to the different patterns of AA concentrations that have been observed after ingestion of whey or casein protein [24,38]. Therefore, casein has been termed as "slow", and whey has been termed as "fast" protein [39,40].

In general, the slowly absorbed casein protein would promote a more sustained and prolonged postprandial protein deposition by an inhibition of protein breakdown without excessive increase in amino acid concentration. By contrast, a fast whey protein stimulates protein synthesis but also oxidation. This impact of amino acid absorption speed on protein metabolism is true when proteins are given alone, this might be blunted in more complex meals that could affect gastric emptying (lipids) and or insulin response (carbohydrates) [41]. Additionally the more prolonged anabolic effects of casein seems to be effective in resting condition while after training the ingestion of one single dose of whey protein has been proposed as to be more effective to stimulate anabolic responses in resistance trained individuals [5,25].

Amino acid profile of whey and casein protein supplements

Based on human AA requirements, digestibility and their bioavailability, similar to eggs protein, both whey and casein protein have been classified as high quality proteins [31]. Considering both the protein digestibility corrected AA score (PDCAAS) and the recently developed digestible indispensable AA score (DIAAS), casein and whey protein fractions contain higher amount and proportion of essential amino acids (EAA) compared to other vegetable protein sources such as soy or rice [42]. Nevertheless, in addition to their different digestive patters, some special physiological effects have also been attributed to their particular AA composition [43]. Figure 1 compares the AA compositions of the whey and casein protein fractions [24].

Data from Figure 1 indicates that when the same amount of casein or whey protein are consumed, whey provide more than 3% of EAA and higher amount of Cysteine, and Leucine. Cysteine is thought to play a key role in the regulation of whole body protein metabolism,

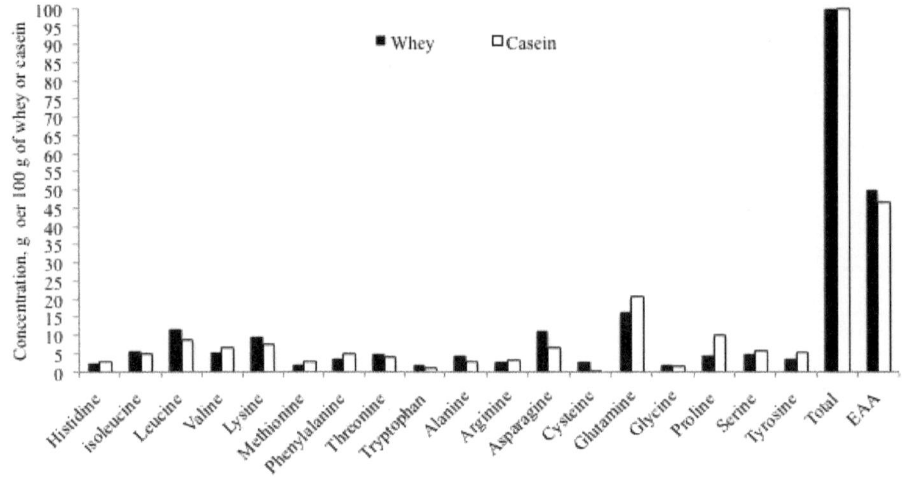

Figure 1: Comparison between whey and casein amino acid profile.

acting as a potent anticatabolic and antioxidant agent [45]. Cysteine supplementation has been shown to promotes glutathione synthesis, and shifts whole body nitrogen disposal in favor of preserving the muscle amino acid pool [45].

Leucine, one of the Branched Chain Amino acid (BCAA) is a key essential AA to trigger a potent increase in protein synthesis when a minimum amount of 1 g or 2 g per meal is consumed by young or elderly people respectively [46].

On the other side, whey protein contains lower quantities of Methionine, Glutamine, Arginine and Tyrosine. Additionally both whey and casein contain lower or trace amount of Taurine, which is a conditionally essential amino acid, involved in a number of physiological processes including cell membrane stabilization, neural excitability or sensibility for nutrient intake into the cell. Even when is the most abundant free amino acid in excitable tissue such as muscle heart and brain it is not used to build protein but has important functions as insulin mimetic, cellular hydration and protein synthesis stimulation [47].

As the above mentioned amino acids have important neuronal and metabolic functions, in order to maximize the nutritional proprieties of the whey protein extract, a high quality based whey protein product could be fortified with the addition of peptides of L-Glutamine, L-Arginine, L-Taurine, L-Methionine and L-Tyrosine [14,31]. For example, glutamine accounts for 30-35% of the amino acid nitrogen in the plasma being the most abundant amino acid in blood. L-glutamine fulfills a number of biochemical needs. It operates as a nitrogen shuttle, taking up excess ammonia and forming urea. It can act as a powerful anticatabolic agent contributing for the production of other AAs, glucose, nucleotides, protein, and glutathione [42]. Arginine is a semi-essential AA, involved in numerous areas of human biochemistry, including ammonia detoxification, hormone secretion, and immune modulation. L-arginine is the main physiological precursor of nitric oxide that plays an important regulatory role by increasing blood flow to the muscles and modulating muscle contraction, glucose and AAs uptake by the muscle [30]. Methionine is an essential AA associated with the methyl donor reactions for the synthesis of epinephrine, creatine, melatonin, glutathione, the polyamines spermine and spermidine, as well as the AAs L-cysteine and taurine, all of which play vital roles in human health [48]. Tyrosine in addition to support phenylalanine levels, is essential for the production of catecholamine neurotransmitters, including dopamine, norepinephrine, and epinephrine. Tyrosine is the precursor for the hormones thyroxine and triiodothyronine by the thyroid gland and grow hormone by the pituitary [49]. There is some evidence that supplementation with L-tyrosine can lead to an increase in dopamine that in turn may lead to an improvement in mood state [50].

Although, each protein source has unique attributes that may convey specific nutritional advantages compared to the others (general health benefits, body weight management, gaining lean body mass, enhancing muscle recovery after exercise or stimulating muscular protein synthesis) the degree by which each source of protein can stimulate these process are related to different factors involving digestion rates, divergent AA profiles, pattern of ingestion and the metabolic state (rest or exercise) related to the timing of ingestion [39,40].

Documented Effects of Whey Protein Supplement to Optimize Resistance-Training Responses

Whey protein extract, because of its increased bioavailability and solubility, and its higher percentage content of EAA including BCAAs, specifically Leucine, has been proposed as the best optimal form of protein for strength and power athletes [17,45,51]. Although several studies have analysed the effect of whey protein supplementation on resistance training performance and outcomes only some of them have focused on resistance trained individuals [12,17,23,24,26,38,52,53].

Cribb et al., [45] reported higher significant improvements in LBM, strength and loss of body fat in a group of recreational bodybuilders who supplemented their diet with the addition of 1.5 g /kg/d of hydrolyzed whey protein isolate compared to other group who ingested the same amount of casein during a supervised 10-week resistance training program. The 1.5 g/kg/d supplement dose was divided into smaller equal servings and consumed throughout the day (e.g. breakfast, lunch, immediately after training, and dinner).

Kraemer et al., [53], analysed the effects of 14 days supplementation period in 10 resistance trained males who were exposed to three different supplementation protocols: 20 g of whey protein isolate, 20 g of soy protein isolate or 20 g of carbohydrates. Each participant completed all three conditions separated by a two weeks wash out period. Lower cortisol and higher total testosterone levels were measured from 5 to 30 min after performing a squat protocol involving 6 sets of 10 repetitions at 80% 1RM followed by the whey protein supplementation period compared to when participants were exposed to soy or placebo. In addition, whey supplementation might also attenuate the normal increase of cortisol observed after carbohydrate condition.

Tang et al. [17] reported positive effects of 10 g of whey protein combined with 21 g of fructose, to induce a 2-fold rise in muscle protein synthesis in young well resistance trained men, over 4 h, after performing 4 sets of 8–10 repetitions at 80% 1RM for the leg press and leg extension exercises.

As whey protein contains about 50% of EAA, 10 g of whey high quality extract would provide circa 5 g of EAA [24]. If we consider that 20 g of whole egg protein, containing 8.6 g of EAA including 2 g or Leucine, have been necessary to maximally stimulate muscle and albumin protein synthesis after a lower-body resistance exercise in young men it may be possible that even when 10 g of whey protein were sufficient to elicit significant increases of muscle protein synthesis, a higher dose (≈17 g) would be necessary to achieve the optimal maximal response beyond which a marked stimulation of whole-body AA oxidation with no further increase in muscle protein synthesis would occur in young resistance trained males [10].

High-quality proteins extract, such as whey, stimulate muscle protein synthesis in proportion to the amount of EAA and specifically Leucine administered per serving [38]. Norton and Wilson suggest that optimal protein intake per meal should be based on the amount of leucine provided by the source of protein consumed [54]. Thus, the presence of the relative amount of the EAA including Leucine is of cornerstone importance for determining the amount of protein to be ingested in every meal. In fact when the amount of EAA and Leucine are equated the effects on muscle protein synthesis and training outcomes seems to be similar regardless of which protein source is consumed [12,54]. Joy et al. [12], observed no differences of ingesting either 48 g of isolate protein extracted from rice or whey during 8 weeks of daily ondulated periodized resistance training program on short term recovery (Ratings of perceived recovery, soreness, and readiness) or training-induced adaptations (increase lean body mass, muscle mass, strength and power and decrease fat mass) in 24 resistance trained young males. Even when the absence of control group did not allow the authors to conclude how beneficial whey or rise proteins supplementation would be compared to resistance training alone, based on previous investigations it could be possible to say that regardless of the source, between 17 to 20 g of high quality protein (200 to 250 mg/kg) providing 8 to 10 g of EAA (90 to 110 mg/kg) and about 2 g of Leucine (20 to 25 mg/kg) would be necessary to elicit an optimal muscle protein synthesis response in young strength trained individuals after performing a typical resistance training workout [10,17]. As a consequence, when ingested others plant-based protein extracts such as soy or rice containing less proportion of EAA and leucine, in order to obtain similar results, higher doses should be administered. However, larger protein ingestion entail also higher caloric intake greater digestion time (slower release of AA to the periphery), and increased AA oxidation and ureagenesis because more proportion of AA would be converted to urea rather than used for protein synthesis [5].

Summarizing the previous information, even when the need of EAA and Leucine could be satisfied from different protein sources, whey protein extract seems to be more efficient, on a gram per gram basis.

Whey protein combined with carbohydrates, other proteins sources, amino acid and/or creatine

Added carbohydrates to whey protein extract have been shown to enhance cellular hydration, glycogen resynthesis and reduce muscle protein breakdown which then magnifies the increase in net protein balance and/or lessen the immunosuppressive effects of exercise compared to the ingestion of whey protein or AA alone [8,55,56]. These positive effects are in part related to a more powerful insulin secretion [54]. With regard to resistance training, the ingestion of 40 g of whey protein with 120 of sucrose, honey powder or maltodextrine (1:3 protein to carbohydrate ratio) following a typical resistance training workout involving 9 exercises of 3 sets per 10 rep at 70% 1RM, did significantly influence glucose and insulin responses without significantly altering markers of anabolism, catabolism or immunity during the first two hours of recovery [18].

Multinutrients supplements containing whey protein, carbohydrates, amino acids, and other natural compounds such a creatine may optimize recovery time and training induced adaptation [19-21,57-59].

Kerksick et al. [20] reported significant greater increases in fat free mass in 36 resistance-trained men after combining a 10 weeks strength training program with the ingestion of 40 g whey plus 8 g casein and 2 g of carbohydrates compared to both a carbohydrate-placebo and a similar multinutrient containing only 40 g of whey enriched with 3 g of BCAAs, 5 of glutamine and 2 g of carbohydrates. Supplements where ingested within 2 hours after workout during training days or at the morning on non-training days. Authors concluded that co-ingestion of blend high quality whey and casein proteins mix may be an effective means to promote higher improvements on body composition in resistance-trained individuals compared to the ingestion of only one protein source.

As stated previously whey and casein possess different patterns of amino acid release, which has been shown to greatly affect the extracellular amino acid concentrations and the resulting levels of protein synthesis and breakdown [60]. Differences in digestion rates would cause a more sustained increase in blood amino acid levels, resulting in greater muscle amino acid uptake [39]. Casein tends to inhibit protein catabolism when consumed at rest and has a slight, but relatively long increase in protein synthesis. The pattern of amino acid delivery with casein appears to lead to better leucine balance (net protein state) than whey at rest [5]. Conversely, after a typical resistance training workout whey protein have shown to stimulates a greater acute (0-3 h post-exercise) rise in muscle protein synthesis compared with the same amount of casein and is still highly effective for stimulating muscle protein synthesis over 3-5 h post-exercise [60-62]. Thus, possibly when both types of proteins sources are combined, in addition to a more favorable AA muscle blood-flow after workout, a higher aminoacidemia would be sustained along the day. As the stimulation of protein synthesis may be largely depend on the availability of the extracellular concentration of AA, for resistance trained practitioners, the co-ingestion of fast (whey) and slow (casein) high quality protein extract would elicit a more powerful anabolic and effective stimulus compared to only one source.

Cribb et al. [21] examined the effects of 11 weeks of resistance training program combined with whey protein and/or creatine monohydrate (both separately and in combination) on body composition, muscle strength, and muscular hypertrophy in a group of recreational male bodybuilders. Participants were dived in 4 groups: whey protein; whey protein plus creatine monohydrate; carbohydrates and carbohydrates plus creatine monohydrate. Supplementation with whey protein, whey protein plus creatine monohydrates and carbohydrates plus creatine monohydrate resulted in greater hypertrophy responses and strength gains compared to the ingestion of only carbohydrates. Additionally, the consumption of a creatine monohydrate in conjunction with whey proteins or carbohydrates provides similar benefits that in addition were greater than those obtained from carbohydrates or whey protein alone. In the line with the previous investigation, Cooper et al. [59] reported greater possibilities for improving 1 RM bench press (78%) and upper and lower body muscular endurance (49%) when a group of resistance trained males who performed a 12 weeks resistance-training program ingested 2 serving of 60 g per day of a multinutrient containing 21 g of carbohydrate, 30 g of whey protein, 4.7 g of fat, 5.1 g of creatine, 5.1 g of glutamine and 1.5 g HMB instead of a carbohydrate-placebo.

Summarizing the previous information, in addition to the synergic effects of adding carbohydrates, in order to optimize the positive effects of whey protein for improving resistance training adaptation, combining other protein sources such as casein and specifically the addition of creatine monohydrate would be appropriate. On the other hand, the additional benefits on resistance training outcomes resulted from the addition of other AA or proteins derivatives such as glutamine, BCAAs or HMB remain to be elucidated.

Whey protein supplementation protocol: the nutrient-timing strategy

Unfortunately there is no conclusive evidence about what time point and dose are optimal for the ingestion of protein or amino acid-carbohydrate supplement for optimizing muscular adaptations to exercise. Many studies have provided positive results for ingesting high quality protein before, during, immediately after or several hours (1 to 3-5 h) post exercise for promoting increases in protein synthesis [58]. With regard to the most convenient nutrition-time-protocol for improving resistance training outcomes, Cribb and Hayes reported significantly greater increases in lean body mass, strength and hypertrophy after 10 weeks of resistance training in a group of trained males who ingested a multinutrient contained glucose, whey isolate, creatine monohydrate and fat just before and after workout compared to another group which consumed the same dose before breakfast and just prior retiring to bed [26].

The optimal feeding strategy to maximally enhance recovery and anabolic response to resistance exercises should also consider the serving size and feeding distribution before, during and after workout. West et al., [25] observed greater muscular protein synthesis for 5 h of recovery in 8 recreationally trained males when consuming a 25 g single-bolus-dose of whey protein after performing 8 sets of 8-10 repetitions of a bilateral leg extension compared to the same amount of proteins ingested as repeated, small pulsed drinks (10 doses of 2.5 g of whey protein every 20 min). In another similar study, Burke et al. [63] observed different patterns of aminoacidemia in 12 resistance trained males who ingested 25 g of whey protein enriched with 5 g of Leucine or placebo before performing 1 set x 8-10 repetition at 80% 1RM in a single leg extension exercise. Supplements were administered in a single-bolus-dose (45 min before) or as a series of 15 small-pulsed drinks, (of approximately 33 mL each) starting 45 min before and ended 2 h after completed the training. Although similar increases in muscle protein synthesis (near 250% respect to placebo) were observed over 5 h after exercise, in the early phase of recovery the pulsed strategy produced higher AA and insulin concentration.

If we assume that between 17 to 20 g of high quality protein providing 8 to 10 g of EAA are necessary to maximally stimulates muscle protein synthesis after exercises, considering that a typical resistance training workout enhance muscle protein synthesis for at least 24 h; in order to maximize the anabolic effects of feeding it should be necessary to maintain a frequent protein ingestion, not only during the periworkout period but also along the day [64,65]. Because muscle protein synthesis becomes refractory to persistent aminoacidemia in order to maintain an optimal protein synthesis stimulation, between 5 to 6 meals providing 17 to 20 g of high quality protein should be recommended [54]. In line with this rationale, Areta et al., [66] examined the effects of three different protein feeding distributions over a 12 h recovery period in 24 resistance trained male who performed 4 sets of 10 repetitions at 80% 1RM with 3 min rest between sets followed by the ingestion of 80 g of whey protein isolate. Participants were divided in three groups: Pulse (ingested 8 servings of 10 g every 1.5 h); Intermediate (ingested 4 servings of 20 g every 4 h) and bolus (ingested 2 servings of 40 g every 6 h). Results showed higher myofibrillar protein synthesis stimulation for the intermediate protocol (4 intakes of 20 g) compared to both pulse (8 servings of 10 g) and bolus (2 servings of 40 g). Possibly 10 g of whey protein is not enough and resulted in some suboptimal stimulation of the protein synthesis. In contrast, larger but less frequent servings of 40 g, even if should be appropriate to maximally stimulate muscle protein synthesis, represent a suboptimal ingestion pattern due to irreversible amino acid oxidation of the excess ingested protein and possible the lack of anabolic stimulus between intakes (>5 h).

In summary as the cell membrane is highly sensitive to the internal and external (blood) rise of AA concentration, frequent meals (every 3 to 5 h) containing 17 to 20 g or high quality protein would potentiate and maintain a long lasting and optimal muscular protein synthesis stimulus. Additionally, with the aim to maximize the anabolic response of resistance training workout a higher protein intake (bolus) should be provided immediately after training. Figure 2 depicts the theoretical optimal protein-feeding pattern protocol starting 3 h before (small intakes ≈10 g) and ending 6 h after training (higher intakes ≈ 20 g).

It is important to note that even when high quality whey protein extract would be an appropriate option for ingesting during training and just after workout others protein sources including those coming from regular food such as eggs, meet, cheese etc can be used along the different daily meals [67].

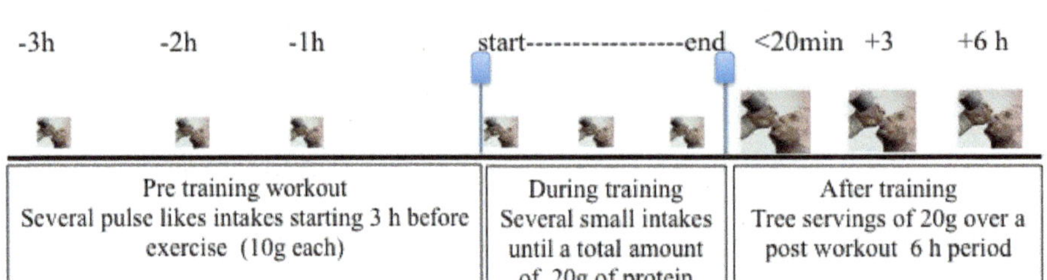

Figure 2: Proposed ideal protocol of protein feeding for the periworkout hours.

Contraindications and Precautions Related to Whey Protein Extract Ingestion

To date, no severe adverse reactions have been reported following administration of whey protein extracts. Although some individuals, who are hypersensitive to milk proteins, can experience allergy symptoms including possible serious ones (in this case is strongly recommended to avoid whey proteins containing products). Other dairy-sensitive individuals are lactose-intolerant. Most whey proteins are processed to remove lactose and finished whey products only contain trace amounts. De-lactosed whey, produced from crystallizing a majority of the lactose out and recovering the remaining whey, is appropriate for lactose-intolerant individuals [28].

Conclusions and Final Recommendations

The optimal protocol for administering a supplement containing high quality whey protein still needs to be determined. However in order to stimulate a more powerful anabolic response, frequent meals (every 3 to 5 h) containing 17 to 20 g of high quality protein (200 to 250 mg/kg) providing 8 to 10 g of EAA (90 to 110 mg/kg) and about 2 g of Leucine (20 to 25 mg/kg) seems appropriate for eliciting optimal muscular responses and adaptations in resistance training practitioners.

Co-ingestion of whey protein and carbohydrates in 1:3 ratio would helps glycogen restoration and inhibits protein catabolism, creating synergistic effects with the EAA, particularly leucine, for optimizing recovery process after resistance training workout [68].

Special attention should be given to the periworkout hours where the ingestion of small amount of whey protein (≈10 g) under a pulse like protocol should began 3 h before and continue through the training session. A higher protein intake (≈20 g) would be recommended immediately post workout and possibly at 3 and 6 h after training. In addition, combined whey with others protein sources such as casein and specifically with creatine monohydrate (0.1 g/kg/d), would be appropriate for improving recovery process and the anabolic responses induced by resistance training in athletes [69].

Most available studies have analysed the results based on serial biopsies of only one muscle and limited training conditions (low volume and number of exercises) that are substantially different from what athletes actually perform.

Future research may explore the responses of regular resistance training practitioners under most realistic training condition, using others timing strategies and possibly higher proteins doses than what is currently being recommended.

References

1. American Dietetic Association; Dietitians of Canada; American College of Sports Medicine, Rodriguez NR, Di Marco NM, Langley S (2009) American College of Sports Medicine position stand. Nutrition and athletic performance. Med Sci Sports Exerc 41: 709-731.
2. Campbell B, Kreider RB (2008) Conjugated linoleic acids. Curr Sports Med Rep 7: 237-241.
3. Layman DK, Shiue H, Sather C, Erickson DJ, Baum J (2003) Increased dietary protein modifies glucose and insulin homeostasis in adult women during weight loss. J Nutr 133: 405-410.
4. Volek JS, Forsythe C (2008) Very-Low Carbohydrate Diets, Chapter 25, in Essential of Sports Nutrition and supplements, J Antonio, Kalman D, Stout JR, Greenwood M, Willoughby DS, et al. (Eds.), Humana Press. 581-603.
5. Bilsborough S, Mann N (2006) A review of issues of dietary protein intake in humans. Int J Sport Nutr Exerc Metab 16: 129-152.
6. Paddon-Jones D, Sheffield-Moore M, Zhang XJ, Volpi E, Wolf SE, et al. (2004) Amino acid ingestion improves muscle protein synthesis in the young and elderly. Am J Physiol Endocrinol Metab 286: E321-328.
7. Børsheim E, Tipton KD, Wolf SE, Wolfe RR (2002) Essential amino acids and muscle protein recovery from resistance exercise. Am J Physiol Endocrinol Metab 283: E648-657.
8. Tipton KD, Wolfe RR (2001) Exercise, protein metabolism, and muscle growth. Int J Sport Nutr Exerc Metab 11: 109-132.
9. Elliot TA, Cree MG, Sanford AP, Wolfe RR, Tipton KD (2006) Milk ingestion stimulates net muscle protein synthesis following resistance exercise. Med Sci Sports Exerc 38: 667-674.
10. Moore DR, Robinson MJ, Fry JL, Tang JE, Glover EI, et al. (2009) Ingested protein dose response of muscle and albumin protein synthesis after resistance exercise in young men. Am J Clin Nutr 89: 161-168.
11. Zhan S, Ho SC (2005) Meta-analysis of the effects of soy protein containing isoflavones on the lipid profile. Am J Clin Nutr 81: 397-408.
12. Joy JM, Lowery RP, Wilson JM, Purpura M, De Souza EO, et al. (2013) The effects of 8 weeks of whey or rice protein supplementation on body composition and exercise performance. Nutr J 12: 86.
13. Shing CM, Hunter DC, Stevenson LM (2009) Bovine colostrum supplementation and exercise performance: potential mechanisms. Sports Med 39: 1033-1054.
14. Etzel MR (2004) Manufacture and use of dairy protein fractions. J Nutr 134: 996S-1002S.
15. Campbell B, Kreider RB, Ziegenfuss T, La Bounty P, Roberts M, et al. (2007) International Society of Sports Nutrition position stand: protein and exercise. J Int Soc Sports Nutr 4: 8.
16. Kreider RB, Wilborn CD, Taylor L, Campbell B, Almada AL, et al. (2010) ISSN exercise & sport nutrition review: research & recommendations. J Int Soc Sports Nutr 7: 7.
17. Tang JE, Manolakos JJ, Kujbida GW, Lysecki PJ, Moore DR, et al. (2007) Minimal whey protein with carbohydrate stimulates muscle protein synthesis following resistance exercise in trained young men. Appl Physiol Nutr Metab 32: 1132-1138.
18. Kreider RB, Earnest CP, Lundberg J, Rasmussen C, Greenwood M, et al. (2007) Effects of ingesting protein with various forms of carbohydrate following resistance-exercise on substrate availability and markers of anabolism, catabolism, and immunity. J Int Soc Sports Nutr 4: 18.
19. Willoughby DS, Stout JR, Wilborn CD (2007) Effects of resistance training and protein plus amino acid supplementation on muscle anabolism, mass, and strength. Amino Acids 32: 467-477.
20. Kerksick CM, Rasmussen CJ, Lancaster SL, Magu B, Smith P, et al. (2006) The effects of protein and amino acid supplementation on performance and training adaptations during ten weeks of resistance training. J Strength Cond Res 20: 643-653.
21. Cribb PJ, Williams AD, Hayes A (2007) A creatine-protein-carbohydrate supplement enhances responses to resistance training. Med Sci Sports Exerc 39: 1960-1968.
22. McGregor RA, Poppitt SD (2013) Milk protein for improved metabolic health: a review of the evidence. Nutr Metab (Lond) 10: 46.
23. Hulmi JJ, Kovanen V, Selänne H, Kraemer WJ, Häkkinen K, et al. (2009) Acute and long-term effects of resistance exercise with or without protein ingestion on muscle hypertrophy and gene expression. Amino Acids 37: 297-308.
24. Reitelseder S, Agergaard J, Doessing S, Helmark IC, Lund P, et al. (2011) Whey and casein labeled with L-[1-13C]leucine and muscle protein synthesis: effect of resistance exercise and protein ingestion. Am J Physiol Endocrinol Metab 300: E231-242.
25. West DW, Burd NA, Coffey VG, Baker SK, Burke LM, et al. (2011) Rapid aminoacidemia enhances myofibrillar protein synthesis and anabolic intramuscular signaling responses after resistance exercise. Am J Clin Nutr 94: 795-803.
26. Cribb PJ, Hayes A (2006) Effects of supplement timing and resistance exercise on skeletal muscle hypertrophy. Med Sci Sports Exerc 38: 1918-1925.
27. Snyder BS, Haub MD (2007) Whey, Casein, and Soy Proteins. Chapter 8, in Sports Nutrition Fats and Proteins, JA Driskell (Edr.), CRC Press 143-163.
28. Marshall K (2004) Therapeutic applications of whey protein. Altern Med Rev 9: 136-156.

29. Wong CW, Watson DL (1995) Immunomodulatory effects of dietary whey proteins in mice. J Dairy Res 62: 359-368.

30. Cockburn E, Stevenson E, Hayes PR, Robson-Ansley P, Howatson G (2010) Effect of milk-based carbohydrate-protein supplement timing on the attenuation of exercise-induced muscle damage. Appl Physiol Nutr Metab 35: 270-277.

31. Hoffman JR, Falvo MJ (2004) Protein- Which is the best? J Sports Sci Med 13: 118-130.

32. Bucci LR, Unlu L (2000) Protein and amino acid supplements in exercise and sport., in Energy yielding macronutrients and energy metabolism in sports nutrition, I Wolinsky, Driskell JA, (Edr.), CRC Press: Boca Raton, FL. 191-212.

33. Manninen AH (2004) Protein hydrolysates in sports and exercise: a brief review. J Sports Sci Med 3: 60-63.

34. Calbet JA, MacLean DA (2002) Plasma glucagon and insulin responses depend on the rate of appearance of amino acids after ingestion of different protein solutions in humans. J Nutr 132: 2174-2182.

35. Holmer-Jensen J, Mortensen LS, Astrup A, de Vrese M, Holst JJ, et al. (2013) Acute differential effects of dietary protein quality on postprandial lipemia in obese non-diabetic subjects. Nutr Res 33: 34-40.

36. Bounous G, Gervais F, Amer V, Batist G, Gold P (1989) The influence of dietary whey protein on tissue glutathione and the diseases of aging. Clin Invest Med 12: 343-349.

37. Dangin M, Boirie Y, Garcia-Rodenas C, Gachon P, Fauquant J, et al. (2001) The digestion rate of protein is an independent regulating factor of postprandial protein retention. Am J Physiol Endocrinol Metab 280: E340-348.

38. Tipton KD, Elliott TA, Cree MG, Wolf SE, Sanford AP, et al. (2004) Ingestion of casein and whey proteins result in muscle anabolism after resistance exercise. Med Sci Sports Exerc 36: 2073-2081.

39. Paul GL (2009) The rationale for consuming protein blends in sports nutrition. J Am Coll Nutr 28 Suppl: 464S-472S.

40. Tipton KD (2011) Efficacy and consequences of very-high-protein diets for athletes and exercisers. Proc Nutr Soc 70: 205-214.

41. Yang Y, Churchward-Venne TA, Burd NA, Breen L, Tarnopolsky MA, et al. (2012) Myofibrillar protein synthesis following ingestion of soy protein isolate at rest and after resistance exercise in elderly men. Nutr Metab (Lond) 9: 57.

42. FAO United Nations Expert Consultation (Ed), (2011) Dietary protein quality evaluation in human nutrition: Auckland, New Zealand

43. Dangin M, Guillet C, Garcia-Rodenas C, Gachon P, Bouteloup-Demange C, et al. (2003) The rate of protein digestion affects protein gain differently during aging in humans. J Physiol 549: 635-644.

44. Hildebrandt W, Hamann A, Krakowski-Roosen H, Kinscherf R, Dugi K, et al. (2004) Effect of thiol antioxidant on body fat and insulin reactivity. J Mol Med (Berl) 82: 336-344.

45. Cribb PJ, Williams AD, Carey MF, Hayes A (2006) The effect of whey isolate and resistance training on strength, body composition, and plasma glutamine. Int J Sport Nutr Exerc Metab 16: 494-509.

46. Breen L, Phillips SM (2011) Skeletal muscle protein metabolism in the elderly: Interventions to counteract the 'anabolic resistance' of ageing. Nutr Metab (Lond) 8: 68.

47. Hall WL, Millward DJ, Long SJ, Morgan LM (2003) Casein and whey exert different effects on plasma amino acid profiles, gastrointestinal hormone secretion and appetite. Br J Nutr 89: 239-248.

48. Calder PC, Yaqoob P (2004) Amino acids and immune function Chapter 19 in Metabolic and Therapeutic Aspects of Amino Acids in Clinlcal Nutrition, LA Cynober, (Edr.), CRC Press LLC 305-320.

49. Di Pasquale MG (2008) Examples of Useful Nutritional Supplement Formulations Chapter 13, in Amino Acids and Proteins for the Athlete: The Anabolic Edge, MG Di Pasquale, (Edr.), CRC Press 397-426.

50. Lemon PWR (2011) Protein and Amino Acid, chapter 5, in Sport and Exercise Nutrition, SA Lanham-New, Stear, SJ, Shirreffs, SM Collins, AL, (Eds.), Wiley-Blackwell, USA 41-50.

51. Battermann W (1986) Whey protein for athletes Deutsche Milchwirtschaft, 37: 1010-1012.

52. Tipton KD, Elliott TA, Cree MG, Aarsland AA, Sanford AP, et al. (2007) Stimulation of net muscle protein synthesis by whey protein ingestion before and after exercise. Am J Physiol Endocrinol Metab 292: E71-76.

53. Kraemer WJ, Solomon-Hill G, Volk BM, Kupchak BR, Looney DP, et al. (2013) The effects of soy and whey protein supplementation on acute hormonal reponses to resistance exercise in men. J Am Coll Nutr 32: 66-74.

54. Norton L, Wilson GJ (2009) Optimal protein intake to maximize muscle protein synthesis. AgroFood industry hi-tech, 20: 54-57.

55. Burke LM, Hawley JA, Wong SH, Jeukendrup AE (2011) Carbohydrates for training and competition. J Sports Sci 29 Suppl 1: S17-27.

56. Costa R JS, Walters R, Bilzon J LJ, Walsh NP (2011) Effects of immediate postexercise carbohydrate ingestion with and without protein on neutrophil degranulation. Int J Sport Nutr Exerc Metab 21: 205-213.

57. Kerksick CM, Leutholtz B (2005) Nutrient administration and resistance training. J Int Soc Sports Nutr 2: 50-67.

58. Kerksick C, Harvey T, Stout J, Campbell B, Wilborn C, et al. (2008) International Society of Sports Nutrition position stand: nutrient timing. J Int Soc Sports Nutr 5: 17.

59. Cooper R, Naclerio F, Larumbe-Zabala E, Chassin C, Allgrove A, et al. (2013) Effects of a Carbohydrate-Protein-Creatine Supplement on Strength Performance and Body Composition in Recreationally Resistance Trained Young Men. JOEP online, 16: 72-85.

60. Biolo G, Maggi SP, Williams BD, Tipton KD, Wolfe RR (1995) Increased rates of muscle protein turnover and amino acid transport after resistance exercise in humans. Am J Physiol 268: E514-E520.

61. Bohé J, Low JF, Wolfe RR, Rennie MJ (2001) Latency and duration of stimulation of human muscle protein synthesis during continuous infusion of amino acids. J Physiol 532: 575-579.

62. Moore DR, Tang JE, Burd NA, Rerecich T, Tarnopolsky MA, et al. (2009) Differential stimulation of myofibrillar and sarcoplasmic protein synthesis with protein ingestion at rest and after resistance exercise. J Physiol 587: 897-904.

63. Burke LM, Hawley JA, Ross ML, Moore DR, Phillips SM, et al. (2012) Preexercise aminoacidemia and muscle protein synthesis after resistance exercise. Med Sci Sports Exerc 44: 1968-1977.

64. Kim PL, Staron RS, Phillips SM (2005) Fasted-state skeletal muscle protein synthesis after resistance exercise is altered with training. J Physiol 568: 283-290.

65. Phillips SM, Tipton KD, Aarsland A, Wolf SE, Wolfe RR (1997) Mixed muscle protein synthesis and breakdown after resistance exercise in humans. Am J Physiol 273: E99-107.

66. Areta J, Burke LM, Ross ML, Camera DM, West DD, et al. (2013) Timing and distribution of protein ingestion during prolonged recovery from resistance exercise alters myofibrillar protein synthesis. J Physiol 591: 2319-2331.

67. La Bounty PM, Campbell BI, Wilson J, Galvan E, Berardi J, et al. (2011) International Society of Sports Nutrition position stand: meal frequency. J Int Soc Sports Nutr 8: 4.

68. Ziegenfuss TN, Landis J, Lemieux RA (2010) Protein for Sports-New Data and New Recommendations. Strength Cond J 32: 65-70.

69. Cooper R, Naclerio F, Allgrove J, Jimenez A (2012) Creatine supplementation with specific view to exercise/sports performance: an update. J Int Soc Sports Nutr 9: 33.

13

Effect of Tai Chi Exercise on Immune Function in Middle-aged and Elderly Women

Jing Liu[1,2]*, Peijie Chen[3], Ru Wang[3], Yonghong Yuan[4], and Chunying Li[5]*

[1]*Department of Martial Arts, Shanghai University of Sport, Shanghai 200438, China*
[2]*Department of Psychology, School of Kinesiology, University of Michigan, Ann Arbor, MI, 48109, USA*
[3]*Department of Sports Medicine, Shanghai University of Sport, Shanghai 200438, China*
[4]*Department of Sports Leisure, Shanghai University of Sport, Shanghai 200438, China*
[5]*Department of Biochemistry & Molecular Biology, Wayne State University School of Medicine, Detroit, Michigan 48201, USA*

Abstract

Objective: The purpose of this study was to investigate the effect of Tai Chi (TC) exercise on immune functions among middle-aged and elderly women, and to evaluate the relationship between immune modulation of Natural Killer T (NKT) cells and Dendritic Cells (DCs) and T Helper (Th) 1 /Th2 immune response.

Methods: Sixty healthy middle-aged and elderly women were randomly assigned into 2 groups: Tai Chi (TC) group (n=30) and control (CON) group (n=30). Subjects in TC group participated in TC exercise for 6 months, 60 minutes a day, four times a week. Meanwhile, subjects in CON group maintained their normal physical activity levels during the whole study period. Peripheral blood samples were collected right before, and after 4 and 6 months of the exercise program, and the sampled were analyzed within 24 hours after collection.

Results: After the 6-month TC exercise program, the percentage of $CD4^+$ T lymphocytes, the $CD4^+$:$CD8^+$ ratio, and the percentage of NK and NKT cells in TC group significantly increased ($p<0.05$). The percentage of interferon-γ (IFN-γ) producing T cells increased significantly after 4 months ($p<0.01$) and 6 months ($p<0.05$) of exercise. The percentage of interleukin-4 (IL-4) producing T lymphocytes also demonstrated an increase after 4 months ($p<0.05$) and 6 months ($p>0.05$) of exercise. The percentage of $CD123^+$ DCs and $CD11c^+$ DCs also significantly increased after the 6-month program ($p<0.01$), with the percentage of $CD11c^+$ cells increasing much more dramatically than $CD123^+$ DCs. However, the CON group did not show any significant changes in these parameters.

Conclusion: Regular TC exercise favors the development of Th1 immune responses in middle-aged and elderly women. TC-induced changes in Th1 and Th2 immune responses are associated with the immune modulation of NKT cells and DCs and their reciprocal interactions.

Keywords: Physical activity; Immunology; Immunosenescence; Aging; Female

Introduction

Immunosenescence is the steady degeneration of the immune system that occurs with age in humans and animals [1]. Multiple aspects of the immune response are severely disregulated by aging, among which the T cell immune response is the most dramatically affected. T cell-mediated production of cytokines Interleukin (IL)-2 and Interferon (IFN)-γ decreases significantly with age. The amount of IFN-γ decreases along with the activity of T Helper 1 (Th1) cells and the amount of IL-4 and IL-10 increases along with the activity of T Helper 2 (Th2) cells [2,3], resulting in a decreasing ratio of Th1/Th2 in elderly people. The decrease in the numbers of Natural Killer (NK) cells and Natural Killer T (NKT) cells contributes to the deleterious immune response in the elderly, and the number of myeloid Dendritic Cells (DCs) also progressively declines with age [4].

Aging is also associated with decreased physical activity. Exercise can profoundly influence health, and there is mounting evidence that the mechanisms behind these effects are related, in part, to the impact of exercise on immune function [5]. It has been shown that the numbers of circulating T cells and their functions are influenced by brief periods of exercise [6,7]. Hinton et al. [8] reported significant changes in the composition of the total lymphocyte cultures immediately post-exercise: increased numbers of $CD56^+$ NK cells and $CD8^+$ T cells and decreased numbers of T-helper cells ($CD4^+$), in male endurance-trained runners after an interval running session of 15×1-min intervals at 95% VO_2 max. A decrease in mitogen-stimulated T cell proliferation and T cell production of IL-2 and IFN-γ was reported immediately after acute, intensive exercise [9]. In fact, the volume of exercise has been shown to be a critical element in inducing a positive or negative effect on the immune response [5,10]. It has been shown that moderate exercise enhances T cell function and decreases respiratory infections [11]. Although many components of the immune system are known to exhibit various changes depending on the stage and type of exercise, the long-term effects of regular moderate exercise on immune responses remain incompletely understood.

Tai Chi (TC) is a traditional Chinese martial art with a long history. It usually consists of TC Chuan and TC Weapon (for example, TC Sword, TC Spear, TC Broa dsword). TC has gained popularity in Western countries in recent years for its recognized positive effects on health in the elderly [12]. TC incorporates slow-moving, gentle physical activity, balance, and weight shifting, with meditation, relaxation, deep

***Corresponding authors:** Jing Liu, Ph.D., Department of Martial Arts, Shanghai University of Sport, 588 Qing Yuan Huan Road, Shanghai 200438, China, E-mail: liujing_j3@163.com

breathing, and imagination. Reported benefits of TC include increased balance and decreased incidence of falls, increased strength and flexibility, reduced pain and anxiety, improved self-efficacy, improved sleep, and enhanced cardiopulmonary function [12]. TC has also been shown to significantly increase the ratio of $CD4^+$ *vs.* $CD8^+$, significantly increase $CD4^+/CD25^+$ regulatory T cell number [13] reduce the levels of HbA1c in type II diabetes and enhance the Th1 response [14] and increase varicella-zoster virus specific cell-mediated immunity [15], significantly increased the numbers and activity of natural killer cells in the peripheral blood [3]. To our knowledge, there haven't been any studies as to whether TC could promote the amelioration of the age-induced Th1/Th2 immune imbalance.

The purpose of this study was to investigate the effect of TC on the subsets of T cells, NK cells, NKT cells and DCs, and the cytokines IFN-γ and IL-4 producing T cells, in aged 50–65 women who had practiced TC for six months. Our hypothesis was that TC induces a Th1-type immune response in elderly people, ameliorating the age-induced immune imbalance. By evaluating the relationships between TC exercise and T lymphocyte immune function, we sought to elucidate the role that TC exercise plays in reversing the age-associated imunosenescence.

	CON group (N=30)		TC group (N=30)	
	Pre	Post	Pre	Post
Age (yr)	55 ± 2.74	-	54 ± 3.54	-
Body Weight (kg)	62.14 ± 12.77	62.33 ± 11.86	64.41 ± 10.09	63.93 ± 11.26
Height (cm)	165.28 ± 1.95	165.42 ± 1.87	164.33 ± 2.09	164.97 ± 1.77
BMI (kg/m²)	23.96 ± 0.87	23.34 ± 0.93	24.19 ± 0.79	23.99 ± 0.68
Body Fat (%)	28.82 ± 7.61	28.72 ± 6.34	29.07 ± 6.33	29.02 ± 5.69

Table 1: Characteristics of all subjects in both CON and TC groups before and after 6 months of TC exercise training. CON group: control group; TC group: Tai Chi exercise group; Pre: pre-exercise program; Post: 6-month after exercise program; BMI: body mass index.

Materials and Methods

Subjects

Sixty women, aged 50–65, were recruited by advertising for the study, and randomly divided into 2 groups: Tai Chi (TC) exercise group (n=30) and non-exercise control (CON) group (n=30). Table 1 shows the physical characteristics of the study subjects, and both groups were of similar age and body composition. Body mass and Body Mass Index (BMI) did not demonstrate any significant changes during the whole study period in either TC group or CON group. Exclusion criteria included angiocardiopathy (cardiopulmonary illness), autoimmune disorder, metabolic disorder, malignancies actively being treated with chemotherapy, hormone replacements (such as the use of corticosteroids), and acute illness from infection, and major surgery during the preceding 6 months. All subjects had no TC training experience before. Written informed consent was obtained from all participants upon enrollment, and the protocol was reviewed and approved by the institutional review board of Shanghai University of Sport. The subjects in the CON group were instructed not to participate in any formal exercise but simply to maintain their normal levels of physical activity as usual for the whole 6-month study period, and they kept diaries to record their daily activities.

TC exercise program

All subjects in TC group participated in TC Chuan (24 forms;

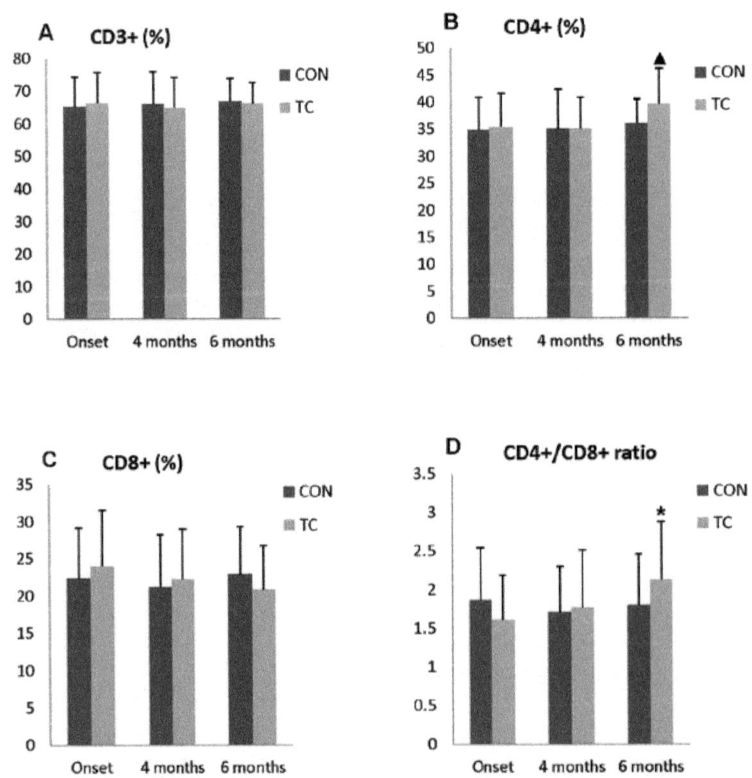

Figure 1: Comparison of the percentages of T lymphocyte $CD3^+$ (**A**), and their subsets $CD4^+$ (**B**) and $CD8^+$ (**C**) in the peripheral blood, as well as $CD4^+/CD8^+$ ratio (**D**) at the onset, 4 months and 6 months during the study period in control (CON) group and Tai Chi (TC) exercise group. Data are presented as Mean ± SEM. *P* values were analyzed by Student's paired *t*-test (*n*=3subjects per group). * $p<0.05$ as compared with onset of the same group▲$p<0.05$ as compared with 4 months of the same group.

Supplementary figure 1 for TC techniques) and TC Sword (42 forms) exercise for 6 months, 4 sessions a week. They were supervised and instructed by an experienced TC teacher who has practiced TC for 18 years. Each TC session lasted 60 minutes consisting of a 10 minutes warm up, a 40 minutes practice, and a 10 minutes cool down. The subjects in TC group spent 3 months in learning and practicing all forms of TC Chuan and TC Sword, and then continued to practice for another 3 months. All TC subjects kept diaries to record details.

Blood sampling and analysis

Blood sampling: At the onset, 4-month, and 6-month during the study period, peripheral venous blood (5 ml) of each subject in both groups was collected in an anticoagulant heparin tube. Blood samples were analyzed within 24 hours of collection. Blood was collected between 7 am–9 am in the morning after a 12 hours overnight fast (only water was allowed). On the day of blood collection, subjects did not carry out any TC exercise. All subjects refrained from any exercise for at least 24 hours before the blood collection/sampling.

Analysis of T cell subset, NKT cells, and NK cells

Flow cytometric analysis for T cells: Peripheral blood (100 l) was incubated with anti-human CD4-fluorescein isothiocyanate (FITC), anti-human CD8-phycoerythrin (PE), as well as anti-human CD3-peridinin chlorophyll protein (PerCP)-Cy5 antibodies (Immunotech Co.) in the dark for 15 minutes. Then haemolysis fixative agent (0.5 ml) (Beckman Coulter) was added for another 10 minutes, followed by the addition of Isoton II diluent (0.5 ml) (Beckman Coulter). $CD3^+$, $CD4^+$, and $CD8^+$ cells were measured using fluorescence detection by flow cytometry.

Flow aytometric analysis for NK/NKT cells: Peripheral blood (100 μl) was stained with anti-human CD3-FITC, anti-human CD16-PE, and anti-human CD56-PE antibodies (Beckman Coulter, California, USA). After staining, red blood cells were lysed with OptiLyse C Lysing Solution (Beckman Coulter). Finally, cells were analyzed using a Coulter EPICS XL Flow Cytometer (Beckman Coulter) with System IITM software. NK cells were defined as $CD3^-CD16^+CD56^+$ cells, and NKT as $CD3^+CD16^+CD56^+$ cells [16].

Analysis of IFN-γ and IL-4 producing $CD3^+CD4^+$ T cells

Ten μl of PMA (1 μg/ml), 8 μl of ionomycin (50 μg/ml) and 6.8 μl of monensin fluid (0.1 mg/ml; Sigma Chemical Co.) were added to peripheral blood (200 μl) along with RPMI-1640 media (200 μl), and incubated for 4 to 6 hours at 37°C in a 5% CO2 incubator. Monoclonal anti-CD3-PerCP (20 μl) and anti-CD4-FITC antibodies (20 μl; Beckman Coulter) were then added and the mixture was incubated for another 15 minutes. After the incubation, cell suspension of each sample was divided into three 100-l aliquots, and all samples were treated with fixation/permeabilization reagents according to the manufacturer's instructions (Beckman Coulter). Intracellular cytokines in each aliquot were stained using PE-conjugated mAbs against IL-4, IFN-γ, or an isotype control (Beckman Coulter) for 30 minutes. The samples were washed with PBS and the supernatant was discarded. The cell pellet was resuspended in PBS and analyzed by flow cytometry. All incubations (except PMA-activation and incubation) were performed at room temperature in the dark.

Analysis of $CD123^+$ and $CD11c^+$ dendritic cells by direct immunofluorescence staining of whole blood

Monoclonal antibodies: PE-conjugated anti–IL-3 receptor α chain (CD123), PE-conjugated anti-CD11c, PerCP-conjugated anti–HLA-DR, and FITC-conjugated lineage cocktail 1 (lin 1), as well as PE- and PerCP-conjugated isotype control murine mAbs were obtained from BD (San Jose, CA). The lin 1 contains monoclonal antibody clones against CD3 (T cells), CD14 (monocytes/macrophages), CD16 (natural killer cells), CD19 (B cells), CD20 (B cells), and CD56 (natural killer cells). Sensitive detection of DCs was achieved by exclusion of cells positive for CD3, CD14, CD16, CD19, CD20, or CD56 using Lineage Cocktail 1 (FITC-conjugated Ab mixture against CD3, CD14, CD16, CD19, CD20, and CD56). Thereafter, myeloid and lymphoid DCs (DC1s and DC2s, respectively) were detected using PE-conjugated Ab against CD11c and CD123, respectively.

Flow cytometric analysis: Peripheral blood cells obtained from the subjects were analyzed by three-color flow cytometry. To minimize selective cell loss during the preparation procedure, the cells were first stained with mAbs followed by lysing the erythrocytes. Briefly, aliquots (100 μl) of peripheral blood were incubated with a mixture of anti-lin mAbs (BD Biosciences), a PerCP-conjugated anti-HLA-DR mAb, and either a PE-conjugated anti-CD11c mAb to detect myeloid DC or a PE-conjugated anti-CD123 mAb to detect plasmacytoid DC, or a PE-conjugated isotype control (BD Biosciences) in the dark at room temperature for 15 min (Supplementary table 1). Then 2 ml of FACS lysing solution (BD) was added, vortexed, and incubated for 10 minutes to lyse the erythrocytes. The mixture was centrifuged at 300×g for 5 minutes, and the supernatant was discarded. The mixture was then vortexed gently with 1 ml of wash buffer, centrifuged again as described above, and the supernatant was discarded. Thereafter, the mixture was vortexed and resuspended in 300 μl of 1% paraformaldehyde for 10 min, and then washed and analyzed on a flow cytometer. Identical flow cytometric settings were used for the acquisition of all samples enabling the expression of cell surface molecules on different samples to be directly compared. All incubations were performed at room temperature in the dark. DCs were defined as the cells positive for PerCP-conjugated anti-HLA-DR mAb and negative for FITC-conjugated lin 1. Anti-CD11c or anti-CD123 mAb conjugated with PE was used for further identification of the mDC and pDC subsets.

Statistical analysis

All data were expressed as means ± SEMs, and $p<0.05$ was set as the criterion for significance. The Statistical Package for Social Sciences (SPSS Inc, USA; version 12.0) was used for statistical analysis. Data were analyzed using one-way Analysis Of Variance (ANOVA), and the independent samples t-tests were applied to assess differences between control group and TC group before exercise program. Paired-samples *t*-tests were only used to assess differences of variables between pre-exercise and 4-month, as well as between pre-exercise and 6-month.

Results

Effect of TC exercise on T lymphocytes and their subsets

As shown in Figure 1, the percentages of T lymphocytes ($CD3^+$) and their subsets ($CD4^+$ and $CD8^+$) in the peripheral blood before exercise program (at onset) did not show any significant inter-group differences between CON and TC groups. Six-month TC exercise program significantly increased the percentage of $CD4^+$ T (Th) lymphocytes and the $CD4^+$:$CD8^+$ ratio ($p<0.05$; Figures 1B and 1D), while no significant change in the percentages of $CD3^+$ or $CD8^+$ T cells was observed (Figures 1A and 1C). Within the TC exercise group, the difference was significant in the $CD4^+$:$CD8^+$ ratio at 6-month of TC exercise compared with the ratio at the onset ($p<0.05$; Figure 1D). There was also a significant difference in the percentage of $CD4^+$ T lymphocytes at

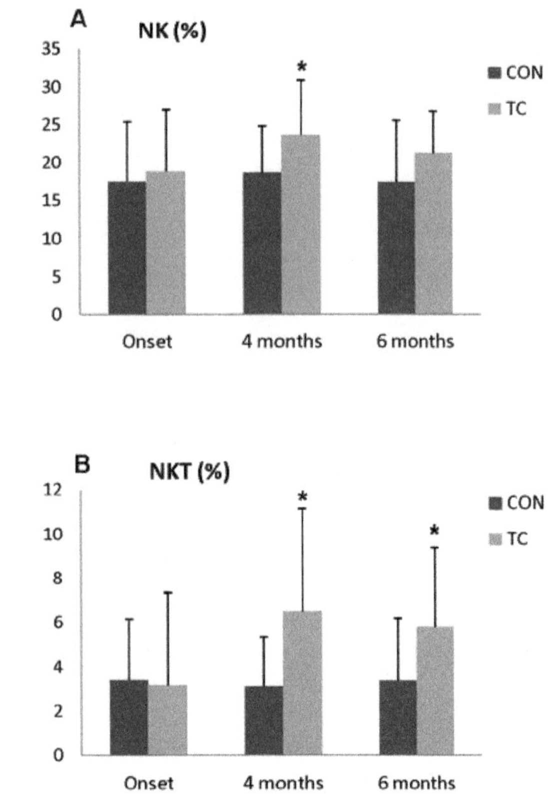

Figure 2: Comparison of NK (**A**) and NKT (**B**) cell percentages in the peripheral blood at the onset, 4 months and 6 months during the study period in control (CON) group and Tai Chi (TC) exercise group. Data are presented as Mean ± SEM. * $p<0.05$ as compared with onset of the same group.

6-month compared with at 4-month of TC exercise ($p<0.05$; Figure 1B). However, the percentages of T lymphocytes ($CD3^+$) and their subsets ($CD4^+$ and $CD8^+$) in CON group did not demonstrate any changes during the whole study period (onset; 4 months; and 6 months).

Effect of TC exercise on NK and NKT cells

Figure 2 shows the changes in the percentages of NK cells and NKT cells in the peripheral blood in both CON and TC groups. The percentages of NK cells and NKT cells before exercise program (at onset) did not show any inter-group differences between CON and TC groups. Following TC exercise program, the percentages of both NK and NKT cells significantly increased at 4 months compared with at the onset ($p<0.05$; Figures 2A and 2B). At 6 months of TC exercise program, the percentages of both NK and NKT cell decreased slightly compared with at 4-month, but the percentage of NKT cells at 6-month was still significantly higher than at the onset ($p<0.05$; Figure 2B). The percentages of NK cells and NKT cells in CON group did not demonstrate any significant changes during the whole study period (onset; 4 months; and 6 months).

Effect of TC exercise on cytokines IL-4 and IFN-γ producing $CD4^+$ T cells

Figure 3 shows the changes in the percentages of IFN-γ producing $CD4^+$ T cells (Th1) and IL-4 producing $CD4^+$ T cells (Th2) in both CON and TC groups. The percentages of both IFN-γ and IL-4 producing $CD4^+$ T cells before exercise program (at onset) were not significantly different between CON and TC groups (Figure 3). However, TC exercise program significantly increased both IFN-γ and IL-4 producing $CD4^+$ T cells (Figure 3). There was significant difference in the proportion of IFN-γ ($p<0.01$; Figure 3A) and IL-4 ($p<0.05$; Figure 3B) producing T cells at 4-month of TC exercise compared with at the onset. IFN-γ producing T cells also demonstrated a significantly higher percentage at 6-month than at the onset ($p<0.05$; Figure 3A). The percentages of IFN-γ and IL-4 producing $CD4^+$ T cells in CON group did not show any significant changes during the whole study period (onset; 4 months; and 6 months).

Effect of TC exercise on $CD123^+$ DCs and $CD11c^+$ dendritic cells

As shown in figure 4, the percentages of both $CD123^+$ (plasmacytoid) DCs and $CD11c^+$ (myeloid) DCs before TC exercise program (at onset) were not significantly different between CON and TC groups. However, after the 6 months of TC exercise program, the percentage of both $CD123^+$ (plasmacytoid) DCs and $CD11c^+$ (myeloid) DCs significantly increased (Figure 4). There was significant increase in the percentages of $CD11c^+$ DCs ($p<0.01$; Figure 4 A) and $CD123^+$ DCs ($p<0.01$; Figure 4B) at 6 months of TC exercise compared with at the onset. There was also significant increase in the percentage of $CD11c^+$ DCs ($p<0.01$; Figure 4A) and $CD123^+$ DCs ($p<0.01$; Figure 4B) at 6-month compared with at 4-month of TC exercise. The number of $CD11c^+$ DCs (myeloid) (Figure 4A) increased much more dramatically than that of $CD123^+$ DCs (plasmacytoid) (Figure 4B). The percentages of both $CD123^+$ (plasmacytoid) DCs and $CD11c^+$ (myeloid) DCs in CON group did not show any changes during the study period (onset; 4 months; and 6 months).

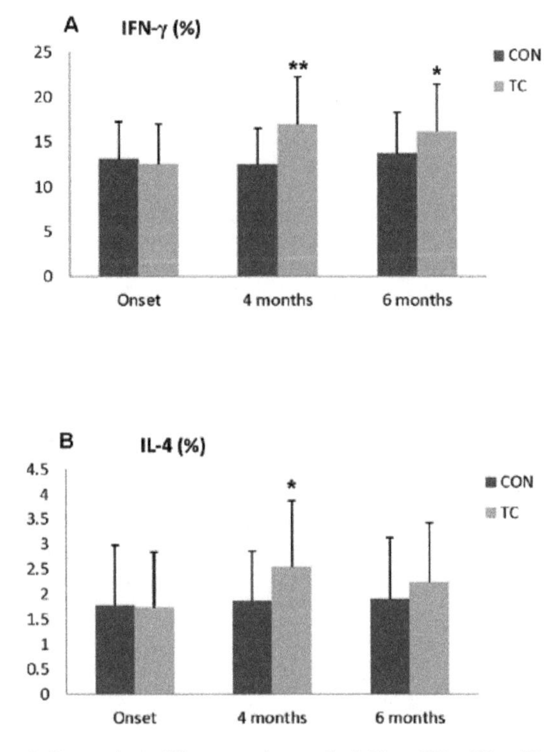

Figure 3: Comparison of the percentages of cytokines IFN-γ (**A**) and IL-4 (**B**) producing CD4 T cells in the peripheral blood at the onset, 4 months and 6 months during the study period in control (CON) group and Tai Chi (TC) exercise group. Data are presented as Mean ± SEM. * $p<0.05$, ** $p<0.01$ as compared with onset of the same group.

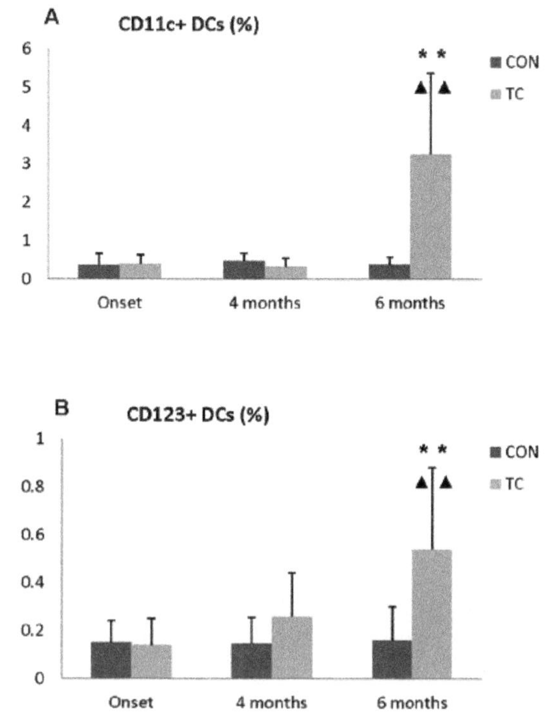

Figure 4: Comparison of the percentages of $CD11c^+$ (**A**) dendritic cells (DCs) and $CD123^+$ (**B**) DCs in the peripheral blood at the onset, 4 months and 6 months during the study period in control (CON) group and Tai Chi (TC) exercise group. Data are presented as Mean ± SEM. ** $p<0.01$ as compared with onset of the same group; ▲▲ $p<0.01$ as compared with 4 months.

Discussion

The human immune system demonstrates degenerative changes with advancing age [17], especially T cells which demonstrate prominent age-related alterations in distribution and function, such as declined number of circulating Th cells, NKT cells, and DCs, decreased production of Th1 cytokines (IFN-γ) and increased production of Th2 cytokines (IL-4) with aging [2,4,3]. However, the findings of our present study demonstrated that after a 6-month TC exercise program, the percentages of $CD4^+$ T lymphocytes, NK cells, NKT cells, and DCs, along with the $CD4^+$:$CD8^+$ ratio and cytokines IFN-γ and IL-4 producing T cells, significantly increased in middle-aged and elderly women.

Many studies have reported exercise-induced changes in the immune function [5]. Changes in exercise-induced immune functions are associated with the exercise type, intensity, and the duration of both the exercise and any intermissions [5]. It was observed that the number of $CD4^+$ T cells decreased while the number of $CD8^+$ T cells significantly increased, resulting in a decreased $CD4^+$:$CD8^+$ ratio, in seven middle- and long-distance runners undergoing four-week intensive training after 36 hours of rest [18]. After a bout of strenuous and prolonged exercise (>1.5 h), the number of circulating T lymphocytes decreased below pre-exercise levels for several hours after exercise, with a decreased $CD4^+$/$CD8^+$ ratio [19]. Excessive training can cause significant drop in NK cell number, leading to immune suppression [20]. However, our present work and some previously published studies showed that moderate physical exercise improved immune function [21,22]. A 6-month supervised exercise training program led to nominal increases in some aspects of immune function in previously sedentary elderly [22]. While others reported that NK cell activity increased by 33% after moderate intensity training for 16 weeks in the elderly population [23], and increased by 57% in a group of middle-aged women after six weeks of moderate intensity exercise training (60% VO_2 max) [24]. Yeh et al. [14] reported that after 12 weeks of TC exercise, transcription factor T-bet as well as expression of Th1/Th2/T regulatory (Treg) cells significantly increased in type 2 diabetes patients. So far, there have been no studies reporting changes in the age-induced Th1/Th2 immune imbalance after regular long-term Tai Chi exercise. The results of our present study demonstrated for the first time that regular TC exercise appears to favor improvement of Th1 immune responses in middle-aged and elderly women and the percentage of NKT cells and $CD11c^+$ DCs significantly increased after 6-month regular TC exercise as compared to the control group.

Th1 cytokines, of which IFN-γ is typical, support cell-mediated inflammatory reactions by activating cytotoxic and inflammatory functions; while Th2 cytokines, of which IL-4 is typical, support humoral immune responses [25]. Th1 and Th2 cytokines are mutually inhibitory for the differentiation and effector functions of the reciprocal phenotype [26]. IFN-γ selectively inhibits proliferation of Th2 cells, and IL-4 and IL-10 inhibit cytokine synthesis by Th1 cells [26]. A number of studies have shown that physical exercise affects Th1 and Th2 immune responses as well as the balance between these responses. Excessive or exhaustive exercise has been reported to induce exercise-related immunosuppression via altering the Th1/Th2 balance by decreasing the percentage of circulating Th1 lymphocytes, with increase or no change in Th2 cells; and also by decreasing IFN-γ production and increasing IL-4 production resulting in a decreased IFN-γ/IL-4 ratio [6,27-29]. However, 2-month endurance training of moderate intensity promoted IFN-γ production in moderately trained athletes [30], and 6 months of moderate combined (endurance and resistance) training increased spontaneously CD28 expressing Th cells and mitogen-stimulated IFN-γ producing Th1 cells in elderly subjects [31]. Consistent with these findings, our present study showed that after 6-month regular TC exercise, the percentages of IL-4 and IFN-γ producing T cells significantly increased, and IFN-γ producing T cells were up-modulated more dramatically than IL-4 producing T cells. These results suggest that long-term TC exercise can up-regulate Th cell-mediated immune responses and promote the switch of the focus of the immune system from humoral immunity to cell immunity, resulting in a higher Th1-type immune response (Th1 dominance) and therefore enhancing anti-viral function. However, the mechanism by which TC modulates the Th immune responses and the Th1/Th2 balance remains unclear.

CD1d-restricted NKT cells expressing both invariant T-cell receptors and NK cell receptors are an important immunoregulatory subset of T lymphocytes, and they play an important role not only in immune defense and surveillance, but also in regulating the immune balance [16]. Activated NKT cells are involved in immune differentiation of Th1 and Th2 cells, and in the switch of the immune response in the opposite direction, i.e., towards a Th1-type response [16]. Most recently, we investigated the relationship between NKT cells and the Th1/Th2 lymphocyte imbalance after overtraining and excessive exercise, and showed that -galactosylceramide played an important modulatory role in the exercise-induced Th1/Th2 lymphocyte imbalance, which may correlate with NKT immunoregulatory cells [32]. It was reported that not only the NKT cell function depends on stimulation and the microenvironment in the initial stages of the immune response, but also the NKT activation signal is transmitted by the specific type of APCs, such as DCs [33].

DCs are the most important and potent APCs, priming the primary immune response [34]. Two distinct DC subsets, myeloid DCs (mDC, also called Type 1 DCs, DC1), and plasmacytoid DCs (pDC, also called Type 2 DCs, DC2) that may produce different outcomes after their interaction with T lymphocytes, have been identified in humans [34,35], DC1 (identified as $CD11c^{+}CD123^{-}$) subsets induce Th1 cell differentiation by the secretion of IL-12. DC2 (identified as $CD11c^{-}CD123^{+}$) subsets secrete mainly IL-10, which induces initial T cells to differentiate into Th2 cells, resulting in immune tolerance. On the basis of these distinct properties of the DC subtypes, mDCs and pDCs are considered to be specialized APCs inducing a Th1 and Th2 response, respectively. Exercise has been reported to induce a significant increase in DC numbers and modulate myeloid DC differentiation and maturation in rats [36,37]. The findings of our present study demonstrated that TC exercise promotes $CD11c^{+}$ DCs and $CD123^{+}$ DCs, with the change in $CD11c^{+}$ DCs being more dramatic, suggesting that TC exercise facilitates the induction of Th1 cell differentiation.

As the most powerful APCs, DCs can activate resting NKT cells *in vivo*, present antigen peptide and provide a co-stimulus signal for NKT cell sensitization, activation and amplification [38]. It was shown that DCs produce high levels of co-stimulus molecules to activate T cells, after combining DCs and T cells to mediate the Th1 response by secreting large amounts of IL-12, helping to eliminate tumors [39]. Others reported that exogenous or endogenous IL-12 induces a progressive decrease in the number of liver NKT cells producing IL-4, thus supporting the development of Th1 immune responses [38]. However, immature DCs do not induce Th cell differentiation, and IFN-γ mainly induces immature DC differentiation to DC1 cells. The increased percentage of NKT cells enhanced IFN-γ secretion, promoting DC1 production and possibly favoring the development of Th1 immune responses. Therefore, NKT cells and DCs demonstrate reciprocal interactions and cooperatively regulate Th immune differentiation. Our results suggested that TC-induced changes in the Th1 and Th2 immune responses were related to immune modulation of NKT cells and DCs, and their reciprocal interactions with each other.

In conclusion, our present study has shown that a six-month regular TC exercise program significantly improved immune function in middle-aged and elderly women. The $CD4^{+}$:$CD8^{+}$ ratio showed a significant increase, and the percentages of NKT cells, $CD11c^{+}$ DCs and $CD123^{+}$ DCs, as well as the percentages of cytokine IFN-γ producing T cells were also significantly increased. The percentage of $CD11c^{+}$ DC was increased more dramatically than that of $CD123^{+}$ DC. We conclude that regular TC exercise can improve age-associated immune imbalance and promote the development of Th1 immune responses, and these changes may be related to the immune modulation of NKT cells and DCs and their reciprocal interactions with each other. Therefore, regular TC exercise has beneficial effects of reversing the age-associated immunosenescence in middle-aged and elderly people.

Acknowledgements

The authors thank Dr. Lai Wei (National Eye Institute, and National Center for Complementary and Alternative Medicine, National Institutes of Health, USA) for critically reading the manuscript. This study was supported by grants from the Shanghai Pujiang Program, the Shanghai Natural Science Foundation (No. 07ZR14103) and the Shanghai Leading Academic Discipline Project (No. T0902). Appreciation is also extended to all participating staff and subjects, whose cooperation made this study possible.

References

1. Pawelec G, Solana R (1997) Immunosenescence. Immunol Today 18: 514-516.
2. Alberti S, Cevenini E, Ostan R, Capri M, Salvioli S, et al. (2006) Age-dependent modifications of Type 1 and Type 2 cytokines within virgin and memory CD4+ T cells in humans. Mech Ageing Dev 127: 560-566.
3. Ernst DN, Weigle O, Hobbs MV (1995) Aging and lymphokine gene expression by T cell subsets. Nutr Rev 53: S18–S25.
4. Della Bella S, Bierti L, Presicce P, Arienti R, Valenti M, et al. (2007) Peripheral blood dendritic cells and monocytes are differently regulated in the elderly. Clin Immunol 122: 220-228.
5. Gleeson M (2007) Immune function in sport and exercise. J Appl Physiol 103: 693-699.
6. Lancaster GI, Halson SL, Khan Q, Drysdale P, Wallace F, et al. (2004) Effects of acute exhaustive exercise and chronic exercise training on type 1 and type 2 T lymphocytes. Exerc Immunol Rev 10: 91-106.
7. Zaldivar F, Wang-Rodriguez J, Nemet D, Schwindt C, Galassetti P, et al. (2006) Constitutive pro- and anti-inflammatory cytokine and growth factor response to exercise in leukocytes. J Appl Physiol 100: 1124-1133.
8. Hinton JR, Rowbottom DG, Keast D, Morton AR (1997) Acute intensive interval training and in vitro t-lymphocyte function. Int J Sports Med 18: 130-135.
9. Gleeson M, Bishop NC (2005) The T cell and NK cell immune response to exercise. Ann Transplant 10: 43-48.
10. Shore S, Shinkai S, Rhind S, Shephard RJ (1999) Immune responses to training: how critical is training volume? J Sports Med Phys Fitness 39: 1-11.
11. Davis JM, Murphy EA, Brown AS, Carmichael MD, Ghaffar A, et al. (2004) Effects of moderate exercise and oat beta-glucan on innate immune function and susceptibility to respiratory infection. Am J Physiol Regul Integr Comp Physiol 286: R366-372.
12. Li JX, Hong Y, Chan KM (2001) Tai chi: physiological characteristics and beneficial effects on health. Br J Sports Med 35: 148-156.
13. Yeh SH, Chuang H, Lin LW, Hsiao CY, Eng HL (2006) Regular tai chi chuan exercise enhances functional mobility and CD4CD25 regulatory T cells. Br J Sports Med 40: 239-243.
14. Yeh SH, Chuang H, Lin LW, Hsiao CY, Wang PW, et al. (2009) Regular Tai Chi Chuan exercise improves T cell helper function of patients with type 2 diabetes mellitus with an increase in T-bet transcription factor and IL-12 production. Br J Sports Med 43: 845-850.
15. Irwin MR, Pike JL, Cole JC, Oxman MN (2003) Effects of a behavioral intervention, Tai Chi Chih, on varicella-zoster virus specific immunity and health functioning in older adults. Psychosom Med 65: 824-830.
16. Kronenberg M, Gapin L (2002) The unconventional lifestyle of NKT cells. Nat Rev Immunol 2: 557-568.
17. Weiskopf D, Weinberger B, Grubeck-Loebenstein B (2009) The aging of the immune system. Transpl Int 22: 1041-1050.
18. Nieman DC, Pedersen BK (1999) Exercise and immune function. Recent developments. Sports Med 27: 73-80.
19. Berk LS, Ton SA, Nieman DC, Eby EC (1986) The suppressive effect of stress from acute exhaustive exercise on T-lymphocyte helper/suppressor ratio in athletes and non-athletes. Med Sci Sports Exerc 18: 706–710.
20. Mackinnon LT, Hooper S (1994) Mucosal (secretory) immune system responses to exercise of varying intensity and during overtraining. Int J Sports Med 3: S179-183.
21. Nieman DC (1994) Exercise, upper respiratory tract infection, and the immune system. Med Sci Sports Exerc 26: 128-139.
22. Woods JA, Ceddia MA, Wolters BW, Evans JK, Lu Q, et al. (1999) Effects of 6 months of moderate aerobic exercise training on immune function in the elderly. Mech Ageing Dev 109: 1-19.
23. Crist DM, Mackinnon LT, Thompson RF, Atterbom HA, Egan PA (1989) Physical exercise increases natural cellular-mediated tumor cytotoxicity in elderly women. Gerontology 35: 66-71.
24. Nieman DC, Nehlsen-Cannarella SL, Markoff PA, Balk-Lamberton AJ, Yang H, et al. (1990) The effects of moderate exercise training on natural killer cells and acute upper respiratory tract infections. Int J Sports Med 11: 467-473.
25. Mosmann TR, Sad S (1996) The expanding universe of T-cell subsets: Th1, Th2 and more. Immunol Today 17: 138-146.
26. Fiorentino DF, Bond MW, Mosmann TR (1989) Two types of mouse T helper

cell. IV. Th2 clones secrete a factor that inhibits cytokine production by Th1 clones. J Exp Med 170: 2081-2095.

27. Haahr PM, Pedersen BK, Fomsgaard A, Tvede N, Diamant M, et al. (1991) Effect of physical exercise on in vitro production of interleukin 1, interleukin 6, tumour necrosis factor-alpha, interleukin 2 and interferon-gamma. Int J Sports Med 12: 223-227.

28. Lakier Smith L (2003) Overtraining, excessive exercise, and altered immunity: is this a T helper-1 versus T helper-2 lymphocyte response? Sports Med 33: 347-364.

29. Steensberg A, Toft AD, Bruunsgaard H, Sandmand M, Halkjaer-Kristensen J, et al. (2001) Strenuous exercise decreases the percentage of type 1 T cells in the circulation. J Appl Physiol 91: 1708-1712.

30. Mueller O, Villiger B, O'Callaghan B, Simon HU (2001) Immunological effects of competitive versus recreational sports in cross-country skiing. Int J Sports Med 22: 52-59.

31. Shimizu K, Kimura F, Akimoto T, Akama T, Tanabe K, et al. (2008) Effect of moderate exercise training on T-helper cell subpopulations in elderly people. Exerc Immunol Rev 14: 24-37.

32. Ru W, Peijie C (2009) Modulation of NKT cells and Th1/Th2 imbalance after alpha-GalCer treatment in progressive load-trained rats. Int J Biol Sci 5: 338-343.

33. Wesley JD, Robbins SH, Sidobre S, Kronenberg M, Terrizzi S, et al. (2005) Cutting edge: IFN-gamma signaling to macrophages is required for optimal Valpha14i NK T/NK cell cross-talk. J Immunol 174: 3864-3868.

34. Banchereau J, Briere F, Caux C, Davoust J, Lebecque S, et al. (2000) Immunobiology of dendritic cells. Annu Rev Immunol 18: 767-811.

35. Rissoan MC, Soumelis V, Kadowaki N, Grouard G, Briere F, et al. (1999) Reciprocal control of T helper cell and dendritic cell differentiation. Science 283: 1183-1186.

36. Chiang LM, Chen YJ, Chiang J, Lai LY, Chen YY, et al. (2007) Modulation of dendritic cells by endurance training. Int J Sports Med 28: 798-803.

37. Liao HF, Chiang LM, Yen CC, Chen YY, Zhuang RR, et al. (2006) Effect of a periodized exercise training and active recovery program on antitumor activity and development of dendritic cells. J Sports Med Phys Fitness 46: 307-314.

38. Pinzon-Charry A, Maxwell T, López JA (2005) Dendritic cell dysfunction in cancer: a mechanism for immunosuppression. Immunol Cell Biol 83: 451-461.

39. Villadangos JA, Heath WR (2005) Life cycle, migration and antigen presenting functions of spleen and lymph node dendritic cells: limitations of the Langerhans cells paradigm. Semin Immunol 17: 262-272.

Estimates of Critical Power and Anaerobic Work Capacity from a Single, All-Out Test of Less than 3-Min

Bergstrom HC[1]*, Housh TJ[1], Zuniga JM[2], Camic CL[3], Traylor DA[1], Lewis RW[1], Schmidt RJ[1] and Johnson GO[1]

[1]*Department of Nutrition and Health Sciences, University of Nebraska-Lincoln, USA*
[2]*School of Allied Health, Western New Mexico University, USA*
[3]*Department of Health & Physical Education, University of Wisconsin- Platteville, USA*

Abstract

The purpose of this study was to determine if Critical Power (CP) and Anaerobic Work Capacity (AWC) could be estimated from a single, all-out test of less than 3-min. Twenty-eight subjects (mean ± SD: age 23.3 ± 3.3 years, body mass 71.6 ± 16 kg) performed an incremental cycle ergometer test to exhaustion to determine peak oxygen consumption rate and heart rate peak. The 3-min all-out test was used to determine the criterion and six estimated values of CP and AWC. The criterion critical power (CP_{180}) and anaerobic work capacity (AWC_{180}) values were determined from the 3-min all-out test and were expressed as 30-s averages (155-180-s). The six estimated CP and AWC values were calculated from 30-s averages at decreasing 10-s intervals from 145 to 170-s (CP_{170} and AWC_{170}), 135 to 160-s (CP_{160} and AWC_{160}), 125 to 150-s (CP_{150} and AWC_{150}), 115 to 140-s (CP_{140} and AWC_{140}), 105 to 130-s (CP_{130} and AWC_{130}), and 95 to 120-s (CP_{120} and AWC_{120}). Mean differences, total error, constant error, standard error of the estimate, and correlations were used to compare the criterion to the estimated CP and AWC values. The results of the present study indicated that 150-s was the shortest test duration that resulted in non-significant differences between the criterion (CP_{180} and AWC_{180}) and estimated CP (CP_{150}) and AWC (AWC_{150}) values. The subsequent validation analyses showed that there were close agreements for the estimated CP_{150} and AWC_{150} versus the criterion (CP_{180} and AWC_{180}) values. Therefore, the current findings indicated that estimates of CP and AWC were not affected by shortening the test by 30-s. Reducing the length of the test to 2.5 minutes provides a less strenuous, yet valid protocol for estimating CP and AWC.

Keywords: Critical Power (CP); Anaerobic Work Capacity (AWC); All-out test

Introduction

The Critical Power (CP) test provides estimates of two parameters: CP and Anaerobic Work Capacity (AWC). Theoretically, CP represents the highest sustainable power output, while AWC is a measure of the total work that can be performed utilizing only stored energy sources within the muscle including Adenosine Triphosphate (ATP), phosphocreatine, glycogen, and the oxygen bound to myoglobin [1-3]. Critical power and AWC have been used to examine the effectiveness of exercise training programs [2,4-6], predict endurance exercise performance [5,7-9], examine the mechanisms of fatigue [4,10,11], describe the effects of prior exercise on performance [12,13], assess the exercise capacity of patients with COPD (chronic obstructive pulmonary disease) [14], determine the efficacy of nutritional supplements [15-19], examine fatigue thresholds [2,3,6,9,20,21], and demarcate the heavy from severe exercise intensity domains [9,21].

The original model of Moritani et al. [2] required three or four exhaustive workbouts on a cycle ergometer to estimate CP and AWC. One objective of exercise testing is to minimize the stress on the subject, while obtaining valid results [22]. Therefore, to improve its practicality, previous studies [10,21] have examined and modified the original CP test of Moritani et al. [2]. For example, Housh et al. [10] reported that instead of three or four workbouts, only two exhaustive workbouts were needed to accurately estimate CP and AWC. Recently, Vanhatalo et al. [21] showed that the 3-min all-out test, proposed by Burnley et al. [12], could be used to estimate CP and AWC. The protocol of Vanhatalo et al. [21], however, requires the measurement and analysis of expired gas samples during an incremental test to exhaustion on an electronically braked cycle ergometer, to determine the power output used for the 3-min all-out test [12,21]. Therefore, Bergstrom et al. [23] proposed that CP and AWC could be estimated from the 3-min all-out test and a single workbout by setting the resistance according to the subject's body weight. While both of the 3-min all-out tests of Vanhatalo et al. [21] and Bergstrom et al. [23] reduced the amount of time required to estimate CP and AWC, the demanding nature of an all-out test of 3-min duration may affect the motivation of the subjects to provide a maximal effort throughout the test and limit its application depending on the fitness level of the subjects.

Previous studies have suggested that it may be possible to estimate CP and AWC from an all-out test that is shorter than 3-min. For example, it has been suggested [24] that anaerobic work capacity reaches its maximum value within 2 min of all-out exercise. In addition, Burnley et al. [12] indicated that the power output at 2-min was not significantly different from the power output at the end of the 3-min all-out test. Thus, if the length of the test could be reduced, it would provide a less strenuous protocol to estimate CP and AWC. Therefore, the purpose of this study was to determine if accurate estimates of CP and AWC could be obtained from an all-out test of less than 3-min. Based on previous studies [12,24], we hypothesized that the all-out test could be shortened to 2-min without affecting the CP or AWC.

Methods

Subjects

Twenty-eight subjects (14 male and 14 female, mean ± SD: age

***Corresponding author:** Haley C Bergstrom, M.S., Department of Nutrition and Health Sciences, 110 Ruth Leverton Hall, University of Nebraska-Lincoln, Lincoln, NE 68583-0806
E-mail: hbergstrom@unlserve.unl.edu

23.3 ± 3.3 years, body mass 71.6 ± 16 kg, height 175.3 ± 10.2 cm) volunteered for this study. The subjects were moderately trained [22], and none were competitive cyclists. According to the American College of Sports Medicine [22], moderate training includes aerobic activity performed for a minimum of 30 min five times a week. Specifically, the subject's physical activities included running (n = 20), cycling (n = 14), and recreational sports (n = 6). This study was approved by the University Institutional Review Board for Human Subjects and all subjects completed a health history questionnaire and signed a written informed consent document before testing.

Procedures

Determination of $\dot{V}O_2$ peak and gas exchange threshold: Each participant performed an incremental test to exhaustion on a calibrated Lode (Corval V3, Groningen, the Netherlands) electronically-braked cycle ergometer at a pedal cadence of 70 rev·min^{-1}. The ergometer seat height was adjusted so that the subject's legs were near full extension at the bottom of the pedal revolution. Toe clips were used to maintain pedal contact throughout the test. All participants wore a nose clip and breathed through a 2-way valve (Hans Rudolph 2700 breathing valve, Kansas City, MO, USA). Expired gas samples were collected and analyzed using a calibrated TrueMax 2400 metabolic cart (Parvo Medics, Sandy, UT, USA). The gas analyzers were calibrated with room air and gases of known concentration prior to all testing sessions. The O_2, CO_2, and ventilatory parameters were expressed as 30-s averages [25]. The participants were fitted with a Polar Heart Watch system to record heart rate (Polar Electro Inc., Lake Success, NY). The test began at 50 W and the power output was increased by 30 W every 2 min until voluntary exhaustion or the subject's pedal rate fell below 70 rev·min^{-1} for more than 10 seconds, despite strong verbal encouragement. The $\dot{V}O_2$ peak was defined as the highest $\dot{V}O_2$ value in the last 30 s of the test that met two of the following three criteria [25]: 1) 90% of age-predicted maximum heart rate; 2) respiratory exchange ratio >1.1; and 3) a plateau of oxygen uptake (less than 150 mL·min^{-1} in $\dot{V}O_2$ over the last 30 s of the test).

The Gas Exchange Threshold (GET) was determined using the V-slope method described by Beaver et al. [26]. The GET was defined as the $\dot{V}O_2$ value corresponding to the intersection of two linear regression lines derived separately from the data points below and above the breakpoint in the $\dot{V}CO_2$ versus $\dot{V}O_2$ relationship.

Critical power 3-min all-out test: Critical power was determined on the calibrated Lode electronically-braked cycle ergometer, using the procedures of Vanhatalo et al. [21]. To be consistent with the terminology of Moritani et al. [2], the term CP was used to represent the End Power (EP) and AWC was used to represent work done above end power (WEP) as described by Vanhatalo et al. [21]. Each subject completed a warm-up at 50 W for 5-min followed by 5 min of rest. The test began with unloaded cycling at 90 rev·min^{-1} for 3 min followed by a 3 min all-out effort at the determined resistance. The participants were instructed to increase the pedaling cadence to 110 rev·min^{-1} in the last 5 s of the unloaded phase and then maintain the cadence as high as possible throughout the 3 min test. The resistance for the test was set using the linear mode of the electronically-braked cycle ergometer (linear factor = power/cadence^2). The linear factor was calculated as the power output halfway between $\dot{V}O_2$ peak and GET (GET + 50% Δ) divided by a cadence of 70 rev·min^{-1} squared [12,21]. Thus, the linear factor was equal to GET + 50% Δ / (70 rev·min^{-1})^2. To prevent pacing and ensure an all out effort, the participants were not made aware of the elapsed time and strong verbal encouragement was provided. The criterion measure of CP (CP_{180}) was the average power output over the final 30-s (155-s to 180-s) of the test and the criterion measure of AWC (AWC_{180}) was calculated as the integral of the power versus time relationship above CP [21]. Six estimated values of CP (CP_{170}, CP_{160}, CP_{150}, CP_{140}, CP_{130}, CP_{120}) and AWC (AWC_{170}, AWC_{160}, AWC_{150}, AWC_{140}, AWC_{130}, AWC_{120}) were also calculated from 30-s averages at decreasing 10-s time intervals from 170-s to 120-s (i.e., the estimates were calculated from 30-s averages from 145 to 170-s, 135 to 160-s, 125 to 150-s, 115 to 140-s, 105 to 130-s, and 95 to 120-s).

Statistical analyses: Mean differences among the criterion and estimated CP and AWC values were compared with separate one-way repeated measures ANOVAs at an alpha of $p < 0.05$. *Post-hoc* comparisons were performed using paired *t*-tests at a Bonferroni corrected alpha of $p < 0.0071$ (0.05/7) (Table 1). Separate zero-order correlation matrices were used to determine the relationships among the criterion and estimated CP and AWC values (Tables 2 and 3). Further validation analyses were based on the evaluation of the criterion versus estimated CP and AWC via calculations of the total error (TE $= \sqrt{\sum[criterion - estimated]^2 / n}$), constant error (CE = criterion – estimated), standard error of the estimate (SEE (Standard Error of the Estimate) = SD $\sqrt{1-r^2}$), correlations between CE and criterion values, and the similarity between the standard deviations of the criterion and estimated values (Table 4). In addition, the data have been presented using the method of Bland and Altman [27]. The analyses were conducted using Statistical Package for the Social Sciences software (v.19.0. SPSS Inc., Chicago, Illinois, USA).

The following criteria were used in the present study to evaluate the results of the validation analyses: (a) the mean values for the criterion CP and AWC should not be significantly different from the estimated values; (b) there should be close similarity between the TE and SEE; (c) there should be no significant correlation between the CE and the criterion measures; (d) there should be a high correlation between the criterion and estimated values; (e) there should be close agreement between the standard deviation values of the criterion and estimated values.

Results

The mean (± SD) $\dot{V}O_2$ peak for the subjects in this study was 42.2 ± 7.1 mL·kg^{-1}·min^{-1} and the maximal power output for the incremental test to exhaustion was 231 ± 51 W. In addition, the GET (27.7 ± 5.2 mL·kg^{-1}·min^{-1}) occurred at 66% of $\dot{V}O_2$ peak and 60% of maximal power output (139 ± 37 W).

A one-way repeated measures ANOVA indicated that there were no significant differences among CP_{180} (187 ± 47 W), CP_{170} (189 ± 49 W), CP_{160} (191 ± 50 W), CP_{150} (192 ± 51 W), and CP_{140} (193 ± 51 W) (Table 1). In addition, no significant differences were found among AWC_{180} (10.2 ± 3.4 kJ), AWC_{170} (9.9 ± 3.5 kJ), AWC_{160} (9.7 ± 3.4 kJ), and AWC_{150} (9.5 ± 3.3 kJ) (Table 1). Thus, 150-s was the shortest test duration that resulted in non-significant differences between both the criterion (CP_{180} and AWC_{180}) and estimated CP (CP_{150}) and AWC (AWC_{150}) values (Figure 1). Therefore, the subsequent validation analyses were performed between the estimated CP_{150} and AWC_{150} values versus the criterion values (CP_{180} and AWC_{180}) (Table 4). The SEE and TE values for CP were 9 W and 10 W, respectively. The SEE and TE values for AWC were 1.2 kJ and 1.4 kJ, respectively. The TE represented 5.5% and 13.7% of the mean values for the CP_{180} and AWC_{180} values, respectively. In addition, there were non-significant ($p > 0.05$) correlations for the CE versus CP_{180} (r = -0.24) and the CE versus AWC_{180} (r = 0.27) (Figures 2 and 3). The CP_{180} was highly

Time (s)	180	170	160	150	140	130	120
CP (W)	187 ± 47	189 ± 49	191 ± 50	192 ± 51	193 ± 51	196 ± 52*	199 ± 54*
AWC (kJ)	10.2 ± 3.4	9.9 ± 3.5	9.7 ± 3.4	9.5 ± 3.3	9.3 ± 3.1†	9.0 ± 3.0†	8.8 ± 3.1†

significantly different from CP_{180} at a Bonferroni corrected alpha of $p < 0.0071$ (0.05/7)
† significantly different from AWC_{180} at a Bonferroni corrected alpha of $p < 0.0071$ (0.05/7)

Table 1: Mean (± SD) values for six estimated (170-s, 160-s, 150-s, 140-s, 130-s, and 120-s) and criterion (180-s) measures of Critical Power (CP) and Anaerobic Work Capacity (AWC).

	CP_{180}	CP_{170}	CP_{160}	CP_{150}	CP_{140}	CP_{130}	CP_{120}
CP_{180}	1.00						
CP_{170}	1.00	1.00					
CP_{160}	0.99	1.00	1.00				
CP_{150}	0.98	0.99	1.00	1.00			
CP_{140}	0.98	0.98	0.99	1.00	1.00		
CP_{130}	0.97	0.97	0.98	0.98	1.00	1.00	
CP_{120}	0.96	0.96	0.97	0.97	0.99	1.00	1.00

Table 2: Correlation matrix for Critical Power (CP) among the estimated (CP_{170}, CP_{160}, CP_{150}, CP_{140}, CP_{130}, CP_{120}) and criterion (CP_{180}) values.

	AWC_{180}	AWC_{170}	AWC_{160}	AWC_{150}	AWC_{140}	AWC_{130}	AWC_{120}
AWC_{180}	1.00						
AWC_{170}	0.98	1.00					
AWC_{160}	0.96	0.99	1.00				
AWC_{150}	0.93	0.97	0.99	1.00			
AWC_{140}	0.91	0.93	0.97	0.98	1.00		
AWC_{130}	0.88	0.89	0.93	0.94	0.98	1.00	
AWC_{120}	0.79	0.81	0.84	0.86	0.92	0.96	1.00

Table 3: Correlation matrix for Anaerobic Work Capacity (AWC) among the estimated (AWC_{170}, AWC_{160}, AWC_{150}, AWC_{140}, AWC_{130}, and AWC_{120}) and criterion (AWC_{180}) values.

	Constant Error (CE)	Stadard Error of the Estimate (SEE)	Total Error (TE)
CP_{150} vs. CP_{180}	-5 W	9 W	10 W
AWC_{150} vs. AWC_{180}	0.7 kJ	1.2 kJ	1.4 kJ

Table 4: Validation analyses (n = 28) for the estimated critical power (CP_{150}) and anaerobic work capacity (AWC_{150}) values versus the criterion CP_{180} and AWC_{180}.

correlated with the estimated CP_{150} (r = 0.98) (Table 2). There was also a high correlation (r = 0.93) between AWC_{180} and the estimated AWC_{150} (Table 3). Furthermore, the standard deviations for the CP_{180} (47 W) and AWC_{180} (3.4 kJ) values were similar to those of the estimated CP_{150} (51 W) and AWC_{150} (3.3 kJ) values.

Discussion

The results of the present study, as well as those of previous studies [12,24], suggested that it is possible to estimate CP and AWC from a single, all-out workbout of less than 3 minutes duration. For example, Burnley et al. [12] indicated that there was no significant change in power output over the last minute of the 3-min test (120 to 180-s) and suggested that it may be possible to estimate CP from a shorter test. During the 3-min all-out test, Burnley et al. [12] found that the power output at 120-s was only 5 W (2%) greater than the power output at 180-s. Furthermore, when 30-s averages were considered, Burnley et al. [12] reported that average power outputs after 135-s were not significantly different from the final power output. In addition, Medbø et al. [24] found that the treadmill analog of AWC for cycle ergometry called the Anaerobic Running Capacity (ARC), was equal to the maximal accumulated oxygen deficit (oxygen deficit = the difference between oxygen demand and oxygen uptake) during exhaustive running for 2-min at supramaximal intensities. Thus, Medbø et al. [24] suggested that anaerobic stores were exhausted and, therefore, ARC would not change significantly after 2-min of an all-out test. The current findings indicated that there were no significant differences between the estimated CP_{150} and AWC_{150} and the criterion CP_{180} and AWC_{180} values, respectively. These non-significant differences were evaluated as 30-s averages beginning at 2-min and, thus, supported the findings of Burnley et al. [12] and Medbø et al. [24]. Therefore, the results of the present study indicated that the 3-min all-out test could be shortened to 2.5-min without affecting the estimated values for CP and AWC. Reducing the length of the test by 30-s, results in a less strenuous protocol to estimate CP and AWC.

The results of the validation analyses in the present study provided additional support for shortening the all-out test from 3 to 2.5-min. For example, the power output at CP_{150} was only 2.7% (CE = -5 W) greater than the power output at CP_{180} and the AWC_{150} value was 6.9% (CE = 0.7 kJ) lower than the AWC_{180} value. In addition, there were high correlations between CP_{150} and CP_{180} (r = 0.98), as well as AWC_{150} and AWC_{180} (r = 0.93). Furthermore, the SD values for CP_{150} and AWC_{150} (51W and 3.3 kJ, respectively) were 4 W greater and 0.1 kJ less than the SD values for CP_{180} and AWC_{180} (47 W and 3.4 kJ, respectively). Thus, these findings indicated that there were close agreements between the estimated and criterion CP and AWC values.

The SEE for CP_{150} and AWC_{150} were 4.8% and 11.8% of the mean CP_{180} and AWC_{180}, respectively. The TE for CP_{150} and AWC_{150} were 5.5% and 13.7% of the mean CP_{180} and AWC_{180}, respectively. The differences between the estimated and criterion SEE and TE values were 1 W and 0.2 kJ for CP and AWC, respectively. In the present study, the close similarity between the SEE and TE was due, primarily, to the small CE values.

Bland and Altman plots [27] were used to describe the distributions of the CE versus criterion (CP_{180} and AWC_{180}) values (Figures 2 and 3). Figures 2 and 3 indicated that the CE values remained stable across the criterion measures. Furthermore, the correlation coefficients (r) for the CE values versus CP_{180} and AWC_{180} were not significantly different from zero at r = -0.24 and r = 0.27, respectively. Thus, the current findings indicated that the magnitude of the CE values were not affected by the subject's levels of CP or AWC.

Conclusions

The 3-min all-out test has been proposed as a less time consuming alternative to the original multiple exhaustive workbout model of Moritani et al. [2] for estimating CP and AWC. The demanding nature of this test, however, limits its practicality. Thus, we examined the accuracy of CP and AWC estimates from shorter test durations. The results of the present study showed that there were no significant mean differences and close agreements between CP_{150} and CP_{180}, as well as between AWC_{150} and AWC_{180}. Therefore, the current findings indicated that estimates of CP and AWC were not affected by shortening the test by 30-s. Reducing the length of the test provides a less strenuous, yet valid protocol for estimating CP and AWC. Future studies should examine the metabolic responses and times to exhaustion at CP determined from the 2.5-min all-out test and validate the 2.5-min protocol against other fatigue thresholds.

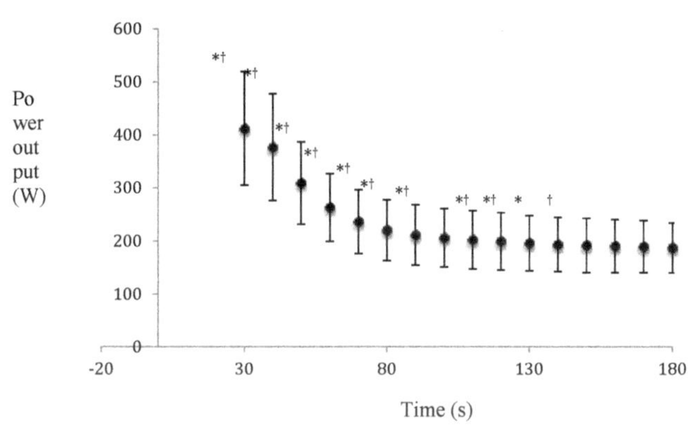

Figure 1: Mean (± SD) 30-s averaged power outputs for all subjects (n = 28) during the 3-min all-out critical power (CP) test. The error bars indicate standard deviations. The asterisks indicate a significant difference in CP estimates from the criterion (CP_{180}) and the crosses (†) indicate a significant difference in anaerobic work capacity (AWC) estimates from the criterion (AWC_{180}). The results indicated that 150-s was the shortest test duration that resulted in non-significant differences between the criterion (CP_{180} and AWC_{180}) and estimated CP (CP_{150}) and AWC (AWC_{150}) values.

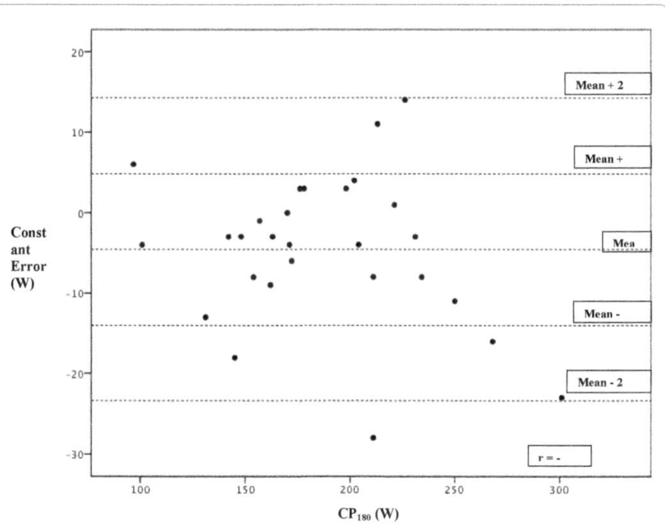

Figure 2: The relationship (n = 28) between constant errorr (CE) and the criterion critical power (CP_{180}) values.

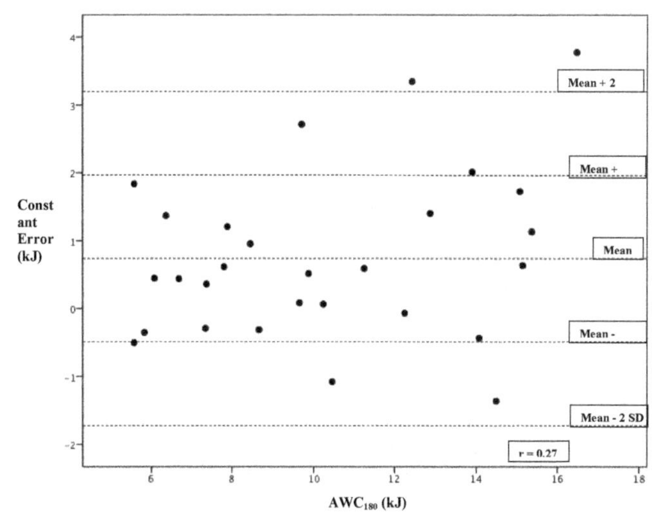

Figure 3: The relationship (n = 28) between constant errorr (CE) and the criterion anaerobic work capacity (AWC_{180}) values.

References

1. Monod H, Scherrer J (1965) The work capacity of a synergic muscular group. Ergonomics 8: 329-338.
2. Moritani T, Nagata A, deVries HA, Muro M (1981) Critical power as measure of physical work capacity and anaerobic threshold. Ergonomics 24: 339-350.
3. Poole DC, Ward AW, Gardner GW, Whipp BJ (1988) Metabolic and respiratory profile of the upper limit for prolonged exercise in man. Ergonomics 31: 1265-1279.
4. Brickley G, Doust J, Williams CA (2002) Physiological responses during exercise to exhaustion at critical power. Eur J Appl Physiol 88: 146-151.
5. Francis JT, Quinn TJ, Amann M, LaRoche DP (2010) Defining intensity domains from the end power of a 3-min all-out cycling test. Med Sci Sports Exerc 42: 1769-1775.
6. Jenkins DG, Quigley BM (1990) Blood lactate in trained cyclists during ergometry at critical power. Eur J Appl Physiol Occup Physiol 61: 278-283.
7. Hill DW, Smith JC (1999) Determination of critical power by pulmonary gas exchange. Can J Appl Physiol 24: 74-86.
8. Housh DJ, Housh TJ, Bauge SM (1989) The accuracy of the critical power test for predicting time to exhaustion during cycle ergometery. Ergonomics 32: 997-1004.
9. McClave SA, LeBlanc M, Hawkins SA (2011) Sustainablility of critical power determined by a 3-minute all-out test in elite cyclists. J Strength Cond Res 25: 3093-3098.
10. Housh DJ, Housh TJ, Bauge SM (1990) A methodological consideration for the determination of critical power and anaerobic work capacity. Res Q Exercise Sport 61: 406-409.
11. Housh TJ, deVries HA, Housh DJ, Tichy MW, Smyth KD, et al. (1991) The relationship between critical power and the onset of blood lactate accumulation. J Sports Med Phys Fit 31: 31-36.
12. Burnley, M, Doust JH, Vanhatalo A (2006) A 3-min all-out test to determine peak oxygen uptake and the maximal steady state. Med Sci Sports Exerc 38: 1995-2003.

13. Vanhatalo A, Jones AM (2008) Influence of prior sprint exercise on the parameters of the 'all-out critical power test' in men. Exp Physiol 94: 255-263.

14. Neder JA, Jones PW, Nery LE, Whipp BJ (2000) Determinants of the exercise endurance capacity in patients with chronic obstructive pulmonary disease: The power-duration relationship. Am J Respir Crit Care Med 162: 497-504.

15. Eckerson JM, Stout JR, Moore GA, Stone NJ, Nishimura K, et al. (2004) Effect of two and five days of creatine loading on anaerobic working capacity in women. J Strength Cond Res 18: 168-173.

16. Eckerson JM, Stout JR, Moore GA, Stone NJ, Iwan KA, et al. (2005) Effect of creatine phosphate supplementation on anaerobic working capacity and body weight after two and six days of loading in men and women. J Strength Cond Res 19: 756- 763.

17. Kendall KL, Smith AE, Graef JL, Fukuda DH, Moon JR, et al. (2009) Effects of four weeks of high intensity interval training and creatine supplementation on critical power and anaerobic working capacity in college-aged men. J Strength Cond Res 23: 1663-1669.

18. Stout JR, Eckerson JM, Housh TJ, Ebersole KT (1999) The effects of creatine supplementation on anaerobic working capacity. J Strength Cond Res 13: 135-138.

19. Vanhatalo A, Jones AM (2009) Influence of creatine supplementation on the parameters of the all-out critical power test. J Exerc Sci Fit 7: 9–17.

20. Jones AM, Wilkerson DP, DiMenna F, Fulford J, Poole DC (2007) Muscle metabolic responses to exercise above and below the "critical power" assessed using 31P-MRS. Am J Physiol Regul Integr Comp Physiol 294: R585-593.

21. Vanhatalo A, Doust DH, Burnley M (2007) Determination of critical power using a 3-min all-out cycling test. Med Sci Sports Exerc 39: 548-555.

22. Thompson WR, Gordon NF, Pescatello LS (2010) American College of Sports Medicine: ACSM's guidelines for exercise testing and prescription (8th ed). Lippincott Williams Wilkins, Philadelphia PA.

23. Bergstrom HC, Housh TJ, Zuniga JM, Camic CL, Traylor DA, et al. (2012) A new single work bout test to estimate critical power and anaerobic work capacity. J Strength Cond Res 3: 656-663.

24. Medbø JI, Mohn AC, Tabata I, Bahr R, Vaage O, et al. (1988) Anaerobic capacity determined by maximal accumulated O_2 deficit. J Appl Physiol 64: 50-60.

25. Day JR, Rossiter HB, Coats EM, Skasick A, Whipp BJ (2003) The maximally attainable VO_2 during exercise in humans: The peak vs. maximum issue. J Appl Physiol 95: 1901-1907.

26. Beaver WL, Wasserman K, Whipp BJ (1986) A new method for detecting anaerobic threshold by gas exchange. J Appl Physiol 60: 2020-2027.

27. Bland JM, Altman DG (1986) Statistical methods for assessing agreement between two methods of clinical measurement. Lancet 1: 307-310.

Effect of Training Surface on Agility and Passing Skills of Prepubescent Female Volleyball Players

Eugenia Gortsila[1], Apostolos Theos[1], Goran Nesic[2] and Maria Maridaki[1]*

[1]*Department of Physical Education & Sports Science, National & Kapodistrian University of Athens, Greece*
[2]*Faculty of Sport and Physical Education, University of Belgrade, Serbia*

Abstract

The purpose of the present study was to investigate the effect of different training surfaces (hard or sand surface) on agility and passing skills of prepubescent female volleyball players. 45 prepubescent girls (age: 11.1 ± 0.5 years) participated in this study and were separated in three groups. Groups S (N=15) and I (N=15) consisted of volleyball players, while group C (N=15) consisted of girls that had no volleyball training experience. All groups participated in a 10-week (3 days/week) volleyball training program that included technical and passing skills exercises. The program of groups S and I also included jumping and sprinting exercises. The training program of group S was conducted on sand surface, while groups I and C trained on hard surface. Measurements of agility (T-test and 505-test) and passing skills were conducted on both hard and sand surface before, in the middle (5th week) and after the end of the training program for groups S and I. Group C was tested only on hard surface before and after the training period. Data were analyzed using two-way ANOVA for independent samples. Agility T-test and 505-test were significantly ($p<0.001$) improved in all three groups after the 10-week training program. Agility improvement of group S was significantly ($p<0.001$) greater than the other two groups (I and C), regardless of the surface (hard or sand) that the test was executed. Group S achieved greater improvements than the other two groups in passing skills too. All three groups were significantly ($p<0.001$) improved in overhead and forearm passing accuracy after the 10-week training period, but it was group S that achieved the greatest improvement, regardless of the (hard or sand) that the test was executed. In conclusion training on sand surface could be a useful and effective tool for improving agility and passing skills in prepubescent female volleyball players.

Keywords: T-test; 505-test; Sand surface; Overhead pass; Forearm pass

Introduction

Volleyball is a competitive sport played on many different court surfaces depending on whether it is being conducted indoors or outdoors. Thus indoor volleyball is played upon a hard flat surface that is mostly made out of wood or other synthetic materials, while outdoor volleyball is played upon concrete, grass or most commonly sand.

Strength and muscle power of both upper and lower extremities as well as neuromuscular coordination and technical skills are elements that a good volleyball player aims to develop [1]. Several studies have investigated the anthropometric and physiological characteristics of both teenage and adult volleyball players and their impact on volleyball performance [1-5].

Agility is recognized as the ability to maintain and control body's position while rapidly moving and changing directions as a response to a stimulus [6,7]. It seems to be related to athletic abilities like strength, power, speed and balance and it's a determinant of sport performance in field and court sports like volleyball, soccer and rugby [6-8,10,11].

T-test is a well accepted standard agility test that is easy to administer, since it does not require complex equipment and long hours of preparation [11,12]. Pauole et al. evaluated the reliability and validity of the T-test as a measure of leg power, leg speed and agility in college students [13]. T-test performance was highly associated with all three performed skill tests (40-yard dash, counter-movement vertical jump and hexagon test) [13]. Thus T-test appeared to be a highly reliable tool in measuring a combination of physical components including agility, speed and power of lower limbs [13]. Especially in volleyball Barnes et al. showed that countermovement jumping ability is correlated with agility and can be used as a predictor of agility test time [11]. More recently Sassi et al. tried to establish a modified agility T-test and showed that is still highly correlated to countermovement jump and 10m sprint highlighting the significance of agility on sport performance [12].

505-test is also a reliable and valid test for the evaluation of agility in many sports but it requires the use of dual beam electronic timing gates (photocells) [14,15]. Gabbett et al. investigated the relationship among speed, change of direction speed and reactive agility in forty-two rugby league players and showed that 505-test is the most reliable ($r=0.90$, typical error of measurement=1.9%) of all change of direction speed tests conducted in their study [16]. Furthermore they concluded that 505-test simulates the "general" movement patterns in team sports like rugby, basketball and volleyball. In accordance Gabbett reported that 505-test is a reliable and valid test ($r=0.84$, typical error of measurement=1.9%) for the evaluation of agility in female rugby players and concluded that it can be used in both sexes [15].

Technical skills like serving, spiking, setting, blocking and passing accuracy along with tactical skills seem to play a critical role in volleyball performance [17]. Gabbett et al. evaluated the technical skills of junior volleyball players before and after an 8-week skill-based training program [18]. Investigators reported that training induced significant improvements in spiking, setting and passing accuracy and spiking and passing technique. The above mentioned study along with many other volleyball studies were all conducted on hard-court surface and according to our knowledge there is little or no research regarding the influence of different training surfaces on volleyball performance

***Corresponding author:** Maria Maridaki, Associate Professor, Department of Physical Education & Sports Science, National & Kapodistrian University of Athens, Greece, E-mail: mmarida@phed.uoa.gr

[11,18-21]. Furthermore in all the above mentioned studies the physiological and technical characteristics of volleyball players were evaluated on hard- court surface and there are no studies investigating volleyball performance and characteristics on sand surface. Therefore the purpose of the present study was to investigate the effect of different training surfaces (hard or sand surface) on agility and passing skills of prepubescent female volleyball players.

Methods

Participants

Thirty female prepubescent volleyball players took part in this study and were randomly allocated in two groups (Table 1). Group S (N=15) participated in a 10 week training programme on sand surface, while group I (N=15) participated in a same programme on hard surface indoors. Maturity status was also evaluated (Table 1) according to Tanner's scale [22]. None of the girls had experienced menstruation before or reported any menstruation signs during the study.

All participants were randomly recruited from regional volleyball teams of Athens and had a volleyball training experience of at least two years. Participants and their parents were informed on the purposes of the study, the methods and the possible risks involved and informed consents were signed by the children's parents. A third training group (N=15), that served as control (Group C, Table 1) and had no volleyball training experience was recruited from elementary schools and exercised in volleyball three times per week (45 minute-training session) for 10 weeks according to the program of the Greek Ministry of Education.

Procedures

Measurements of agility and passing skills were conducted in groups S and I before the beginning of the 10-week training program, in the middle of it (end of the 5th week) and right after the end of it, while group C conducted agility and skill tests only before and after the end of the 10-week training program. Participants of groups S and I were tested on both hard surface indoors and on the sand, on the same court surfaces that were used for training, while participants of group C were tested only on hard surface indoors.

The 10 week- training program for groups S and I included three 90 minute-training sessions per week separated by at least a 1-day interval and the level of difficulty and complexity of the exercises were gradually increased during the training program (Table 2). Each training session consisted of exercises aiming to improve technical skills in overhead and forearm pass and agility. Weekly training plan was designed according to guidelines described elsewhere [23-25]. T-test and 505 agility tests were used in order to assess agility and time was recorded with the use of photocells [13,14]. For the evaluation of passing skills, overhead passing test and forearm passing test were conducted [26,27]. Participants were fully familiarized with the testing procedure a week before the beginning of the training program and the best out of two trials was recorded for each test [28]. All tests were executed in a random and balanced order and subjects had the chance to fully recover in between tests.

Statistical analysis

Comparisons between and within groups (C, S and I) for agility and passing skills were performed by two-way ANOVA (groups x time) for independent samples. Significant differences between means were determined using Tukey's Post hoc tests. Statistical analysis was performed using the SPSS statistical package (SPSS, v. 17, Chicago, IL). Results are presented as mean ± standard deviation.

Results

Anthropometrical data of the subjects are presented in Table 1 and there was no significant difference between participants in groups S and I in body height ($p = 0.72$), body mass ($p = 0.27$), chronological age ($p = 0.74$) and Tanner stage for pubic hair ($p = 0.80$) and genitals development ($p = 0.84$).

Agility

The changes in agility T-test over the 10-week training program are presented in Table 3. Training induced significant ($p<0.001$)

Groups	Age (years)	Body weight (kg)	Body height (cm)	Tanner Stage (P)	Tanner Stage (G)
S (N=15)	11.2 ± 0.6	40.8 ± 6.8	151.6 ± 7.1	2.3 ± 0.1	2.1 ± 0.1
I (N=15)	11.3 ± 0.6	39.9 ± 6.4	151.3 ± 7.5	2.3 ± 0.1	2.1 ± 0.1
C (N=15)	10.8 ± 0.2	35.4 ± 6.0	147.0 ± 7.4	-	-

Tanner stage (P): Tanner stage for pubic hair

Tanner stage (G): Tanner stage genitals development

Table 1: Subjects anthropometrical characteristics *(mean ± SD).*

	Groups S and I		Group C
Warm-up	15-min general activity		10-min general activity
Main part	15-min speed and jumping exercises	45-min technical and passing skills exercises	30-min technical and passing skills exercises
Cool-down	15-min cool-down and stretching		5-min cool-down and stretching

Table 2: Training program used over the 10 weeks for all three groups.

Groups	Pre-training		5th week		Post-training	
	Hard	Sand	Hard	Sand	Hard	Sand
S	15.3 ± 0.4	18.0 ± 0.5	14.4 ± 0.5*§	16.8 ± 0.6*§	13.2 ± 0.2*§	15.0 ± 0.5*§
I	15.1 ± 0.6	18.1 ± 0.8	14.7 ± 0.6*	17.6 ± 0.7*	14.4 ± 0.6*	17.2 ± 0.7*
C	15.3 ± 1.0				15.1 ± 1.1*	

*p<0.001 from the pre-training value

§p<0.001 from group I

Table 3: Performance time (sec) in agility T-test for all three groups before (pre), in the middle (5th wk) and after the end (post) of the 10-week training program *(mean ± SD).*

improvements of performance time in both groups (S and I) and in both courts (hard and sand surface) even from the 5th week. The % improvement achieved from group S at the end of the training program was significantly greater than the one achieved from group I (Group S=13.8 ± 1.6% vs. group I = 4.9 ± 1.2%, $p < 0.001$). When tested on sand surface the % improvement achieved from group S was even greater (Group S = 16.5 ± 1.7% vs. group I = 4.7 ± 0.9%, $p < 0.001$). Group C also showed a slight but significant improvement over the 10-week training period (1.0 ± 0.4%, $p < 0.001$).

The changes in 505 agility test over the 10-week training program are presented in Table 4. Training induced significant ($p<0.001$) improvements of performance time in both groups (S and I) and in both courts (hard and sand surface) even from the 5th week. The % improvement achieved from group S at the end of the training program was significantly greater than the one achieved from group I (Group S=13.8 ± 0.7% vs. group I=4.7 ± 0.7%, $p<0.001$). When tested on sand surface the % improvement achieved from group S was even greater (Group S=14.4 ± 0.9% vs. group I=4.3 ± 0.8%, $p<0.001$). Group C also showed a slight but significant improvement over the 10-week training period (1.3 ± 1.0%, $p<0.001$).

Passing skills

The changes in overhead passing skills over the 10-week training program are shown in Table 5. All three groups were significantly improved after the training period (Group S=39.7 ± 7.5%, group I=13.5 ± 3.7% and group C=12.0 ± 9.1%, $p<0.001$) with group S showing the greater improvement and differing significantly from the other two groups ($p < 0.001$). When tested on sand surface group S showed even greater improvement (47.9 ± 5.9%) and differed significantly from group I (9.6 ± 6.0%, $p<0.001$).

Forearm passing skills were also significantly ($p<0.001$) improved in all three groups after the 10-week training period (Table 6). The % improvement of group S was 56.6 ± 7.5% and differed significantly ($p<0.001$) from the other two groups (Group I=16.9 ± 5.1% and group C=11.3 ± 10.5%). When tested on sand surface group S showed a slightly smaller improvement (48.3 ± 9.7%) compared to the % improvement shown on hard surface, but still remained significantly different from group I (12.3 ± 5.2%, $p<0.001$).

Discussion

The main findings of the present study were that a) agility improved significantly more in the S group compared to the I group after the 10-week training program, b) passing skills were also improved significantly more in the S group compared to the I group after the 10-week training program, highlighting the importance of training surface. Factors such as height and body mass are of great importance and have a significant impact on performance while training during the developmental stages of growth and maturity [29,30]. In our study subjects does not differ in any of their anthropometric characteristics neither before nor after the 10-week training program. Therefore differences between groups in agility and passing skills should be attributed to the impact of training surface.

Improvements in speed, power and balance seem to improve agility [6,8,9,16]. In a more recent study Sassi et al. tried to investigate the relationship of agility T-test to the countermovement jump (CMJ) and the 10m straight sprint and therefore they tested 86 subjects [12]. The

Groups	Pre-training		5th week		Post-training	
	Hard	Sand	Hard	Sand	Hard	Sand
S	3.45 ± 0.07	3.55 ± 0.09	3.25 ± 0.12*	3.32 ± 0.10*§	2.98 ± 0.06*§	3.04 ± 0.07*§
I	3.34 ± 0.15	3.50 ± 0.11	3.25 ± 0.12*	3.40 ± 0.11*	3.18 ± 0.14*	3.35 ± 0.11*
C	3.41 ± 0.18				3.36 ± 0.20*	

*p<0.001 from the pre-training value

§p<0.001 from group I

Table 4: Performance time (sec) in 505 agility test for all three groups before (pre), in the middle (5th wk) and after the end (post) of the 10-week training program *(mean ± SD)*.

Groups	Pre-training		5th week		Post-training	
	Hard	Sand	Hard	Sand	Hard	Sand
S	15.0 ± 1.0†	11.5 ± 0.8	18.2 ± 1.0*§	14.2 ± 0.9*§	20.9 ± 0.8*§†	16.9 ± 0.7*§
I	14.9 ± 0.9†	11.9 ± 0.9	15.8 ± 1.1*	12.6 ± 0.9*	16.9 ± 1.1*†	12.9 ± 0.9*
C	8.2 ± 1.8				9.1 ± 2.0*	

*p<0.001 from the pre-training value

§p<0.001 from group I

†p<0.001 from group C

Table 5: Overhead passing skills score for all three groups before (pre), in the middle (5th wk) and after the end (post) of the 10-week training program *(mean ± SD)*.

Groups	Pre-training		5th week		Post-training	
	Hard	Sand	Hard	Sand	Hard	Sand
S	18.6 ± 1.1†	15.3 ± 1.0	22.2 ± 1.4*§	18.9 ± 1.3*§	†29.1 ± 1.0*§	22.7 ± 0.9*§
I	18.2 ± 1.3†	15.3 ± 1.3	19.5 ± 1.6*	16.7 ± 1.6*	†21.3 ± 1.6*	17.2 ± 1.4*
C	8.4 ± 1.7				9.1 ± 1.7*	

*p< 0.001 from the pre-training value

§p< 0.001 from group I

†p<0.001 from group C

Table 6: Forearm passing skills score for all three groups before (pre), in the middle (5th wk) and after the end (post) of the 10-week training program *(mean ± SD)*.

results showed that there is a strong negative correlation between agility T-test and CMJ (r=-0.74) and agility T-test and 10m straight sprint (r=-0.78). Such a strong negative correlation between CMJ and agility was also reported in previous studies [8,11]. In accordance Sekulic et al. reported that speed and power are the most significant predictors of agility, especially in women [10].

In our study the 10-week training program included jumping (CMJ and Squat Jump) and sprinting exercises. Even in the technical skills training part, that was the major part of each training session; all exercises were designed and conducted in a constant move with sudden changes of direction and short sprints (2-3 m). Such a training intervention is supposed to improve jumping ability and power resulting in significant improvements in agility, like the ones we observed in our study in both groups (S and I). In the S group, in particular, the improvement in both agility tests (T-test and 505-test) was significantly greater than the one observed in the I group, regardless of the surface upon which the tests were performed (sand or indoors). The absorption and energy release upon different ground surfaces have been examined by several researchers in the past [31]. Lejeune et al. used oxygen consumption along with video analysis in order to determine the mechanical work and the energy cost of walking and running on sand and on firm surface [32]. The results of this research showed that walking on the sand requires 1.6-2.5 times more mechanical work than walking with the same speed on a hard surface while running on the sand requires 1.15 times more mechanical work than running with the same speed on a hard surface. In accordance, in a recent study Gaudino et al. reported that the energy cost of sprinting on dry, soft sand was 30% greater than the values achieved while sprinting on grass or artificial grass [33].

The above mentioned results lead us to the assumption that the relative intensity of the exercises conducted by the S group on sand surface was higher than the relative intensity of the same exercises conducted by the I group on hard surface indoors. Differences in relative intensity of the exercises induce different training adaptations and therefore may explain the greater agility improvement observed in the S group.

Furthermore a non solid ground, like sand, may evoke changes in the neuromuscular junctions [31]. An unstable surface may lead to repeated losses of balance, which in turn and in order to avoid falling may promote neuromuscular communication and therefore improve balance [34,35]. But as it was mentioned before balance is correlated to agility and any improvements in balance would lead to improvements in agility [10]. Hence the greater agility improvement of group S may be the result of improvements in balance, which occurred due to the non solid of the training surface.

In our study the major part of each training session included exercises aiming to improve technical and more specifically passing skills. In a previous study Gabbett et al. reported significant improvements (40-76%) of overhead passing, forearm passing and attacking after an 8-week training program [18]. In accordance groups S and I improved their forearm and overhead passing skills, after the 10-week training program, but group S showed significantly greater improvement compared to group I. A possible explanation for the above mentioned results could be that subjects in group S increased their arm strength more than subjects in group I during the 10-week training program and therefore managed to perform better in passing skills tests.

Arms seem to significantly contribute to jumping performance and power despite the fact that when running they seem to contribute only 1% to total mass center acceleration and propulsion [36,37]. According to Lees & Barton arms contribute more than 12% in total vertical momentum in case of vertical jumping while even in running Hamner et al. and Pontzer et al. reported that arms counterbalance changes in angular momentum of the legs and reduce torso rotations [37-39]. Therefore arms seem to play a critical role when sprinting or jumping on sand counterbalancing angular momentum and retaining balance.

In the present study training on sand surface could result on greater contribution of the arms to sprinting and jumping and therefore a greater increase on arm strength. When sprinting on sand surface and because of the instability of the ground, there are no changes on stride frequency but there is a significant reduction on stride length and a larger number of surface contacts are needed in order to cover the same distance [33]. Consequently the larger number of strides during sprinting or the lower contribution of plantar flexion during jumping on sand surface would result in more arm swinging movements and possible greater strength gains [31]. Although we did not measure arm strength a possible greater increase of it in group S could explain differences observed in passing skills between groups S and I.

Conclusion

In conclusion the present study showed that training on sand surface could be a useful and effective tool for improving agility and passing skills in prepubescent female volleyball players. Agility was significantly improved in both groups after the 10-week training program, because each training session included sprinting and jumping exercises. Even passing drills during training were conducted in constant movement and included short sprints and changes of direction. The greater % improvement observed in group S should be attributed to the increased energy cost of moving on sand surface and therefore the greater effort needed when sprinting or jumping that possibly induced larger increases in strength compared to group I. The instability of the sand surface also seems to promote improvements of balance, which in turn improve agility. Furthermore, when sprinting and jumping on the sand, arms seem to contribute more to performance result and therefore training on the sand could enhance strength improvements. Although we did not measure arm strength in our study, differences in passing skills between groups should be attributed to possible greater arm strength gains achieved by group S.

References

1. Smith DJ, Roberts D, Watson B (1992) Physical, physiological and performance differences between Canadian national team and universiade volleyball players. J Sports Sci 10: 131-138.
2. Gabbett T, Georgieff B (2005) Physiological characteristics of elite junior volleyball players over competitive season. J Strength Cond Coach 13: 2-7.
3. Gabbett T, Georgieff B (2007) Physiological and anthropometric characteristics of Australian junior national, state, and novice volleyball players. J Strength Cond Res 21: 902-908.
4. Fleck SJ, Case S, Puhl J, Van Handle P (1985) Physical and physiological characteristics of elite women volleyball players. Can J Appl Sport Sci 10: 122-126.
5. Thissen-Milder M, Mayhew JL (1991) Selection and classification of high school volleyball players from performance tests. J Sports Med Phys Fitness 31: 380-384.
6. Little T, Williams AG (2005) Specificity of acceleration, maximum speed, and agility in professional soccer players. J Strength Cond Res 19: 76-78.
7. Sheppard JM, Young WB (2006) Agility literature review: classifications, training and testing. J Sports Sci 24: 919-932.
8. Markovic G, Sekulic D, Markovic M (2007) Is agility related to strength qualities?--Analysis in latent space. Coll Antropol 31: 787-793.
9. Nimphius S, McGuigan MR, Newton RU (2010) Relationship between strength,

power, speed, and change of direction performance of female softball players. J Strength Cond Res 24: 885-895.

10. Sekulic D, Spasic M, Mirkov D, Cavar M, Sattler T (2013) Gender-specific influences of balance, speed, and power on agility performance. J Strength Cond Res 27: 802-811.

11. Barnes JL, Schilling BK, Falvo MJ, Weiss LW, Creasy AK, et al. (2007) Relationship of jumping and agility performance in female volleyball athletes. J Strength Cond Res 21: 1192-1196.

12. Sassi RH, Dardouri W, Yahmed MH, Gmada N, Mahfoudhi ME, et al. (2009) Relative and absolute reliability of a modified agility T-test and its relationship with vertical jump and straight sprint. J Strength Cond Res 23: 1644-1651.

13. Pauole K, Madole K, Garhammer J, Lacourse M, Rozenek R (2000) Reliability and Validity of the T-Test as a Measure of Agility, Leg Power, and Leg Speed in College-Aged Men and Women. Journal of Strength and Conditioning Research 14: 443-450.

14. Draper JA, Lancaster MG (1985) The 505 test: A test for agility in the horizontal plane. Aust. J. Sci Med Sport 17: 15-18.

15. Gabbett TJ (2007) Physiological and anthropometric characteristics of elite women rugby league players. J Strength Cond Res 21: 875-881.

16. Gabbett TJ, Kelly JN, Sheppard JM (2008) Speed, change of direction speed, and reactive agility of rugby league players. J Strength Cond Res 22: 174-181.

17. Häkkinen K (1993) Changes in physical fitness profile in female volleyball players during the competitive season. J Sports Med Phys Fitness 33: 223-232.

18. Gabbett T, Georgieff B, Anderson S, Cotton B, Savovic D, et al. (2006) Changes in skill and physical fitness following training in talent-identified volleyball players. J Strength Cond Res 20: 29-35.

19. Lidor R, Ziv G (2010) Physical and physiological attributes of female volleyball players--a review. J Strength Cond Res 24: 1963-1973.

20. Nikolaidis PT, Ziv G, Arnon M, Lidor R (2012) Physical characteristics and physiological attributes of female volleyball players--the need for individual data. J Strength Cond Res 26: 2547-2557.

21. Schaal M, Ransdell LB, Simonson SR, Gao Y (2013) Physiologic performance test differences in female volleyball athletes by competition level and player position. J Strength Cond Res 27: 1841-1850.

22. Tanner JM (1962) Growth at adolescence. (2nd Edn),bBlackwell Scientific Publications, Oxford.

23. Diallo O, Dore E, Duche P, Van Praagh E (2001) Effects of plyometric training followed by a reduced training programme on physical performance in prepubescent soccer players. J Sports Med Phys Fitness 41: 342-348.

24. Kotzamanidis C (2006) Effect of plyometric training on running performance and vertical jumping in prepubertal boys. J Strength Cond Res 20: 441-445.

25. Witzke KA, Snow CM (2000) Effects of plyometric jump training on bone mass in adolescent girls. Med Sci Sports Exerc 32: 1051-1057.

26. Bartlett J, Smith L, Davis K, Peel J (1991) Development of a valid volleyball skills test battery. J Phys Edu Recr Dance 62: 19-21.

27. Barzouka K, Bergeles N, Hatziharistos D (2007) Effect of simultaneous model observation and self-modeling of volleyball skill acquisition. Percept Mot Skills 104: 32-42.

28. Mirkov DM, Nedeljkovic A, Milanovic S, Jaric S (2004) Muscle strength testing: evaluation of tests of explosive force production. Eur J Appl Physiol 91: 147-154.

29. Claessens AL, Lefevre J, Beunen G, Malina RM (1999) The contribution of anthropometric characteristics to performance scores in elite female gymnasts. J Sports Med Phys Fitness 39: 355-360.

30. Watts PB, Joubert LM, Lish AK, Mast JD, Wilkins B (2003) Anthropometry of young competitive sport rock climbers. Br J Sports Med 37: 420-424.

31. Muramatsu S, Fukudome A, Miyama M, Arimoto M, Kijima A (2006) Energy expenditure in maximal jumps on sand. J Physiol Anthropol 25: 59-61.

32. Lejeune TM, Willems PA, Heglund NC (1998) Mechanics and energetics of human locomotion on sand. J Exp Biol 201: 2071-2080.

33. Gaudino P, Gaudino C, Alberti G, Minetti AE (2013) Biomechanics and predicted energetics of sprinting on sand: hints for soccer training. J Sci Med Sport 16: 271-275.

34. Hewett TE, Paterno MV, Myer GD (2002) Strategies for enhancing proprioception and neuromuscular control of the knee. Clin Orthop Relat Res 402: 76-94.

35. Zech A, Hübscher M, Vogt L, Banzer W, Hänsel F, et al. (2010) Balance training for neuromuscular control and performance enhancement: a systematic review. J Athl Train 45: 392-403.

36. Walsh MS, Böhm H, Butterfield MM, Santhosam J (2007) Gender bias in the effects of arms and countermovement on jumping performance. J Strength Cond Res 21: 362-366.

37. Hamner SR, Seth A, Delp SL (2010) Muscle contributions to propulsion and support during running. J Biomech 43: 2709-2716.

38. Lees A, Barton G (1996) The interpretation of relative momentum data to assess the contribution of the free limbs to the generation of vertical velocity in sports activities. J Sports Sci 14: 503-511.

39. Pontzer H, Holloway JH 4th, Raichlen DA, Lieberman DE (2009) Control and function of arm swing in human walking and running. J Exp Biol 212: 523-534.

Heart Rate Responses during Small-Sided Soccer Games

Evaggelos Manolopoulos[3], Vasilios I. Kalapotharakos[1*], George Ziogas[2], Michalis Mitrotasios[1], Konstantinos S. Spaneas[1] and Savvas P. Tokmakidis[1]

[1]*Department of Physical Education & Sport Science, Democritus University of Thrace, Komotini, Greece*
[2]*Sports Clinic, Thessaloniki, Greece*
[3]*Department of Physical Education & Sport Science, Aristotle University of Thessaloniki, Serres, Greece*

Abstract

The purpose of the present study was to examine the heart rate responses during small-sided games with different number of players. Sixteen professional soccer players were evaluated for body fat (%) using the skin fold thickness at three sites, VO_2max and running velocity at the lactate threshold using an incremental treadmill protocol. %HRmax was measured during four-, five-, six-, seven-, and eight-a side soccer games. The four-a-side game showed significantly ($p<0.05$) higher %HRmax in comparison to the other small-sided games. On the other hand, the %HRmax of the eight-a-side game was significantly lower ($p<0.05$) than three-, four-, five-, six-, and seven-a-side game. The intensity of small-sided games decreases as the number of players increase. The monitoring of heart rate during small-sided games combined with laboratory VO_2max tests is a possible way to define target training intensity zones.

Keywords: Soccer; Intensity; Small-sided games

Introduction

It is common during the daily soccer training to perform games with a limited number of players on each team in a smaller area of the pitch. These small-sided games develop physical abilities, as well as technical and tactical skills [1-3]. As far as physical condition is concerned, small-sided games develop aerobic capacity [1,4-6]. Small sided-games are an equally effective mode of aerobic training as interval running [1] and short duration intermittent running [4]. Other important characteristics of small-sided games training mode are environmental and competitive conditions similar to actual match-play [2,7].

An important research question is how the training intensity, as measured by heart rate (HR) responses, is differentiated among the small-sided games. Previous investigators have shown that the relative pitch size area per player, coach encouragement, the number of players on each side, the number of ball touches and the use of goalkeepers influence the intensity of small-sided games [3,7-9]. Although several studies have examined the effects of the above factors using soccer players of different ages, training experience, level of competition, divisions and National leagues, limited data exists on the influence of each of these factors separately on elite soccer players [1,2,7,9,10]. Elite soccer players present higher physical condition level compared to amateurs and other players from lower divisions, which may affect positively their physical effort during various small-sided games. The knowledge of physical effort during various small-sided games allows coaches and trainers to better control the training process, and develop effective daily and weekly training plan. In this context, it is necessary to develop a better understanding of the drill intensity on elite soccer players as the number of players differentiates the effects of small-sided games with different number of players at the physiological levels.

The purpose of the present study was to examine the heart rate responses during small-sided games with different number of players (four-, five-, six-, seven-, and eight-a-side) in elite professional soccer players. It is hypothesized that heart rate responses should decrease as the number of players increase, from four- to eight-a-side.

Methods

Participants

Sixteen elite Greek professional soccer players participated in the study. All participants belonged to the same club and they had similar soccer training programs. All players were informed of the purpose of the study and gave their informed consent according to the Declaration of Helsinki.

Experimental design

A within subjects experimental design was used to examine the intensity of small-sided games with different number of players (four-, five-, six-, seven-, and eight-a-side) in soccer players. Although, the number of the players, the duration, and the pitch dimensions were different among the five training drills that could affect the research design, this research approach compares the effectiveness of five small-sided games on heart rate responses. The within-subjects design helped to control for subject variability, such as anthropometric and physiological characteristics. Initially, participants were evaluated in endurance characteristics, such as VO_2 max, running velocity at the lactate threshold, and %HRmax at the lactate threshold using an incremental treadmill protocol. Then, their %HRmax was recorded during small-sided games with different number of players (four-, five-, six-, seven, and eight-a-side game) for four weeks.

Soccer players were trained through daily small-sided games with different number of players according to the training's goals (both physical and tactical). The in-season weekly training program included six training sessions in five days, an official match (usually on Sunday), and a free day after the match (on Monday) [11]. Technical staff organized the players into respective teams according to the tactical needs. Four-, five-, six-, seven, and eight-a-side games with the ball always replaced promptly when out of play [7]. Players participated in the small-sided games as part of their normal training and for this reason the order of games was not randomized. All small-sided

***Corresponding author:** Vasilios I. Kalapotharakos, Research Associate, Department of Physical Education & Sport Science, Democritus University of Thrace, 16 Diogenous str., Haidari – P.C. 12461 Athens, Greece
E-mail: vasikal@yahoo.com

games were played outdoors. The size of the pitch and the duration for each small sided game are presented in Table 1 and were according to previous studies [4,5,7]. In every training session, participants were informed of the aim of each small-sided game, and they encouraged maximum effort [7]. The limitations for all small-sided games were: two touches for each player, pass and sprint, and press the ball. The coach provided continuous encouragement during all small-sided games. All training sessions were conducted in the afternoon. No extreme environmental conditions (heat or cold) were observed during data collection. All small-sided games were performed after a 15 min warm-up. Warm-up was not standardized, but it was according to the goals of training. Participants were informed to maintain their normal diet, with emphasis on high fluid and carbohydrate intakes [2,7].

Heart rate was recorded every five seconds during each training session using downloadable, frequency coded heart rate watches (Polar S610, Kempele, Finland). After each training session, the heart rate data were downloaded to a PC, and were analyzed using POLAR software program by the same investigator. The mean percentage of maximum heart rate (% HRmax) of each small-sided game was calculated for each participant during each small-sided game. Each small-sided game was administered at least three times in a four week period. Maximal heart rate for each player was established using a VO_2 max test, as described below. No significant differences were observed in resting HR in all soccer players during the four week data collection period.

Laboratory measures

At the beginning of the first week, all participants were evaluated for body fat, VO_2 max, and running lactate threshold velocity.

Anthropometrics Characteristics: Height was measured to the nearest 0.1 cm using a stadiometer, and body mass was measured to the nearest 0.1 kg. Skin fold thickness was measured at right sites using a Harpenden skinfold calipers. Skin fold sites were chest, abdomen, and thigh. Body fat percentage (%) was calculated according to standard equations [12,13].

VO_2 max and lactate threshold: Expired gas analysis and blood lactate curve analysis were used for determination of VO_2 max and lactate threshold at fixed blood lactate concentration (4 mmol/L), respectively [14-16]. Warm up consisted of a 6 min run at 8 km/h (level treadmill grade) without gas analysis, where heart rate and blood lactate were measured. During this time, the metabolic cart (TrueMax 2400, ParvoMedics) was calibrated using known calibration gases, and volume also was calibrated with a 3-L syringe (Hans Rudolph). Then, the initial speed was set at 10 km/h and it was held constant for 3 minutes. Thereafter, speed was increased by 2 km/h for every 3 minutes until 16 km/h and then speed was increased 2 km/h for every 2 minutes until volitional exhaustion. During testing, expired gases were continuously analyzed using 30-s intervals and at the end of each stage, subjects stopped for 20 seconds for blood lactate determination (Accutrend lactate analyzer, Roche Diagnostics). Analyzers were calibrated each day using known standards. Running speeds (V-4mM) corresponding to fixed whole blood concentration of 4 mmol/l were calculated using linear interpolation [16,17]. Maximal oxygen uptake was determined by attaining at least 3 of the following 4 criteria: RER in excess of 1.10, maximal heart rate within +5% of age-predicted HRmax, a plateau in oxygen uptake despite increase in work rate, and max lactate concentration >8 m mol/l. The highest VO_2 value obtained during the test was considered as the VO_2max. Heart rate was measured throughout the test using a Polar heart rate monitor.

Statistical analysis

Data was analyzed using the SPSS PC program (ver. 14.0) for windows. Mean ± SD were calculated. A repeated measures ANOVA followed by Bonferroni post-hoc test for pair-wise comparisons was applied to examine any differences in %HRmax of soccer players among the five small-sided games (four-, five-, six-, seven-, and eight-a-side). Statistical significance was accepted at $p<.05$.

Results

Anthropometric characteristics, VO_2 max, and running velocity at lactate threshold is presented in Table 2.

A repeated measures ANOVA revealed significant effect of the type of small-sided game (four-, five-, six-, seven-, and eight-a-side) on % HRmax ($F_{4,60}$=129.120, p<0.001, power = 1, η^2 = 0.896). Bonferoni's post-hoc test for pair-wise comparisons revealed that the four-a-side game led to significantly (p<0.05) higher % HRmax in comparison to the other small-sided games (Table 3).

Discussion

The determination of %HRmax in soccer drills is a popular approach to monitor the intensity of small sided game [2,3,6,7,10]. The present study focuses on the influence of different types of small-sided games (four-, five-, six-, seven-, and eight-a side) in the exercise intensity of elite Greek soccer players. The findings of the present study

Small-sided games	Size	Duration
4 vs 4	30m X 40m	4 set X 4 min, 2 min rest
5 vs 5	35m X 45m	4 set X 6 min, 3 min rest
6 vs 6	40m X 50m	3 set X 7 min, 3 min rest
7 vs 7	50m X 60m	3 set X 8 min, 3 min rest
8 vs 8	50m X 60m	3 set X 8 min, 3 min rest

Table1: Size and duration characteristics of small-sided games.

Endurance Characteristics	n=16
Age (y)	25 ± 5
Body Mass (kg)	75.7 ± 5.3
Height (m)	1.79 ± 0.06
Body Fat (%)	9.3 ± 2.1
VO_2max (mL/kg/min)	60.1 ± 2.8
HRmax (bmp)	186.4 ± 8.5
Running Velocity at the LT (km/h)	13.8 ± 0.3

VO_2 max indicates the maximal oxygen uptake; HRmax indicates the maximum heart rate; LT indicates the lactate threshold

Table2: Anthropometric and endurance characteristics of elite Greek soccer players (M ± SD).

Small-sided games	%HRmax (n = 16)
Four-a-side	93.5 ± 1.7*
Five-a-side	90.7 ± 2.5*#
Six-a-side	89.7 ± 2*§
Seven-a-side	88.1 ± 3*#§,†
Eight-a-side	85.3 ± 2.2*#§†

* $p < 0.05$ significant differences between 4 vs. 4 and 5 vs. 5, 6 vs. 6, 7 vs. 7, and 8 vs. 8 small-sided games

# $p < 0.05$ significant differences between 5 vs. 5, and 7 vs. 7, 8 vs. 8 small-sided games

§ $p < 0.05$ significant differences between 6 vs. 6, and 7 vs. 7, 8 vs. 8 small-sided games

† $p < 0.05$ significant differences between 7 vs. 7 and 8 vs. 8 small-sided games

Table3: Percentage of maximum heart rate (% HRmax) during small-sided games with different number of players (M ± SD).

suggest that the intensity of small-sided games, as measured by the %HRmax, decreases as the number of players increase, from four- to eight-a-side.

The higher intensity among the small sided games was observed in four- a side small game compared to five-, six-, seven-, and eight-a side small game. Similarly, Rampinini et al. [7] have reported a significant increase in the intensity of a four- side small game compared to a six-a side small game. Other factors that may contribute to the change of the intensity in small-sided games are the field dimensions, coach encouragement, number of touches and goalpost, pressing, and the presence of goalkeepers [3,5-8,10].

In the present study, the percentage (%) of HRmax during the four-, five-, and six- a side game was 93%, 90% and 89%, respectively. Previous studies have reported lower % HRmax during all of these small-sided games [2,7]. Rampinini et al. [7] have reported 89.4%, 88.8%, and 87% of HRmax in four-, five-, and six-a-side small-sided game, respectively. Little and Williams [2] have found a 90.2%, 89%, 87.8%, and 88.5%, in four-, five-, six-, and eight-a-side small-sided games. It is possible the different results among the present and the previous two studies are attributed to the different training experience of participants [amateur in the study of Rampinini et al. [7]], the rules of the small-sided games [free number of touches in the studies of Rampinini et al. [7] and Little and Williams [2]] and the size of the field [Rampinini et al. [7] and Little and Williams [2]]. Recent studies [3,10] have confirmed these results. Dellal et al. [3] have reported that the number of ball touches authorized per possession affects the soccer player activity, whereas the same research group [10] has found that amateurs covered less total distance with respect to sprinting and high intensity running compared to international players. The field dimensions are an important factor affecting the intensity of small-sided games [6,7]. The higher %HRmax during four-, five- six-, and eight-a-side small-sided games compared to previous studies [Rampinini et al. [7] and Little and Williams [2]] might be attributed to the larger field dimensions used in the present study.

Important endurance parameters are the VO_2 max, the running velocity at the LT, and the %HRmax at the LT [16,18]. Helgerud et al. [19] have suggested that VO_2 max is related to the work rate in a soccer match. The current VO_2 max values (60.1 ml/kg/min) are comparable with VO_2 max values of soccer players from different National leagues [18,20]. Running velocity at the LT and the %HRmax at the LT are important endurance characteristics as well, because the average intensity of a soccer match is close to the anaerobic lactate threshold [21]. Previous studies have reported that the running velocity at the LT is a critical endurance factor among teams with different ranking in the championship [16]. Previous studies from other championships have reported higher running velocity at the LT (14.67 Km/h) in British professional youth soccer players [15], and lower (13 Km/h) in Spanish professional (1st division) soccer players [20].

Except to the evaluation of endurance performance characteristics from the laboratory VO_2 max tests, another significant purpose of them is the determination of individual HR-VO_2 relationship that may better analyze the metabolic demands of the sport specific exercises. Heart rate itself can be considered indicative of the physiological effort and can be used to define target exercise intensity zones. A previous study [22] has reported a practical link between the monitoring of %HRmax at small-sided games combined with the identification of HRmax, %HRmax at lactate threshold, from the laboratory VO_2 max measurements [22]. The validity of HR monitoring to determine the metabolic demands during soccer exercises was high, especially in the range between 80% - 90% of HRmax [22]. So, coaches can monitor the daily training intensity of the soccer drills and can test the produced intensity for increasing endurance performance.

As far as intensity is concerned, the weekly pattern reaches a peak by mid-week and then tapers off in order to obtain peak performance in the match [23]. That is why in the present study high intensity small sided-games (4v4 and 5v5) were organized mid-week (Wednesday and Thursday), whereas lower intensity games were played at the beginning or by the end of the week. This ensures that soccer players were at top fitness level by the end of the week, before the official match.

In conclusion, the monitoring of %HRmax in soccer drills, using heart rate monitors, is a popular approach to determine the intensity of the small-sided game. The intensity of small-sided games, as measured by the %HRmax, decreases as the number of players increase, from four- to eight-a-side. The monitoring of %HRmax at small sided-games combined with the endurance characteristics may evaluate the training intensity of these soccer drills. The usefulness of monitoring the intensity of small-sided games for coaches is to determine the training intensity and to design and plan the daily and weekly training sessions.

Acknowledgements

The authors would like to thank the volunteers for their cooperation.

References

1. Impellizzeri FM, Marcora SM, Castagna C, Reilly T, Sassi A, et al. (2006) Physiological and performance effects of generic versus specific aerobic training in soccer players. Int J Sports Med 27: 483-492.
2. Little T, Williams AG (2006) Suitability of soccer training drills for endurance training. J Strength Cond Res 20: 316-319.
3. Dellal A, Lago-Penas C, Wong del P, Chamari K (2011) Effect of the number of ball contacts within bouts of 4 vs. 4 small-sided soccer games. Int J Sports Physiol Perform 6: 322-333.
4. Dellal A, Chamari K, Pintus A, Girard O, Cotte T, et al. (2008) Heart rate responses during small-sided games and short intermittent running training in elite soccer players: a comparative study. J Strength Cond Res 22: 1449-1457.
5. Hill-Haas SV, Coutts AJ, Rowsell GJ, Dawson BT (2009) Generic versus small-sided game training in soccer. Int J Sports Med 30: 636-642.
6. Hill-Haas SV, Dawson B, Impellizzeri FM, Coutts AJ (2011) Physiology of small-sided games training in football: a systematic review. Sports Med 41: 199-220.
7. Rampinini E, Impellizzeri FM, Castagna C, Abt G, Chamari K, et al. (2007) Factors influencing physiological responses to small-sided soccer games. J Sports Sci 25: 659-666.
8. Mallo J, Navarro E (2008) Physical load imposed on soccer players during small-sided training games. J Sports Med Phys Fitness 48: 166-171.
9. Hill-Haas SV, Dawson BT, Coutts AJ, Rowsell GJ (2009) Physiological responses and time-motion characteristics of various small-sided soccer games in youth players. J Sports Sci 27: 1-8.
10. Dellal A, Hill-Haas S, Lago-Penas C, Chamari K (2011) Small-sided games in soccer: amateur vs. professional players' physiological responses, physical, and technical activities. J Strength Cond Res 25: 2371-2381.
11. Kalapotharakos VI, Ziogas G, Tokmakidis SP (2011) Seasonal aerobic performance variations in elite soccer players. J Strength Cond Res 25:1502-1507.
12. Siri WE (1956) The Gross composition of the body. Adv Biol Med Phys 4: 239-280.
13. Jackson AS, Pollock ML (1985) Practical assessment of body composition. Phys Sportsmed 13: 76-90.
14. Heck H, Mader A, Hess G, Mucke S, Muller R, et al. (1985) Justification of the 4-mmol/l lactate threshold. Int J Sports Med 6: 117-130.

15. McMillan K, Helgerud J, Grant SJ, Newell J, Wilson J, et al. (2005) Lactate threshold responses to a season of professional British youth soccer. Br J Sports Med 39: 432-436.

16. Kalapotharakos VI, Strimpakos N, Vithoulka I, Karvounidis C, Diamantopoulos K, et al. (2006) Physiological characteristics of elite professional soccer teams of different ranking. J Sports Med Phys Fitness 46: 515-519.

17. Nicholson RM, Sleivert GG (2001) Indices of lactate threshold and their relationship with 10-km running velocity. Med Sci Sports Exerc 33: 339-342.

18. Stolen T, Chamari K, Castagna C, Wisloff U (2005) Physiology of soccer: an update. Sports Med 35: 501-536.

19. Helgerud J, Engen LC, Wisloff U, Hoff J (2001) Aerobic endurance training improves soccer performance. Med Sci Sports Exerc 33: 1925-1931.

20. Casajus JA (2001) Seasonal variation in fitness variables in professional soccer players. J Sports Med Phys Fitness 41: 463-469.

21. Bangsbo J (1994) The physiology of soccer – with special reference to intense intermittent exercise. Acta Physiol Scand Suppl 619: 1-155.

22. Esposito F, Impellizzeri FM, Margonato V, Vanni R, Pizzini G, et al. (2004) Validity of heart rate as an indicator of aerobic demand during soccer activities in amateur soccer players. Eur J Appl Physiol 93: 167-172.

23. Bangsbo J, Mohr M, Krustrup P (2006) Physical and metabolic demands of training and match-play in the elite football player. J Sports Sci 24: 665-674.

Resistance Training Supplements and their Potential Benefit

Lawrence D Hayes[1,2], Catherine E Baker[1], Gordon F Bickerstaff[3] and Julien S Baker[2*]

[1]School of Human Sciences, London Metropolitan University, UK
[2]Institute of Clinical Exercise and Health Science, University of the West of Scotland, UK
[3]Department of Biology, University of the West of Scotland, UK

Abstract

Resistance Exercise (RE) is a widely practiced activity both in leisure time and in training periods for competitive athletes. Recent advanced in molecular biology and muscle physiology has elucidated some of the mechanisms that regulate muscle growth. As a result of these biochemical advances, an increased number of supplements claiming to enhance adaptations to Resistance exercise have become available. Essentially, the aim of these supplements is to influence protein synthesis and therefore gradual protein accretion leading to increased muscle size and strength. The aim of this review is to discuss the most commonly consumed supplements associated with RE and make recommendations with regards to timing, volume and combinations of supplementations.

Keywords: Creatine; Protein; Carbohydrate; β-alanine; Weight training

Introduction

Resistance exercise (RE) is one of the most widely practiced forms of physical activity. This type of exercise is often used to enhance athletic performance, augment musculo-skeletal health, and alter body aesthetics. The health benefits of RE are primarily preventative or as a countermeasure to circumstances where muscle weakness compromises optimal function (injury or prolonged inactivity, sarcopenia or musculo-skeletal disorders) however, it can also have a positive effect on skeletal and general metabolic health as well as possible psychological benefits. This review will consider dietary factors that can influence the outcomes of RE, and will review current recommendations for favourable physiological & biochemical adaptation.

Nutrient intake before, during, and after training will support the adaptations that occur in response to the training stimulus [1]. The effect of nutrition on adaptations that arise from training may not be as important as the training itself, but the effect on the final outcome is important. In recent years, the effect of nutrition on training adaptations has received increasing attention, particularly with respect to maximising the benefits of RE. Consequently the nutritional supplements industry has expanded to become a multi-million dollar industry with an array of products for enhancement of both nutritional status and capacity for increased RE. This review will consider current opinion and practical advice on some of the key macronutrients of a standard diet, and the most commonly used supplements associated with RE.

Protein

Proteins are synthesised from 20 amino acid building blocks, and to ensure continuity of the synthesis of a given protein, the amino acids are collected in pools to ensure continuous availability for protein synthesis. The absence of any one amino acid from a pool results in immediate cessation of protein synthesis associated with that pool. To avoid a situation where amino acid shortage causes failure of essential protein synthesis, most proteins in the body are in a state of constant turnover (synthesis and degradation) to facilitate constant top up of amino acid pools. Typically a male body of 70 kg contains about 12 kg of protein, and 200 g of free amino acids. Roughly 120 g of free amino acids are located in skeletal muscle and around 5 g of free amino acids are found in circulation. Backup support is provided by a suite of transaminase enzymes that can both interchange amino acids, and produce amino acids from simple carbohydrates to make up any shortfall in amino acid pools (Figure 1). Of the 20 amino acids, 12 are designated non-essential in adults because they are readily synthesised as required, and 8 are designated essential and must be supplied in the diet (Table 1).

Protein has long been considered the most vital macronutrient to

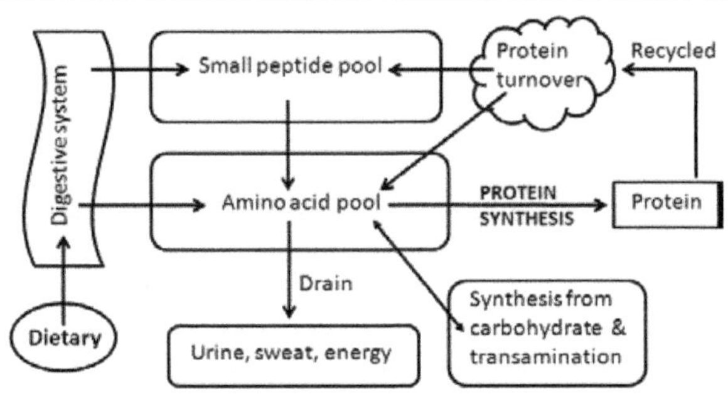

Figure 1: Amino acid pool showing sources of synthesis and degradation.

Non-essential	Essential
Alanine	Arginine *
Asparagine	Histidine
Aspartate	Isoleucine #
Cysteine#	Leucine
Glutamate	Lysine
Glutamine	Methionine
Glycine	Phenylalanine
Proline	Threonine
Serine	Tryptophan
Tyrosine	Valine #

(* only in growing young, not in adults)
(# BCAA branched chain amino acid)

Table 1: Non-essential and essential amino acids.

***Corresponding author:** Julien S Baker, Professor, Institute of Clinical Exercise and Health Science, University of the West of Scotland, Lanarkshire, Scotland, UK
E-mail: jsbaker@uws.ac.uk

facilitate adaptations to RE especially if hypertrophy and strength gains are targeted. In recent times, individuals seeking increased aerobic power and stamina as well as weight loss have become increasingly concerned with the importance of protein in a diet [2,3]. Muscular hypertrophy is a developmental process founded on complex metabolism and signalling events in the body. In normal circumstances the body aims to maintain protein homeostasis by keeping protein anabolism and catabolism in balance. Increased mass of muscle is produced by increased anabolic activity to support synthesis of muscle myofibrillar proteins, and with suitable training regimes, protein homeostasis can be shifted toward adaptations that result in increased muscle mass. A positive change in the relative protein content of muscle requires a shift in major metabolic pathways (including energy) and hormone activity that support anabolic production of protein. A negative change in the relative protein content of muscle can occur when the balance shifts to catabolic activity as in periods of starvation when muscle is actively catabolised to provide amino acids as a source of energy. Exercise and nutrition have strong influences on the relative balance of anabolic and catabolic metabolism of muscle protein [4].

RE and Endurance Exercise (EE) both produce mixed muscle protein synthesis during the subsequent recovery phase and turnover of mixed muscle proteins is increased following RE [5]. Increased supply of amino acids during this time will ensure that amino acid pools are not depleted and will facilitate better muscle protein synthesis after RE [4,6]. This could be achieved with a product supply that creates a temporary hyperaminoacidaemia to increase amino acid delivery to the muscle, transport into the muscle cell, and intracellular amino acid pool top up [7]. Tipton and colleagues reported that increased provision of amino acids was responsible for the elevation of protein synthesis [8]. Kobayashi et al. [9] supported this observation by showing that lower levels of blood amino acids resulted in decreased muscle protein synthesis, and that protein synthesis was restored with restoration of increased blood amino acids. Clearly blood amino acid levels are essential for muscle protein synthesis.

Recent research has focused on the importance of individual amino acids to influence anabolism with leucine receiving most attention [1,10]. Leucine is one of the Branched-Chain Amino Acids (BCAA), and is an essential amino acid. Koopman et al. [10] investigated the effects of additional free leucine to a post exercise recovery drink (carbohydrate vs. carbohydrate and protein vs. carbohydrate, protein and leucine). The addition of leucine resulted in an increased plasma insulin response and increased net protein balance when compared with protein ingestion alone. However, Tipton suggests that additional leucine does not have a greater influence in an already anabolic situation following RE plus protein ingestion, and hypothesised that metabolism and hormone actions are already fully activated by RE and amino acids, including leucine, in whey proteins and therefore, no further activation by free leucine is possible [1,11]. As a result of these findings, it is unclear whether additional leucine supplementation provides any advantage. It is clear that post exercise recovery of muscle protein synthesis does require leucine, but it is likely that dietary or supplemented protein will provide sufficient amounts of leucine to facilitate synthesis.

Research into the optimum timing of protein and amino acid ingestion has also produced equivocal results [3,12]. Tipton et al. reported that protein ingestion pre and post RE both resulted in the change from negative net muscle protein balance to a positive balance [12]. However, the total response to an Essential Amino Acid-Carbohydrate (EAC) solution was greater when consumed immediately pre exercise compared to immediately post. Interestingly, muscle protein metabolism was also elevated for longer when the EAC solution was consumed pre-exercise compared to post. The length of the effect, plus higher blood flow during exercise in the PRE trial, resulted in significantly greater total uptake over the entire study period. A commonly discussed concept in RE and protein ingestion is that of the "metabolic window" (i.e. the 45 min-1 h immediately post RE). It has been suggested that this is the time when consumption of protein is most effective [13]. However, this phenomenon may not be as important as previously thought as Rasmussen et al. demonstrated that the response of muscle to an EAC solution was similar when ingested 1 and 3h following RE [14]. Interestingly, Cribb and Hayes reported greater increases in lean body mass, CSA of type II muscle fibres and 1-repetition maximum (1RM) when ingestion of an EAC was immediately pre and post compared to early morning and late evening suggesting that the timing of protein ingestion can enhance the desired adaptations from RE training [13].

While the importance of protein for muscular adaptation is clear and unquestioned, the amount of protein required is controversial. Protein synthesis is elevated post RE and the amount of protein intake should be sufficient to support the increased level of anabolism. Typically the protein requirement of an individual is based on nitrogen balance, which is generally elevated for athletes compared with sedentary individuals [14]. Many coaches and athletes advocate very high protein intake, up to 4.0 $gkg^{-1}day^{-1}$ [15]. Even the American Dietetic Association, Dieticians of Canada and the American College of Sports Medicine state that protein intake must be > 1.6 $gkg^{-1}day^{-1}$ for gains in muscle mass [16]. There is another school of thought that protein requirements for active individuals are not increased above that of sedentary controls [3,17]. This argument is supported by the fact that exercise increases the turnover and hence efficiency of amino acid utilisation possibly due to reutilisation of amino acids from muscle protein breakdown to re-supply amino acid pools [17,18]. RE trained individuals also exhibit a greater negative net muscle protein balance than untrained volunteers in a fasted state [4]. Tipton proposed that exercise decreases protein requirement. Ratamess and colleagues reported no increased response to a 10 week RE protocol when comparing low (< 1.2 $gkg^{-1}day^{-1}$), moderate (1.21 - 1.90 $gkg^{-1}day^{-1}$), and high (> 1.91 $gkg^{-1}day^{-1}$) protein intake in collegiate football players [1,18]. Ferrara et al. [19] reported similar findings when examining changes in body composition after a high (1.9 $gkg^{-1}day^{-1}$) and normal (1.3 $gkg^{-1}day^{-1}$) protein intake for six months. These findings suggest that high protein intake (> 1.9 $gkg^{-1}day^{-1}$) is unnecessary for gains in muscle mass and that moderate consumption (approximately 1.2 - 1.9 $gkg^{-1}day^{-1}$) appears sufficient. Conversely, Hoffman et al. [20] demonstrated a trend for increased lean body mass with protein supplementation of 2.0 $gkg^{-1}day^{-1}$ compared to 1.2 $gkg^{-1}day^{-1}$ in collegiate football players. The authors also demonstrated a significant increase in 1 RM squat performance after a 12 week RE program on the higher protein intake compared to moderate consumption. Interestingly, Hoffman et al. [20] did not observe any statistical difference in 1RM bench press, wingate performance, body mass, resting testosterone, insulin-like growth factor-1 (IGF1), or growth hormone (GH) between groups. The combination of these findings suggest that elevated protein intake > 2.0 $gkg^{-1}day^{-1}$ may augment strength development in RE trained individuals however the increase above moderate consumption is likely minimal. The purpose of protein ingestion is to top up amino acid pools that will then support protein synthesis, and it should be recognized that such pools are finite, such that when topped up to the maximum then further protein ingestion will not result in increased pool size. Excess amino acids are eliminated from the body and protein intake above moderate consumption may also be potentially harmful as removal of excess amino acids may add stress to the function of the kidneys (Figure 1).

The majority of studies investigating protein consumption on RE adaptations have not used competitive strength/power athletes directly, but instead seek to extrapolate from various populations what strength/power athletes need. This is a weakness in such studies and despite the high internal validity of these studies, their practical application to elite and competitive RE athletes is potentially limited.

It is known that not all proteins are equal as sources of amino acids that will support the synthesis of myofibrillar protein. The biological value of a protein is a measure of the efficiency with which a given protein is absorbed and assimilated into the protein of an organism. Milk and egg white are examples of proteins with high biological value, whereas plant sources have a relatively low value due to absence of some essential amino acids. Wilkinson and colleagues demonstrated that fat-free mass was increased to a greater extent in individuals consuming fluid milk (whey and casein) than when a soya protein beverage was consumed [21]. Numerous studies have reported diverse absorption characteristics of whey (rapidly absorbed) and casein (slowly absorbed) proteins [22]. Tang et al. [6] reported that muscle protein synthesis was elevated in a stepwise manner (whey > soy > casein) after exercise and at rest. These authors suggested that to increase muscle anabolism, a rapid increase in essential amino acids (possibly leucine specifically) is required. Yet, the benefit of one over the other is still unknown with regard to RE. Also important is the relationship between muscle and liver as a significant amount of ingested amino acids can be taken up by the liver and oxidized for fuel or used for other metabolic requirements.

From the evidence reviewed, moderate protein consumption (approximately 1.2-1.9 $gkg^{-1}day^{-1}$) is recommended for individuals partaking in RE for aesthetics or for general health as to date no study has shown favourable anthropometric changes for high consumption over moderate consumption [22]. For elite and competitive athletes higher levels of protein intake may result in weight gain and movement through weight categories, but may be important in supporting and maintaining a high level of protein turnover. Excessively high levels of protein intake will not result in increased protein synthesis due to limitations imposed by amino acid pools, and may be harmful as excess amino acids are removed from the body. With regards to timing of ingestion, immediately pre RE is likely to be more beneficial as this has shown to increase protein synthesis for a longer period than post-RE consumption.

Carbohydrate

Carbohydrate (CHO) supplementation is common in endurance athletes and provides an exogenous source of glucose [23]. Less importance has been placed on the consumption of CHO in RE trained individuals compared with protein. As discussed above, RE stimulates protein synthesis and supply of amino acids can elevate protein synthesis further. It has been suggested that an addition of CHO to a post exercise protein solution may increase muscle anabolism by taking advantage of the resultant insulin response to CHO. An increase in insulin, as a result of glucose ingestion, would counteract the adenosine monophosphate-activated protein kinase (AMPK) activity which promotes glucose and fatty acid oxidisation for energy and inhibits protein synthesis (Figure 2). AMPK promotes energy release and inhibits energy consumption, and protein synthesis is an energy-demanding process [24]. During exercise, metabolism rightly shifts to the catabolic mechanisms that provide energy for muscle activity. Anabolic activity is curtailed and although insulin is a key anabolic hormone in moving glucose into muscle cells via its regulation of GLUT4, the anabolic activity of insulin during exercise is inhibited.

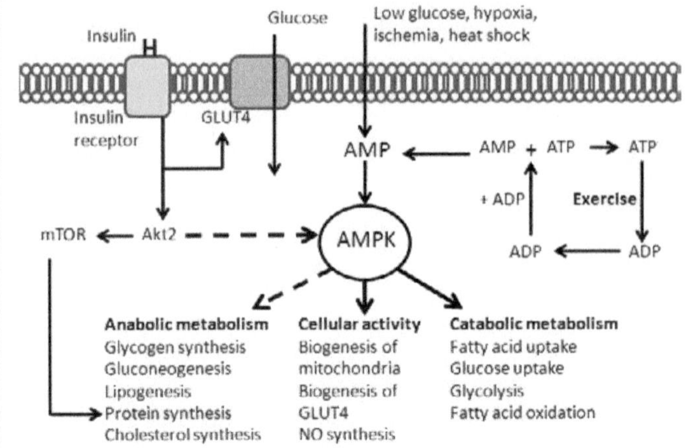

Figure 2: AMPK activity and subsequent metabolic effects.

It is the aim during RE to minimise the reduction in insulin as it has been shown to have significant effect on muscle protein synthesis when adequate amino acid concentrations are available, by reducing protein catabolism [22]. Exercise-induced mRNA transcription and synthesis of proteins is only fully activated when plasma insulin levels are elevated [24]. Elevations in insulin are expected to inhibit AMPK activity, therefore promoting protein synthesis (Figure 2). Insulin exerts its effect on translation through the protein kinase B (Akt2)-mammalian target of rapamycin (mTOR) pathway. This response is critical for increasing muscle protein synthesis and subsequent hypertrophy [25]. The mTOR signal serves to increase protein synthesis by increasing the number of messenger RNA translated per ribosome. Insulin concentrations parallel changes in blood glucose, and the response is enhanced when protein and carbohydrates are ingestion prior to, during, or after a workout [26].

It has previously been reported that insulin in the absence of amino acid availability does not stimulate protein synthesis [27]. Therefore, the ingestion of protein with CHO after exercise should allow insulin to exert its stimulatory effect on muscle, which, according to Ivy and colleagues would likely manifest itself as an interactive effect (i.e. the combined effects of hyperinsulinemia and the exogenous protein would be greater than the sum of their independent effects) [28]. This hypothesis has been both supported and opposed [10,29]. Ivy et al. [28] reported that supplementation with a CHO-protein drink after exercise increased phosphorylation of Akt, mTOR, ribosomal protein S6 and glycogen synthase kinase 3α/β when compared to a placebo. This in turn lead to increased release of amino acid into the blood and would theoretically stimulate muscle protein synthesis however this was not measured directly in the study. Interestingly, Ivy et al. [28] examined phosphorylation of these muscle proteins after repeated sprints on a cycle ergometer. It is therefore unclear if any hypertrophy did occur as this type of exercise may or may not result in muscular growth in already conditioned individuals.

Vollestad et al. [29] suggested that intermittent activities (such as RE) can stimulate significant glycogenolytic effects. MacDougall et al. [30] indeed reported that RE can significantly decrease muscle glycogen stores. Therefore, it is commonly accepted that muscle glycogen is an important fuel for RE and maintenance of these stores may enhance performance. Reductions in muscle glycogen have resulted in decreased isokinetic and isometric force production and accentuated exercise-induced muscle weakness [31]. A study by Haff et al. [32] demonstrated that RE-induced decreases in muscle glycogen can be attenuated by CHO feeding during RE. Haff et al. [32] however, did not report enhanced isokinetic leg extension performance with increased muscle glycogen as a result of CHO supplementation. This result may be a product of the performance test selected as Leveritt and Abernethy reported than decreased muscle glycogen resulted in impaired back squat performance but not isokinetic leg extension [33]. Lambert et al. [34] and Haff and colleagues have reported enhanced RE performance with CHO supplementation over isokinetic and free-weight testing protocols [35,36]. Conversely, Conley et al. [37] and Vincent et al. [38] reported no benefit of CHO supplementation on a RE protocol of high volume. It is important to note that these studies differed significantly in time; studies by Lambert et al. [34] and Haff et al. [35,36] lasted 56, 77, and 57 mins respectively whereas the investigations by Conley et al. [37] and Vincent et al. [38] were much shorter in duration. As exercise bouts lasting less than 41 min rely primarily on muscle glycogen as a fuel source, the increased duration and reliance of exogenous blood glucose may have promoted performance decrements in the three longer duration investigations. It appears from these findings that with increased duration of RE, the probability of decreased performance increases. Notably, these investigations asked participants to perform a RE session of high volumes of work similar to those performed using a hypertrophy protocol. Therefore the effect of CHO supplementation on a strength protocol (sets of 1-6RM) is unknown. The literature suggests that CHO supplementation may be vital to maximise performance of RE when using large-muscle mass free-weight exercise performed with high training volumes and moderate loads as the amount of glycogen used in these exercise appears to be related to the total amount of work and the duration of the RE protocol. More research is required to provide greater understanding of the effect of CHO supplementation on RE. To date no studies have concerned the effect of high/low glycemic CHO on RE, adaptations to chronic CHO supplementation without addition of protein, a dose-response relationship with CHO supplementation (dose), and RE performance (response) or the timing of CHO ingestion (before vs. after RE).

Creatine

Creatine supplementation has been surrounded by controversy since it gained popularity in the early 1990's [39]. Some anecdotal reports have claimed that creatine has a number of health risks, and is an unnecessary practice. However, many athletes and experts in the field have reported that use of creatine not only enhances exercise performance, but is also clinically safe [40]. In the initial stages of intense exercise when Adenosine Triphosphate (ATP) consumption is high, energy to re-phosphorylate adenosine diphosphate (ADP) to ATP (Figure 3) during and following intense exercise is provided by, and is therefore largely dependent on the amount of, phosphocreatine (PCr) stored in the muscle [41]. High-intensity exercise depletes PCr stores and the rate of energy availability diminishes as a result of reduced rate of ATP production. The capacity for maximal-intensity exercise declines and availability of PCr in muscle dictate energy generation until other mechanisms of ATP production take over. It has been hypothesised that increasing muscle creatine content by exogenous supplementation may allow greater training adaptations because of an enhanced quality and volume of work performed as a result of an improved rate of ATP resynthesis during high-intensity exercise.

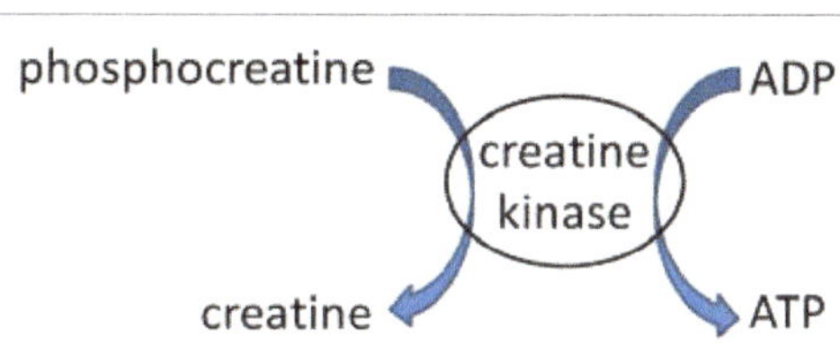

Figure 3: PCr actions.

Creatine is synthesised in liver and pancreas from amino acids arginine, methionine, and glycine with approximately 95% of the body's creatine stored in skeletal muscle [42]. Furthermore, small amounts of creatine can be found in the testes and brain. Approximately two thirds of creatine stored in muscle is stored as PCr and the rest as free creatine. Approximately 1-2% of the creatine pool is broken down per day into creatinine in the skeletal muscle and then excreted in urine [41]. Creatine stores can be replenished by dietary intake containing creatine (meat and fish) or through endogenous synthesis of creatine from arginine, methionine, and glycine. Relatively small amounts of creatine are found in meat and fish and therefore supplementation provides a cost effective and simple means of increasing creatine availability without excessive fat, protein or calorific intake. Tarnopolsky et al. compared 10 g creatine monohydrate and 50 g CHO against 10 g casein protein and 50 g CHO and reported that the creatine group reported a greater increase in fat free mass compared to the protein group [43]. The implications of this suggest that in sports where body weight is unimportant, creatine is a superior supplement than casein protein when combined with CHO to enhance hypertrophy.

Various supplementation protocols have been suggested as effective in increasing muscle stores of muscle creatine. The amount of increase in muscle storage is dependent on creatine levels in the muscle prior to supplementation. Individuals with lower muscle stores may experience storage increases of 20-40% whereas those with relatively high stores may only increase by 10-20% [41]. The extent of the increase in skeletal muscle creatine storage is important as studies have reported performance changes to be correlated to this increase [44]. The most commonly described protocol is known as the "loading" protocol; characterised by ingestion of approximately 5 g four times per day for 5-7 days and 3-5 $g{\cdot}d^{-1}$ thereafter [41]. This protocol has results in an increase of 10-40% in muscle creatine and PCr stores [45]. Further research has demonstrated that a shorter loading period is still beneficial, as is a reduced dosage, particularly if ingested with CHO or protein [45]. Other suggested protocols include those with no loading phase as well as "cycling". Cycling protocols typically consist of "loading doses" for 3-5 days every 3-4 weeks. These protocols have been shown to be effective in increasing strength and hypertrophy [46,47]. It would be interesting to compare these protocols within one research paper to establish optimum strategy and determine whether the strategy or the total creatine consumption is the key factor concerning RE adaptations.

Many forms of creatine currently exist in the marketplace within various formulations. However, few of these have shown any benefit over the traditional creatine monohydrate. Recently, Spillane et al. examined the effectiveness of creatine ethyl ester and reported no additional benefit in muscle strength or anthropometry when compared to creatine monohydrate [48]. Similar findings have been reported for creatine phosphate a creatine/β-hydroxy-β-methlybutyrate (HMB) combination and creatine plus glycerol [42,49,50]. However, the combination of CHO and creatine in a formula has been shown to increase muscle creatine retention with Pittas et al. suggesting only a small amount of CHO is required to optimise insulin-mediated creatine retention [45,51]. These authors also reported that a combination of protein, CHO and creatine was optimum for insulin response and creatine retention. Other recent studies have indicated a potential benefit to RE when combining creatine with protein [52]. From these findings, it appears that combining creatine with protein and/or CHO produces optimal results. Despite the trepidation surrounding creatine supplementation, it appears to be the most effective nutritional supplement in terms of improving lean body mass and anaerobic capacity. With regard to the medical safety of creatine supplementation, no peer-reviewed paper to date has reported any clinically significant side effect other than weight gain as a result of normal creatine intake (< 25 g d^{-1}).

β-Alanine

The dipeptide carnosine is synthesized in human skeletal muscle and has been shown to contribute increased capacity to buffer hydrogen ions (H^+) during intense exercise [53]. It is synthesized within skeletal muscle from histidine and β-alanine. While histidine, a non-essential amino acid (in adults), is found in high concentrations along with carnosine synthetase in skeletal muscle β-alanine, an amino acid derivative, is found in much lower concentrations [54]. Therefore, β-alanine is likely the rate-limiting step in carnosine synthesis [54]. Increased skeletal muscle carnosine levels through β-alanine supplementation have been shown to support the maintaintenance acid-base balance, delay fatigue, and improve exercise performance.

A number of investigations concerning the effect of β-alanine supplementation on EE events suggest that supplementation enhances performance [55]. Less research has been conducted on the efficacy of β-alanine on RE. Hoffman et al. compared supplementation of creatine with a combination of creatine and β-alanine in collegiate football players [56]. Addition of β-alanine appeared to provide a greater training stimulus than creatine alone. Significant improvements were observed for both squat and bench press exercise, lean tissue mass and fat loss in subjects supplementing with both β-alanine and creatine compared with creatine alone. Interestingly, no differences were noted in the magnitude of strength improvements between the groups. In fact, to date, no research suggests that β-alanine supplementation improves maximum strength. Hoffman et al. [56] showed no improvements in 1RM squat exercise after supplementation. Kendrick et al. [57] reported that β-alanine supplementation did not enhance performance of a box squat, bench press, dead lift or isokinetic leg extension at 180° s^{-1}. These results are not entirely surprising as β-alanine supports buffering capacity, and maximal strength is not limited by acidosis. Similarly, Portington et al. [58] also showed that other buffering agents such as sodium bicarbonate also failed to demonstrate any ergogenic effect on strength performance.

The major putative effects of greater buffer capacity are likely to be observed in activities eliciting a high intracellular acidosis. In particular, stronger buffer capacity has been especially ergogenic in multiple bouts of high-intensity short-term exercises interspersed by short recovery intervals [59]. Hoffman et al. [56] showed that β-alanine supplementation did not enhance maximal strength performance but resulted in a ~20% increase in total work volume during RE in well-trained resistance athletes. Conversely, when an exercise protocol elicits a less extreme muscular acidosis (i.e. exercise lasting < 60s or exercises using small muscle groups), no beneficial effects of β-alanine have been observed [59,60].

From the literature concerning β-alanine to date, it is possible to draw the following conclusions: 1) chronic supplementation of β-alanine can enhance performance of multiple bouts of high-intensity short-term exercise interspersed by short recovery; 2) acute supplementation of β-alanine appears not to enhance strength performance and; 3) total work during RE can be increased through β-alanine supplementation even in well-trained athletes.

Caffeine

Caffeine remains the most widely utilised ergogenic aid, and bears a strong evidence base for beneficial use in medium to long duration sports performance. However, the impact of caffeine upon short duration high intensity activity remains unclear; with some studies showing no effect or even a performance decrement with caffeine supplementation [61-63]. Duncan et al. however, reported that number of repetitions completed was higher when caffeine was ingested 60 min pre-RE [64]. This suggests that total work was higher in the caffeine condition. Therefore, if this phenomenon continued over time, RE adaptation would likely be augmented due to a greater stimulus. However, the study by Duncan et al. only concerned one RE bout and therefore, this is purely speculation. Astorino and Roberson suggest that trained athletes may respond more favourably than untrained participants to ergogenic effects of caffeine in resistance training [65]. Moreover, they suggest that RPE and Pain sensation remain unaffected by caffeine supplementation in short term activity. Like many proposed ergogenic supplements, the magnitude of response varies between individuals and this is arguably owing to different rates of metabolism [66]. The exact mechanism of caffeine, as an ergogenic substance, remains unclear although it is believed that the effector is located outside of the muscle cell thus, acute resistance exercise, where metabolism occurs within the cell, in understandably less affected by caffeine ingestion [65].

Nitrates

Dietary nitrates have recently attracted attention as a potential ergogenic aid to sports performance. Although there is some support for their use with endurance activity the efficacy of utilisation in short duration resistance exercise remains unsubstantiated [67-69]. This is perhaps unsurprising given their mechanism of impact via cardiorespiratory efficiency. However, as duration of exercise increases, where muscular endurance becomes an important performance factor, nitrate supplementation may yet prove beneficial. Evidence is beginning to support the use of nitrate supplementation, most often in the form of beetroot juice, for high intensity constant workloads; whilst the support for use in intermittent high intensity work remains equivocal [70]. Interestingly, Kelly and Colleagues observed that nitrate supplementation improved exercise tolerance during exercise at 60, 70, and 80% delta, but not 100% peak power, suggesting that nitrate can improve performance at submaximal intensity but not peak power output [71]. There is some debate as to the primary effector mechanism for the performance gains seen post nitrate supplementation; with suppressed muscular ATP turnover and alterations in mitochondrial efficiency both being posited [69]. Thus, whilst there is no argument for utilising nitrates during resistance training itself, there may be benefits to the athletes involved in resistance training as part of a broader programme for sports performance.

Conclusion

Availability of amino acids is important for protein synthesis associated with hypertrophy and inclusion of CHO may maximise the effect of insulin with creatine also increasing lean body mass. Therefore, a combination of CHO, protein and creatine could be beneficial to consume pre-, during-, and post-exercise to maximise hypertrophy and recovery. However, creatine is not recommended for athletes who compete in events that require acceleration of one's own body mass. Of course, acute program variables of the training protocol (volume, load, rest period length, exercise selection, and exercise order) have the largest impact upon adaptations to resistance exercise and these factors must be optimized to maximize resultant physiological modifications. A number of other factors affect adaptations to RE including age, genetics, gender, timing of training periods, posture as well as cultural and general habits.

References

1. Tipton KD (2008) Protein for adaptations to exercise training. Eur J Sport Sci 8: 107-118
2. Jesudason D, Nordin BC, Keogh J, Clifton P (2013) Comparison of 2 weight-loss diets of different protein content on bone health: a randomized trial. Am J Clin Nutr 98: 1343-1352.
3. Saunders MJ (2007) Coingestion of carbohydrate-protein during endurance exercise: influence on performance and recovery. Int J Sport Nutr Exerc Metab 17 Suppl: S87-103.
4. Phillips SM, Tipton KD, Ferrando AA, Wolfe RR (1999) Resistance training reduces the acute exercise-induced increase in muscle protein turnover. Am J Physiol 276: E118-124.
5. Tipton KD, Witard OC (2007) Protein requirements and recommendations for athletes: relevance of ivory tower arguments for practical recommendations. Clin Sports Med 26: 17-36.
6. Tang JE, Moore DR, Kujbida GW, Tarnopolsky MA, Phillips SM (2009) Ingestion of whey hydrolysate, casein, or soy protein isolate: effects on mixed muscle protein synthesis at rest and following resistance exercise in young men. J Appl Physiol (1985) 107: 987-992.
7. Biolo G, Tipton KD, Klein S, Wolfe RR (1997) An abundant supply of amino acids enhances the metabolic effect of exercise on muscle protein. Am J Physiol 273: E122-129.
8. Tipton KD, Ferrando AA, Phillips SM, Doyle D Jr, Wolfe RR (1999) Postexercise net protein synthesis in human muscle from orally administered amino acids. Am J Physiol 276: E628-634.
9. Kobayashi H, Børsheim E, Anthony TG, Traber DL, Badalamenti J, et al. (2003) Reduced amino acid availability inhibits muscle protein synthesis and decreases activity of initiation factor eIF2B. Am J Physiol Endocrinol Metab 284: E488-498.
10. Koopman R, Beelen M, Stellingwerff T, Pennings B, Saris WH, et al. (2007) Coingestion of carbohydrate with protein does not further augment postexercise muscle protein synthesis. Am J Physiol Endocrinol Metab 293: E833-842.
11. Rennie MJ (2007) Exercise- and nutrient-controlled mechanisms involved in maintenance of the musculoskeletal mass. Biochem Soc Trans 35: 1302-1305.
12. Tipton KD, Rasmussen BB, Miller SL, Wolf SE, Owens-Stovall SK, et al. (2001) Timing of amino acid-carbohydrate ingestion alters anabolic response of muscle to resistance exercise. Am J Physiol Endocrinol Metab 281: E197-206.
13. Cribb PJ, Hayes A (2006) Effects of supplement timing and resistance exercise on skeletal muscle hypertrophy. Med Sci Sports Exerc 38: 1918-1925.
14. Rasmussen BB, Tipton KD, Miller SL, Wolf SE, Wolfe RR (2000) An oral essential amino acid-carbohydrate supplement enhances muscle protein anabolism after resistance exercise. J Appl Physiol (1985) 88: 386-392.
15. Alway SE, Grumbt WH, Stray-Gundersen J, Gonyea WJ (1992) Effects of resistance training on elbow flexors of highly competitive bodybuilders. J Appl Physiol (1985) 72: 1512-1521.
16. American College of Sports Medicine; American Dietetic Association; Dietitians of Canada (2000) Joint Position Statement: nutrition and athletic performance. American College of Sports Medicine, American Dietetic Association, and Dietitians of Canada. Med Sci Sports Exerc 32: 2130-2145.
17. Phillips SM, Moore DR, Tang JE (2007) A critical examination of dietary protein requirements, benefits, and excesses in athletes. Int J Sport Nutr Exerc Metab 17 Suppl: S58-76.
18. Ratamess NA, Hoffman JR, Faigenbaum AD, Mangine GT, Falvo MJ, et al. (2007) The combined effects of protein intake and resistance training on serum osteocalcin concentrations in strength and power athletes. J Strength Cond Res 21: 1197-1203.
19. Ferrara LA, Innelli P, Palmieri V, Limauro S, De Luca G, et al. (2006) Effects of different dietary protein intakes on body composition and vascular reactivity. Eur J Clin Nutr 60: 643-649.
20. Hoffman JR, Ratamess NA, Kang J, Falvo MJ, Faigenbaum AD (2007) Effects of protein supplementation on muscular performance and resting hormonal changes in college football players. J Sports Sci Med 6: 85-92.
21. Wilkinson SB, Tarnopolsky MA, Macdonald MJ, Macdonald JR, Armstrong D, et al. (2007) Consumption of fluid skim milk promotes greater muscle protein accretion after resistance exercise than does consumption of an isonitrogenous and isoenergetic soy-protein beverage. Am J Clin Nutr 85: 1031-1040.
22. Tipton KD, Elliott TA, Cree MG, Wolf SE, Sanford AP, et al. (2004) Ingestion of casein and whey proteins result in muscle anabolism after resistance exercise. Med Sci Sports Exerc 36: 2073-2081.
23. Phillips SM, Sproule J, Turner AP (2011) Carbohydrate ingestion during team games exercise: current knowledge and areas for future investigation. Sports Med 41: 559-585.
24. Ju JS, Gitcho MA, Casmaer CA, Patil PB, Han DG, et al. (2007) Potentiation of insulin-stimulated glucose transport by the AMP-activated protein kinase. Am J Physiol Cell Physiol 292: C564-572.
25. Hawke TJ (2005) Muscle stem cells and exercise training. Exerc Sport Sci Rev 33: 63-68.
26. Hather BM, Tesch PA, Buchanan P, Dudley GA (1991) Influence of eccentric actions on skeletal muscle adaptations to resistance training. Acta Physiol Scand 143: 177-185.
27. Goto K, Nagasawa M, Yanagisawa O, Kizuka T, Ishii N, et al. (2004) Muscular adaptations to combinations of high- and low-intensity resistance exercises. J Strength Cond Res 18: 730-737.
28. Ivy JL, Ding Z, Hwang H, Cialdella-Kam LC, Morrison PJ (2008) Post exercise carbohydrate-protein supplementation: phosphorylation of muscle proteins involved in glycogen synthesis and protein translation. Amino Acids 35: 89-97.
29. Vøllestad NK, Tabata I, Medbø JI (1992) Glycogen breakdown in different human muscle fibre types during exhaustive exercise of short duration. Acta Physiol Scand 144: 135-141.
30. MacDougall JD, Ray S, Sale DG, McCartney N, Lee P, et al. (1999) Muscle substrate utilization and lactate production. Can J Appl Physiol 24: 209-215.
31. Yaspelkis BB 3rd, Patterson JG, Anderla PA, Ding Z, Ivy JL (1993) Carbohydrate supplementation spares muscle glycogen during variable-intensity exercise. J Appl Physiol (1985) 75: 1477-1485.
32. Haff GG, Koch AJ, Potteiger JA, Kuphal KE, Magee LM, et al. (2000) Carbohydrate supplementation attenuates muscle glycogen loss during acute bouts of resistance exercise. Int J Sport Nutr Exerc Metab 10: 326-339.
33. Leveritt M, Abernethy PJ (1999) Effects of carbohydrate restriction on strength performance. J Strength Cond Res 13: 52-57.
34. Lambert CP, Flynn MG, Boone JB, Michaud TJ, Rodriguez-Zayas J (1991) Effects of carbohydrate feeding on multiple-bout resistance exercise. J Apply Sport Sci Res 5: 192-197.
35. Haff GG, Stone MH, Warren BJ, Keith R, Johnson RL et al. (1999) The effect of carbohydrate supplementation on multiple sessions and bouts of resistance exercise. J Strength Cond Res 13: 111-117.
36. Haff GG, Schroeder CA, Koch AJ, Kuphal KE, Comeau MJ, et al. (2001) The effects of supplemental carbohydrate ingestion on intermittent isokinetic leg exercise. J Sports Med Phys Fitness 41: 216-222.
37. Conley MS, Stone MH, Marsit JL, O'Bryant HS, Nieman DC, et al. (1995) Effects of carbohydrate ingestion on resistance exercise. J Strength Cond Res 9: 20.
38. Vincet KR, Clarkson PM, Freedson PS, De-Cheke M (1993) Effect of pre-exercise liquid, high carbohydrate feeding on resistance exercise performance. Med Sci Sport Exerc 25: 194.
39. Balsom PD, Söderlund K, Ekblom B (1994) Creatine in humans with special reference to creatine supplementation. Sports Med 18: 268-280.
40. Poortmans JR, Francaux M (1999) Long-term oral creatine supplementation does not impair renal function in healthy athletes. Med Sci Sports Exerc 31: 1108-1110.
41. Buford TW, Kreider RB, Stout JR, Greenwood M, Campbell B, et al. (2007) International Society of Sports Nutrition position stand: creatine supplementation and exercise. J Int Soc Sports Nutr 4: 6.
42. Peeters BM, Lantz CD, Mayhew JL (1999) Effect of oral creatine monohydrate and creatine phosphate supplementation on maximal strength indices, body composition, and blood pressure. J Strength |Cond Res 13: 3-9
43. Tarnopolsky MA, Parise G, Yardley NJ, Ballantyne CS, Olatinji S, et al. (2001) Creatine-dextrose and protein-dextrose induce similar strength gains during training. Med Sci Sports Exerc 33: 2044-2052.
44. Greenhaff PL, Bodin K, Soderlund K, Hultman E (1994) Effect of oral creatine supplementation on skeletal muscle phosphocreatine resynthesis. Am J Physiol 266: E725-730.

45. Steenge GR, Simpson EJ, Greenhaff PL (2000) Protein- and carbohydrate-induced augmentation of whole body creatine retention in humans. J Appl Physiol (1985) 89: 1165-1171.

46. Willoughby DS, Rosene J (2001) Effects of oral creatine and resistance training on myosin heavy chain expression. Med Sci Sports Exerc 33: 1674-1681.

47. Willoughby DS, Rosene JM (2003) Effects of oral creatine and resistance training on myogenic regulatory factor expression. Med Sci Sports Exerc 35: 923-929.

48. Spillane M, Schoch R, Cooke M, Harvey T, Greenwood M, et al. (2009) The effects of creatine ethyl ester supplementation combined with heavy resistance training on body composition, muscle performance, and serum and muscle creatine levels. J Int Soc Sports Nutr 6: 6.

49. O'Connor DM, Crowe MJ (2007) Effects of six weeks of beta-hydroxy-beta-methylbutyrate (HMB) and HMB/creatine supplementation on strength, power, and anthropometry of highly trained athletes. J Strength Cond Res 21: 419-423.

50. Easton C, Turner S, Pitsiladis YP (2007) Creatine and glycerol hyperhydration in trained subjects before exercise in the heat. Int J Sport Nutr Exerc Metab 17: 70-91.

51. Pittas G, Hazell MD, Simpson EJ, Greenhaff PL (2010) Optimization of insulin-mediated creatine retention during creatine feeding in humans. J Sports Sci 28: 67-74.

52. Cribb PJ, Williams AD, Stathis CG, Carey MF, Hayes A (2007) Effects of whey isolate, creatine, and resistance training on muscle hypertrophy. Med Sci Sports Exerc 39: 298-307.

53. Suzuki Y, Ito O, Mukai N, Takahashi H, Takamatsu K (2002) High level of skeletal muscle carnosine contributes to the latter half of exercise performance during 30-s maximal cycle ergometer sprinting. Jpn J Physiol 52: 199-205.

54. Dunnett M, Harris RC (1999) Influence of oral beta-alanine and L-histidine supplementation on the carnosine content of the gluteus medius. Equine Vet J Suppl : 499-504.

55. Van Thienen R, Van Proeyen K, Vanden Eynde B, Puype J, Lefere T, et al. (2009) Beta-alanine improves sprint performance in endurance cycling. Med Sci Sports Exerc 41: 898-903.

56. Hoffman JR, Ratamess NA, Ross R, Shanklin M, Kang J, et al. (2008) Effect of a pre-exercise energy supplement on the acute hormonal response to resistance exercise. J Strength Cond Res 22: 874-882.

57. Kendrick IP, Harris RC, Kim HJ, Kim CK, Dang VH, et al. (2008) The effects of 10 weeks of resistance training combined with beta-alanine supplementation on whole body strength, force production, muscular endurance and body composition. Amino Acids 34: 547-554.

58. Portington KJ, Pascoe DD, Webster MJ, Anderson LH, Rutland RR, et al. (1998) Effect of induced alkalosis on exhaustive leg press performance. Med Sci Sports Exerc 30: 523-528.

59. Artioli GG, Gualano B, Coelho DF, Benatti FB, Gailey AW, et al. (2007) Does sodium-bicarbonate ingestion improve simulated judo performance? Int J Sport Nutr Exerc Metab 17: 206-217.

60. Hoffman J, Ratamess NA, Ross R, Kang J, Magrelli J, et al. (2008) Beta-alanine and the hormonal response to exercise. Int J Sports Med 29: 952-958.

61. Plaskett CJ, Cafarelli E (2001) Caffeine increases endurance and attenuates force sensation during submaximal isometric contractions. J Appl Physiol (1985) 91: 1535-1544.

62. Woolf K, Bidwell WK, Carlson AG (2008) The effect of caffeine as an ergogenic aid in anaerobic exercise. Int J Sport Nutr Exerc Metab 18: 412-429.

63. Williams AD, Cribb PJ, Cooke MB, Hayes A (2008) The effect of ephedra and caffeine on maximal strength and power in resistance-trained athletes. J Strength Cond Res 22: 464-470.

64. Duncan MJ, Stanley M, Parkhouse N, Cook K, Smith M (2013) Acute caffeine ingestion enhances strength performance and reduces perceived exertion and muscle pain perception during resistance exercise. Eur J Sport Sci 13: 392-399.

65. Astorino TA, Roberson DW (2010) Efficacy of acute caffeine ingestion for short-term high-intensity exercise performance: a systematic review. J Strength Cond Res 24: 257-265.

66. Grant DM, Tang BK, Kalow W (1983) Variability in caffeine metabolism. Clin Pharmacol Ther 33: 591-602.

67. Larsen FJ, Weitzberg E, Lundberg JO, Ekblom B (2007) Effects of dietary nitrate on oxygen cost during exercise. Acta Physiol (Oxf) 191: 59-66.

68. Wilkerson DP, Hayward GM, Bailey SJ, Vanhatalo A, Blackwell JR, et al. (2012) Influence of acute dietary nitrate supplementation on 50 mile time trial performance in well-trained cyclists. Eur J Appl Physiol 112: 4127-4134.

69. Jones AM (2013) Dietary Nitrate: the new magic bullet? Sports Sci Ex 26: 1-5.

70. Vanhatalo A, Bailey SJ, Blackwell JR, DiMenna FJ, Pavey TG, et al. (2010) Acute and chronic effects of dietary nitrate supplementation on blood pressure and the physiological responses to moderate-intensity and incremental exercise. Am J Physiol Regul Integr Comp Physiol 299: R1121-1131.

71. Kelly J, Vanhatalo A, Wilkerson DP, Wylie LJ, Jones AM (2013) Effects of nitrate on the power-duration relationship for severe-intensity exercise. Med Sci Sports Exerc 45: 1798-1806.

Knowledge and Attitude of the Sports Teachers in Central India towards Oro-facial Injuries and the use of Mouth Guard

Kalaskar AR* and Kalaskar R

Government Dental College & Hospital, Nagpur, Maharashtra, India

Abstract

Objective: To evaluate the sports teachers' knowledge and attitude towards sports related oro-facial injuries and the use of mouth guards.

Methods: Certified sports teachers from various schools and colleges of Vidarbha region, Central India were exposed to pre-validated questionnaire containing both open ended and closed ended questions. Data obtained was analyzed and expressed as percentage.

Results: Total 197 sports teachers from 167 schools and colleges participated in the study. Approximately 67.5% of the sport teachers agreed that sports related oro-facial injuries are common and inline skating (58.4%) was the most common sport. Only 8.1% of the sport teachers were having knowledge regarding first aid to oro-facial injuries. All sport teachers agreed that sport related oro-facial injuries can be prevented, but only 10.1% incorporated protective measures in practice to prevent it. Majority of the sports teachers (85.8%) were aware that mouth guard is used as a protective device to prevent oro-facial injuries but only few recommended in their school. Lack of motivation by the school and college administration was the major reason (50%) for non-recommending. Inline skating (54.8%) was the highly recommended sports for mouth guards by sports teachers, followed by boxing and basketball. Only 29.9% of the sports teachers were aware that dentist are the appropriate specialist to approach for mouth guards.

Conclusion: The sports teachers had adequate knowledge regarding the sports related orofacial injuries and the protective devises used to prevent it, but their inappropriate attitude is the main hindrance in the prevention of orofacial injuries.

Keywords: Oro-facial injuries; Mouth guard; Sports teachers; Knowledge; Attitude

Introduction

Oro-facial injuries in children are common during various sports activities. The peak age groups with highest risk of trauma are 8-11 years [1,2]. Utmost care of dentition during this age group is must as the dentition is not fully formed which could affect the child's oro-facial growth, esthetic, psychology and parental economy. Several sports related oro-facial injuries can be life threatening in nature therefore it is mandatory to use protective device. Various basic protective devises such as helmets, face masks and mouth guards are used to reduce the risk of sport related oro-facial injuries. Studies have shown that regular use of mouth guards is of paramount importance in reducing the incidence of oro-facial injuries. In spite of having adequate information about its use there is minimal utilization which results in oro-facial injuries. This points out that more attention and motivation in addition to strict rules is required to reduce the incidence of sports related oro-facial injuries.

Parents have an important role to educate their children and keep a strict vigilance on them regarding use of sport related preventive measures. But their role is taken up by the sports teachers as the children move out from their home campus to school playground or sports academy. Hence it becomes essential to check the sports teachers' knowledge and attitude towards sports related injuries and regular practice of the preventive measures.

Hence a study was planned in Vidarbha region of Central India to evaluate the knowledge, attitude and practice of sports teachers towards oro-facial injuries and use of mouth guards.

Material and Methods

The study was undertaken among the sports teachers of various schools and colleges of Vidarbha region, Central India between June 2015 and December 2015. Only certified sports teacher were included in the study. The written permission was obtained from schools and colleges regarding participation of sport teachers in the survey. The sports teachers were exposed to pre- validated questionnaire which was designed to assess their knowledge and attitude regarding oro-facial injuries and use of mouth guards. The pre- validated questionnaire was distributed by hand delivery system. It consisted of both open ended and closed ended questions. The data obtained was analyzed and expressed as percentage.

Result

A total number of 197 sports teachers from 167 schools and colleges were included in the study. Of these 197 sport teachers, 181(91.8%) were male and 16 (8.12%) were female. Majority of sports teacher were having more than 3 years of teaching experience as a sports teacher. The age of the sport teachers ranged from 22-40 years. Approximately 67.5% of the sport teacher agreed that sports related oro-facial injuries are common and it affects the esthetic and psychology (Table 1). Inline skating (58.4%) was considered the most common sport causing orofacial injuries particularly the laceration type (61.4%) and teeth fracture (25.9%) (Table 2). Only 8.1% of the sport teachers were having knowledge regarding first aid to oro-facial injuries (Table 1). All sport teachers agreed that sport related oro-facial injuries can be prevented

***Corresponding author:** FDr. Ashita R Kalaskar (MDS), Associate professor, Dept. of Oral Diagnosis Medicine & Radiology, Government Dental College & Hospital, Nagpur, Maharashtra, India
E-mail: ashitaradio@ rediffmail.com

	Questions	Yes N (%)	No N (%)
1	Are sport related OFI common?	133 (67.5)	64 (32.5)
2	Does Sport related OFI affects esthetic & psychology?	130 (66.0)	67 (34.0)
3	Do you have knowledge of first aid to OFI?	16 (8.1)	181 (91.9)
4	Can sport related OFI be prevented?	100 (100)	0. 0 (0.0)
5	Can avulsed tooth be replanted?	178 (90.4)	19 (9.6)
6	Are mouth guard used as a protective device to prevent OFI?	169 (85.8)	28 (14.2)
7	Do you recommend mouth guard in your school / institute?	6 (3)	191 (97)

OFI = Oro- facial injuries

Table1: Response of sports teachers to various questions.

Name of sport	N (%)	Type of injury	N (%)
Inline Skating	115 (58.4)	Laceration	121 (61.4)
Basket ball	10 (5.0)	Teeth fracture	51 (25.9)
Football	28 (14.3)	Avulsion	18 (9.1)
Running	17 (8.6)	Any other	7 (3.6)
Cricket	4 (2.0)	Total	**100 (100)**
Boxing	23 (11.7		
Total	**100 (100)**		

Table 2: Distribution of sports causing Oro- facial injuries and type of injury

(Table 1), but only 10.1% practice protective measures to prevent it (Table 3). Nearly 90% of the sports teachers were aware that avulsed tooth can be replanted (Table 1) but very few (5.5%) knew about the best storage medium (Table 4). Majority of the sports teachers (60.4) consider that saline/water is the best storage medium for avulsed tooth (Table 4). Approximately 85.5% of the sports teachers were aware that mouth guard is used as a protective device to prevent oro-facial injuries but only few (3%) recommended in their school (Table 1). Lack of motivation by the school and college administration was the major reason (50%) for non-recommending. Inline skating (54.8%) was the highly recommended sports for mouth guards by sports teachers, followed by boxing and basketball (Table 5). Only 29.9% of the sports teachers were aware that dentist are the appropriate specialist to approach for mouth guards (Table 6).

Discussion

Sports can be fun time or a moment of competition. But such fun or competitions can be marred by the unwanted injuries inflicted during sports activities. In India the reported prevalence of orofacial injuries ranges from 4-35% amongst the adolescents [3,4] as against the prevalence of 15-35% reported in other countries [5,6]. Out of this, the sports related injuries account for one of the major etiological factors (18.1%) for oro-facial injuries [7,8]. This observation indicates that there is some inadequacy in the implementation of protective measures to prevent sports related orofacial injuries. Helmet, face mask and mouth guard are the protective devices used to protect sport related orofacial injuries. Of all the protective measures, mouth guards have a major role in reducing the sports related oro-facial injuries [9]. Studies conducted in Hawaiian [10], Australia [11] and America population have shown reduced oro-facial injuries with the use of mouth guards [12]. Mouth guards an intraoral appliance act as a buffer between oral soft tissue and teeth thus preventing soft tissue and dental injuries [13-15]. Several countries have made the use of mouth guards mandatory during contact and non-contact sports [16]. But in India no such rules are there mandating the use of mouth guard in sports. This might be one of the reasons for ignorance towards strict follow-up of use of protective devices and increased prevalence of sports related oro-facial injuries.

Preventive measures	N (%)
Helmet	5 (2.5)
Chin cap	2 (1.0)
Mouth guard	6 (3.0)
Other	7 (3.6)
No measures	177 (89.9)

Table 3: Measure taken to prevent OFI by sports teachers.

Storage medium	N (%)
Milk	11 (5.5)
Saline/water	119 (60.4)
Oral cavity	7 (3.6)
Dry	41 (20.8)
Don't know	19 (9.7)
Total	197 (100)

Table 4: Knowledge about best storage media.

Name of sports	N (%)
Inline Skating	108 (54.8)
Basket ball	12 (6.1)
Football	00 (0.0)
Running	6 (3.0)
Cricket	00 (0.0)
Boxing	71(36.1)
Total	197 (100)

Table 5: Highly recommended sports for mouth guards by school teachers.

Name of specialist	N (%)
Dentist	59 (29.9)
Physiotherapist	112 (56.9)
Pharmacist	1 (0.5)
Physician	4 (2.0)
Others	21 (10.7)
Total	197 (100)

Table 6: Distribution of appropriate specialist for mouth guard preparation.

Sports teachers have not only the responsibility of educating the sports persons about protective devises but also help them in motivating for its regular use. Studies have shown that although the sports teachers have adequate knowledge of protective devices, few imply it in their regular practice [17,18]. Similar results have been observed by the present study, wherein only 3% of the sports teachers recommended the use of mouth guards. Interestingly majority said that the reason for non- recommendation was the lack of motivation by the school and college administration. This might be attributed to financial constraints or their inappropriate attitude. Other reasons were, lack of knowledge regarding availability of the appliance or non-compliance of the students either due to decreased efficiency in the sports due to mouth guard use, poor esthetics or ignorance. Negligence on the side of teachers could also be a possible reason for non-recommendation.

Risk of orofacial injuries is influenced by the type of sports. Contact sports and sports involving collision have been associated with higher risk of orofacial injuries. Studies done in Chandigadh [17] and Banglore [19] have reported boxing with the highest risk of orofacial injuries. In the present study inline skating was reported to have the highest risk of orofacial injuries followed by football (14.3%) and boxing (11.7%). This observation is in accordance with the studies conducted in Switzerland and Germany [20]. The possible reason for increased risk of orofacial injuries in inline skating might be due to the fact that this sport is associated with high speed and an imbalance at any time could lead to injuries. Also it is not obligated like other sports (boxing, hockey) to wear mouth guard especially at amateur level. Therefore a serious consideration is required in this aspect as in central parts of India inline skating is becoming one of the popular sports and is practiced by many people of different age groups. Therefore educating sports persons for the use of mouth guards in this particular sport is the need of hour. Similar views were expressed by the sports teachers of the present study, majority of whom recommended skating as the sport highly requiring mouth guard use.

Soft tissue lacerations, abrasions, tooth intrusions, avulsions and crown-root fractures are the most commonly reported orofacial injuries whereas zygoma, mandibular and alveolar fractures are less commonly observed [8,21]. This data is in accordance with the data reported in the current study.

Sports are such activities which can any time be associated with emergency requiring first aid. In the present study 91% of the teachers were unaware of the first aid provided after orofacial injuries. Similar observations were also reported in studies conducted in developing countries like Saudi [22] and Morocco [23]. Lack of knowledge of first aid among the sports teachers is a matter of great concern. Basic knowledge of first aid helps in preventing major loss or permanent damage to orofacial structures which otherwise would contribute to unesthetics and related psychological changes in children. This fact was accepted by majority (66%) of the sports teacher in the current study. Therefore basic training of the first aid should be given to all sports teachers which could be a part of their curriculum or consultation from a dentist.

Avulsed tooth has to be replanted as early as possible. To preserve the vitality of periodontal ligament cells of the avulsed tooth, Hanks balanced salt solution is the most recommended storage medium. Other preferred storage media are coconut water, milk white egg and ORS [24]. A review study conducted by Emerich et al. [25] reported similar observations and proposed 'Save-a-Tooth boxes' containing an isotonic transport medium, which can maintain the viability of an avulsed tooth for up to 72 hours. In the present study 90.4% sports teachers agreed that avulsed tooth can be replanted and according to majority (60.4%) saline or water should be used as the storage media for the avulsed tooth. This indicates inadequate knowledge regarding the storage medium used. Although sports teacher had inadequate knowledge about the first aid and storage medium, they were aware that the tooth can be re-implanted. This difference in the knowledge could be attributed to the different factors such as; previous experience regarding treatment of avulsed tooth or information from media which might be in the form of newspaper or interviews of specialists.

Dentists are the appropriate specialist to fabricate mouthguard and to educate sports person, sports teachers and parents regarding the regular use of mouthguard. But surprisingly the specialists recommended by most of the sports teachers (56.9%) were the physiotherapists. The possible explanation for this observation could be the lack of knowledge, motivation, negligence on the part of sports teachers and unavailability of mouth guard in this region.

Sports teachers play an important role in educating, instructing and motivating the sports persons about the precautions taken during the sports activities. Also they are the ones to make the school or college managements understand the need of protective devises. Hence evaluating and updating their knowledge is essential to decrease the incidence of orofacial injuries. The present study reflects inappropriate attitude of sports teachers towards orofacial injuries. There is an urgent need to educate sports teacher, children and parents regarding traumatic dental injuries and its associated complication including psychological trauma. Educational tools such as educational programmes, posters or pamphlets can be used to educate the society. Secondly a dentist should be appointed at every sports institution; who will not only take prophylactic care but will also provide therapeutic care.

Secondly mouth guard should be made mandatory in sports activities in India. This act will definitely change the attitude of the parents, sports persons and sports teachers towards appropriate use of protective devises, which will help in reducing the incidence of sport related orofacial injuries.

Conclusion

The present study showed that although sports teachers had adequate knowledge regarding the sports related orofacial injuries and the protective devises used to prevent it, very few teachers recommended it. This inappropriate attitude on their part is the main hindrance in the prevention of orofacial injuries. Mandating the use of mouth guard for sports activities and periodic motivation in various forms could be of immense help to reduce the occurrence of orofacial injuries.

References

1. Rodd HD, Chesham DJ (1997) Sports-related oral injury and mouthguard use among Sheffield school children. Community Dent Health 14: 25-30.
2. Petti S, Tarsitani G (1996) Traumatic injuries to anterior teeth in Italian schoolchildren: prevalence and risk factors. Endod Dent Traumatol 12: 294-297.
3. Baldava P, Anup N (2007) Risk factors for traumatic dental injuries in an adolescent male population in India. J Contemp Dent Pract 8: 35-42.
4. Gupta S, Kumar-Jindal S, Bansal M, Singla A (2011) Prevalence of traumatic dental injuries and role of incisal overjet and inadequate lip coverage as risk factors among 4-15 years old government school children in Baddi Barotiwala Area, Himachal Pradesh, India. Med Oral Patol Oral Cir Bucal 1: e960-965.
5. Hargreaves JA, Matejka JM, Cleaton-Jones PE, Williams S (1995) Anterior tooth trauma in eleven-year-old South African children. ASDC J Dent Child 62: 353-355.
6. Kalaskar RR, Tawani GS, Kalaskar AR (2013) Paediatric traumatic dental injuries in hospital of central India. A 2.5 year retrospective review. IJRID 3:1-10.
7. Kumamoto DP, Maeda Y (2004) A literature review of sports-related orofacial trauma. Gen Dent 52: 270-280.
8. Heintz WD (1968) Mouth protectors: a progress report. Bureau of Dental Health Education. J Am Dent Assoc 77: 632-636.
9. CDHA. (2005) CDHA Position paper on sports mouthguards. Canadian journal of dental hygiene 39: 1-18.
10. Finch C, Braham R, McIntosh A, McCrory P, Wolfe R (2005) Should football players wear custom fitted mouthguards? Results from a group randomised controlled trial. Inj Prev 11: 242-246.
11. Labella CR, Smith BW, Sigurdsson A (2002) Effect of mouthguards on dental injuries and concussions in college basketball. Med Sci Sports Exerc 34: 41-44.
12. Shultz SJ, Valovich TC, Zinder SM (2005) Mouthguard use. In: Sports medicine handbook. Indianapolis (IN): National Federation of State High School Associations pp: 91-94.
13. Ranalli DN (2002) Sports dentistry and dental traumatology. Dent Traumatol 18: 231-236.
14. Heintz W (1975) The case for mandatory mouth protectors. Phys Sportsmed 3: 61-63.
15. Beachy G (2004) Dental Injuries in Intermediate and High School Athletes: A 15-Year Study at Punahou School. J Athl Train 39: 310-315.
16. Knowlton R, Kracher CM, Smith WS (2003) Sports-Related Dental Injuries and Sports Dentistry.
17. Lehl G (2005) Perceptions of Chandigarh sports coaches regarding oro-facial injuries and their prevention. J Indian Soc Pedod Prev Dent 23: 67-70.

18. Onyeaso CO, Adegbesan OA (2003) Knowledge and attitudes of coaches of secondary school athletes in Ibadan, Nigeria regarding oro-facial injuries and mouthguard use by the athletes. Dent Traumatol 19: 204-208.

19. Neeraja G, Bharadwaj S, Shah K, Subramaniam P (2014) Knowledge, attitude, and practices regarding oro-facial injuries and oro-facial protective devices among physical instructors in Bangalore. J Int Oral Health 6: 1-6.

20. Fasciglione D, Persic R, Pohl Y, Filippi A (2007) Dental injuries in inline skating - level of information and prevention. Dent Traumatol 23: 143-148.

21. Kvittem B, Hardie NA, Roettger M, Conry J (1998) Incidence of orofacial injuries in high school sports. J Public Health Dent 58: 288-293.

22. Al-Obaida M (2010) Knowledge and management of traumatic dental injuries in a group of Saudi primary schools teachers. Dent Traumatol 26: 338-341.

23. Toure B, Benoist FL, Faye B, Kane AW, Kaadioui S. (2011) Primary School Teachers' Knowledge Regarding Emergency Management of Avulsed Permanent Incisors. J Dent (Tehran) 8: 117-122.

24. Poi WR, Sonoda CK, Martins CM, Melo ME, Pellizzer EP, et al. (2013) Storage media for avulsed teeth: a literature review. Braz Dent J 24: 437-445.

25. Emerich K, Kaczmarek J (2010) First aid for dental trauma caused by sports activities: state of knowledge, treatment and prevention. Sports Med 40: 361-366.

Anti-Doping Systems in Sports are Doomed to Fail: A Probability and Cost Analysis

Aaron Hermann* and Maciej Henneberg

School of Medical Sciences, University of Adelaide, University of Adelaide, Adelaide, South Australia, Australia

Abstract

Objective: Doping in sports now seems to be more widespread despite testing. The objective is to assess the effectiveness and cost effectiveness of the current anti-doping system.

Methods: A probability and cost analysis was performed. Using calculations based on official world-level data of positive doping test results, sensitivity and frequency of testing in 93 categories of sport, and estimates of numerical characteristics (frequency, window of detectability, test predictability)

Results: A low probability of doping detection was demonstrated; 0.029 for doping once a week by a single random test with average sensitivity (40%) and window of detectability of 48 hours. With 12 tests a year probability of detection of continuous doping is ~33%. To detect 100% of doping in one year 16-50 tests per athlete must be done costing ~$25,000.

Conclusion: Testing is not economically viable for effective detection. Changes are thus required to the current system to combat sophisticated doping techniques.

Keywords: WADA; Statistics; Ineffective; Policy; Cost analysis; Probability; Doping; Cheats

Introduction

The year 1968 saw the International Olympic Committee's (IOC) first true attempt to combat doping in sport [1]. A number of international sporting organisations had attempted to address the issue of doping in sports before this point, one notable example being the International Association of Athletic Federations (IAAF). These early attempts however proved to be little more than hopeful, as they lacked a key component necessary for such anti-doping systems; anti-doping testing. Similarly, even the IOC's early attempts were, it can be argued, ambitious but ultimately lacked substance. It is well known that early anti-doping testing was, at best, rudimentary and, perhaps, did little more than keep up the appearance of combatting the issue of doping. The IOC's decision to finally introduce measures to curb doping, was in response to numerous doping related deaths and controversies. Whilst, these attempts were ambitious, in many ways they simply have not lived up to the promise they once had. Numerous high profile scandals, such as East Germany [2], China [3], and more recently Lance Armstrong and US Postal [4] only revealed years after the fact, have shown the fragility of the anti-doping system both past and present.

It has been suggested by a number of different peoples in the sporting arena, including officials, athletes, and scientists, that the current (and past) anti-doping systems are both ineffective and inefficient. Furthermore, current doping detection statistics, in some sports, under represent the true extent of doping in sports [5]. This demonstrates that there is a need for an assessment of various factors influencing the success of anti-doping systems. There has been considerable work produced on the factors influencing an athlete's decision to dope [6,7], the reasons behind doping [8,9], and consequences of doping [8,10]. However, little work has been produced to actually assess the factors within the sporting and anti-doping system which may influence the effectiveness and efficiency of anti-doping testing. It is true that the anti-doping system as a whole can be argued as to also include the education of anti-doping, the programs in place to attempt to deter doping etc. However, it should be pointed out that it can also be argued that testing and the science behind the testing leading to detection or not, is the primary tool in anti-doping. Education is definitely of help, but without a means to find any wrong doing education alone would not prevent doping. As such this paper primarily focuses on testing as the pivotal element of the anti-doping system. Therefore, one must ask the question, despite the apparent efforts of sporting bodies for almost a century, why does doping continue to be a problem? Why is it that even today when testing is widespread, random out-of-competition testing is performed, prohibited lists are updated regularly and experts are consulted on the systems to be used, why do these problems persist? Perhaps this is simply because irrespective of the system in place some people will always want to cheat. Or perhaps the problems lie within the anti-doping system itself, an inherent flaw within this paper sets out to investigate this question, to assess the current anti-doping system and to determine if there are indeed issues with its very structure, or rather if factors of the real world impact its efficiency and effectiveness.

To elaborate, one key component of the current anti-doping system is test sensitivity. There seems to be some debate on this area and it tends to be a somewhat contentious issue amongst scientists. The success rate of anti-doping testing has been reported in some cases to be less than 10%, and on average less than 50% [11,12]. Whilst this figure is not definitive on the balance of probabilities, based on the available information, this seems to be a reasonable estimate. This is but one example of the issues in anti-doping systems, upon further investigation the issues appear to expand exponentially. Current testing systems are influenced by numerous factors of the sporting world that simply cannot be restrained by theoretical frameworks and the best hopes of policy formers. Test success rates, doping techniques aimed at deliberate circumventing of testing (e.g. micro-dosing), and in some cases minimalistic sample collection due to economic restraints are all examples of the real world (and evolving nature) of sports and doping, that makes inflexible rules on paper fail in everyday life. Consequently anti-doping practices are less effective in their mission than one

***Corresponding author:** Aaron Hermann, University of Adelaide, University of Adelaide, Adelaide, South-Australia, Australia
E-mail: aaron.hermann@adelaide.edu.au

would hope; the simple reality of it is that not all dopers are caught; the issues with US Postal are testament to this fact. If one then adds to these factors the additional evolving factors of the sporting world, window of detection and randomization of selection for testing, one begins to get the picture as to the current state of doping detection; a less than optimal system. The aim of this research is, therefore, to assess the extent to which the current anti-doping systems are effective and efficient in their task of deterring, preventing and detecting anti-doping infringements. Unlike other papers, this research does not focus solely on the psychology of the athlete, the fear or threat factor, or even a discussion of issues with punishment as a means of deterrent. Rather this paper analyses the effectiveness and efficiency of anti-doping systems with the assistance of statistics and realities of human biology. Moreover, this paper seeks to assess whether the realities of the sporting world and athletes action manage to invalidate the anti-doping practices or demonstrate inherent flaws in the system. The reasons being, that if such issues do exist in the current system and these issues are able to be demonstrated, perhaps this will aid policy makers and organizations to amend the legislation. The eventual end result of this research is hopefully to ensure a fairer sporting environment for all participants, through the creating of policies that are both more efficient and effective in detection and prevention.

Anti-doping policies and realities

It is prudent to begin with an outline of some of the key arguments as to the existence of anti-doping systems and furthermore, the opinions of the current level of success and issue of these policies as far as they exist.

Of the assortment of factors argued as being the reasons behind the creation and existence of anti-doping, the three most commonly included reasons are, 1) athlete's health, 2) fairness and equality, and 3) sports should be a representation of a person's natural abilities. Many of the international policies in sports contain some or all of these points as justification of their existence, the WADA Code [13] and UNESCO International Convention against Doping in Sport [14] are two such examples. What is more, there is also the inclusion of such terms as 'with the potential to' enhance etc. "potential" is such an ambiguous term it is no doubt that there is much debate on the issue.

Human health: To begin with the health argument, the WADA code [13] lists health as (one of) the 'fundamental rationale's for the world anti-doping code'. The UNESCO International Convention against Doping in Sport [14], states it is "Concerned by the use of doping by athletes in sport and the consequences thereof for their health' in its preamble. It is well reported that some doping agents do indeed have harmful effects, if not though their use then through their abuse [10,15]. Beastall et al. demonstrated the deadly outcome of injection of insulin in a healthy adult. Despite this, however, there is ample evidence that suggests that a number of substances listed on the WADA prohibited list have little to no evidence that they can cause harm. One such example can be seen in the recently banned Xenon gas. Some research [16] claims that it is in fact beneficial to human health and may provide 'long term benefit' with regard to strokes. In fact, many of the substances which are now abused as doping agents began their life as medicaments. Similarly, vitamins in sports are not banned substances. It is often argued that vitamins are necessary in order for athletes to be able to compete at the highest level, implying that without them athletes would not be able to recover as quick or perform as well (does this not sound like performance enhancing?). Vitamins are deemed safe, yet abuse of vitamins can be as harmful as the abuse of banned doping substance. There is ample evidence to support the idea that high doses of some vitamins can indeed result in negative health effects [17-19].

Fairness and equality: Similar arguments can be found with fairness and equality. These two concepts are often argued as being the backbone of anti-doping policy, the reason for its existence and the primary mission of the policies. It is often difficult to define exactly what the meanings of these terms are. They differ from person to person, depending on their own sets of values and morals. Furthermore, they are in effect intangibles; they have no physical substance and are often fluid in nature. Perhaps, however, one of the most useful definitions of what fairness and equality is and to a larger extent morality in sport can be found in the works of Kuchler, who defines it as accepting the 'opponent as a partner', 'keeping in the rules', values victory no higher than their attitudes to opponents, refuses dishonour and inequality, and goes about it all good-heartedly [20].

Yet it can be said that sports, by its very nature, are not fair or equal. Athletes are never provided with the same opportunities to advance and compete. Athletes from third world nations or developing nations are automatically at a disadvantage be it because of dietary reasons, economic, or even access to training and opportunities to perform. Similarly, there is segregation between genders/sex and age. One could ask, if an athlete wants to compete with others of any background, sex or age and meet the performance requirements should they not be able to, without first gaining permission, and hoping permission will be granted. It is as if the very structure of sports promotes the idea that it is not a right but rather a privilege that one must earn and fight for. If this is the case, then it goes against everything claimed, not only by anti-doping policies but, also against the very spirit of sports.

Natural abilities: Finally, the notion that sports should be a representation of a person's natural abilities. This concept is self-explanatory. However, like the previous two concepts there is much debate about it being touted as one of the primary reasons for anti-doping policy. To begin with, there is a question of what exactly constitutes natural abilities. Moreover, there is the debate about what constitutes an alteration of a person's natural abilities. Much like the arguments outlined previously with regard to vitamins and doping practices, one must assess what constitutes enhancement and an alteration. Take vitamins again as an example. There would be those that consider the benefits that vitamins bestow upon an athlete (recovery, dietary supplementation etc.) as an indication that their performance is no longer natural. This is because, without these supplements, the athletes would not be able to perform at the high level, or at least not as long as they do and it would take longer to regain the chance of performing at this level again. Similarly as an example, there is the before mentioned argument of Xenon. One of the reasons this practice is banned is because it can be used as a form of performance enhancement. Yet it should be pointed out that Xenon is argued as performance enhancing; it simulates the effects of EPO doping. Its use is argued to stimulate Hypoxia Inducible Factors (HIF) particularly HFI-1α and as such it benefits the athlete in the same way as EPO doping. Yet it should be said that similar gains can be achieved through altitude training. Altitude training is, however, not a banned practice. If the aim of anti-doping is to preserve the fairness and natural abilities of an athlete, should not this form of training also be deemed to be altering the performance of the athlete and as such be banned? Similar arguments can be made for the use of caffeine, headache tablets, sleeping tablets and any assortment of proteins or other similar dietary supplements. These items are not banned, and are commonly used by athlete to help recover, sleep, block pain etc. all of which they would not 'naturally' be able to do without the use of the pharmaceutical or supplementary items.

Effectiveness according to some experts

There has also been some recent argument by some high level athletes that, despite the current anti-doping systems, even if they are effective, testing is at best rare. To elaborate, Chris Froome criticised the lack of anti-doping testing over a two week period during a key training camp for himself and two other high level cycling athletes [21,22]. Similarly in 2011 it was reported by Gerard Vroomen (2009-2010 head of Cervelo Test Team cycling), that 'I have not heard of a rider being tested for the biological passport between the end of the 2010 Tour and April 2011' [23]. This was later supported by Michael Ashenden a member of the UCI passport panel that stated 'It's correct that the observation made by Gerard Vroomen matches with my experience. I have noticed a significant gap between tests in some of the profiles I have reviewed' [24]. This would therefore indicate that despite the justification behind anti-doping policies, their goals are less likely to be achieved if they are not even being performed, irrespective of the issues surrounding the system.

This seems to indicate that there is much controversy as to the justification of anti-doping policies. This is especially true given the fact that the systems, as they currently operate, place a large number of restrictions on the personal liberties and privacy of athletes. Examples of which can be seen with the whereabouts requirement [25] (14.V.18), biological passport [26] (14.VI.120) and the rules governing urine collection [27] (7.2.4.). In fact Kayser, Mauron and Miah [28] suggested that 'current anti-doping measures potentially introduce problems of greater impact than are solved'. Their paper critically assesses current anti-doping policies and concludes that they are in many ways based on a weak foundation. Naturally one would expect by this point in the development of anti-doping systems, the systems (as they currently are) would be finely tuned to ensure that they are effective and efficient in their goals. Furthermore, that they are successful in deterring doping and detecting it when it does occur. The realities are however, unfortunately quite different. There are factors inherent in the sporting systems and the testing practices as they exist that impact the success of anti-doping.

Window of detection

Window of Detection is in reference to the time frame in which a substance remains detectable in a human body before it is broken down/absorbed and it is no longer possible to detect if an illegal substance has been used. Extant literature would seem to indicate that this figure, using the current testing at the disposal of WADA and anti-doping agencies worldwide, would range from as little as 12 hours to a maximum of 120 hours. On the lower end of this scale 12-24 hours. Research conducted by Bidlingmaier, Wu, & Strasburger [29] showed that more contemporary forms of hGH, when administered by subcutaneous methods, return to baseline within 20 hours maximum following administration. They further outline that in some cases the window of these agents, when administered intramuscularly may even be as low as 8 hours. This has serious consequences for detection, particularly when coupled with the apparently increasing method of micro doping. Moreover, micro doping especially with recombinant human erythropoietin (rHuEPO) have been shown to fall into this low window of detectability also [30,31]. It was reported by Asheden et al. [30] that micro dosing reduced the window of detection of rHuEPO to as little as 12 hours. What this means is that should an athlete decide to dope immediately before long distance endurance event, such as the Le Mans 24 hour race, then by the time they are finished any trace of the substance would be removed. More concerning is the combination of these two pieces of research, micro doping with hGH. If intramuscular administration of hGH already has a window of 8 hours micro doping will reduce this further. This means that doping immediately before a race; particularly an endurance event, such as a cycling stage, would mean that the agent would be undetectable well before the end of the event.

It has been found that for the more commonly found doping agents such as steroids and regular doses of rHuEPO that a greater window of detection is obtained, 48-72 hours [31-33]. The plasticizer di-(2-ethylhexyl) phthalate (DEHP) (not a doping agent but argued as being evidence of blood doping) can also be grouped into this category. Research by Monfort, et al. [34] demonstrated that these metabolites remain in the system only up to 48 hours after infusion.

Finally, even some of the more 'traditional' substances of doping such as hGH when applying contemporary techniques of detection still have a somewhat limited window. It has been reported by Erotokritou-Mulligan, et al., [11] that the use of markers such as type 3 pro-collagen (P-III-P) for the detection of hGH may increase the window of detection to around 120 hours.

It should be pointed out that there is some research which demonstrates a longer window of detection of around 18-20 days. This research relates to some forms of methyltestosterone metabolite M2 [35] and oxandrolone metabolite 17β-hydroxymethyl-17α-methyl-18-nor-2-oxa-5α-androsta-13-en-3-on (OX M1) [36]. Yet it should be pointed out that other metabolites of methyltestosterone [35] and the 'parent drug oxandrolone and its isomer epioxandrolone' were only detectable for about 3days, which supports the findings of other research and justifies the use of the estimated figures in this research. However, in order to provide a more comprehensive view of the situation, calculations for these figures can be found in the proceeding sections.

Test sensitivity

Test sensitivity refers to the accuracy of testing. That is to say, if for example 100 tests were performed on samples with doping agents in them what percentage of them are likely to be classified as containing doping agents. It is next to impossible to have any technique that is 100% accurate, in any and all cases of chemical testing there is some margin for error; false positives are an example of common errors that are known to occur. Upon closer inspection of the literature, which is at times apprehensive to outline the exact percentages of accuracy, one begins to obtain a clearer image of the current situation.

The highest rates of success of doping detection have been reported as being between 60% and 80% success rate. It has been reported by Powrie et al., [37] that these levels could be obtained with cases of the more classical doping substance of hGH, when using N-terminal extension peptide of procollagen type III markers for detection, so contemporary techniques for classical problems. Yet other papers have reported far less encouraging results. Erotokritou-Mulligan et al., [11] reported that other forms of growth hormones such as hGH even when combined with the use of Insulin Growth Factor-1 (IGF-I) and P-III- P only resulted in a success rate of 40%. Worse still (and perhaps a worst case scenario) were the findings by Graham et al., [12], who reported that tests, conducted on both non-steroidal hormones and hGH, in some cases resulted in a successful detection rate of only 10%. This is extremely concerning for those in the fight against doping. These figures would seem to indicate that a majority of testing is at best hit or miss. Thus perhaps many doped athletes are slipping through the cracks.

Doping regime

Doping regime is in reference to the actual frequency of doping as performed by athletes deciding to partake in the practice. Given the illegality of doping, and the potential for criminal prosecution in some counties including Austria (Gesamte Rechtsvorschrift für Anti-Doping-Bundesgesetz, 2007) [38], France (Code du sport, 2012) [39] and Italy (Disciplina della tutela sanitaria delle attività sportive e della lotta contro il doping, 2000) [40], there is considerable apprehension by some athletes to reveal exactly the doping methods and frequencies used. Given this, information is limited, but some evidence does still exit. Graham et al. [12] reported that the doping regime of an anonymous UK champion was continuous, multiple times per week, that is to say regular doses when 'required' to ensure maximal performance. Further information is either lacking or ambiguous, but it is safe to say that given the intellect of athletes, some will be using doping agent intermittently so to attempt to ensure evasion of detection.

Predictability of testing

Test predictability is the likelihood that an athlete choosing to partake in doping is able to predict when the anti-doping sample will be required. To elaborate, if an athlete chooses to dope, it is highly unlikely they will do so without some level of thought going into both the decision to dope and the decision as to when to use the banned substances. In the case of the latter, the decision as to when to use, will be based in part on the likelihood that they will be tested or not within the window of detectability period. This likelihood can be argued as being primarily based on the past rates of anti-doping sample collection. That is to say how frequently they and other athletes around them have been selected for sample collection. The literature does not and more than likely is not able to list the figures for an athlete's belief of when they will be tested and so alternative source data must be used to make this determination. As such reference to the statistics available from various nation anti-doping agencies (NADA) and the world anti-doping agency is needed to make this determination. These sources demonstrate vastly differing numbers relating the amounts of testing performed on various athletes in their care. It has been reported that these figures range from 2 through to 24 tests a year [39-44]. These figures are dependent on a number of factors. These include the athlete in question, their rates of success in the events they compete, policies of the NADA, and more than likely the economic realities and resources available to the NADA. What this indicates is that the athlete in question is able to make approximate estimates on when they are likely to be tested, for example during a major competition, or before, or more generally when in a month they are likely to receive an out-of-competition test. All of which contributes to their decision making process and as such the predictability of testing.

Method

This research contains two different approaches to assessing the current effectiveness of the anti-doping system; these being a probability and a cost analysis of the current system of testing.

Probability analyses are a useful tool to attempt to gain a better view of probable outcomes based on a set of uncertainties. They are often used, along with costs analyses, as a useful tool for assessment of effectiveness in health system research [43-47]. The initial step required was to conduct research into the factors influencing the successfulness of anti-doping testing using the current system. This was performed by examining extant literature on the topic. Information pertaining to factors involved in anti-doping testing and doping practices used by athletes was collected from official documents by anti-doping agencies, academic papers, media releases etc. Sources are quoted in the information that follows. It was found that an assortment of factors influence the probability doping will be detected, and as such it was necessary to attempt to quantify these factors. Anti-doping testing does not always result in a positive detection even if and athlete may be engaging in doping. The factors relate to the sporting world impact the actual real life test success. These factors were determined to be as follows based on the literature as outlined previously; a) window of detection, b) test sensitivity, c) doping regime, and d) predictability of testing.

Given the realities, certain conclusions can be made as the necessary parameters to make up the formula to asses probability of success of the anti-doping system. Each of these influences can be considered a variable contributing to the probability of doping detection in a single test. The realities are, a) the window of detection is limited, b) sensitivity of tests is mostly low, c) doping substances may be used intermittently by athletes to help avoid detection, and also d) athletes may guess when a test will occur. The total probability of detection will be a product of probabilities of the four contributing variables, window of detection (W), test sensitivity (S), doping regime (D), and predictability of testing (T). Given this, the second step was to construct a formula demonstrating the likelihood of detection of doping, based on these factors. This formula is as follows:

$P= W\times S\times D\times T$

Where:

W= window of detection in hours expressed as a fraction of a week assuming week or 168 hours = 1

S= test sensitivity

D= how often doping occurs, 1.0 being continuous use and fractions indicating intermittent use

T= test predictability per person per week, expressed as the number of tests that could be expected per year divided by the number of weeks in the year (52).

For example a test with a window of detection of 24 hours i.e. 0.14 in a week, with 40% test sensitivity with a person continuously doping i.e. 1.0 in each week, and predictability of 0.25 because random tests occur on average once a month will produce an overall probability of 0.014 of a random test to be successful. This means that the probability of a random test to be unsuccessful is 0.986, close enough to certainty in most situations.

This concept is depicted graphically in Figure 1 and demonstrates

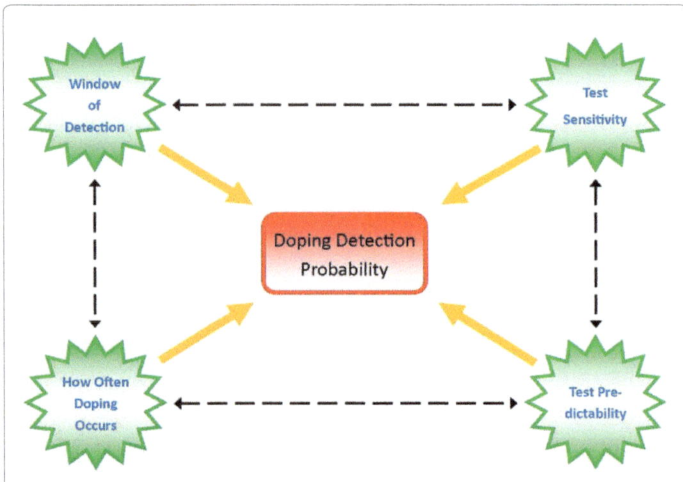

Figure 1: Graphic representation of the factors influencing the probability of detection and their relationship to one another.

the relationship between the four elements and their influence on the probability of doping detection. It shows that each element affecting the probability of doping detection also has an impact on each other element. For example, the window of detectability impacts an athlete's doping regime and test predictability. As too does test sensitivity. An athlete's doping regime is also impacted by the test predictability, and so on (Figure 1).

There are a number of reasons why the literature is apprehensive to reveal definitive numbers pertaining to some of these variables. These reasons include, but are not limited to, the clandestine nature of doping, the lack of dedicated research into each of these components, and apprehension of publication of controversial findings with regard to doping, to name but a few. Thus a range of estimates was used. The estimates used for this research are found in table 1, and are based on the findings in the literature as outlined previously (Table 1).

Similarly, a majority of the substances relate to Androgenic Anabolic Steroid (AAS) and Growth Hormone (GH). EPO, blood doping and stimulants are used and can all be very effective methods of doping. Unfortunately given the somewhat contemporary origins of some of these substances, the lack of funding for doping research in some cases and the general clandestine nature of doping, research in these area's does not provide sufficient information to make a reliable assumption.

Variable	Estimated Values	Drug Types
Window of detectability	12 – 24 hours 48 – 72 hours 120 hours	hGH, micro doping rHuEPO common agents, rHuEPO, DEHP new techniques for old agents
Test sensitivity	10% 40% 60-80%	non-steroidal hormones and hGH hGH (with IGF-I, P-III-P) hGH (N-terminal extension peptide of procollagen type III)
Doping Regime	1.0 (continuous) 0.5 (intermittent)	
Test predictability (tests per year)	2 6 9 12 24	

Table 1: Doping probability formula parameters, estimates and drug types.

The odds of detection per year were calculated as the inverse of the probability of detection in a single test multiplied by the number of tests during a year. The odds of detection in the entire career were based on the assumption of a career of 15 year duration with the annual probabilities unchanging. Thus these odds were an inverse of 15 times the probability of detection per year times the number of tests per year.

The final step in this research was to conduct a cost analysis. This was done in order to attempt to ascertain the feasibilities of anti-doping testing given the realities of the sporting world. A cost analysis is a useful tool for this as it takes into consideration economic realities from numerous sources and can help paint a more complete and tangible picture of what really is happening in reference to real world economics. Cost (and economics) analyses of doping are useful tools when it comes to assessing sports related expenses, and have been used by a number of internationally renowned experts in sports as a tool for assessing efficiency [48-50].

The analysis for this research was a two-step process. Firstly it was necessary to determine the amount of testing needed to, in all probability, actually detect doping when it occurs. Following this these numbers were then assessed in light of the costs associated with standardized urine testing, with figures available from the Australian Sports Anti-Doping Authority. More details relating to these figures are outlined in the relevant sections following.

Results and Discussion

Odds of doping detection

A series of calculations have been performed using values as established from the literature as were outlined previously in the methods section, these calculations can be seen in Table 2. The column entitled Sport with detection rate matching odds, is an indication of

Window of Detection(hrs)	Test Sensitivity	Doping Regime (weekly)	Test predictability per person per week	Probability of detection in a single test	Number of tests (per year)	Odds of escaping detection	Odds of escaping detection in 15yrs career	Sport with detection rate matching odds
12	0.4	1	0.25	**0.0071**	12	12:1	1:1	
18	0.4	1	0.25	**0.0107**	12	8:1	1:1	
48	0.4	1	0.25	**0.0286**	12	3:1	0:1	
72	0.4	1	0.25	**0.0429**	12	2:1	0:1	
120	0.4	1	0.25	**0.0714**	12	1:1	0:1	
12	0.4	1	0.038	**0.0011**	2	461:1	31:1	
18	0.4	1	0.038	**0.0016**	2	307:1	20:1	
48	0.4	1	0.038	**0.0043**	2	115:1	8:1	Sailing, Athletics
72	0.4	1	0.038	**0.0065**	2	77:1	5:1	Basketball, Archery, Cycling, Rugby
120	0.4	1	0.038	**0.0109**	2	46:1	3:1	
12	0.8	1	0.038	**0.0022**	2	230:1	15:1	
18	0.8	1	0.038	**0.0033**	2	154:1	10:1	Aquatics, Sailing
48	0.8	1	0.038	**0.0087**	2	58:1	4:1	Basketball, Cycling

72	0.8	1	0.038	**0.0130**	2	38:1	3:1	
120	0.8	1	0.038	**0.0217**	2	23:1	2:1	
12	0.1	1	0.038	**0.0003**	2	1842:1	123:1	
18	0.1	1	0.038	**0.0004**	2	1228:1	82:1	
48	0.1	1	0.038	**0.0011**	2	461:1	31:1	
72	0.1	1	0.038	**0.0016**	2	307:1	20:1	
120	0.1	1	0.038	**0.0027**	2	184:1	12:1	Shooting
12	0.1	0.5	0.038	**0.0001**	2	3684:1	246:1	
18	0.1	0.5	0.038	**0.0002**	2	2456:1	164:1	
48	0.1	0.5	0.038	**0.0005**	2	921:1	61:1	
72	0.1	0.5	0.038	**0.0008**	2	614:1	41:1	Bobsleigh
120	0.1	0.5	0.038	**0.0014**	2	368:1	25:1	
12	0.4	0.5	0.038	**0.0005**	2	921:1	61:1	
18	0.4	0.5	0.038	**0.0008**	2	614:1	41:1	Bobsleigh
48	0.4	0.5	0.038	**0.0022**	2	230:1	15:1	Fencing
72	0.4	0.5	0.038	**0.0033**	2	154:1	10:1	Aquatics. Athletics
120	0.4	0.5	0.038	**0.0054**	2	92:1	6:1	Cycling, Rugby
12	0.4	0.5	0.25	**0.0036**	12	23:1	2:1	
18	0.4	0.5	0.25	**0.0054**	12	16:1	1:1	Bridge
48	0.4	0.5	0.25	**0.0143**	12	6:1	0:1	Bodybuilding
72	0.4	0.5	0.25	**0.0214**	12	4:1	0:1	
120	0.4	0.5	0.25	**0.0357**	12	2:1	0:1	
12	0.5	0.5	0.5	**0.0089**	24	5:1	0:1	
18	0.5	0.5	0.5	**0.0134**	24	3:1	0:1	
48	0.5	0.5	0.5	**0.0357**	24	1:1	0:1	
72	0.5	0.5	0.5	**0.0536**	24	1:1	0:1	
120	0.5	0.5	0.5	**0.0893**	24	0:1	0:1	
12	0.4	0.5	0.125	**0.0018**	6	93:1	6:1	Triathalon
18	0.4	0.5	0.125	**0.0027**	6	62:1	4:1	Equestrian, Rugby
48	0.4	0.5	0.125	**0.0071**	6	23:1	2:1	Boules, Billiards, Motorcycle Racing, Powerlifiting
72	0.4	0.5	0.125	**0.0107**	6	16:1	1:1	Bridge, Sambo
120	0.4	0.5	0.125	**0.0179**	6	9:1	1:1	
12	0.4	1	0.125	**0.0036**	6	47:1	3:1	Weightlifiting, Rollersport, Golf
18	0.4	1	0.125	**0.0054**	6	31:1	2:1	Airsports
48	0.4	1	0.125	**0.0143**	6	12:1	1:1	Muay Thai
72	0.4	1	0.125	**0.0214**	6	8:1	1:1	
120	0.4	1	0.125	**0.0357**	6	5:1	0:1	
12	0.4	0.5	0.188	**0.0027**	9	41:1	3:1	Weightlifiting

18	0.4	0.5	0.188	**0.0040**	9	28:1	2:1	Morocycle racing
48	0.4	0.5	0.188	**0.0107**	9	10:1	1:1	
72	0.4	0.5	0.188	**0.0161**	9	7:1	0:1	
120	0.4	0.5	0.188	**0.0269**	9	4:1	0:1	
12	0.4	1.0	0.188	**0.0054**	9	21:1	1:1	Kickboxing
18	0.4	1.0	0.188	**0.0081**	9	14:1	1:1	Muay Thai
48	0.4	1.0	0.188	**0.0215**	9	5:1	0:1	Bodybuilding
72	0.4	1.0	0.188	**0.0322**	9	3:1	0:1	
120	0.4	1.0	0.188	**0.0537**	9	2:1	0:1	

Table 2: Probabilities of doping detection.

Discipline	Adverse Analytical Findings %	Discipline	Adverse Analytical Findings %
Aikido	0.00	Hockey	1.32
Air sports	3.09	Judo	1.13
Archery	1.47	Kendo	0.00
Athletics	0.78	Kickboxing	4.97
Baseball	1.99	Motorcycle racing	4.15
Basketball	1.45	Muay Thai	8.11
Biathlon	0.00	Netball	0.83
Billiards	4.24	Powerboating	0.00
Bobsleigh	0.16	Powerlifting	4.88
Bodybuilding and fitness	18.09	Rowing	0.23
Boxing	1.94	Rugby	1.39
Bridge	6.00	Skiing	0.71
Cycling	1.19	Sleddog	3.70
Darts	2.70	Weightlifting	2.42
Football	0.48	Wrestling	1.23
Golf	2.04	Wushu	1.68

Table 3: Adverse Analytical Findings % for an assortment of sports [41].

those sports which have a detection rate which coincides to the figures provided by WADA and its adverse analytical findings (Table 3). It was decided to use the WADA adverse analytical finding (AAF) figures instead of Anti-Doping Rule Violation (ADRV) figures as this research relates to the detection of doping agents not justifications of how they entered the athletes' system and thus subsequent legal and ethical considerations (Table 2).

If one were to therefore use a set of commonly encountered values (W= 48, S = 0.4, D=1 and T=0.25) to calculate a probability of doping detection in one random test, one gets p= 0.029; meaning that in a single test there is only approximately a 2.9% chance of doping being detected.

When this is then extrapolated to yearly detection, if one were to select 12 tests a year as an average, then this results in a detection rate of approximately 34% or an odds ratio of 3:1. This indicates that there is in fact a 66% chance of a doped athlete not being detected, quite good odds for someone willing to take a risk. This calculation is based on an assumption that tests are done completely randomly without prior warning and without predictability. Where an exact date of a test is predictable, the risk of detection would decline even further, even with 12 tests per year. Similarly, if one incorporates the extended window of detection of 21 days, one obtains the following, 21 days x 0.4 sensitivity, intermittent doping of 0.5, and predictability of 0.125, resulting in an overall probability of 0.075 meaning that even in this case there is only a 7.5% chance of being detected in a single test or 92.5% chance of escaping detection. Assuming continuous doping this figure comes down to 85% that is still far away from 50/50 risk taking.

This makes the risk potentially psychologically acceptable to the "doper" [51]. To elaborate, it would seem less likely that an athlete who feels that they have a high probability of getting caught would partake in doping. On the other hand athletes who feel that there is a high probability they will escape detection would be more likely to engage in doping. This is because they may well feel that the result of doping would bring significant rewards without significant risk, the notion of a cost-risk ratio. It can be argued that despite the inherent flaws in the anti-doping systems, this is one feature that provides the most benefit, the impression that anti-doping is effective. Even if it is not, the sheer power of an athlete believing it is may in some cases deter them from engaging. This is the notion of cost-risk ratio, the idea that athletes weigh up the costs of the likelihood of getting caught and the consequence if they do vs. the benefits if they don't. It would seem that as the current anti-doping systems are structured and the problems associated with detection, some athlete may see the benefits significantly outweighing the risks.

However, similarly to this notion of fear and deterrence, there is another element of anti-doping testing which contributes to its effectiveness but is not directly related to success of detection. This concept relates back to Foucault's Panopticon [52] and more recently the work by Haggerty and Ericson's [53] on surveillant assemblage. This notion presents the idea that the panopticon (or other forms of surveillance) results in a decline of undesirable behaviours. One could say it is a form of negative reinforcement. This concept having its origins in a theoretical prison system, purports that an inmate watched or believing they are watched (even if they are not) are less likely to engage in negative behaviors. This, as it relates to sports, would seem to be reasonable, for even if anti-doping is not effective per se, perhaps the mere existence of testing may deter some athletes from doping for fear they might possibly be caught as they are always being watched. There are, however, two problems that exist here. Firstly, some people prefer the notion of being watched, the idea that it is more of a challenge to 'beat the system'. Secondly, in some areas of the world, capital punishment still exists for certain crimes. Some states of the United States are one such example. Moreover, the United States, being one the world's, most technologically advanced nations have ample systems of surveillance of its citizens in place, not only video but there are also numerous organizations which exist to this end. Despite this reality, crimes are still committed; murders are still committed, even with the death penalty in place and constant surveillance. The thought that simply watching someone will eliminate the darker sides of human nature is both unrealistic and delusional. It may, in some limited cases, work, but if someone is determined enough to cheat they will find a way despite all the surveillance and punishments possible.

What the above results indicate is that by using current statistics it would seem that the likelihood of being caught doping is somewhere between 0.1 and 10% in a single test. To put this in perspective, the most complete and considered official current statistics pertaining to adverse analytical findings are provided by the World Anti-Doping Agency [54]. These findings, per sport, range anywhere from 0 to about 18% [41]. This would seem to indicate that given the findings of this research, the extent to which doping occurs is very high. Theoretically, using these figures, if one were to assume that 100% of athletes dope, because of the limited window of detection, low test sensitivity and infrequent testing, it is likely to have result in 2.9% of adverse findings only. To elaborate, according to the calculations, if W= 0.29 (48hours), S = 0.4, D=1 and T=0.25, one obtains a 2.9% chance of doping detection in a single test. Therefore if one was to then again refer to the statistics available from WADA a sport with an adverse analytical finding of 2.9% (such as is closely the case with darts) would seem to indicate that given these conditions a vast majority of athletes in that sport were engaged in doping. Assuming tests were completely random and every athlete doped regularly, then the percentage of positive test findings (adverse analytical findings) would be low, roughly corresponding to actual data published by WADA.

This indicates two things. 1) That doping is far more widespread than official figures would lead one to believe and 2) That the current system of anti-doping testing is inadequate to eliminate doping. This supposition is supported by a number of officials [55] in the sporting arena, some athletes [56] and numerous others involved in sports including academics [28,57]. It should be noted that scientific literature does not always quote specific examples. For this reason they must be searched for in websites and popular literature. This is why such examples were used above. Illicit activities can hardly be researched systematically and this is why formal scientific literature does not provide relevant information. As outlined previously it can be said that it appears as though anti-doping policies are in place more for reasons of perceptions and deterrence through fear then for any effective and efficient scientific merit. This lends further support for the assertions by Hermann & Henneberg, [58] as to the relationship both perceptions and image has to modern sports, their participants and anti-doping.

Rates of doping

Table 3 demonstrates current WADA statistics relating to adverse analytical results.

Whilst it should be pointed out that, by WADA's own admission, these data are not entirely complete; they do still provide a reasonable approximation of the extent of findings in each discipline. When the figures in Table 3 are compared to the calculations in Table 2, Table 4 can be thus derived.

Sport	Adverse Analytical Findings	Corresponding doping characteristics if all athletes dope		
		Window of Detection	Test Accuracy	Dosage
Air Sports	3.09	18	40%	Continuous
Archery	1.47	48	40%	Continuous
Baseball	1.99	48	40%	Continuous
Bobsleigh	0.16	72	10%	Interval
Cycling	1.19	48	80%	Continuous
Football	0.48	48	40%	Interval
Rowing	0.23	48	10%	Continuous

Table 4: Actually reported adverse analytical findings and corresponding possible doping characteristics under assumption that all athletes in a given sport apply doping.

These comparisons demonstrate the assumptions under which the current doping rates would represent a mere portion of the actual doping rates. Continuous or intermittent in Table 4 are based on those in Table 2. Cycling can be used as one such example; WADA statistics indicate a 1. 19 % adverse analytical test result for the sport. If we then use the assumption that there is an 48 hour window of detection of the agents used, a 80% accuracy of testing, doping agents are used continuously and athletes can predict testing in a week knowing that they will be tested about 3 times a year, this allows the possibility to calculate that about 100% of cyclists would be participating in doping. This is done in the following manner, 48 hour window (48/168=0.286) × Sensitivity of 0.84× continuous regime (1.0) × test predictability 0.0576 = 1.32%. If WADA statistics indicate that in cycling just over 1.0% adverse analytical findings are made then this indicates that a significantly higher proportion of athletes in the sport are participating in doping and due to restrictions of the anti-doping system are simply not getting detected. Whilst it is unrealistic to suggest that all cyclists are using doping agents, the suggestion does remain that the figures do not truly represent actual rates of doping. Similar, are the results seen with baseball. Whilst it should be pointed out that this sport historically did not conform to the WADA guidelines for anti-doping testing they still performed some anti-doping tests, some of which are indeed used by other sports. The results are similar to that of cycling. These conclusions are supported by findings of the Mitchell Report which stated that 'the use of steroids in Major League Baseball was widespread' [59]. Moreover, the same report acknowledged the fact that not all substances are detectable (in the case of the Mitchell Report the researchers were referring to hGH) [59]. It also concluded that 'Baseball does not need and cannot afford to engage in a never-ending search for the name of every player who ever used performance enhancing substances' [59]. This could be argued as indicating two things. Firstly, that doping use in Baseball was so widespread it would be next to impossible to make a complete list. Second, perhaps that given the nature of doping detection, clandestine nature of doping and the opposition faced by the researchers [59] such an investigation would be next to impossible.

Testing requirements

The fact that tests are not working well is illustrated by WADA's recent decision to increase the length of doping bans from 2 to 4 years when the 2015 code comes into force in 2015 [60] with the aim of increasing the deterrent effect of the penalty. In law enforcement this practice it is usually performed when detection of a wrongdoing is ineffective. Some research, however, has claimed that increasing the

Sport	Tests Needed	Approximate Cost
Air Sports	43	€ 25,112.00
Archery	22	€ 12,848.00
Baseball	50	€ 29,200.00
Bobsleigh	50	€ 29,200.00
Cycling	16	€ 9,344.00
Football	30	€ 17,520.00
Rowing	43	€ 25,112.00

Table 5: Doping testing needed (per year per athlete) to reliably detect doping. Based on current WADA figures and doping characteristics as outlined in table 4, and examples of costs per year (using urine tests) per athlete for reliable detection of doping.

penalty for a wrongdoing will have no impact on the criminal behavior [61,62]. On the other hand it could be argued that this increase was to attempt to combat the perceived unfairness of current bans, which could result in Olympic athletes not missing a single Olympics. This, however, would depend on when the ban was passed out. Furthermore, professional sports being what they are currently, it is unlikely that a top level professional athlete after missing 2 seasons would be at the same level of fitness as before, especially race fitness. As such a ban of 2 years would still have an effect on their actual success rate. 4 years may amplify this effect, but one must be careful that if the athlete is to be given a second chance, the length of suspension is not too long.

As such this research demonstrates that a new approach to anti-doping policy is needed. Given the current realities of doping in professional sports, the question remains, what regime is required to begin to combat doping?

Table 5 depicts the number of tests needed per year to detect doping effectively. This was calculated using the figures and assumptions provided in Table 2. The number of tests needed was calculated as an inverse of T (predictability) required to achieve 100% detection with given windows of detection, continuity/intermittency of use and test reliabilities. The results of Table 5 indicate that the number of doping tests in many sports will need to be unrealistically increased in order to effectively combat doping. Indications are such that should anti-doping testing remain unchanged legislation would need to be modified to accommodate the realities of doping. One interesting point worth investigating in Table 5 is the number of yearly tests needed per athlete to detect doping (with relative effectiveness) in cycling. The theoretical figures would seem to indicate 16 tests per year would be sufficient to do so. Currently in cycling, either through the UCI, or the national anti-doping agencies, some athletes would no doubt already submit this many samples. One would normally expect that the most successful and high profile athletes would normally be the ones that would be subjected to such a large number of tests a year. This, however, may be questionable, given the statements outlined previously by Chris Froome and the lack of testing he and other top cyclists experienced. Even if this was an isolated case and testing over that small period was lacking, and throughout the rest of the year testing is extensive why then are many doping cases in cycling being revealed only through self-admission rather than positive tests? One possible argument can be seen with the revelations in the Lance Armstrong case there are a number of other factors which play a role in successful detection. These factors are such that they cannot be easily quantified. These factors include third party involvement, warnings of upcoming testing, role of money etc. It should also be pointed out that if athletes are able to manipulate tests then this would make it even harder to detect doping. This does not necessarily mean tampering with sample collection, or tampering with the samples after collection (which still may occur despite measures taken to prevent this), but rather for example athletes may take doping agents immediately after testing, knowing that it is unlikely they will be tested again soon. If athletes can partly predict when tests are going to occur and/or can manipulate testing then it will lower probability of detection in a single test and this strengthens this papers argument. There may also be specific effects of the method of doping or testing that would deviate somewhat from the simple calculations.

The cost of effective anti-doping

If one then focuses on the testing required per year, per athlete, for effective detection, the next step is to then extrapolate this into real world financial figures. Put simply, it is necessary to make a cost determination of such an increase in the testing regime and thus a determination of the cost of an effective and efficient means of doping detection.

Furthermore, reference again to Table 5, one can also see the total cost per athlete per year of doping tests needed to reliably detect doping , is on average €21,190.86 (USD 28,676.30). This is an average based upon the number of tests needed which ranges from 16 to 50 depending on the discipline. This uses approximate urine test cost figures as available through Australian Sports Anti-Doping Authority (ASADA) [63] of about €584 (AU$738, USD 692.59) per test (blood and EPO testing costs are higher). Urine tests were chosen as they are most commonly used test for doping detection and the least expensive. Other testing, such as blood testing, has higher costs associated with it and therefore any calculations would produce greater costs/numbers. There is some argument that blood testing required for the Athletes Biological Passport (ABP) is cheaper, but given the added difficulties in analysis and collecting blood samples, the trained staff needed etc. it seems that in the long run even ABP blood testing would cost more than urine. The lower figures were used in the calculations simply to demonstrate that even at the lowest level the costs associated with effective testing would amount to an astronomical figure. The approximate total cost per year for all athletes in a given nation to be subject to such tests, is subject to the nation in question. If one is to take as an example Germany, and one refers to their website for appropriate data relating to the testing pool, one begins to see the scale. Current data shows that Germany's athletes number around the 4000 [42], this however, does not including the national testing pool of athletes). Given these figures the total funds would need to exceed 84 Million Euros (€84,763,428.57 or about USD$114,715,721.16). The German National Anti-Doping Associations total annual revenue was €4,570,062 (USD 6,184,576.60) for the year ending 2010 [42], this would result in a €80,193,366.57 (USD 108,514,946.82) shortfall.

What is more, this figure incorporates only the actual cost of tests, it does not take into account the additional costs associated with anti-doping testing. These would include, but not be limited to, hiring sample collection staff, collection materials, Out of Competition travelling for collection, physical resources etc. Therefore, what this shows is that the level of testing needed to effectively detect doping is economically unfeasible. Whilst it is likely true that some of the cost of testing will be borne by the national federations themselves, it does, however, seems highly unlikely that all the levels of funding needed for complete testing will be available given economic realities. Sports may be a lucrative area but there are still realities about real world economics and financing that demonstrate that despite the figures involved, the level of funding needed to make an effective testing regime is infeasible.

Biological passport and forensic testing

One cannot assert to having fully addressed the ineffectiveness of the current anti-doping system without addressing the existence and usage of both the Athlete Biological Passport (ABP) [64] and an assortment of forensic methods such as hair testing. WADA outlines the ABP as,

The fundamental principle of the Athlete Biological Passport (ABP) is to monitor selected variables ('biomarkers of doping') over time that indirectly reveal the effect of doping, as opposed to the traditional direct detection of doping by analytical doping controls.

In effect the ABP is a tool for keeping track of the changing variables in human physiology. Unlike conventional testing it does not directly determine the existence of doping substances in the body system but instead considers its indirect consequences. This method is often argued as being the next generation in anti-doping testing; a more effective test, one with greater potential than conventional testing [64-66]. Yet there is ample evidence that supports the notion that, like conventional testing, the ABP is far from perfect and as such supports the supposition that current anti-doping is ineffective.

To begin with, there is the debate surrounding indirect testing. It is true that in some cases doping can be detected without directly discovering the substance in the blood. This is done through indirect blood or urine biomarkers [65-67]. However, these same markers can also be an indication of an assortment of other causes from illness, medical assistance, training techniques, physiological uniqueness of an individual etc [68,69]. It does not in every case indicate the use of banned substances. Despite this the athlete still needs to, in effect, prove their innocence. An additional issue with the ABP can be found in the research by Ashenden, Gough, Garnham, Gore & Sharpe [70]. Their research involved the intravenous injection of recombinant human erythropoietin (rhEPO) into 10 subjects for up to 12 weeks. Results of the study found that in microdose amounts EPO was undetectable in the ABP. If the ABP at present is not even detecting what it was introduced to detect then one can quite clearly conclude that it is ineffective.

Further issues with the ABP have been reported in areas one may not normally expect to be such a major factor contributing to ineffectiveness. Banfi [71] has reported the ABP may be affected by an assortment of factors such as:

'Quality control of the instruments is not completely assured. Analytical variability is not appropriately considered in the program. The seasonal changes of the hematological parameters, due to training and competitions, are not calculated. Statistical analysis, based on a Bayesian-like program, not available to the scientific community, does not follow the classical decision making approach of medicine and science.'

All of these factors indicate that at present the ABP has its shortfalls and may in fact currently not be an effective tool for anti-doping, or at least not to the level it should be.

Furthermore, a number of key international experts in the area of cycling have criticised yet another issue with the ABP. As outlined previously, both Gerard Vroomen former head of Cervelo TestTeam and international anti-doping expert Michael Ashenden reported a lack of testing with regard to the ABP. This lack of testing demonstrates that the current system is ineffective; be that because testing is inaccurate, imprecise or simply not occurring (perhaps due to economic reasons). These could explain the drop in extreme blood values in cyclists since the introduction of the ABP. If there are long periods of no testing then of course the more extreme values are likely to be missed.

It has also been argued that there has been more Anti-Doping Rule Violations (ADRVs) in cycling since the introduction of the ABP. Even if there are more ADRVs in cycling, the actual number of athletes sanctioned because of the ABP remains extremely low. In this regards can it be said that the ABP is having the desired effect? If athletes who are under the ABP are being found to have questionable results, and as such brought up on charges for anti-doping violations, but still are not being sanctioned, then is the program really helping the state of affairs or simply making them worse ?.

In the case of modern forensic testing, there is still some debate as to tests' effectiveness. WADA for example still has not certified the use of forensic testing methods, such as hair analysis, in their anti-doping systems. There are some issues with hair testing. Unlike urine or blood, hair is not always present and available for testing. This can be because of baldness or shaving by the athlete. Similarly, it is simply not possible to detect all the same substances as urine or blood testing does. Or is the decision not to sanction hair testing due to the cost? Would it not cost significantly more (at present) to undertake such analyses? More research is required to ascertain the effectiveness and efficiency of various forms of forensic testing, but the reality is at present that these techniques are not used (for whatever reason) and as such cannot be said to be part of the current anti-doping system. There is one case worth mentioning, the case of Richard Gasquet. In order to clear his name, he ordered an independent hair analysis to determine the presence of cocaine in his system. This was accepted by the Court of Arbitration in Sport (CAS). The reality remains this acceptance was not issued by WADA nor the International Tennis Federation (ITF), and what is more, the test was negative. Gasquet later admitted use but argued it was inadvertent and no fault of his own, this was accepted by the CAS [72]. Overall this brings into question the effectiveness of the hair testing.

Limitation and Future Research

In November 2013 WADA's Foundation Board meeting [73] decided on the introduction of a Steroidal Module into the ABP. This method of profiling may change the effectiveness of the current anti-doping testing. At this point there is too little evidence to determine its current effectiveness and so more testing and time is needed. One can, however, say that if the same problems arise with the Steroidal Module as with haemoglobin; the same scientific issues and ethical issues are involved, then the findings of this research will be strengthened. Similarly if WADA decided to confirm the use of hair and/or similar forensic testing methods, further research will be needed to assess how this may change the effectiveness of anti-doping testing. One key limitation to this research is the difficulty finding specific figures relating the four variables for the formula. The clandestine nature of doping made obtaining exact figures impossible and as such estimates were used. Exact figures would ensure a more complete picture could be painted.

Conclusion

The primary conclusion that can be drawn from this research is that the current system of anti-doping is, given the realities of the sporting world, ineffective at reaching the desired goals. This is assuming the primary goal of the anti-doping system is to eliminate doping, irrespective of whether this is because of the athletes health, fairness and equality or natural ability arguments. Furthermore, it would seem that should the current system of anti-doping remain, significant increases would need to be made in the testing levels; this in turn would require a significant increase in revenue for anti-doping collection and testing. This may be economically impossible and thus other solutions to the ubiquitous problem of doping may need to be sought, outside of individual scientific tests. The alternative is to invest additional funds into the development of more advanced, efficient and effective tests for the detection of doping. If it were possible to increase the test reliability, the window of detectability and the range of substances that could be detected, this would mean the increase of the number of tests could be more modest. Such an increase may well be affordable. On the other hand, this would still not eliminate the issues with test predictability or corruption and as such further demonstrates the current system needs work in order to become both efficient and effective in deterring and punishing doping. The ABP appears to be the solution to the problem but further analysis reveals that it has its shortcomings just like chemical testing. Overall it would seem that the current system, as it stands, needs to be reconsidered and reworked in order to be effective and efficient.

Acknowledgments

This work was funded in part by University of Adelaide Postgraduate Scholarship and Wood Jones Bequest to the University of Adelaide.

References

1. World Anti-Doping Agency (2012) a brief history of anti-doping.
2. Franke W, Berendonk B (1997) Hormonal doping and androgenization of athletes: a secret program of the German Democratic Republic government. Clin Chem 43: 1262–1279.
3. Jeffery N (2008) Systematic Chinese doping scams exposed.
4. United States Anti-Doping Association.
5. Cycling News (2011) Howman: Reform needed in anti-doping fight.
6. Petróczi A (2007) Attitudes and doping: a structural equation analysis of the relationship between athletes' attitudes, sport orientation and doping behaviour. Substan Abuse Treat Prevent Policy 2: 34.
7. Lentillon-Kaestner V, Carstairs C (2010) Doping use among young elite cyclists: a qualitative psychosociological approach. Scand J Med Sci Sports 20: 336–345.
8. Houlihan B (2002) Dying To Win: Doping In Sport and the Development of Anti-Doping Policy. (2nd edn.) Council of Europe, Strasbourg.
9. Ehrnborg C, Rosén T (2009) The psychology behind doping in sport. Growth Horm IGF Res 19: 285–287.
10. Kohler M, Thevis M, Schänzer W, Püschel K (2008) Gesundheitsschäden und Todesfälle durch Doping. Rechtsmedizin 18: 177–182.
11. Erotokritou-Mulligan I, Bassett E, Kniess A, Sönksen P, Holt R (2007) Validation of the growth hormone (GH)-dependent marker method of detecting GH abuse in sport through the use of independent data sets. Growth Horm IGF Res, 17: 416–423.
12. Graham M, Davies B, Grace F, Kicman A, Baker J (2008) Anabolic Steroid Use: Patterns of use and detection of doping. Sports Med 38: 505-525.
13. http://www.wada-ama.org/Documents/World_Anti-Doping_Program/WADP-The-Code/WADA_Anti-Doping_CODE_2009_EN.pdf .
14. UNESCO (2005) International Convention against doping in sport.
15. Beastall G, Gibson I, Martin J (1995) Successful suicide by insulin injection in a non-diabetic. Med Sci Law 35: 79–85.
16. Sheng S, Lei B, James M, Lascola CD, Venkataraman TN, et al. (2012) Xenon neuroprotection in experimental stroke: interactions with hypothermia and intracerebral haemorrhage. Anesthesiology 117:1262-1275.
17. Barness L (1977) Nutritional Aspects of Vegetarianism, Health Foods, and Fad Diets. Nutrition Reviews 35: 153-157.
18. Albanes D, Heinonen O, Taylor P, et al.(1994) Alpha-Tocopherol, Beta-Carotene Cancer Prevention Study Group- The effect of vitamin E and beta carotene on the incidence of lung cancer and other cancers in male smokers. N Engl J Med 330:1029-1035.
19. Omenn G, Goodman G, Thorquist M, Balmes J, Cullen MR, et al. (1996) Effects of a combination of betacarotene and vitamin A on lung cancer and cardiovascular disease. N Engl J Med 334: 1150-1155.
20. Kuchler W (1969) Sportethos. Eine moraltheologische Untersuchung des im Lebensbereich Sport lebendigen Ethos als Beitrag zu einer Phänomenologie der Ethosformen. Int Rev Sociol Sport 10:156.
21. https://twitter.com/chrisfroome/status/471701898731749376.
22. http://www.bbc.com/sport/0/cycling/27616069.
23. http://gerard.cc/2011/08/10/biological-passport/.
24. http://www.cyclingnews.com/news/vroomen-and-ashenden-criticise-lack-of-biological-passport-testing.
25. http://www.uci.ch/Modules/BUILTIN/getObject.asp?MenuId=MjI0NQ&ObjTypeCode= FILE&type=FILE&id=NDc3MDk&LangId=1.
26. http://www.uci.ch/Modules/BUILTIN/getObject.asp?MenuId=MjI0NQ&ObjTypeCode=FILE&type=FILE&id=NDc3MDk&LangId=1.
27. World Anti-Doping Agency (2010) Guidelines for Urine Sample Collection.
28. Kayser B, Mauron A, Miah A (2007) Current anti-doping policy: a critical appraisal. BMC Medical Ethics 8: 2.
29. Bidlingmaier M, Wu Z, Strasburger C (2000) Anti-doping systems in sports are doomed to fail: a probability and cost analysis Test method: GH Baillieare's Clinical Endocrinology and Metabolism 14: 99-109.
30. Ashenden M, Varlet-Marie E, Lasne F, Audran M (2006) The effects of microdose recombinant human erythropoietin regimens in athletes. J Euro Hemt Assoc 91:1143-1144.
31. Lundby C, Achman-Andersen N, Thomsen J, Norgaard A, Robach P (2008) Testing for recombinant human erythropoietin in urine: problems associated with current anti-doping testing. J Appl Physiol 105: 417–419.
32. Breidbach A, Catlin D, Green G, Tregub I, Truong H (2003) Detection of recombinant human erythropoietin in urine by isoelectric focusing. Clin Chem 49: 901-907.
33. Mørkeberg J (2012) Detection of Autologous Blood Transfusions in Athletes: A Historical Perspective. Transfus Med Rev 26: 199-208.
34. Monfort N, Ventura R, Platen P, Hinrichs T, Brixius K, et al. (2012) Plasticizers excreted in urine: indication of autologous blood transfusion in sports. Transfusion 52: 647–657.
35. Gómez C, Pozo O, Marcos J, Segura J, Ventura R (2012) Alternative long-term markers for the detection of methyltestosterone misuse. Steroids 78: 44–52.
36. Guddat S, Fußhöller G, Beuck S, Thomas A, Geyer H, et al. (2013) Synthesis, characterization, and detection of new oxandrolone metabolites as long-term markers in sports drug testing. Anal bioanal chem 405: 8285-8294.
37. Powrie J, Bassett E, Rosen T, Jørgensen J, Napoli R, et al. (2007) Detection of growth hormone abuse in sport. Growth Horm IGF Res 17: 220-226.
38. Bundesgesetz über die Bekämpfung von Doping im Sport (Anti-Doping-Bundesgesetz 2007-ADBG (2007).
39. Code du sport - Version consolidée au 6 août 2014.
40. Disciplina della tutela sanitaria delle attività sportive e della lotta contro il doping (2000), Parlamento Italiano, pubblicata nella Gazzetta Ufficiale n. 294 del 18 dicembre 2000.
41. World Anti-Doping Agency (2010) Laboratory Statistics Report.
42. http://www.nadabonn.de/fileadmin/user_upload/nada/Downloads/Jahresberichte/NADA_Annual_Report_2010.pdf.
43. http://www.usada.org/athlete-test-history.
44. http://www.uci.ch/templates/UCI/UCI5/layout.asp?MenuId=MjI0NQ&LangId=1.
45. Packer A (1967) Applying cost-effectiveness concepts to the community health system. Operat Res 16: 227-253.
46. Epstein S (1980) Implications of Probability Analysis on the Strategy Used for Noninvasive Detection of Coronary Artery Disease. Am J Cardiol 46: 491-499.
47. Sobel D (1995) Rethinking Medicine: Improving Health Outcomes with Cost-Effective Psychosocial Interventions. Psychosom Med 57:234-244.
48. Haugen K (2004) The Performance-Enhancing Drug Game. J Sports Econom 5: 67.
49. Haugen K, Nepusz T, Petróczi A (2013) The Multi-Player Performance-Enhancing Drug Game. PLoS ONE 8: e63306.

50. Maennig W (2014) Inefficiency of the Anti-Doping System: Cost Reduction Proposals. Substance Use & Misuse 49: 1201–1205.

51. Atkinson J (1957) Motivational determinates of risk-taking behaviour. Psychol Rev 64: 359-372.

52. Foucault M (1977) Discipline and Punish: The Birth of the Prison. Vintage, New York, USA.

53. Haggerty K, Ericson R (2000) The surveillant assemblage. British J Sociol 51: 605–622.

54. http://www.wada- ama.org/en/Resources/Testing-Figures/ADO-Testing-Figures/.

55. https://www.facebook.com/Frontal21/posts/140559992625539?stream_ref=5.

56. Hamilton T (2013) The Secret Race: Inside the Hidden World of the Tour de France - Doping, Cover-Ups, and Winning at All Costs, Transworld Publishers Ltd, U.K.

57. Conte V (2008) Interview with BBC Sport, in Conte labels Olympics 'a fraud.

58. Hermann A, Henneberg M (2012) The Doping Myth: 100 m sprint results are not improved by 'doping'. Int J Drug Policy 24: 110–114.

59. http://files.mlb.com/mitchrpt.pdf.

60. http://www.wada-ama.org/Documents/World_Anti-Doping_Program/WADP-The-Code/Code_Review/Code%20Review%202015/WADC-2015-draft-version-2.0.

61. Tsebelis G (1990) Penalty has no Impact on Crime: A Game-Theoretic Analysis. Rationality Society 2: 255-286.

62. Tsebelis G (1993) Penalty and Crime: Further Theoretical Considerations and Empirical Evidence. J Theoret Politics 5: 349-374.

63. Australian Sports Anti-Doping Authority (2012) Fees.

64. World Anti-Doping Agency (2014) Athletes Biological Passport.

65. Robinson N, Saugy M, Vernec A, Sottas P (2011) The Athlete Biological Passport: An Effective Tool in the Fight against Doping. Clin Chem 57: 830–832.

66. Sottas P, Robinson N, Rabin O, Saugy M (2011) The Athlete Biological Passport. Clin Chem 57: 969–976.

67. Zorzoli M (2011) The Athlete Biological Passport from the perspective of an anti-doping organization. Clin Chem LabMed 49:1423–1425.

68. Sanchis-Gomar F, Martinez-Bello V, Gomez-Cabrera M, Vina J (2011) Current limitations of the Athlete's Biological Passport use in sports. Clin Chem Lab Med 49:1413–1415.

69. Hailey N (2012) A false start in the race against doping in sport: concerns with cycling's biological passport. Duke Law J 61: 393-432.

70. Ashenden M, Gough C, Garnham A, Gore C, Sharpe K (2011) Current markers of the Athlete Blood Passport do not flag microdose EPO doping. Europ J Appl Physiol 111: 2307–2314.

71. Banfi G (2011) Limits and pitfalls of Athlete's Biological Passport. Clin Chem LabMed 49:1417–1421.

72. CAS 2009/A/1926 International Tennis Federation v. Richard Gasquet, CAS 2009/A/1930 WADA v. ITF & Richard Gasquet.

73. World Anti-Doping Agency (2013) WADA Foundation Board Announces Outcomes at November Meeting.

Partial Knee Joint Denervation for Knee Pain

A. Lee Dellon*

Department of Plastic Surgery and Neurosurgery, Johns Hopkins University, USA

Abstract

Knee pain is transmitted via peripheral nerves. Once a medical or orthopedic surgical musculoskeletal approach has failed to relieve this chronic problem, then a partial kneedenervation should be considered. In 1994 the medial and lateral retinacular nerveswere described, and these are the main source for knee joint pain. A nerve block ofeach of these nerves followed by observation of increased stair climbing and kneelingwith a decrease in the visual analog scale of > 5 predicts a 90% success rate for partial knee denervation. This approach, pioneered by Dellon, is applicable to patients withpersistent pain after partial or total knee arthroplasty, and to those with sports injuriesand pain after ligament reconstruction, and for those too young for joint replacement.This review includes description of the neuroanatomy, the nerve block technique, thesurgical approach and the results of Dellon's partial knee denervation over the pasttwenty years.

Keywords: Knee pain; Knee arthroplasty; Neuroma resection; Denervation

Introduction

This is a review that highlights a fact which Orthopedic Surgery continues to underappreciate: Joint pain can be of neural origin!

All perception of knee pain must be mediated via the nervous system. Yet the Orthopedic approach to knee pain is traditionally, and universally, and almost exclusively, musculoskeletal. While the musculoskeletal system is the natural starting point for the evaluation of knee pain, once musculoskeletal etiologies have been eliminated or treated, persistent knee pain should then be considered of neural origin. Once a neural etiology is being considered, the Orthopedic Surgeon may wish to proceed with diagnostic nerve blocks, or refer the patient to Pain Management for peripheral nerve blocks, in addition to management of anxiety and chronic pain with neuropathic pain medications. Appropriate nerve blocks will diagnose which nerves are transmitting the pain, permitting a plan for interruption of this painful transmission.

The approach described is to consider knee pain that exists after musculoskeletal or patellofemoral treatment of the knee to be of neural origin. The physician caring for these patients must consider whether the pain is coming from direct damage to the cutaneous nerves about the knee, such as a neuroma of the infrapatellar branch of the saphenous nerve, or whether the pain is coming from an injury to one of the nerves arising within the knee joint structures themselves. A further source of knee pain due to nerve injury is an injury to a nerve far away from the knee, like the lateral femoral cutaneous nerve. The concept of partial joint denervation will be presented as an approach where those joint afferents that transmit a pain message are interrupted, thereby stopping the pain, and preserving the musculoskeletal components of the joint.

At the outset, it must be clear that only sensory nerves are being divided, and that the knee joint is being partially denervated. A Charcot-type joint is not created because the deafferentation of this weight-bearing joint is partial instead of total. It must be stated clearly that a partial knee denervation should only be done for a patient in whom traditional orthopedic approaches have provided a stable knee, with strong ligamentous support and normal patellofemoral tracking.

It is the purpose of this review to describe the peripheral neuroanatomy related to perception of knee pain, the performance of nerve blocks required to diagnose this etiology, the surgical approach for partial knee denervation, and the results of partial knee denervation.

Peripheral Neuroanatomy of the Knee Joint

While it is intuitively clear that a joint is innervated, the exact pathways of this innervation curiously are frequently omitted from the classic and even many of the newer anatomy texts. For the human knee, the innervation pattern was not described until 1994 [1].

The innervation of the human knee joint is remarkably constant. On the medial aspect, the femoral nerve branch that innervates the vastus medialis continues past its motor point and exits deep and distal to the vastus medialis (Table 1). At this point it lies deep to the medial retinaculum and becomes related to the medial recurrent geniculate artery and vein. This nerve was termed the medial retinacular nerve. These structures, nerve and vessels continue directly adjacent to the vastus medialis and superficial to the synovium to enter the ligamentous structures of the medial knee. These fibers also continue towards

Tibiofemoral
Cutaneous: (From anterolateral to medial, then posterior)
1. Lateral femoral cutaneous
2. Anterior femoral cutaneous
3. Medial cutaneous nerve of the thigh
4. Infrapatellar branch of saphenous nerve
5. Posterior femoral cutaneous nerve
Joint: (From anterolateral to medial, then posterior)
1. Lateral retinacular nerve
2. Terminal branch of innervation of vastus intermedius
3. Medial retinacular nerve
4. Popliteal plexus from sciatic nerve
Patellofemoral
1. Lateral retinacular nerve
2. Terminal branch of innervation of vastus intermedius
3. Medial retinacular nerve
Proximal Tibiofibular
1. Recurrent genicular branch of common peroneal nerve

Table 1: Innervation of & around the human knee joint.

***Corresponding author:** A. Lee Dellon, Professor, Department of Plastic Surgery and Neurosurgery, Johns Hopkins University,1122 Kenilworth Dr, suite 18, Towson,Baltimore, Maryland, USA
E-mail: ALDellon@Dellon.com

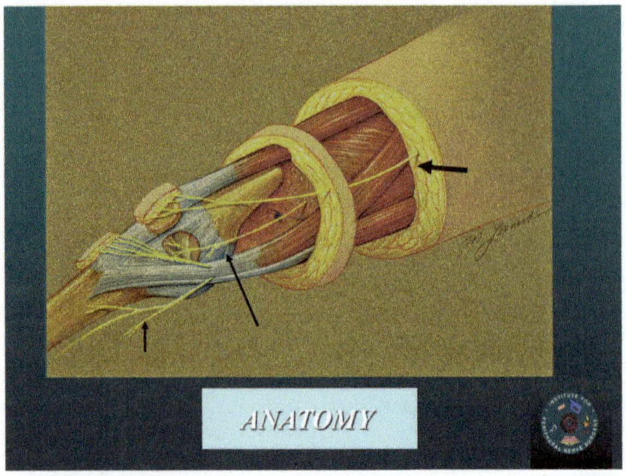

Figure 1: Medial view of the innervation of the knee. The skin overlying the patella is innervated by the medial cutaneous nerve of the thigh, a branch of the saphenous nerve (thick arrow). The medial joint structures are innervated by a branch of the femoral nerve, the medial retinacular nerve, which, after innervating the vastus medialis, continues distal and then anterior to this muscle, to enter the ligamentous structures of the knee joint (long thin arrow). This nerve lies superficial to the synovium and deep to the medial retinaculum. The saphenous nerve's infrapatellar and distal branches are shown in their most common variation (short thin arrow). The nerve to the patellar skin is from the medial cutaneous nerve of the thigh (short thick arrow). (With permission, Dellon.com).

the midline of the knee to innervate the undersuface of the patella (Figure 1). On the lateral aspect, a branch of the sciatic nerve leaves the popliteal fossa, travels laterally and anteriorly, to emerge deep to the biceps tendon and enter the space beneath the lateral retinaculum. In this location the nerve is adjacent to the recurrent lateral recurrent geniculate artery and vein. This nerve was termed the lateral retinacular nerve. These structures, the nerve and vessels, are immediately distal to the vastus lateralis and superficial to the synovium. The nerve enters the ligamentous structures of the lateral knee, and travels to the midline to innervate the undersurface of the patella (Figure 2). Anteriorly, another source of innervation is derived from the femoral nerve innervation of the vastus intermedius. This nerve continues on the surface of the periosteum to innervate the tissues around the pre-patellar bursa. This nerve can be termed the nerve to the prepatellar space (Figure 1). Finally, posteriorly, branches from the sciatic nerve enter the posterior knee joint capsule to provide innervation. These nerves can be termed the popliteal plexus (Figure 2).

While many patients complain of "knee pain", they may be pointing or referring to the joint distal to the knee, laterally, which is the articulation between the fibular head and the tibia. This proximal tibiofibular joint space is likely to be injured by fractures of the fibular, lateral tibial plateau fractures, and surgery related to a high tibial osteotomy or a Maquet procedure (repositioning of the tibial tuberosity). This space is innervated by the recurrent genicular branches of the common peroneal nerve (Figure 2). As the common peroneal nerve travels from the popliteal fossa to the fibular head, it gives off a small, about 1mm diameter, nerve that may enter this space posterior to the fibular head. The common peroneal nerve will give off a second branch to this space immediately as it curves anterior to the fibular head, at the junction with the fibular neck. This branch, too, is about 1 mm diameter. The next branch of the common peroneal nerve goes to the tibialis anterior, a critical motor branch. In the operating room, the only way to identify the branch to the joint is to stimulate this little branch electrically. The branch to the joint will have no motor function elicited when stimulated. This is critical to do. This little branch often looks like epineurium.

Peripheral Neuroanatomy of the Skin around the Knee Joint

The saphenous nerve is a branch of the femoral nerve and arises from the femoral nerve in the proximal thigh. Its cutaneous branches to the skin below the knee are well described and lie in location to be injured directly either from a medial ankle endoscopy portal or the midline incisions used for many surgical approaches to the knee. These branches can be directly injured by blunt trauma as well (Figure 2). Less well-recognized is the nerve to the skin overlying the patellar itself. This is a branch of the femoral nerve, and may include sensory contribution from the obturator nerve joining within Hunter's canal, and is termed the medial cutaneous nerve of the thigh (Figure 2). It approaches from the medial aspect of the knee compared to the vertical approach taken by the anterior femoral cutaneous nerves [1]. Even less well-appreciated is that the saphenous nerve can be compressed in the distal thigh within Hunter's canal. This is called the adductor canal syndrome, and is rare in the absence of direct trauma to this region. Entrapment of the saphenous nerve in this location can present as medial knee pain [2,3]. The skin lateral to the patellar is innervated by the terminal branches of the lateral femoral cutaneous nerve [4,5]. Entrapment or injury to this nerve in the hip area, for example after anterior approaches to total hip arthroplasty or bone graft harvesting, may present as lateral knee pain, especially if the lateral femoral cutaneous nerve is within the inguinal next to the anterior superior iliac crest.

Clinical Evaluation of Knee Pain of Neural Origin

The history of knee pain is critical to obtain. Knee pain does not arise de novo.

Something happened. There will be a history of some type of sports event, over use activity, new activity, or actual direct injury to the knee

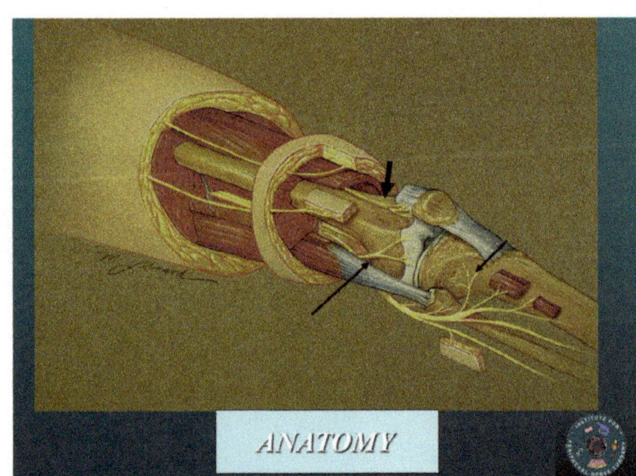

Figure 2: Lateral view of the innervation of the knee. The skin in this area represents the terminal branches of the lateral femoral cutaneous nerve. The lateral joint structures are innervated by a branch of the sciatic nerve that comes from the popliteal fossa, goes deep to the biceps tendon to enter the joint, the lateral retinacular nerve (long thin arrow). The nerve passes just distal to the vastus lateralis, and then lies superficial to the synovium and deep to the lateral retinaculum as it enters the joint. The branches of the sciatic nerve to the posterior knee joint capsule are shown next to the femur posteriorly. The branch to the pre-patellar bursa is shown on the anterior surface of the femur as it exists the vastus intermedius. The innervation of the proximal tibiofibular joint is shown as branches proximal and distal to the fibular head, arising from the common peroneal nerve (short arrow). The terminal branch of the nerve to the vastus intermedius innervates the prepatellar space (short thick arrow). (with permission, Dellon.com).

(Table 2). The knee injury can be blunt or open. Knee surgery should be considered as an iatrogenic source of this trauma. Many patients with knee pain due to musculoskeletal problems awake from their reconstructive knee surgery to have a different pain or paralysis. These are known complications of knee surgery, and should be recognized as such, and referred for appropriate treatment in a timely manner. The history of whether the pain is made worse by certain positions of the body or leg, or is made worse by certain activities is important in arriving at a correct diagnosis. Certainly, most knee pain unrelated to structural impairment will be relieved by non-operative treatment. But when pain persists beyond a reasonable time frame of three to six months, then the history is most consistent with pain of neural origin.

The physical examination is directed to identifying one or more sources of neural origin for the pain. First try to distinguish if any skin territories are dysesthetic, i.e., painful when touched lightly. If so, outline them. The most common distribution is that of the infrapatellar branch of the saphenous nerve, and the second is the skin over the patella itself. These areas might be numb, indicating loss of sensation (Figure 3). Once the pattern is identified, the examination continues proximally, along the course of the given nerve, looking for a trigger spot, which is either a true end-bulb neuroma or an in-continuity nerve lesion. The hypothesis is made that this nerve or these nerves are the source of the cutaneous pain, and a diagnostic nerve block will be required to confirm this hypothesis. A combination of 1% xylocaine and 0.5% Marcaine is mixed 50:50, without epinephrine, and 5 cc is injected into each site for the nerve block. These blocks are done along the course of the involved cutaneous nerve (Figure 4). Then the physical examination is directed to the joint afferents. Palpation is done deeply to the spot located just distal to the vastus medialis muscle, through the medial retinaculum to elicit pain from the medial retinacular nerve. Palpation is next done deeply to the spot located just distal to the vastus

Aging
1. Osteoarthritis in patient not a candidate for total knee arthroplasty
2. Osteoarthritis in patient not wanting a contralateral total knee arthroplasty
Injury
3. Sports-related, with normal MRI, not responding to sports medicine Rx
4. Work-related, with normal MRI, not responding to pain management
Iatrogenic
1. Sports-related, s/p operative approach to ligamentous/osseous reconstruction
2. Work-related, s/p operative approach to ligamentous/osseous reconstruction

Table 2: Indications for partial knee denervation.

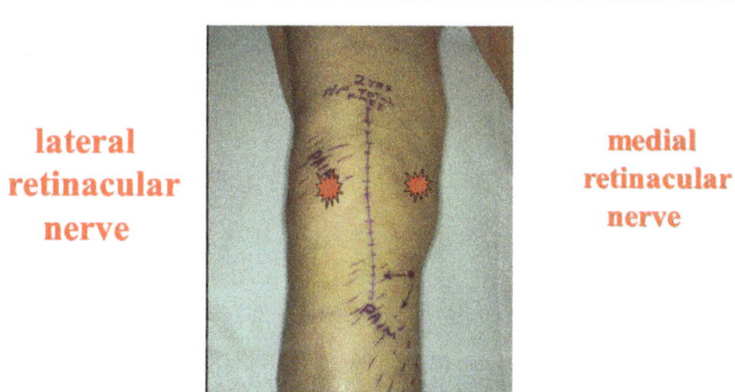

Figure 3: Demonstration of the sites to palpate a tender medial and lateral retinacular nerve in the patient with joint pain. Shaded areas are areas of cutaneous dysesthesia representing the medial cutaneous nerve of the thigh at the patella and the infrapatellar branch of the saphenous nerve laterally. The red areas are the sites to palpate for tenderness of the medial and the lateral retinacular nerves, and will be the sites for the nerve blocks.

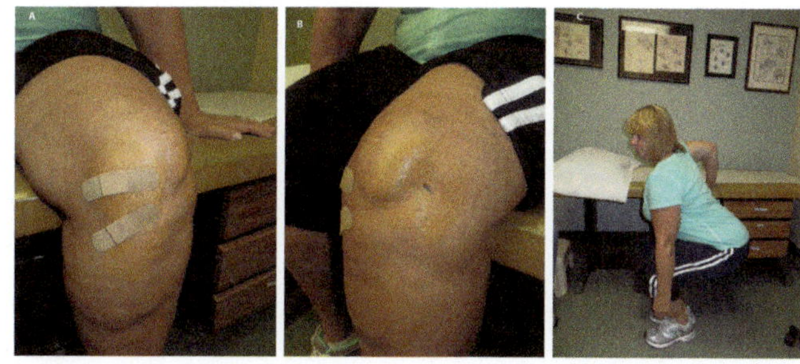

Figure 4: Demonstration of the site to use for a local anesthetic to block the suspected joint and cutaneous afferents in the patient with knee pain. A) The upper band aid is over the site for the medial retinacular nerve, just distal to the vastus medialis, and the lower one is over the tender site of the infrapatellar branch of the saphenous nerve at the pes anserinus. B) The ink mark is the site of pain over the lateral retinacular nerve. If the patient complains of just medial knee pain, and there are two medial trigger points, just these are blocked and the patient is asked to walk and relate where any residual pain is located. Remember that the medial and lateral retinacular nerves overlap anteriorly, and usually both must be blocked to relieve anterior knee pain. C) Patient is seen squatting after the block relieved the knee pain.

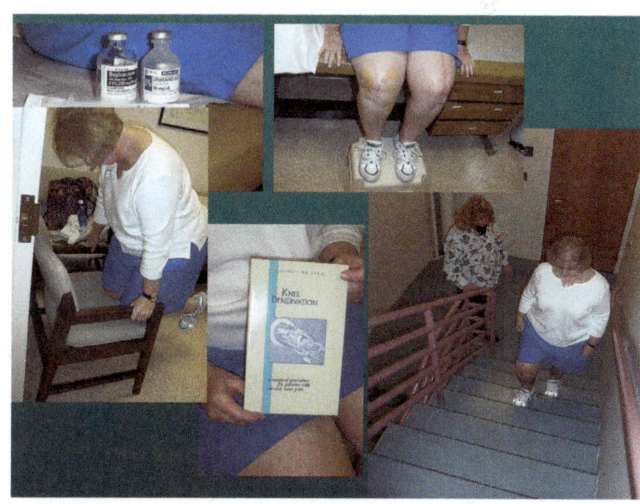

Figure 5: After the nerve block, there should be improved physical activity with less pain, as noted by the patient climbing the stairs and kneeling on a padded chair.

lateralis muscle, through the lateral retinaculum to elicit pain from the lateral retinacular nerve. The hypothesis is made the knee joint pain is due to an injury to one or both of the joint afferents, and a diagnostic nerve block will be required to confirm this hypothesis (Figure 4).

The medial cutaneous nerve to the thigh and the medial retinacular nerve can be blocked at the same spot.

Ten minutes following the nerve blocks, the patient is instructed to walk in the hallway, climb and descend a few steps, and even to kneel on a padded chair (Figure 5). A reduction of 5 points on a visual analog scale, say from 10 to 5, where 10 represents the worst pain, is confirmation that sufficient relief of pain has occurred to permit surgery for partial knee denervation and resection of cutaneous neuromas to proceed. For some patients a reduction in pain of 50% maybe sufficient, but this usually means that there are more nerves involved in the pain mechanism.

If the nerve blocks above have not reduced the pain level to less than five, or the blocks were not effective, the physical examination should go on to include other more rare sources for the nerve pain. In the patient with a knee replacement, the remaining pain may well be from an anterior femoral cutaneous nerve to be found in the proximal portions of the incision, or another branch of the infrapatellar saphenous nerve, which can have many branches, including more distal branches.

Finally, the groin should be examined to search for a Tinel sign over the lateral femoral cutaneousnerve. The patient will be noted to sit with leg extended at the hip. The mid-thigh should be examined to search for a Tinel sign over Hunter's adductor canal. This is best done with the patient supine, and the effected leg externally rotated at the hip, leaving the knee bent. This stretches the adductor muscle group over the saphenous nerve. Then just a gentle palpation over the canal produces a distally radiating painful response.

If the pain is below the knee joint, and laterally located, examine for tenderness in the proximal tibiofibular joint space, and if this is present, a nerve block can be done directly into this space without blocking the common peroneal nerve.

If pain is accompanied by complaints of the leg "giving out" or the foot dragging, or a "foot drop", the motor function of the common peroneal nerve must be evaluated by manual muscle testing. The common peroneal nerve must be palpated or percussed at the fibular neck, with tenderness, even without distal radiation, being considered a positive sign for nerve entrapment. Electrodiagnostic testing should be done to evaluate the common peroneal nerve and the presence of an L4/L or L5/S1 radiculopathy.

Operative Technique

The operative techniques for partial knee denervation given below have been published previously [6-9]. In general, a tourniquet is not needed. Leaving blood in the region permits the small vein on the nerves to the knee joint and to the skin to be identified more easily. Operative loupes of 3.5 x power are used. The bipolar coagulator is used set on a low level to start. Intravenous antibiotic prophylaxis is given prior to starting the procedure. A femoral nerve block is not done due to the risk of injury to the femoral nerve, but rather local anesthetic with epinephrine is infiltrated into the skin edges of the incisions at the start of the surgical procedure. Each nerve to be resected is injected with this local anesthetic prior to cauterization and resection to "shield" the central nervous system form the pain impulses when the nerve is resected. The dressing is xeroform gauze over the incision, then sterile 4 x 4 inch gauze, held in place with kling, and covered with a stockinette.

Finally the concept of minimizing the risk of recurrent neuroma pain must be understood. Since the sensory nerves remain alive once divided, due to their nucleus being intact in the dorsal root ganglion, nerve regeneration will occur in every joint afferent or cutaneous afferent that is divided. Alteration of the micro-environment of the nerve by implanting the proximal end of a divided sensory nerve into an innervated motor environment results in the absence of formation of a true neuroma [10]. Implanting a sensory nerve into an innervated muscle, after resecting the painful neuroma or after interruption of that nerve function by division of that nerve, results in predictable pain relief without recurrent neuroma for upper [11] and lower extremity peripheral nerves [12-14]. The location chosen to place the divided nerve will be explained for each operation described below.

Lateral Knee Denervation

An incision is outlined lateral to the patellar beginning over the distal muscle belly of the vastus lateralis. This muscle sometimes has a slight distal split in the muscle and you must be sure to be distal to the most distal portion of the vastus lateralis muscle. Then the iliotibial band (lateral retinaculum) is divided longitudinally for about 1.5 cm. Immediately adjacent to the muscle belly will be the small recurrent vessels and a 1 to 1.5 mm nerve, going from beneath the iliotibial band (biceps tendon) and across the synovium, and into the lateral joint and infrapatellar structures. This nerve is first infiltrated with Marcaine 0.5% down beneath the iliotibial band, then the nerve and vessels are cauterized towards the patella to prevent bleeding, and then placed under traction and cauterized deep beneath the iliotibial band, to prevent bleeding. The portion between the two cauterized sites is sent to pathology to confirm that a nerve was indeed resected. The iliotibial band (lateral retinaculum) is reconstructed with two figure-of-eight sutures of 2-0 braided non-absorbable material (Figure 6).

Medial Knee Denervation

An incision is outlined medial to the patellar beginning over the distal muscle belly of the vastus medialis. Then the thin medial retinaculum is divided longitudinally for about 1.5 cm. Immediately adjacent to the muscle belly will be the small recurrent vessels and a 1 to 1.5 mm nerve, going from beneath the vastus medialis and across the synovium, and into the medial joint and infrapatellar structures. This nerve is dissected proximally beneath the retinaculum until it exists from beneath the muscle. This nerve is first infiltrated with Marcaine 0.5% down beneath the vastus medialis, then the nerve and vessels are cauterized towards the patella to prevent bleeding, and then placed under traction and cauterized deep beneath the vastus medialis, to prevent bleeding. The portion between the two cauterized sites is sent to pathology. The medial retinaculum is reconstructed with two figure-of-eight sutures of 3-0 braided non-absorbable material (Figure 7).

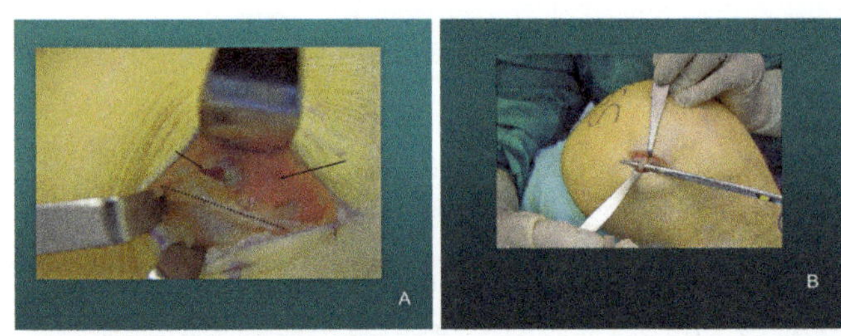

Figure 6: Lateral Knee Denervation. A) Incision is shown, lateral to patella, centered over the tender site shown in Figure 3. Vastus lateralis is shown (short arrow). The iliotibial tract is incised (dotted line) to demonstrate the lateral retinacular nerve (long arrow) adjacent to the lateral recurrent geniculate vessels. B) The lateral retinacular nerve is illustrated. C) The nerve is first infiltrated with local anesthetic, and the cauterized distally and proximally, and then divided proximally below the level of the iliotibial band so that the nerve drops into the popliteal fossa.

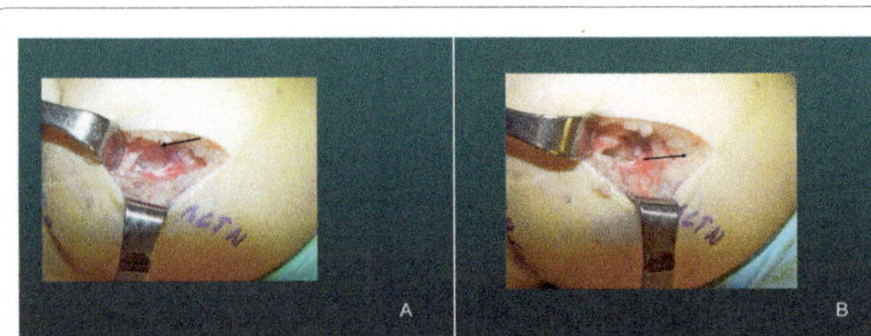

Figure 7: Medial Knee Denervation. A) Incision is shown, medial to patella, centered over the tender site shown in Figure 3. The medial retinaculum is opened. The arrow points to the medial retinacular nerve adjacent to the recurrent medial recurrent geniculate vessels. B) The nerve has been resected. The arrow points to the direction in which, beneath the medial retinaculum, the nerve has been implanted into the vastus medialis muscle. C) Closure of the medial retinaculum is shown.

Resection Infrapatellar Branch of Saphenous Nerve

The saphenous nerve exits Hunter's canal in the distal thigh to become the medial cutaneous nerve of the thigh and the infrapatellar branch of the saphenous nerve and the distal saphenous nerve. The infrapatellar branch crosses the insertion of the adductor tendons into Gurdy's tubercle beneath the deep fascia. There may already be two branches at this level. Ultimately, several terminal branches cross from medial to the lateral across the region of the tibial tuberosity to innervate the lateral knee skin. The skin proximal to this laterally is the terminal zone of innervation of the lateral femoral cutaneous nerve. Whereas the numbness is lateral, the damage to the nerve usually occurs in the axial line of the knee from an incision or medially from a scope portal. The site of theTinel sign is around Gurdy's tubercle. The incision is longitudinal across the Tinel sign. The dissection goes deep to the fascia where the one or more branches are noted by the blood in the vein that accompanies the nerve branch. A thorough search proximally and distally must be done for more than one branch. This is the most common location for a missed remaining painful nerve. The nerve is infiltrated with Marcaine 0.5% proximally, the distal end cauterized to minimize bleeding, a segment resected for pathology, and the proximal end dissected. There is usually a clear tunnel where this nerve has transversed along or through the sartorius or other adductor muscle or tendon. The proximal end of the divided nerve, after cauterization to prevent bleeding, is turned blindly into these muscles and implanted there, proximal to the popliteal crease (Figure 8).

Resection of Medial Cutaneous Nerve of the Thigh

This nerve goes to the skin overlying the patella. This skin is traditionally shown as being innervated by an anterior femoral cutaneous nerve coming vertically down the leg. However, the skin is innervated by a branch of the saphenous and approaches this region medially. Indeed the same tender location for the medial retinacular nerve is the location for this nerve. The clinical clue is that the skin of the patella is dysesthetic. The nerve block medially will block both of these nerves. The incision used to approach the medial retinacular nerve is used. In the immediate subcutaneous tissue will be blood in the small vein that accompanies this nerve. Cauterize the nerve distally, and dissect the proximal end medially across the surface of the vastus medialis. Inject the nerve with 0.5% Marcaine proximally. Open a small window into the fascia of the vastus medialis. Implant the proximal end of the nerve loosely into this muscle (Figure 9).

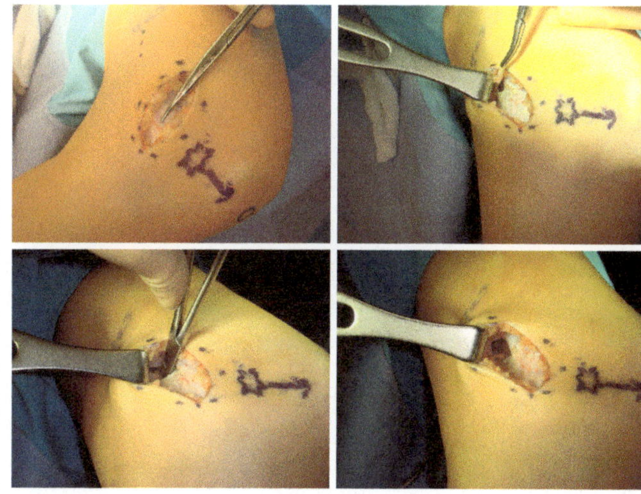

Figure 9: Resection of the Medial Cutaneous Nerve of the Thigh. A 23 year old with a direct injury to the knee resulting in pain over the patellar region. A) Site of Tinel and nerve block that eliminated the pain. B) Medial cutaneous nerve of the thigh demonstrated by the scissors' tips in the subcutaneous plane. This is superficial to the medial retinaculum. C) The nerve has been divided distally and dissected proximally. Here it is held by the clamp. D) A window is made in the fascia over the vastus medialis into which the proximal end of the nerve will be implanted (E).

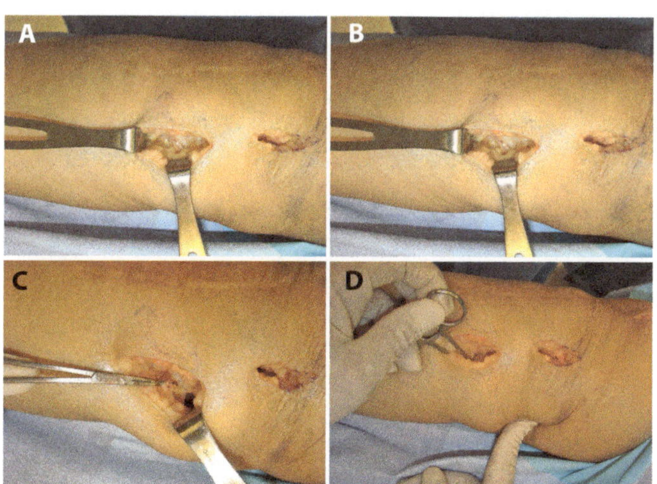

Figure 8: Resection of the Infrapatellar Branch of the Saphenous Nerve. A) Woman 9 years after total knee arthroplasty whose knee is shown from medial aspect demonstrating sites of pain over the anterior femoral cutaneous nerve (proximally), over the medial cutaneous nerve of the thigh (and medial retinacular nerve), and over the infrapatellar branch of the saphenous nerve. B) The infrapatellar branch is noted overlying Gurdy's tubercle. C) The nerve is infiltrated with local anesthetic prior and then D) cauterized and divided. E) The proximal end of the nerve is dissected and implanted into an adductor muscle medially (location denoted by finger at the popliteal fossa. F) A search must be made proximally for other infrapatellar branches. One is shown here in the incision used to resect the medial cutaneous nerve of the thigh and the medial retinacular nerves.

Author's Results

The first group of patients selected for partial knee denervation were chosen from patients who had already had a total knee arthroplasty but who still had persistent pain for greater than 6 months unrelated to loosening, malalignment, or infection[6]. In that study, the Orthopedic Surgeons did a pre-op Knee Society Function Score and range of motion and pain assessment on the 15 patients. I independently did the partial knee denervation, and the Orthopedic Surgeons did the post-operative assessment. A total of 45 nerves were resected in 15 patients: both the medial and lateral retinacular nerve and the infrapatellar branch of the saphenous nerve were removed in each patient. All patients reported subjective improvement in the immediate postoperative period. This improvement was maintained at a mean follow-up of 12 months. It was concluded that selective knee denervation is indicated in the management ofpersistent knee pain of neuroma origin after total knee arthroplasty.

The next series to be reported included 70 patients [7]. Some of these patients also had persistent knee pain after total knee replacement, but now the indications were extended to those with chronic pain after knee trauma, or tibial osteotomy. In patients with nontotal knee arthroplasty pain, arthrosis, synovitis, ligamentous instability, and meniscal derangement had been excluded as a source of pain. Sixty of the 70 (86%) patients were satisfied with the denervation procedure as judged by direct questioning and a reduction in their preoperative pain visual analog score of 5 or more points. The average Knee Society score improved from a preoperative mean of 51 points (range, 40-62 points) to a follow-up mean of 82 points (range, 15-100 points). Forty-nine of 70 (70%) patients had final Knee Society objective scores greater than 80. There was no difference in patient satisfaction whether the followup period was less than 2 years or more than 2 years. It was concluded that partial knee denervation is indicated in the management of intractable knee pain after exhaustion of traditional approaches to any structural or infectious etiologies and after successful selective nerve block.

In the year 2000, a series of 344 patients were reviewed [8]. Of these patients, 255 had a previous total knee arthroplasty and 89 patients had knee trauma. Most patients had several nerves removed. No patient had only one nerve removed. All patients required removal of the medial and the lateral retinacular nerves, and most required removal also of the medial cutaneous nerve of the thigh and the infrapatellar branch of the saphenous nerve. Nerves least often removed were the anterior femoral cutaneous and the distal saphenous nerve. About one half of the patients, especially if there had been knee trauma required a neurolysis of the common peroneal nerve. The proximal tibiofibular joint required denervation in patients with fractures of the fibula, or those who had a Marquet procedure of patellofemoral tracking, or a high tibial osteotomy or a tibial plateau fracture. The results for the whole series were that 70% had an excellent result, 20% had a good result, 5% had some improvement, and 5%were not improved. No patient was neurologically downgraded or made worse. No knee implant or hardware was exposed. No patient had to be hospitalized to treat infection.

A review of knee denervation patients on our office computer from January of 2001 through December of 2013 includes 232 additional patients. Each patient has not been reviewed at this time. The overall experience remains the same as that obtained in our 2000 data review.

The main contra-indicationto a partial knee denervation would be the presence of an unstable knee. Without the presence of mechanical stability, relieving pain would lead to ambulation on an unstable knee with the likelihood of falling. Other relative contra-indications are those of surgery in general, such as infection, bleeding and anesthetic risk. In the person who has already had a total knee arthroplasty, there is also the risk of having an implant become infected. To the best of my knowledge, this has not happened yet.

Other Clinical Studies

Despite the earlier work done on partial wrist denervation,[15-18] and extended to the shoulder [19,20] and ankle, [21-23] the Orthopedic community has been hesitant to accept the concept that knee pain can be of neural origin. There have been very few studies published related to partial knee denervation, and except by someone trained by me [24-27] In the reports from Germany, between May of 1995 and June of 1999, 45 knees were partially denervated using the "Dellon technique". This work was in a trauma center in Murnau and the study included both patients with direct knee injury as well as those with knee reconstruction for osteoarthritis who had joint replacement. The report included 34 patients, 11 with bilateral knee pain, whose age ranged from 25 to 86 with a mean of 34 years. In the post-operative time frame from 6 to 18 months, 70% of the patients reported "a reduction in pain", and after 4 years, 50% "still confirmed a positive result". Complications included one hematoma and two seromaswhich resolved with conservative management.

A recent study, from Turkey, evaluated the innervation of the patella in 30 knees of 15 formaldehyde-fixed cadavers [28]. A nerve from the vastus medialis, which is the nerve described above, [1]entering the patella "superomedially", and a nerve "from the vastus lateralis, entering the patella superolaterally" were identified. The origin of these was not described, and their superolateral nerve "from the vastus lateralis" is probably the nerve described above that originates from the sciatic nerve, crosses in front of the vastus lateralis [1]. I would interpret their anatomic study in the fixed cadavers as confirming our observations reported in 1994. These authors then went on to confirm that these nerves are patellar pain afferents, by performing a local anesthesia block in 32 knees of 20 patients with patellofemoral pain [28]. They observed a significant difference between the visual analogue scale (VAS) scores before and after local anesthetic injections ($p<0.01$). Again, I would interpret their observations to confirm that knee pain can be of neural origin from the medial and the lateral retinacular nerves, as described above. A recent meta-analysis of prophylactically denervating the patella with a unipolar cautery at the time of total knee arthroplasty and patellar resurfacing demonstrated a significant reduction in anterior knee pain compared to patients having the same procedure but without an attempt to remove the terminal branches of the medial and lateral retinacular nerves [29]. This approach also probably removes the terminal branches of the nerve to the quadratus intermedius that innervates the pre-patellar bursa.

References

1. Horner G, Dellon AL (1994) Innervation of the human knee joint and implications for surgery. Clin Orthop Relat Res 221-226.
2. Morganti CM, McFarland EG, Cosgarea AJ (2002) Saphenous neuritis: a poorly understood cause of medial knee pain. J Am Acad Orthop Surg 10: 130-137.
3. Ducic I, Dellon L, Larson EE (2005) Treatment concepts for idiopathic and iatrogenic femoral nerve mononeuropathy. Ann Plast Surg 55: 397-401.
4. Nahabedian MY, Dellon AL (1995) Meralgia paresthetica: etiology, diagnosis, and outcome of surgical decompression. Ann Plast Surg 35: 590-594.
5. Aszmann OC, Dellon ES, Dellon AL (1997) Anatomical course of the lateral femoral cutaneous nerve and its susceptibility to compression and injury. Plast Reconstr Surg 100: 600-604.
6. Dellon AL, Mont MA, Krackow KA, Hungerford DS (1995) Partial denervation for persistent neuroma pain after total knee arthroplasty. Clin Orthop Relat Res 145-150.
7. Dellon AL, Mont MA, Mullick T, Hungerford DS (1996) Partial denervation for persistent neuroma pain around the knee. Clin Orthop Relat Res 216-222.
8. Dellon AL, Mont MA, Hungerford DS (2000) Partial Denervation for the Treatment of Painful Neuromas Complicating Total Knee Arthroplasty. Insall and Scott Surgery of the Knee 5: 1772-1786.
9. Dellon, AL (2010) Knee Pain of Neural Origin, in Knee Disorders: Surgery, Rehabilitation, Clinical Outcomes. Elsevier 42: 1096-1115.
10. Mackinnon SE, Dellon AL, Hudson AR, Hunter DA (1985) Alteration of neuroma formation by manipulation of its microenvironment. Plast Reconstr Surg 76: 345-353.
11. Dellon AL, Mackinnon SE (1986) Treatment of the painful neuroma by neuroma resection and muscle implantation. Plast Reconstr Surg 77: 427-438.
12. Dellon AL, Aszmann OC (1998) Treatment of superficial and deep peroneal neuromas by resection and translocation of the nerves into the anterolateral compartment. Foot Ankle Int 19: 300-303.
13. Kim J, Dellon AL (2001) Pain at the site of tarsal tunnel incision due to neuroma of the posterior branch of the saphenous nerve. J Am Podiatr Med Assoc 91: 109-113.
14. Kim J, Dellon AL (2001) Neuromas of the calcaneal nerves. Foot Ankle Int 22: 890-894.
15. Dellon AL, Seif SS (1978) Anatomic dissections relating the posterior interosseous nerve to the carpus, and the etiology of dorsal wrist ganglion pain. J Hand Surg Am 3: 326-332.
16. Dellon AL, Mackinnon SE, Daneshvar A (1984) Terminal branch of anterior interosseous nerve as source of wrist pain. J Hand Surg Br 9: 316-322.

17. Dellon AL (1985) Partial dorsal wrist denervation: resection of the distal posterior interosseous nerve. J Hand Surg Am 10: 527-533.

18. Dellon AL, Horner G (1993) Partial Wrist Denervation: Problems in Plastic and Reconstruction Surgery: The Wrist. Philadelphia, Lippincott 252-266.

19. Aszmann OC, Dellon AL, Birely BT, McFarland EG (1996) Innervation of the human shoulder joint and its implications for surgery. Clin Orthop Relat Res 202-207.

20. Dellon AL (2004) Anterior Shoulder Denervation. Clin Exper Plast Surg 36: 175-180.

21. Rab M, Ebmer J, Dellon AL (2001) Innervation of the sinus tarsi and implications for treating anterolateral ankle pain. Ann Plast Surg 47: 500-504.

22. Dellon AL (2002) Denervation of the sinus tarsi for chronic post-traumatic lateral ankle pain. Orthopedics 25: 849-851.

23. Dellon AL, Barrett SL (2005) Sinus tarsi denervation: clinical results. J Am Podiatr Med Assoc 95: 108-113.

24. Nahabedian MY, Mont MA, Hungerford DS (1998) Selective denervation of the knee: experience, case reports, and technical notes. Am J Knee Surg 11: 175-180.

25. Nahabedian MY, Johnson CA (2001) Operative management of neuromatous knee pain: patient selection and outcome. Ann Plast Surg 46: 15-22.

26. Fromberg G (2000) Die selective Denervation des Kniegelenks. Arthrosemanagement Knie 2: 13-19.

27. Fromberg, G, Hempfling H (2000) Die selective Denervation des Kniegelenks: Technik nach Dellon. Neue Techniken der Arthroskopie 27: 379-383.

28. Maralcan G, Kuru I, Issi S, Esmer AF, Tekdemir I, et al. (2005) The innervation of patella: anatomical and clinical study. Surg Radiol Anat 27: 331-335.

29. Li T, Zhou L, Zhuang Q, Weng X, Bian YJ (2014) Patellar Denervation in Total Knee Arthroplasty Without Patellar Resurfacing and Postoperative Anterior Knee Pain: A Meta-Analysis of Randomized Controlled Trials. J Arthroplasty pii: S0883-5403(00066-00067).

Relationship between Functional Capacities and Performance Parameters in Soccer

Goran Sporis[2]*, Zoran Milanovic[1], Nebojsa Trajkovic[1], Marko Erceg[3] and Dario Novak[2]

[1]*Faculty of Sport and Physical Education, University of Nis, Nis, Serbia*
[2]*Faculty of Kinesiology, University of Zagreb, Zagreb, Croatia*
[3]*Faculty of Kinesiology, University of Split, Split, Croatia*

Abstract

Aim of this study was to determine the relationship between functional capacities and skills performance among young soccer player. The research was conducted on a sample of 22 players aged U-14, members of the elite junior soccer club. Players were tested for aerobic capacities (Soccer specific endurance tests, Beep test), anaerobic capacities (Sprint test, Repeated sprint test, 300 meter run test) and skill performace in phase of attack and defense. Anaerobic capacity of players explain 37% of the variance ($p = 0.03$) for defensive tactical elements, while the set of functional aerobic variables (Hoff test, $p = 0.18$; beep test, $p = 0.93$) has explained 37% ($p = 0.03$) of defensive players ability. Set of predictors of functional anaerobic variables (Sprint test, Repeated Sprint Ability, 300 meter run test) explain 32% ($p = 0.04$) criteria, while the set of predictors of functional aerobic variables (Hoff test, 20m multi-stage shuttle run test) explain 26% ($p = 0.03$) criteria. On the basis of the research we can conclude that there is a strong correlation between the players' performance and tactical skill, whether it is a tactical-technical element of the phase of attack or defense. Therefore, coaches need to develop both components to achieve desired results in the competition games.

Keywords: Repeated sprint ability; Skill; Hoff test; Aerobic capacities

Introduction

Soccer has apart from aerobic endurance, that is represented by distance covered [1] a tremendous need for the type of anaerobic work like sprints, acceleration, duel games that have a direct impact on the final outcome [2]. Although soccer is dominated by the activities of aerobic character, key situations during the match takes place under anaerobic conditions [3-5]. Lower aerobic activity among players leads to early fatigue, which directly affects the decline in technical skills of players [6].

Technique or sport-specific technical skill takes great part in the development of talented young players of many team sports including soccer [7]. Tactical skills include technical elements applied in different situations such as a variety of gross movements, measures and procedures carried out with the aim of solving certain tasks in the course of the game. However, as soccer belongs to polystructural sports, physiological and technical skills are both important for performance [8]. Despite recent attempts [9] data on the importance of the technical components of the young players are practically unexplored [10]. Their role during the game may have a decisive impact on the final outcome of the match. It must be emphasized that success in soccer certainly depends on how the individual functional, motor and technical skills fit into the whole in order to obtain a coherent team. There are studies that analyze the impact of and correlation between specific tactical techniques and structural elements and performance of the soccer team [11-13].

The current methodology requires specific training exercises that will include tactical, technical and physical capabilities of players. Hoff, Wisloff, Engen, Kemi, Helgerud [14] have shown that the polygon within which the players perform dribbling with the ball and play in a small space satisfies the same conditions of intensity and endurance training to enhance the intensity of 90-95% maximum heart rate for 3 to 5 minutes. According to that fact it can be seen how the endurance training in a soccer game should be organized so that it is more like a soccer match.

Aerobic capacity significantly affects the technical performance and tactical decisions. Helgerud, Engen, Wisloff, Hoff [15] showed that an increase in maximal oxygen (for 5 ml / kg / min) and running economy (7%), significantly affects players performance during the game. To be successful in soccer, endurance is of great importance, but what a top player must own is a good basic level of skills and sense of timing. Correlation between functional capacity and technical elements as in the defense phase as well in the attack phase according to the author's knowledge has not yet been sufficiently explored, although this field is extremely important because these skills during the game permanently intertwined with the players. Aim of this study was to determine the relationship between functional capacities and skills performance among young soccer player.

Methods

Subjects

The research was conducted on a sample of 22 (mean age 13.19±0.32; height 166.04 ± 6.00 cm; body mass 55.19 ± 9.41 kg) players aged U-14, members of the elite junior club. All subjects were given parental consent to access testing. Each of the participants could leave the testing protocol if they wanted. The protocol of this study was approved by the Ethical Committee of the Faculty of Kinesiology, University of Zagreb and according to the revised Declaration of Helsinki. Each player had at least 4 years of training experience, corresponding to 2 hour training sessions, and at least one competition per week.

Testing procedure

Each athlete performed a standardized 15 minute warm-up

***Corresponding author:** Goran Sporis, PhD Assist, Faculty of Kinesiology, Horvacanski zavoj 15, 10000 Zagreb, Croatia
E-mail: gsporis@kif.hr

consisting of general movements and dynamic and static stretching before the testing. Players underwent physical tests assessments in an outdoor stadium. During the test air temperature ranged from 22°C to 25°C. It began at 10 am and finished by 1 pm. Players were instructed not to be involved in strenuous exercise for at least 48 hours before the fitness testing session and consume their normal pre-training diet before the testing session. None of the subjects were injured 6 months before the testing. There was no supplement addition regarding the nutrition of players. In addition, subjects were not taking exogenous anabolic-androgenic steroids and other drugs that might be expected to affect physical performance or hormonal balance. After the general warm-up, players performed assessments of sprint ability (sprint test), repeated sprint ability and soccer specific ability in random order. Sprint test, repeated sprint test, 300 meters run test run and soccer-specific test were performed on the same day in the morning between 10 and 13h for all participants. After 3 days testing was done in the test 20-m multi-stage shuttle run test how the accumulation of fatigue of previous tests would not be reflected in the results. Measurements were taken on Tuesday morning because the athletes had rested after the weekend match. The testing session began with anthropometric measurements. Testing for sprint, repeated sprint, 300 meters run test, soccer-specific test and functional capacity was carried out in 3 days. Sprint test was measured with 3 particles, and the mean was taken as the true value, which was used in data processing. Tests for assessment repeated sprint abilities, anaerobic capacity, soccer-specific capacity and functional capacity were measured with only 1 particle. On the first day, subjects were tasted in the following order of tests: sprint test, repeated sprint test, 300 meters run and soccer specific test. Recovery between the tests in each subject was in a 1:10 ratio (work: rest ratio). After that all subjects had one day rest period. 20 meter multi-stage shuttle run test was performed on the third day to avoid the accumulation of fatigue.

Functional capacities

Sprint test protocol: The fastest sprint assessed with the seven-sprint protocol [16] was the measure of running speed. The test consists of seven separate sprints (each section is 34.2m including slalom sprint) with a break of 25 seconds between each sprint during which participants can walk or jogging to the starting line (Figure 1). Verbal feedback is given to each respondent for 5, 10, 15, 20 and 25 seconds of recovery. Photoelectric cell timing system (Globus Ergo Tester Pro, Codognè, Italy) was used to measure each sprint interval and recovery time with an accuracy of 0.001 seconds. This system was positioned on the opposite side of the test field at start and finish line (Figure 1). Photoelectric cell was conected with PC and software for digital measure. The subjects started with her head immediately behind the "start" line.

Repeated sprint test: Each subject performed twelve repetitions maximum sprint section of 20 meters. Pause between each sprint is 20 seconds, during which time the participants jog or walk to the starting line. This test was chosen because it is the best way to simulate conditions that occur during a soccer match [17,18]. Verbal feedback is given to each participant for 5, 10, 15, 20 and 25 seconds of recovery. Photoelectric cell timing system (Globus Ergo Tester Pro, Codognè, Italy) was used to measure each sprint interval and recovery time with an accuracy of 0.001 seconds. This system was positioned on the opposite side of the test field at start and finish line. Photoelectric cell was conected with PC and software for digital measure. The subjects started with her head immediately behind the "start" line.

300 meter run test: This test is used to assess anaerobic capacity because the anaerobic capacity is the first determinant of performance in maximal all-out efforts eliciting exhaustion between 30 and 60 s [19]. The test is performed on open track length of 400m and the time is recorded manually. Each participant was told to run the section as fast as possible.

Soccer specific endurance tests: The track for the performance was proposed for the first time by Hoff, Wisloff, Engen, Kemi, Helgerud [14] for training purposes. The Hoff test, or circuit as it's often called, includes multiple changes in direction, ball lifting and dribbling in reverse (Figure 2). Recent studies [14] have shown that the Hoff test possesses criterion validity and sensitivity to aerobic fitness development in youth soccer players. His work has shown that this program can be used as a part of regular training to improve fitness. As proposed by Hoff, Wisloff, Engen, Kemi, Helgerud [14] the player moved a soccer ball through the track by dribbling. They then move around the next set of cones. Between point A and B the players turn and dribble backwards while controlling the ball. The purpose of the test was to cover the maximum distance during a 10 minute period. Depending on the exact layout of the course, the total distance covered is about 290m. Five subjects were tested at a time. Four days before the first Hoff test, the subjects performed a pre-test in order to get used to the testing pace so as to obtain maximum performance during the experiment.

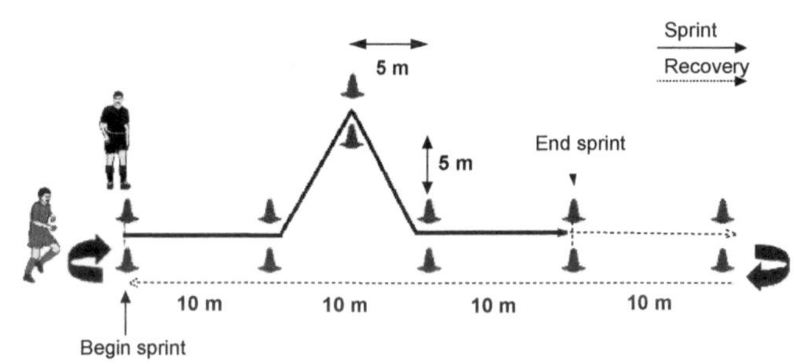

Figure 1 : Diagram of sprint test protocol

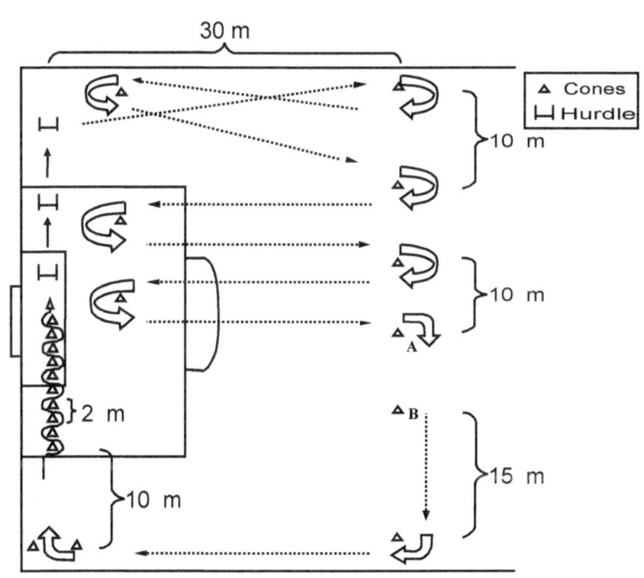

Figure 2: Hoff test

20-m multi-stage shuttle run test: The 20-m shuttle run test is a field test that predicts aerobic fitness (VO_{2max}) and has been shown to be a reliable and valid indicator of aerobic power in various populations [20]. This test was conducted as previously described by Davis, Brewer, Atkin [20]. The main reason for the use of this test for the evaluation of aerobic fitness in the present study, and for its great popularity among soccer coaches, is that the back and forward runs performed in the test mimic the movement pattern of soccer. Players run between lines 20 feet distant in the pace of them sets the "beep" signal from the compact disc (20-m Shuttle Run Test CD, Australian Sports Commission). Tempo running is progressively increasing every minute. The total distance covered is being marked for each player and represents the end result of the test. The objective of the test was to perform as many shuttles as possible; the score corresponded to the total meters covered until the athlete was no longer able to maintain the required speed. Each subject's VO_2 was derived by the formula, y = 6.0x - 24.4, where y equals the predicted VO_{2max} and x equals the maximum speed achieved [20].

Soccer skills

Ten soccer experts assessed the importance of tactical techniques that define the structure of soccer. A soccer coach, an expert advisor, a top player or a college professor teaching soccer at the Faculty of Kinesiology, a coach of a soccer team competing in the European Football Club championships, a coach or a member of expert staff of the national soccer team participating in the European Championships or World Cups, a footballer from a team competing in the European Football Club championships or a member of the national team participating in the European Championship or World Cup were regarded experts in the research study. Relying on their own experience and using the assessment system with values ranging from 0 to 5 the experts graded the impact of tactical techniques on the properties (attributes) of soccer, attack and defense. Competitive match (11 vs. 11) was played on a regular sized synthetic grass soccer pitch over 2 halves each lasting 30 minutes (10- minute interval). Match air temperature and relative humidity were 22.8 ± 1.8°C and 40 ± 9.8%, respectively. We were filmed the match and then analyzed every tactical and technical elementsfor each player.

Variables to assess the real quality of players in the transition phase of attack and in the positioning attack: ball control, passing skills, advancing with ball, play without ball, success in attack transition, ability to play in multiple positions in attack, success in break game phases in attack, shots during active play.

Variables to assess the real quality of players in the transition phase of defense and positioning defense: The level of pressure in the defense, assist in defense, take possession of the ball, success during breaks in defense, success in the defense transition, ability to play in multiple positions in defense, preventing shots, success in offside traps.

Statistical analysis

The statistical Package for Social Studies SPSS (v17.0., SPSS Inc., Chicago, IL) was used for statistical analysis. Prior to the factor analysis, the normality of the distribution of variables was examined by the Kolmogorov-Smirnov test. The objectivity of the expert group in the process of assessing the importance of the tactical techniques of attack and defense was established for every variable and expressed as Chronbach's alpha. The condensed expert assessment results were expressed as the arithmetic mean. To determine the relation between functional capabilities and players performance multiple regression analyzes was applied. In addition, we have applied factor analysis with varimax rotation to determine the latent structure of the applied structure of instruments (quality players in attack and defense). Latent structure for the set of variables was separately determined for players in attack, and especially for the defense. Relying on their own experience and using the assessment system with values ranging from 0 to 5 the experts graded the impact of tactical techniques on the properties (attributes) of soccer, attack and defense. The statistical significance was set at $p<0.05$.

Results

All the variables had normal distribution. Factor structure of the variables (Table 3) has showed that anaerobic variables contribute significantly (p = 0.03) in determining the game capabilities in defense phase. The same significance was observed among the aerobic variables (p = 0.03) so we can conclude that aerobic and anaerobic components have an equal share in the defense phase. Anaerobic capacity of players explain 37% of the variance (p = 0.03) for defensive tactical elements, while the set of functional aerobic variables (Hoff test, p = 0.18; beep test, p = 0.93) has explained 37% (p = 0.03) of defensive players ability.

Table 3 show that both coefficients of multiple correlation factors for technical quality of players in attack were statistically significant. Based on the coefficient of determination it can be concluded that a set of predictors of functional anaerobic variables (Sprint test, Repeated Sprint Ability, 300 meter run test) explain 32% (p = 0.04) criteria, while the set of predictors of functional aerobic variables (Hoff test, 20m multi-stage shuttle run test) explain 26% (p = 0.03) criteria. However, individually only the values obtained by Hoff test statistically present a significant factor in the attack phase (p = 0.05), while the defense phase values obtained by this test does not represent a statistically significant factor (p = 0.18). Other variables do not individually show a statistically significant value in the phase of the defense and attack. The results show that it is necessary to possess a good aerobic and anaerobic capacity so that they together influence the tactical and technical manifestation of the defense and attack phase.

	Factor
Ball control	-0.75
Passing skills	-0.86
Advancing with ball	-0.88
Play without ball	-0.71
Success in attack transition	-0.85
Ability to play in multiple positions in attack	-0.87
Success in break game phases in attack	-0.86
Shots during active play	-0.75
Expl.Var	5.28
Prp.Totl	0.66

Table 1: Factorial analysis in the transition phase of attack and in the positioning attack.

	Factor
The level of pressure in the defense	-0.91
Assist in defense	-0.94
Take possession of the ball	-0.92
Success during breaks in defense	-0.81
Success in the defense transition	-0.89
Ability to play in multiple positions in defense	-0.92
Preventing shots	-0.88
Success in offside traps	-0.77
Expl.Var	6.23
Prp.Totl	0.78

Table 2: Factorial analysis in the transition phase of defense and positioning defense.

	ATTACK		Adjusted			DEFENSE		Adjusted		
	β	p	R	R^2	p	β	p	R	R^2	p
Sprint test protocol	-0.05	0.87				0.29	0.36			
Repeated Sprint Ability	-0.47	0.20	0.56	0.32	0.04	0.01	0.97	0.61	0.37	0.03
300 meter run test	-0.04	0.90				0.34	0.29			
Hoff test	-0.47	0.05	0.51	0.26	0.03	-0.29	0.18	0.61	0.37	0.03
20m multi-stage shuttle run test	-0.01	0.97				-0.02	0.93			

Table 3: Multiple regression analyzes in the phase of defense and attack.

For the success in technical and tactical elements of attack and defense in soccer the most important factor is to have a dimension factor for energy regulation and control of movement. The energy component is important in the movement of players with equal representation of both aerobic and anaerobic capacity ($p = 0.03$ vs. $p = 0.03$) in defense, ($p = 0.03$ vs. $p = 0.04$) in attack, while the movements of a player with the ball present the significance of both components with the preponderance of one or another (Table 1, 2).

Discussion and Conclusion

Generally speaking, we can only state that the aerobic and anaerobic capacities of players are equally important for their actions in the stage of defense and attack. But almost all the variables, if we look at individually, Sprint test ($p = 0.87$), Repeated Sprint Ability ($p = 0.20$), the 300 meters run test ($p = 0.90$), 20 m multi-stage shuttle run test ($p = 0.97$), not impact the tactical movements because they are statistically insignificant. The only test that showed a statistical significance individually was Hoff test ($p = 0.05$) which is understandable because it contains elements which required great technical ability of players. This test has specific aerobic nature and it is designed especially for soccer players [14]. However, its significance is reflected only in the phase of the attack. The explanation lies in the fact that we have isolated at the stage of attack variables such as: ball control, passing skills, advancing with ball that are part of the test [14]. Defensive assignments were predominantly without ball so it is understandable why this specific test showed no statistically significant correlation ($p = 0.18$) with defensive assignments.

The importance of aerobic fitness in soccer is reflected in the fact that movement is mainly dominated by the aerobic activities [18]. Tactical element of attack and defense are taking place under conditions of constant alternation of aerobic and anaerobic activity [21]. When performing a quick attack and counterattack (stage attacks) among players with or without the ball comes to the accumulation of lactate, which eliminates the over-intensity aerobic activity [18]. Therefore, good aerobic fitness is desirable and from this research it could be seen that they can influence the technical abilities of players in both the technical skills and tactical characteristics of defense phase ($p = 0.03$) and stage attacks ($p = 0.03$). Sprint abilities of football players are extremely important because they take place every 90 seconds and usually the sprint lasts 2-4 seconds [3]. Percentages on the activity of anaerobic character during soccer match is 1-11% with the effective time of the game (the time when the ball is in possession of) almost 0.5-3% [3,15]. Although we can see that the anaerobic capacity is less represented, their role is reflected in key situations, both in the defense and in attack phase. Our results have shown that the players must have the ability to multi-dimensional manifestation of anaerobic activity (sprint performance, repeated sprint performance and run performance), as observed individually these abilities do not affect the defensive and offensive elements. The importance of short sprints (Sprint test protocol) and repeated sprint ability should be especially emphasized during the match because the players perform from 1000-1400 mainly short activities, changing every 2-4 seconds [3]. In our research, we see that these values of repeated sprint ability is much more important in tactical elements of the attacks ($p = 0.20$) than in the defense phase ($p = 0.97$). The smallest impact of the attack phase has been showed in a variable 300 meter run test ($p = 0.90$) which can be attributed to time players during a game not required for expression of high-intensity activity on such a large distance but the greatest number of sprint action ends in the range of 20-40 meters.

The limitation of this research was a lack of sprint 5, 10, 20 and 30m, because they are mostly the distance at which players perform sprinting during the game. So that future research should examine how they influence the technical characteristic and tactical skill elements.

On the basis of the research we can conclude that there is a strong correlation between the players' performance and tactical skill, whether it is a tactical-technical element of the phase of attack or defense. Players in soccer must possess a comprehensive aerobic and anaerobic capabilities how would their joint actions affect the technical characteristics and tactical skills. Therefore, coaches need to insist on the all round fitness training and their actions should be reflected in the technical abilities of players. The high level of functional ability, aerobic or anaerobic is a prerequisite for successful execution of technical-tactical skills in the process of defense and attack. The results of this study show us the complexity of functional abilities since they viewed themselves; do not affect the performance of the technical elements but only integrally.

References

1. Kemi OJ, Hoff J, Engen LC, Helgerud J, Wisloff U (2003) Soccer specific testing of maximal oxygen uptake. J Sports Med Phys Fitness 43: 139-144.
2. Little T, Williams AG (2005) Specificity of acceleration, maximum speed, and agility in professional soccer players. J Strength Cond Res 19: 76-78.
3. Bangsbo J, Norregaard L, Thorsoe F (1991) Activity profile of competition soccer. Can J Sports Sci 16: 110-116.
4. Ben Abdelkrim N, El Fazaa S, El Ati J (2007) Time-motion analysis and physiological data of elite under-19-year-old basketball players during competition. Br J Sports Med 41: 69-75.
5. Sporis G, Vuleta D, Vuleta D, Milanović D (2010) Fitness profiling in handball: physical and physiological characteristics of elite players. Coll Antropol 34: 1009-1014.
6. Sporis G, Ruzic L, Leko G (2008) The anaerobic endurance of elite soccer players improved after a high-intensity training intervention in the 8-week conditioning program. J Strength Cond Res 22: 559-566.
7. Malina RM, Cumming SP, Kontos AP, Eisenmann JC, Ribeiro B, et al. (2005) Maturity-associated variation in sport-specific skills of youth soccer players aged 13-15 years. J Sports Sci 23: 515-522.
8. Fernandez-Gonzalo R, De Souza-Teixeira F, Bresciani G, Garcıa-Lopez D, Hernandez-Murua JA, et al. (2010) Comparison of technical and physiological characteristics of prepubescent soccer players of different ages. J Strength Cond Res 24: 1790-1798.
9. Rostgaard T, Iaia FM, Simonsen DS, Bangsbo J (2008) A test to evaluate the physical impact on technical performance in soccer. J Strength Cond Res 22: 283-292.
10. Castagna C, D'Ottavio S, Abt G (2003) Activity profile of young soccer players during actual match play. J Strength Cond Res 17: 775-780.

11. Bishovets A, Gadjiev G, Godik M (1993) Computer analysis of the effectiveness of collective technical and tactical moves of footballers in teh matches of 1988 Olympics and 1990 World Cup. In T Reilly, J Clarys A Stibbe (eds) Science and Football II. E & FN Spon, London.

12. Yamanaka K, Hughes M, Lott M (1993) An analysis of playing patterns in the 1990 World Cup for association football. In T Reilly, J Clarys, A Stibbe (eds) Science and Football II. E & FN Spon, London.

13. Hughes M (1996) Notational Analysis. In T Reilly (Ed), Science and soccer. E & FN Spon, London.

14. Hoff J, Wisloff U, Engen LC, Kemi OJ, Helgerud J (2002) Soccer Specific Aerobic Endurance Training. Br J Sports Med 36: 218-221.

15. Helgerud J, Engen LC, Wisløff U, Hoff J (2001) Aerobic endurance training improves soccer performance. Med Sci Sports Exerc 33: 1925-1931.

16. Bangsbo J (1994) Fitness Training for Football: A scientific approach. HO+Storm, Bagsverd.

17. Reilly T (1994) Motion characteristics. In: Football (Soccer). B Ekblom (ed) Blackwell Scientific Publications, London.

18. Stolen T, Chamari K, Castagna C, Wisloff U (2005) Physiology of soccer. Sports Med 35: 501–536.

19. Calbet JA, De Paz JA, Garatachea N, Cabeza De Vaca S, Chavarren J (2003) Anaerobic energy provision does not limit Wingate exercise performance in endurance-trained cyclists. J Appl Physiol 94: 668-676.

20. Davis JA, Brewer J, Atkin D (1992) Pre-season physiological characteristics of English first and second division soccer players. J Sports Sci 10: 541-547.

21. Milanovic Z, Trajkovic N, Barisic V, Dujic I, Ljubicic M, et al. (2011) Discriminant analysis of soccer tactical elements in the phases of attack and defense determined by cluster analysis. Homosporticus 13: 12-20.

Effects of Resistance Exercise on Intramuscular Oxygenation and Muscle Fiber Composition

Fumio Aita[1], Shukoh Haga[2], Shogo Sato[3], Takuya Sakurai[3*], Kazuki Esaki[4], Takafumi Hamaoka[5], Masao Mizuno[6], Koji Toshinai[7], Hiromi Miyazaki[8], Tohru Takemasa[9], Noboru Hashimoto[10], Junetsu Ogasawara[3], Toshihito Katsumura[11], Takako Kizaki[3] and Hideki Ohno[3]

[1]*Edosaki Sohgoh High School, Inashiki, Japan*
[2]*Institute of Health and Sport Science, University of Tsukuba, Tsukuba, Japan*
[3]*Department of Molecular Predictive Medicine and Sport Science, Kyorin University, School of Medicine, Mitaka, Japan*
[4]*Faculty of Education, Shiga University, Ohtsu, Japan*
[5]*Faculty of Sports and Health Science, Ritsumeikan University, Kusatsu, Japan*
[6]*Faculty of Education, Hokkaido University, Sapporo, Japan*
[7]*Faculty of Medicine, University of Miyazaki, Miyazaki, Japan*
[8]*Division of Traumatology, National Defense Medical College Research Institute, Tokorozawa, Japan*
[9]*Graduate School of Comprehensive Human Sciences, University of Tsukuba, Tsukuba, Japan*
[10]*Department of Judo Therapy, Faculty of Health Science, Tokyo Ariake University of Medical and Health Science, Kotoh-ku, Japan*
[11]*Department of Sports Medicine for Health Promotion, Tokyo Medical University, Shinjuku-ku, Japan*

Abstract

Determining the oxygenation level of skeletal muscle is an effective non-invasive method of evaluating its physiological changes. Nevertheless, the relationship between muscle fiber composition and intramuscular oxygenation is still unclear. In the present study we examined the differences in muscle fiber composition and their relationship to muscle oxygenation levels by comparing power lifters (Training group), who regularly engaged in muscular resistance training, with ordinary healthy people (Control group). The vastus lateralis muscle oxygenation level was measured via near infrared continuous wave spectroscopy, and muscle tissues were collected and used for histochemical analyses in order to calculate muscle fiber compositions. When the rate of decrease in muscle oxygenation after performing a single squat at 50 and 80% of the participants' maximal lifting weight (MLW) was examined, the rate of decrease was significantly higher at 80% of MLW than at 50% of MLW in Training group, and was significantly higher in the Training group than in the Control group. Moreover, after performing multiple squat movements at 80% of MLW, compared with the Control group, the Training group showed a significant delay in the time it took for their muscle oxygenation level to recover to 50% of its original level at resting time ($T_{1/2}$). A significant correlation between the occupancy of Type IIa fiber and $T_{1/2}$, or between an average cross-sectional area of muscle fibers and $T_{1/2}$ was noted. The present study demonstrated that in the Training group, in a cross-sectional area of Type IIa fiber that had increased, the decreased muscle oxygenation level due to performing squat exercises exhibited a delay in recovery at the resting time, suggesting that the amount of oxygen consumption was increased in the Training group because the cross-sectional area of Type IIa fiber was larger, compared with the Control group.

Keywords: Resistance training; Muscle oxygenation; Near infrared continuous wave spectroscopy; Muscle fiber composition

Introduction

Skeletal muscle is composed of several types of muscle fibers such as Type I, Type IIa, and Type IIx, all of which differ in contractile and metabolic characteristics. Skeletal muscle is referred to as a "plastic" tissue because it adapts to exercise. In fact, the exercise-induced stimulation from muscular resistance increases muscle mass and strength, changes muscle composition and improves muscle function. This process is thought to be the after-effect of hypertrophy of muscle fiber size, an increase in muscle fiber number, accretion of connective tissue around muscle fiber, or some combination of these [1].

Recently, the effects of hypoxia on muscle structure and function have been investigated. Resistance training under local hypoxia reportedly induces muscle hypertrophy (Type II fiber) and increases muscle strength [2-5]. Also, it has been suggested that under hypoxia, low-intensity resistance training, which is generally thought not to induce muscle hypertrophy, can induce muscle hypertrophy [6,7]. On the other hand, hypoxia-induced intramuscular environmental changes are synergistically developed by resistance exercise [8]. A muscle contraction-induced rise in intramuscular pressure excretes blood and results in the flow of more blood after relaxation. Thus, the ischemic interval is dependent upon the length of the muscle contractile time. Therefore, the extension of an ischemic interval induced by resistance training attracts hypoxia and affects muscle structure and function.

Examination of muscle oxygenation levels is thought to be effective as a non-invasive method of evaluating physiological changes in skeletal muscle caused by exercise. Near infrared continuous wave spectroscopy (NIRcws) has been used to evaluate the kinetics of skeletal muscle oxygenation during various types of exercise non-invasively and continuously [9-11]. In fact, some studies have examined the relationship between changes in exercise intensity and muscle oxygenation level by having participants perform squat exercises [12-15]. For example, muscle oxygen recovery kinetics appeared to be influenced by differences in the intensity and volume of exercise [12]. Nevertheless, in addition to exercise intensity and volume, little is known about factors that affect changes in muscle oxygenation. In the present study, we hypothesized that muscle fiber composition affected intramuscular oxygenation because of differences in oxygen consumption and oxidation capacity of each muscle fiber type. Therefore, we investigated differences in muscle

***Corresponding author:** Takuya Sakurai, Department of Molecular Predictive Medicine and Sport Science, Kyorin University, School of Medicine, 6-20-2 Shinkawa, Mitaka, Tokyo 181-8611, Japan
E-mail: sakutaku@ks.kyorin-u.ac.jp

fiber compositions and their relationship with muscle oxygenation levels were evaluated via NIRcws between powerlifters (Training group) and ordinary healthy people (Control group).

Materials and Methods

Participants

Thirteen healthy male adults participated in the study: 7 powerlifters for the Training group and 6 healthy graduate students and working adult volunteers for the Control group. The powerlifters belonged either to a powerlifting club at the University of Tsukuba in Japan or to a powerlifting association in Japan, and had entered a powerlifting competition. The average length of competitive experience in powerlifting of the Training group was 8.0 ± 2.8 years. All the participants had almost the same age, weight, BMI, and skinfold thickness, except for height (Table 1). The study was conducted with the participants who agreed to participate after having received sufficient explanation on the purpose, method, safety, and problems of this study. Experimental procedures were approved by the Ethics Committee of the Institute of Health and Sport Science, University of Tsukuba, Japan.

Protocol for measuring

The protocol of this research is shown in Figure 1. After a muscle biopsy, the participants were given time to recover until muscular activities could be done smoothly. We determined the maximal lifting weight (MLW) of each participant in advance and calculated relative exercise loads at 50 and 80% of their MLW. The determination of the MLW for the powerlifters was based on their best records in a powerlifting competition. On the other hand, for determinations of MLW for the Control group, we measured each of 6 repetition maximum (RM) loads during a squat exercise. A 6RM load is known to be reliable (Intra-class correlation coefficient > 0.95) and can be an alternative to a 1RM load determination [16]. The 1RM load can be estimated from a 6RM load using the following conversion equation: 1RM load=6RM load / 85% [17].

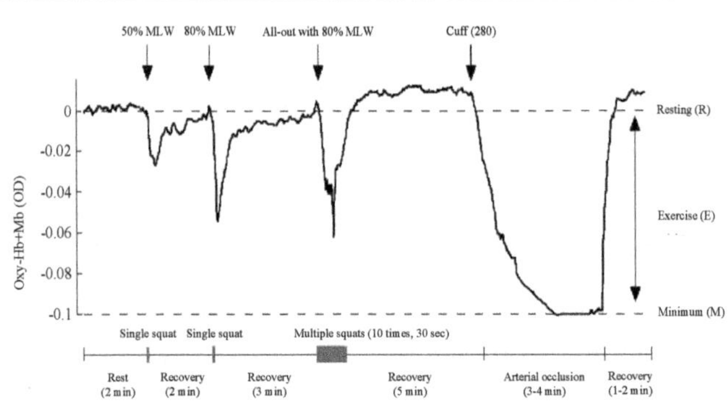

Figure 1: Experimental protocol of the muscle oxygenation during a squat exercise

Relative muscle oxygenation was determined by assigning the resting oxy-Hb+Mb value (R) (100%) and the minimum oxy-Hb+Mb value (M) obtained from arterial occlusion (0%). Muscle oxygenation (%) was expressed by using algebraic expression, i.e., muscle oxygenation (%) = (M-E)/(M-R)×100. MLW = maximal lifting weight.

The participants took a standing posture in the squat rack (NISHI Athletic Goods Co., Ltd., Tokyo, Japan) after resting on a chair for 2 minutes. Each participant assumed their exercise posture 10 seconds before the start of the exercise. At the moment when they were given a signal, they started a squat movement at 50% of their MLW. Next, after confirming that the muscle oxygenation level had recovered to the resting level (almost 2 min), the participants performed a squat at 80% of their MLW. Finally, after sufficient recovery time (almost 3 min), the participants performed multiple squats at 80% of their MLW until exhaustion (almost 10 times, 30 sec). We judged subjects as being in an exhausted state when failure to perform the squat exercise (failure to stand, decreases in knee flexion angle, stagger, and so on) was observed. Because the Control groups lacked sufficient experience in squat exercises, assistants with sufficient knowledge and experience, supervised the exercise performances of the Control group to avoid accidents during exercise. Moreover, immediately after each squat movement, assistants on both sides of a participant lifted the barbell by hand so that the participant could be in the recovery period in a relaxed condition. This was done to avoid the influence of muscle oxygenation during the recovery process in participants after the exercises. Five minutes after the completion of all the exercises, arterial occlusion was performed.

Evaluation of oxygenation levels in skeletal muscle

NIRcws is used as the measurement of oxygen concentration in tissues by utilizing the absorbance characteristics of hemoglobin and myoglobin at the near infrared region. To measure NIRcws, we used Omron's near-infrared spectroscopy device (HEO-100, Kyoto, Japan). This device uses a two-wavelength method of two near infrared wavelengths (760 and 850 nm) as the basis of measurement [18]. Its probe is composed of two LEDs, which emit two near infrared wavelengths, photo diode, and photodetection amplifier. The probe was attached to the vastus lateralis muscle of the right thigh, which was the same part where the muscle biopsy was conducted. Near-infrared light of 760 and 850 nm wavelengths emitted from the light source was injected into the muscle tissue and changes in oxygenation levels of skeletal muscle were measured based on the amount of light that reached the photodetector sensor after being absorbed by oxyhemoglobin and oxymyoglobin (oxy-Hb+Mb), as well as deoxyhemoglobin and deoxymyoglobin (deoxy-Hb+Mb). A relative value of skeletal muscle oxygenation cannot be calculated by the measurement of oxy-Hb+Mb using NIRcws. Therefore, following the arterial occlusion method ≥ 280 mmHg of pressure was applied to the thigh cuffs until the oxy-Hb+Mb showed the minimal value [19-21]. The minimal oxy-Hb+Mb value was determined when the oxy-Hb+Mb value had reduced (almost 2 min) and maintained a steady state for 1-2 min. The relative value of skeletal muscle oxygenation was calculated with the following formula, using the minimum value obtained (M), the value obtained at resting (R), and the value obtained during exercise (E):

(Formula) Muscle oxygenation (%) = (M-E)/(M-R)×100.

The distance between the light source of the probe and the photodetector used was 3 cm. Therefore, the depth of measurement was assumed to be 1 to 2 cm below the skin surface [21-23]. Based on the fact that the thigh skinfold thickness in subjects tested in this

	Age (yr)	Height (cm)	Weight (kg)	BMI (kg/m²)	Skinfold thickness (cm)	Training experience (yr)
Control group (N=6)	33.2 ± 5.1	171.4 ± 0.7	71.4 ± 1.9	24.3 ± 0.7	0.5 ± 0.1	-
Training group (N=7)	30.0 ± 4.8	165.5 ± 2.2*	68.7 ± 4.4	25.1 ± 1.4	0.4 ± 0.1	8.0 ± 2.8

Values are means ± SE. BMI = body mass index; skinfold thickness = thickness of skin and tissue at the place of NIRcws probe. *$p < 0.05$ vs. Control group.

Table 1: Characteristics of subjects.

experiment averaged 0.4 ± 0.1 cm for the Training group and 0.5 ± 0.1 cm for the Control group, respectively, it could be assumed that the oxygen levels measured were derived mainly from skeletal muscle.

Muscle biopsy

A physician who specialized in exercise physiology conducted the muscle biopsies. Dexterity with vastus lateralis muscle was the focus of this experiment. Skin was sterilized with an anti-bacterial preparation (Isodine) and then muscle tissue (20~30 mg) was sampled under local anesthesia (1% xylocaine). Two specimens of muscle tissue were sampled for histochemical analysis. The muscle tissue was rapidly embedded in a compound (TISSUE-TEK, Miles Co., Elkhart, USA) and instantly frozen in 2-methylbutane (isopentane; WAKO, Osaka, Japan), then maintained with liquid nitrogen. Frozen samples were stored at -80°C until moments before use.

Histochemical analysis

A continuous cross-section (10 μm) of muscle tissues was obtained by cryostat (OF/FAS5030; Bright Instrument, Cambridgeshire, UK) at -20°C. The sections were subjected to myosin-ATPase stain (pre-incubation; pH 10.3 and 4.6) [2,24]. The sections were photographed using a photomicrographic camera (Nikon M-35FA, Nikon, Tokyo, Japan). According to methods established by Brooke and Kaiser each sample of muscle fiber was separated into either Type I or Type II (Type IIa, Type IIx, and Type IIc) fiber, and the % of Fiber Type was calculated. Each type of muscle fiber from the same sample was randomly traced and calculated as to mean fiber area per fiber with respect to each of the types using image analysis software [3,25]. Based on those values, the muscle fiber cross-sectional area per capillary vessel (i.e., Diffusion index between capillary vessel and muscle fiber and muscle fiber type area distribution) was also calculated. On the other hand, other sections were subjected to amylase-PAS stain (pre-incubation; 0.5% α-amylase) for visualization of capillaries [26]. The number of capillaries around the fiber type and the number of capillaries per unit area (1000 μm^2) for each fiber type were calculated.

Statistical analysis

The numerical values obtained are indicated as means ± SE. An unpaired t-test was applied to compare the data between the two groups. Furthermore, Pearson's correlation analysis was conducted to examine the correlation between different measured values. The level of statistical significance was set at less than 5 percent.

Results

Changes in muscle oxygenation level caused by performing squat exercises

Figure 2A shows the changes in muscle oxygenation after performing a single squat at 50% of MLW. Muscle oxygenation in both groups decreased with the start of the squat movement, and after reaching the lowest peak value, it tended to gradually recover to the original level at resting (Figure 2A). The lowest peak value during the decrease in muscle oxygenation was 84.3 ± 5.6% for the Control group and 68.1 ± 8.1% for the Training group, respectively (Figure 2A). Similar results were obtained after performing a single squat at 80% of the participants' MLW (Figure 2B). The muscle oxygenation level observed immediately after exercise was 89.8 ± 5.7% for the Control group and 84.0 ± 3.1% for the Training group, respectively (Figure 2B). The lowest peak value during the decrease in muscle oxygenation was 65.1 ± 9.8% for the Control group and 58.3 ± 9.2% for the Training group, respectively (Figure 2B). On the other hand, during the multiple squats, a muscle oxygenation level

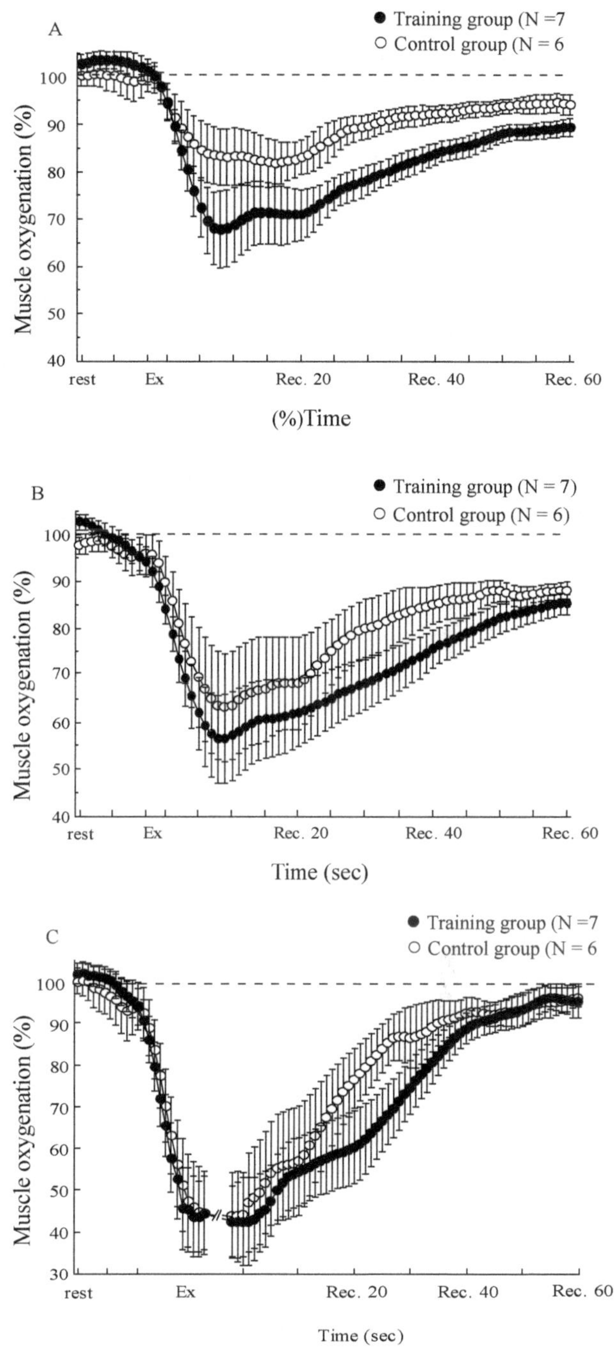

Figure 2: Changes in muscle oxygenation level caused by performing squat exercises

Changes in muscle oxygenation during one trial squat exercise with 50% (A) and 80% (B) of MLW and a recovery period in the Training (close circle) and Control (open circle) groups is shown. Values are means ± SE. Rec=Recovery. C: Changes in muscle oxygenation during squat exercises to exhaustion with 80% of MLW and recovery period in the Training (close circle) and Control (open circle) groups. Values are means ± SE. Rec = Recovery.

at 80% of the participants' MLW decreased in a linear fashion followed by a stable condition in both groups (Figure 2C). After performing the movement, recovery to the original level at resting was time-dependent (Figure 2C). However, although the Control group's recovery time of muscle oxygenation was quick (especially between 10 and 25 seconds), the Training group showed a more gradual recovery rate during the same time period, which indicated a delay in recovery (Figure 2C).

Changes in the rate of decrease in muscle oxygenation level caused by performing a single squat

With the results shown in Figures 2A and 2B, the rate of decrease in muscle oxygenation after performing a single squat at 50 and 80% of the participants' MLW was examined (Figure 3). At both loads, the rate of decrease in muscle oxygenation after performing a squat was significantly higher ($p<0.05$) in the Training group than in the Control group. The rate of decrease in muscle oxygenation in the Training group was significantly higher ($p<0.01$) at 80% of MLW than at 50% of MLW.

Changes in recovery time of muscle oxygenation after multiple squats

After performing multiple squats at 80% of the participants' MLW until exhaustion, recovery of muscle oxygenation was slower in the Training group than in the Control group (Figure 2C). The time it took for the muscle oxygenation level to recover to 50% of its original value at rest ($T_{1/2}$) was examined. As a result, the delay in recovery was significantly longer ($p<0.05$) in the Training group than in the Control group (Figure 4).

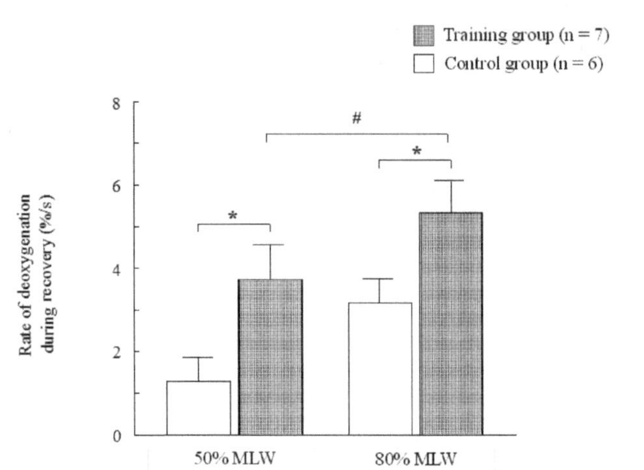

Figure 3: Changes in the rate of deoxygenation obtained during recovery

Rate of deoxygenation obtained during recovery (%/s) after both one trial squat exercise (50% and 80% of MLW) was calculated. Values are means ± SE. *p<0.05 vs. Control group; # p<0.01 vs. 50% of MLW in Training group.

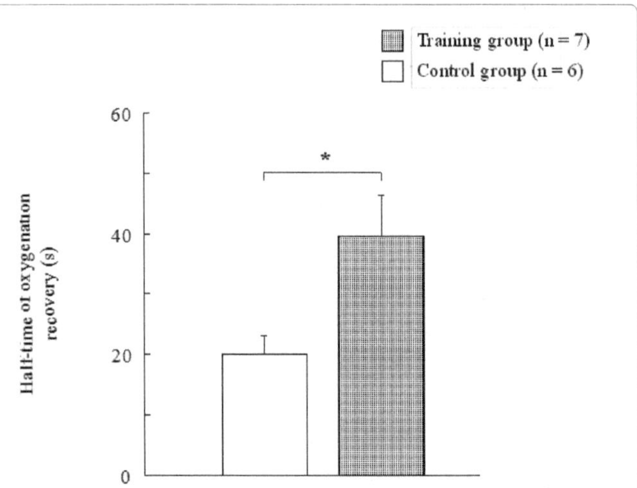

Figure 4: Changes in half-time of oxygenation recovery after squat exercises

Half-time of oxygenation recovery ($T_{1/2}$) after squat exercises to exhaustion with 80% of MLW was calculated. Values are means ± SE. *p<0.05 vs. Control group.

(A) Fiber type composition (%)			
Fiber type	Control group N = 6	Training group N = 7	P-value
Type I	41.7 ± 3.9	47.8 ± 6.9	NS
Type IIa	33.9 ± 3.8	41.1 ± 6.4	NS
Type IIx	23.6 ± 3.6	10.0 ± 4.5	NS
Type IIc	0.8 ± 0.4	1.0 ± 0.7	NS
(B) Fiber type area distributuion (%)			
Fiber type	Control group N = 6	Training group N = 7	P-value
Type I	41.9 ± 4.4	44.8 ± 6.7	NS
Type IIa	36.7 ± 4.1	45.7 ± 7.0	NS
Type IIx	20.8 ± 2.9	8.7 ± 3.9	0.05
Type IIc	0.7 ± 0.4	0.8 ± 0.6	NS
(C) Fiber type cross-sectional area (μm²)			
Fiber type	Control group N = 6	Training group N = 7	P-value
Type I	4708 ± 376	5672 ± 287	NS
Type IIa	5099 ± 459	6880 ± 481	0.05
Type IIx	4207 ± 447	3004 ± 1087	0.05
Type IIc	2034 ± 911	1447 ± 939	NS
Mean	4012 ± 548	4251 ± 697	NS
(D) Number of capillaries around fiber type			
Fiber type	Control group N = 6	Training group N = 7	P-value
Type I	4.8 ±0 .4	5.6 ± 0.3	NS
Type IIa	4.4 ± 0.5	5.4 ± 0.2	NS
Type IIx	3.9 ± 0.5	2.3 ± 0.8	NS
Type IIc	1.2 ± 0.6	1.9 ± 1.2	NS
Mean	3.6 ± 0.5	3.8 ± 0.6	NS

Values are meals ± SE

P-values denote level of significance between Training and Control groups

Table 2: Morphological characteristics of vastus lateralis muscle in Training and Control groups.

	Control group N = 6	Training group N = 7	P-value
Mean area (μm²)	4781 ± 397	6153 ± 377	0.05
Number of capillaries around muscle fiber	4.5 ± 0.5	5.3 ± 0.1	NS
Number of capillaries per muscle fiber	2.3 ± 0.2	2.7 ± 0.1	0. 05
Number of capillaries per unit area	451.7 ± 32.2	415.6 ± 21.3	NS
Diffusion index (μm²)	2108 ± 146	2289 ± 119	NS

Values are meals ± SE

P-values denote level of significance between Training and Control groups

Table 3: Mean Cross Sectional area of the vastus lateralis muscle in both groups.

Muscle fiber composition

As shown in Table 2A, the proportion of Type I and IIa fibers was not significantly different between both groups. The area distribution of Type IIx fiber was significantly lower ($p<0.05$) in the Training group than in the Control group (Table 2B). The cross-sectional area of Type IIa fiber was significantly higher ($p<0.05$) in the Training group than in the Control group, but that of Type IIx fiber was significantly lower ($p<0.05$) in the Training group than in the Control group (Table 2C). The number of capillary vessels around each muscle fiber was not significantly different between the groups.

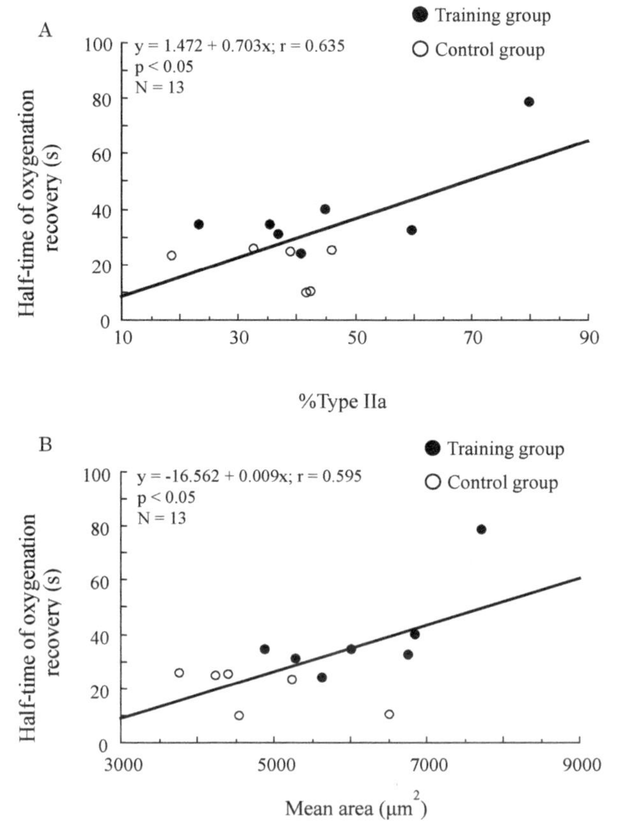

Figure 5: The relationship of the ratio of Type IIa fibers and mean cross-sectional area of muscle fiber with half-time of oxygenation recovery

A: Relationship between the % Type IIa fibers and half-time of oxygenation recovery ($T_{1/2}$) after squat exercises to exhaustion with 80% of MLW in Control and Training groups. Close and open circles indicate Training (N=7) and Control (N=6) groups, respectively. B: Relationship between the mean area of muscle fiber (μm²) and half-time of oxygenation recovery ($T_{1/2}$) after squat exercises to exhaustion with 80% of MLW in Control and Training groups. Close and open circles indicate Training (N=7) and Control (N=6) groups, respectively.

Table 3 shows the morphological characteristics of the vastus lateralis muscles. The mean value for the cross-sectional area of muscle fiber was significantly higher ($p<0.05$) in the Training group than in the Control group. Furthermore, the number of capillary vessels per muscle fiber was also higher ($p<0.05$) in the Training group than in the Control group. However, the number of capillary vessels per unit area was similar for both groups. Likewise, there was no difference in the diffusion index between the groups.

The relationship between the ratio of Type IIa fibers and $T_{1/2}$, and between the cross-sectional area of muscle fiber and $T_{1/2}$ after multiple squats

Finally, we examined the relationship of the ratio of Type IIa fibers and mean cross-sectional area of muscle fiber (μm²) with $T_{1/2}$. Significantly positive correlations were observed both between the ratio of Type IIa fibers and $T_{1/2}$ (Figure 5A), and between the mean cross-sectional area of muscle fiber and $T_{1/2}$ (Figure 5B).

In the present study, a decrease in muscle oxygenation that depended on exercise intensity was observed after performing a single squat exercise for both the Training and the Control groups, even though the muscle fiber compositions were different between the two groups. However, this decrease was more remarkable in the Training group than in the Control group. Furthermore, the rate of decrease in muscle oxygenation was significantly higher in the Training group than in the Control group. In addition, in the Training group, the decreased muscle oxygenation level due to performing multiple squat exercises showed a delay in recovery at resting time, and as the ratio of the Type IIa muscle fiber increased, this phenomenon became more significant.

Discussion

The decrease in muscle oxygenation level in the Training group was significantly higher at 80% of the participants' MLW than at 50% of the participants' MLW. Also, even though it was not statistically significant, the Control group appeared to show a higher rate of decrease in muscle oxygenation at 80% of MLW than at 50% of MLW. The physiological reactions of the vastus lateralis muscle in the right thigh caused by performing a squat included a constriction of arterioles and blood capillaries due to an increase in intramuscular pressure associated with muscular contraction, microcirculatory dysfunction, and decreased peripheral muscle blood flow. These reactions appeared to become stronger as the exercise load increased.

The changes in the types of muscle fibers recruited were associated with the changes in the capacity of oxygen consumption by mitochondria, which brought about changes in muscle oxygenation. Oxygen consumption of mitochondria is thought to be governed by ADP, Pi, NADH, and oxygen concentration and oxygen consumption by mitochondria increases according to an increase in the intensity of exercise [27,28]. In fact, Haga et al. [21] have reported that, when a high intensity exercise is performed, oxygen consumption by mitochondria increases and muscle oxygenation decreases from the beginning of the exercise. It can be assumed that the higher rates of decreases in muscle oxygenation observed at 80% of the participants' MLW in both groups were partly associated with the changes in the types of muscle fiber recruited due to the increase in exercise load. In both groups, activities employing Type I fiber might be significant at 50% of the participants' MLW. However, changes were seen in the rate of decrease in muscle oxygenation at 80% of MLW. It can be assumed that this occurred because activities employing Type IIa fibers, which have a relatively higher capacity of oxygen consumption than Type IIx fibers, were also prompted during the exercise performed at 80% of MLW.

On the other hand, the rate of decrease in muscle oxygenation after performing a single squat movement at both loads was significantly higher in the Training group than in the Control group. We may assume that the amount of oxygen consumption increased in the Training group because the cross-sectional area of skeletal muscle is larger in the Training group compared to the Control group, leading to more increased muscle oxygenation. $T_{1/2}$ after performing multiple squats at 80% of the participants' MLW until exhaustion showed a significant delay in the Training group. The recovery time of muscle oxygenation level after exercise reflects the synthesis of phosphocreatine that decreased due to exercise and oxygen transport to mitochondria, as well as the speed of oxidative ATP resynthesis [22]. Therefore, this time factor is considered to be an index of the aerobic capacity of skeletal muscle [18].

To search for the causes underlying the differences in the recovery time of muscle oxygenation between the Control and Training groups, we further examined the muscle fiber composition in both groups. The results of this study suggest that with resistance training, increases in occupancy depend on the number and size of Type I and IIa fibers that result from the migration caused not only by an increase in the number and size of Type I and IIa fibers, but also by a decrease in the number and size of Type IIx fibers. It is well known that an increase in the amount of physical activity transitions into a slow-twitch type of muscle fiber, and, conversely, a decrease in the amount of physical activity transitions into a fast-twitch type of muscle [29]. Since subjects in the Training group of this study had habitually performed squat exercises, their Type I and IIa fibers were mainly stimulated and hypertrophied according to the "Principle of size" [6,30]. Furthermore, it is accepted that high-intensity endurance training and sprint training promote the migration of the Type II fiber subtype (decrease in Type IIx fiber and increase in Type IIa fiber) which is the opposite effect of detraining [16,31-33]. Actually, cast immobilization and bed rest is known to decrease the cross-sectional area of Type I fibers and conversely increase that of Type IIx fibers [34]. These reports demonstrate that the amount of physical activity that is defined by either intensity or endurance can be associated with the resultant transition to fiber type. Moreover, in the present study, because an increase in the cross-sectional area of Type IIa fiber was observed in the Training group, and there was significantly positive correlations between the ratio of Type IIa fibers and $T_{1/2}$. One of the reasons for the delay in oxygenation recovery in the Training group is thought to be due to increased cross-sectional area of the Type IIa fiber.

The present study also showed that resistance training relatively, but not significantly, increased the number of capillary vessels around Type I and IIa fibers, and conversely decreased that around Type IIx fibers. The results from this study agreed with those from Schantz [26]. However, it is an accepted fact that intramuscular hypoxia induces the growth of capillary vessels and angiogenesis [35]. In particular, endurance training is known to increase the capillary plexus [24]. Additionally, since the endurance training-induced formation of the capillary plexus is recognized as being much higher under a hypoxic environment than under a low ground environment exercise-induced hypoxic stimulus to muscle tissue should contribute to the growth of the capillary plexus [36].

In summary, in the present study, we compared the differences in muscle fiber compositions and their relationship with muscle oxygenation levels between powerlifters, who regularly engaged in muscular resistance training, and ordinary healthy people. As a result, the present study demonstrates that habitual muscular resistance training increases the cross-sectional area of Type IIa fibers, but exhibits a delay in recovery of decreased muscle oxygenation level due to performing squat exercises. These results suggest that habitual muscular resistance training increases the amount of oxygen consumption because the cross-sectional area of Type IIa fiber is larger, compared to that found in ordinary healthy people.

Acknowledgements

This work was supported, in whole or in part, by the Grants-in-Aid for Specific Project Research from the Ministry of Education, Culture, Sports, Science and Technology of Japan, and the grant of THE DESCENTE AND ISHIMOTO MEMORIAL FOUNDATION FOR THE PROMOTION OF SPORTS SCIENCE.

References

1. MacDougall JD, Sale DG, Alway SE, Sutton JR (1984) Muscle fiber number in biceps brachii in bodybuilders and control subjects. J Appl Physiol Respir Environ Exerc Physiol 57: 1399-1403.
2. Moritani T, Sherman WM, Shibata M, Matsumoto T, Shinohara M (1992) Oxygen availability and motor unit activity in humans. Eur J Appl Physiol Occup Physiol 64: 552-556.
3. Sundberg CJ (1994) Exercise and training during graded leg ischaemia in healthy man with special reference to effects on skeletal muscle. Acta Physiol Scand Suppl 615: 1-50.
4. Takarada Y, Nakamura Y, Aruga S, Onda T, Miyazaki S, et al. (2000) Rapid increase in plasma growth hormone after low-intensity resistance exercise with vascular occlusion. J Appl Physiol (1985) 88: 61-65.
5. Takarada Y, Sato Y, Ishii N (2002) Effects of resistance exercise combined with vascular occlusion on muscle function in athletes. Eur J Appl Physiol 86: 308-314.
6. Beachle TR, Earle RW (2000) Essentials of strength training and conditioning. Human Kinetics, Champaign, Illinois.
7. Trappe SW, Costill DL, Fink WJ, Pearson DR (1995) Skeletal muscle characteristics among distance runners: a 20-yr follow-up study. J Appl Physiol (1985) 78: 823-829.
8. Takarada Y, Ishii N (1998) Resistance training under hypoxia. J Health Phys Edu Recreation 48: 36-42.
9. Ozyener F (2002) Evaluation of intra-muscular oxygenation during exercise in humans. Journal of Sports Science and Medicine 1: 15-19.
10. Quaresima V, Lepanto R, Ferrari M (2003) The use of near infrared spectroscopy in sports medicine. J Sports Med Phys Fitness 43: 1-13.
11. Hamaoka T, McCully K, Chance B, Iwane H (1994) Noninvasive measures of muscle metabolism. In: Exercise and Oxygen Toxicity. Sen C, Packer L, and Hanninen O, Elsevier Science, (Eds.), Amsterdam, 481-510.
12. Hoffman JR, Im J, Rundell KW, Kang J, Nioka S, et al. (2003) Effect of muscle oxygenation during resistance exercise on anabolic hormone response. Med Sci Sports Exerc 35: 1929-1934.
13. Hoffman JR, Im J, Kang J, Maresh CM, Kraemer WJ, et al. (2007) Comparison of low- and high-intensity resistance exercise on lipid peroxidation: role of muscle oxygenation. J Strength Cond Res 21: 118-122.
14. Rittweger J, Moss AD, Colier W, Stewart C, Degens H (2010) Muscle tissue oxygenation and VEGF in VO-matched vibration and squatting exercise. Clin Physiol Funct Imaging 30: 269-278.
15. Spiering BA, Kraemer WJ, Hatfield DL, Vingren JL, Fragala MS, et al. (2008) Effects of L-carnitine L-tartrate supplementation on muscle oxygenation responses to resistance exercise. J Strength Cond Res 22: 1130-1135.
16. Wong del P, Tan EC, Chaouachi A, Carling C, Castagna C, et al. (2010) Using squat testing to predict training loads for lower-body exercises in elite karate athletes. J Strength Cond Res 24: 3075-3080.
17. Baechle TR, Earle RW (2008) Essentials of strength training and conditioning (3rdedn). Human Kinetics, Champaign, IL, 641.
18. Hamaoka T, Albani C, Chance B, Iwane H (1992) A new method for the evaluation of muscle aerobic capacity in relation to physical activity measured by near infrared spectroscopy. Med Sport Sci 37: 421-429.
19. Bae SY, Hamaoka T, Katsumura T, Shiga T, Ohno H, et al. (2000) Comparison of muscle oxygen consumption measured by near infrared continuous wave spectroscopy during supramaximal and intermittent pedalling exercise. Int J Sports Med 21: 168-174.
20. Chance B (1992) Noninvasive approaches to oxygen delivery and cell bioenergetics in functioning muscle. Clin J Sport Med 2: 132-138.
21. Haga S, Bae SY, Hamaoka T, Katsumura T, Toshinai K, et al. (1998) Oxidative metabolism in skeletal muscle measured during supramaximal exercise in sprinter and active control groups by near infrared continuous wave spectroscopy. Adv Exerc Sports Physiol 4: 57-64.
22. Chance B, Dait MT, Zhang C, Hamaoka T, Hagerman F (1992) Recovery from exercise-induced desaturation in the quadriceps muscles of elite competitive rowers. Am J Physiol 262: C766-775.
23. Hamaoka T, Mizuno M, Katsumuea T, Osada T, Shimomitsu T, et al. (1998) Correlation between indicators determined by near infrared spectroscopy and muscle fiber types in humans. Jpn J Appl Physiol 28: 339-344.
24. Saltin B, Gollnick PD (1993) Skeletal muscle adaptability. In Handbook of Physiology, Skeletal muscle, Significance for metabolism and performance. Am Physiol Soc 555-631.
25. Brooke MH, Kaiser KK (1970) Three "myosin adenosine triphosphatase" systems: the nature of their pH lability and sulfhydryl dependence. J Histochem Cytochem 18: 670-672.
26. Schantz P (1983) Capillary supply in heavy-resistance trained non-postural human skeletal muscle. Acta Physiol Scand 117: 153-155.

27. Chance B, Leigh JS Jr, Kent J, McCully K, Nioka S, et al. (1986) Multiple controls of oxidative metabolism in living tissues as studied by phosphorus magnetic resonance. Proc Natl Acad Sci U S A 83: 9458-9462.

28. Mahler M (1985) First-order kinetics of muscle oxygen consumption, and an equivalent proportionality between QO2 and phosphorylcreatine level. Implications for the control of respiration. J Gen Physiol 86: 135-165.

29. Wada M, Katsuta S (1989) Muscle fiber performance. Jpn J Sports Sci 8: 62-68.

30. Sale DG (1987) Influence of exercise and training on motor unit activation. Exerc Sport Sci Rev 15: 95-151.

31. Andersen P, Henriksson J (1977) Capillary supply of the quadriceps femoris muscle of man: adaptive response to exercise. J Physiol 270: 677-690.

32. Allemeier CA, Fry AC, Johnson P, Hikida RS, Hagerman FC, et al. (1994) Effects of sprint cycle training on human skeletal muscle. J Appl Physiol (1985) 77: 2385-2390.

33. Glass DJ (2005) Skeletal muscle hypertrophy and atrophy signaling pathways. Int J Biochem Cell Biol 37: 1974-1984.

34. Häggmark T, Eriksson E, Jansson E (1986) Muscle fiber type changes in human skeletal muscle after injuries and immobilization. Orthopedics 9: 181-185.

35. Hudlicka O, Brown M, Egginton S (1992) Angiogenesis in skeletal and cardiac muscle. Physiol Rev 72: 369-417.

36. MacDougall JD (1994) Morphological changes in human skeletal muscle following strength training and immobilization. Champaign, IL, 269-288.

The Impact of Inhaled Salbutamol on Repeated Sprint Ability in Pre-Fatigued Soccer Players

Dickinson J[1], Hu J[2], Chester N[2], Loosemore M[3], and Whyte G[2]

[1]*Endurance Research Group, University of Kent, Chatham Maritime, UK*

[2]*Research Institute for Sport and Exercise Sciences, Liverpool John Moores University, Liverpool, UK*

[3]*The Institute of Sport, Exercise and Health, University College London, London, UK*

Abstract

Objectives: Investigate the ergogenic effect of inhaling up to 1600 µg of salbutamol on intermittent running performance in pre-fatigued soccer players.

Methods: In a single blind randomised repeated measures design seven male and six female soccer players volunteered to participant. All participants were regularly playing competitive soccer and had no history of asthma. Following familiarisation sessions participants visited the exercise physiology laboratory on three occasions to complete an intermittent running protocol followed by twelve 17.5 m sprints. Prior to each trial participants inhaled either: placebo, 800 µg inhaled salbutamol (SAL800) or 1600 µg inhaled salbutamol (SAL1600). Following completion of the sprints a sample from the first urine passed was analysed for salbutamol concentration. A repeated measures ANOVA was used to compare the mean sprint time, maximal sprint power, peak blood lactate post sprints and post sprint salbutamol urine concentration between conditions.

Results: Mean sprint time, maximum power, maximum velocity, peak HR and peak blood lactate during the 17.5 m sprints were not significantly different between treatments in soccer players. There was no significant difference between male and female players in urine drug concentration following SAL800 (mean + SD; 201.47 + 294.47 $ng.ml^{-1}$ vs. 180.2 + 102.15 $ng.ml^{-1}$) or SAL1600 (739.24 + 549.21 $ng.ml^{-1}$ vs. 879.58 + 633.14 $ng.ml^{-1}$). Three players urine drug concentrations were above the WADA decision limit set at 1200 $ng.ml^{-1}$.

Conclusions: Inhaling up to 1600 µg inhaled salbutamol did not significantly improve repeated sprint performance. However, inhalation of 1600 µg may result in a urine concentration above the current WADA upper limit and decision limit leading to a positive test. Athletes should ensure they use inhaled salbutamol at therapeutic doses to avoid the risk of breaching the WADA decision limit.

Keywords: Anti-doping; WADA code; Asthma; Treatment; Athlete care; Abuse; Adverse analytical finding

Introduction

Between 2002 and 2010, International Olympic Committee (IOC) established the requirement that athletes present evidence of current asthma or exercise induced bronchoconstriction (EIB) through the Therapeutic Use Exemption (TUE) process. The weight of evidence supports the improved health care of athletes following the introduction of the TUE [1,2]. In contrast, there is limited evidence to suggest inhaled doses of β_2-agonist have significant ergogenic effects according to a study by Pluim et al. The current List of banned substances and methods allows athletes to inhale up to 1600 µg salbutamol without the requirement of a TUE [3].

To date, there are no published studies examining the impact of inhaled short acting β_2-agonists on team game performance. Whilst athletes are usually prescribed 200 - 400 µg of inhaled salbutamol, our experience suggests that athletes are often instructed to take salbutamol on an 'as needed basis' that could be interpreted as an ability to inhale an unlimited amount of salbutamol to combat respiratory symptoms. Given the global importance of team games such as Soccer it is imperative that the performance impact of inhaled short acting β_2-agonists be examined to justify their position on the WADA list of prohibited substances.

The purpose of this study was to examine the ergogenic effect of inhaling 800 µg and 1600 µg of salbutamol versus placebo repeated sprint performance in pre-fatigued soccer players. Furthermore, to investigate the impact of prior exercise and gender on urine salbutamol concentrations following inhalation of the WADA recommended upper limit of 1600 µg of Salbutamol.

Materials and Method

Ethical approval for this study was provided by the Liverpool John Moores University Local Ethics Committee (ethics no: 09E18GW). Seven male (mean + SD; age 23.1 + 3.9 years; weight 72.9 + 4.3 kg; height 177.0 + 4.7 cm) and six female (21.3 + 1.4 years; weight 63.9 + 5.8 kg; height 162.3 + 4.7 cm) soccer players volunteered and provided written and verbal informed consent. All players played regular competitive 11 a-side soccer at least once a week and trained specifically for soccer at least twice a week. All participants were free from asthma and EIB. This was confirmed by the presentation of a negative Eucapnic Voluntary Hyperpnoea challenge [4]. On three separate occasions players were required to complete a 52 minute intermittent running

***Corresponding author:** Dr. John Dickinson, School of Sport and Exercise Sciences, University of Kent, Medway Building, Chatham Maritime, Kent, ME4 4AG, UK
E-mail: J.W.Dickinson@kent.ac.uk

protocol followed by twelve, 17.5 m sprints. Each trial was completed in a temperate environment (18°C and 40% relative humidity). Each trial was separated by 7 days. Fifteen minutes prior to the initiation of each intermittent run players inhaled one of the following treatments, via a pocket chamber, in a randomised single blind design:

Treatment 1: 16 inhalations of placebo (PLA)

Treatment 2: 8 inhalations of 100 µg salbutamol, 8 inhalation of placebo (SAL800)

Treatment 3: 16 inhalations of 100 µg salbutamol (SAL1600)

Maximal flow volume loops were recorded at baseline, 10 minutes post-treatment inhalation and 5 minutes post-simulated soccer match. A 90 ml urine sample was obtained between 30 and 180 minutes following the cessation of the twelve 17.5 m sprints.

The intermittent running protocol involved players completing 52 minutes of an adapted version of a validated soccer game performance treadmill test [5,6]. The test was conducted on a motorised treadmill (Pulsar, h/p/cosmos, Germany). The players were asked to complete five LOW and two HIGH intensity stages (Figure 1). The female low and high intensity stages were 10% slower than the male speeds. The stages were completed in the following order LOW, LOW, HIGH, LOW, LOW, HIGH, LOW. Between each stage there was a one minute stationary period (Figure 1).

Fifteen minutes following the soccer specific intermittent running protocol participants completed twelve 17.5 m sprints with a 10 s recovery between each sprint. This test is an adaption of the Repeated Anaerobic Sprint Test (RAST), which involves 6×35 m sprints [7]. The players completed the 17.5 m sprints on a non-motorised treadmill (Force Treadmill System, Woodway, SA). For each sprint the following variables were recorded: time, peak power and peak velocity. HR was monitored during the sprints and peak HR across all the twelve sprints was recorded. Consistent verbal encouragement was given to the players during each sprint. Players were encouraged to complete the sprints as fast as they could.

Three maximal flow-volume loops were measured at baseline, ten minutes after inhalation of PLA, SAL800 and SAL1600, and five minutes after the soccer specific intermittent running protocol. On each occasion maximal flow volumes were measured according to the European Respiratory Society (ERS) criteria [8].

Prior to the commencement of each trial players were asked to provide a urine sample in order to void them of urine, after which the placebo or salbutamol was administered as described above. Players were instructed to collect the first sample of urine passed following completion of the laboratory-based tests in line with in-competition anti-doping procedures as outlined in the World Anti-Doping Code International Standard for Testing [9]. Consumption of water during this period was encouraged ad libitum to ensure diuresis. From the sample provided by each subject a 20 ml aliquot of urine was stored at -80°C until analysis.

All urinalysis was performed at HFL Sport Science (Fordham, UK) an independent drug surveillance laboratory and former WADA-accredited laboratory. Sample preparation involved the addition of 200 ng of Salbutamol-D3 (NMI) as an internal standard to 1 ml of urine. Following the addition of 2 ml of 0.1M phosphate buffer pH 6.8 and 100 µl of *E. Coli* enzyme (β-glucuronidase) solution the mixture was incubated overnight at 37°C. Strata XC 60 mg solid phase extraction cartridges (Phenomenex, Macclesfield, UK) were conditioned with 3 ml of methanol followed by 3 ml of reagent grade water. Following centrifugation at 3500 rpm for 5 min the samples were applied to the cartridges. The cartridges were then washed with 3 ml of 0.1M acetate buffer pH 9.0 followed by 3 ml of reagent grade water, 3 ml of 0.1M HCl, 3 ml of methanol and 3 ml of diethyl ether. The cartridges were then dried for 5 min for vacuum and samples were eluted into glass vials with two, 1 ml of basic drug elution solvent (160 ml ethyl acetate, 34 ml propan-2-ol and 6 ml 34% ammonia solution). Samples were then evaporated to dryness at ambient temperature using a centrifugal vacuum concentrator (Genevac Ltd, Ipswich, UK) and reconstituted in 10 µl of isopropanol followed by 200 µl of basic reconstitution solution (495 ml of 0.1 acetic acid mixed with 5 ml Benzyldimethylphenyl Ammonium). Samples were centrifuged at 3000 rpm for 10 min prior to LCMS submission. Samples were injected onto a Thermo Scientific Accela HPLC system coupled to a Thermo Scientific LTQ Orbitrap Discovery Mass Spectrometer (Thermo Fisher Scientific, Waltham, USA). Chromatographic separation was performed on a Waters Atlantis T3 column (2.1×100 mm, particle size 3 µm; Waters Ltd, Elstree, UK) at 35°C. The mobile phase was a gradient system of 0.1% acetic acid aqueous solution containing uracil (300 ng.ml^{-1}) and 0.1% acetic acid in acetonitrile containing uracil (300 ng.ml^{-1}) set at a flow rate of 0.4 ml.min^{-1}.

The urine salbutamol concentrations reported correspond to the sum of the free and glucuronide conjugates. The samples were analysed over the calibration range of 10-2000 ng.ml^{-1}. Samples with salbutamol concentrations greater than the upper limit of quantification were diluted with blank human urine prior to analysis. The lower limit of

a) b)

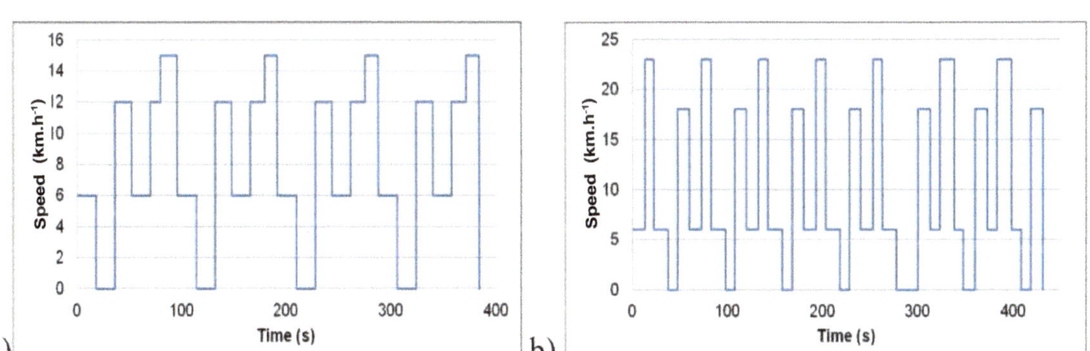

Figure 1: Low (a) and high (b) intensity phases of the male soccer specific treadmill run.

quantification was accepted as the lowest standard on the calibration curve (10 ng.ml^{-1}).

Male and female data were analysed together. Mean sprint time to complete the twelve, 17.5 m sprints under each of the treatments was analysed by a repeated measures ANOVA. Similar analyses were undertaken for peak power, peak velocity and peak HR. Repeated measures ANOVA were used to compare FEV1, FVC, PEF and FEF25-75. A p value of <0.05 was deemed significant for all analysis.

Results

All seven male and six female players completed the football specific run and twelve, 17.5 m sprints under each condition. No participant reported any adverse symptoms from inhaling either 800 or 1600 µg salbutamol.Under each of the three treatments no significant difference was observed in mean sprint time (PLA 4.74+0.65s; SAL800 4.65+0.55 s; SAL1600 4.74+0.53 s; p=0.35), peak power (PLA 1641.7+492.0 W; SAL800 1681.7+524.0 W; SAL1600 1738.8+499.9 W; p=0.40), peak velocity (PLA 4.99+0.66 m.s^{-1}; SAL800 5.00+0.70 m.s^{-1}; SAL1600 5.01+0.68 m.s^{-1}; p=0.51), peak HR (PLA 182.6+5.1 b.min^{-1}; SAL800 184.6+4.5 b.min^{-1}; SL1600 183.4+4.54 b.min^{-1}; p=0.22) or, peak lactate (PLA 11.55+2.16 mmol.l^{-1}; SAL800 12.45+2.59 mmol.l^{-1}; 13.52+2.3 mmol.l^{-1}; p=0.06).

Maximal lung function did not significantly alter between treatments at baseline, 10 minutes after inhalation of treatment or 5 minutes after the completion of the football specific run.

Following inhalation of 800 µg and 1600 µg of salbutamol and completion of a football-specific running protocol and twelve, 17.5 m sprints under temperate (20°C, 40% RH) ambient conditions the cohort reported mean (± SD) urine drug concentrations of 250.91 + 234.51 ng.ml^{-1} and 804.02 + 568.46 ng.ml^{-1}, respectively (see figure 2). Whilst mean (+ SD) urine drug concentrations following inhalation of 800 µg of salbutamol was 301.47 + 294.47 ng.ml^{-1} in males compared to 180.12 + 102.15 ng.ml^{-1} in females there was no significant difference according to sex (Figure 2). Likewise, there were no significant sex differences in urine drug concentrations following inhalation of 1600 µg of salbutamol in male 739.24 + 549.21 ng.ml^{-1} and female 879.58 + 633.14 ng.ml^{-1} players. Nevertheless there was a high degree of inter-individual differences in urine drug concentrations amongst male and female participants. Whilst mean urine drug concentrations did not breach the WADA urinary threshold for salbutamol two male and three female players recorded urine drug concentrations that exceeded the threshold (1000 ng.ml^{-1}), of which, three cases were above the WADA decision limit set at 1200 ng.ml^{-1}.

Discussion

The results from the current study suggest that inhaling up to 1600 µg of salbutamol does not result in an improvement in repeated sprint performance in pre-fatigued soccer players. Despite this, our results demonstrate that it is possible for athletes to present with a salbutamol urine concentration above 1000 ng.ml-1 following inhalation of up to 1600 µg of salbutamol.

Previous studies focused on inhaled salbutamol have generally employed non-specific performance trials such as running to exhaustion or physiological markers of performance [10]. Few of the previous studies have demonstrated any improvement following the inhalation of acute doses of up to 800 µg Salbutamol on running time to exhaustion, O2max, peak power, 20 km cycling time-trial and total work during a 30 s Wingate test [10]. Dickinson et al. [11] reported no improvement in 5 km running time trial performance following inhalation of 1600 µg salbutamol. Elers et al. [12] suggested inhaling an acute dose of up to 4000 µg salbutamol resulted in no improvement in cycling time to exhaustion or oxygen kinetics. Accordingly, from a performance perspective the current WADA guidelines permitting athletes to inhale up to 1600 µg in a single day appear appropriate as there is no resultant improvement in performance in non-asthmatic athletes. Furthermore, there also appears to be no improvement in strength, power or endurance when none asthmatic athletes inhale 1600 µg Salbutamol on a daily basis for 6 weeks [13]. However, in contrast to our findings a recent study has suggest there may be an improvement in swimming sprint performance and maximal contraction of the quadriceps femoris if inhaled salbutamol is taken in combination with inhaled long acting β2-agonists [14]. In addition, oral salbutamol taken acutely and over a two week period has been shown to improve peak power output on repeated cycling sprint performance [15]. However, Hostrup et al. [15] did report β2-adrenergic stimulation was blunted in the second and third sprints. In our study we used a soccer specific running protocol to induce fatigue in our participants prior to the 17.5 m sprints. It may be possible that the preceding soccer specific treadmill run impacted on the potential for inhaled salbutamol to improve individual sprint and repeated sprint performance. Future studies investigating repeated sprint performance may benefit from inhaling salbutamol directly before the sprinting protocol.

The current WADA regulations impose a urinary salbutamol threshold of 1000 ng.ml-1for salbutamol [3]. This regulation is to distinguish legitimate therapeutic use from misuse. Supporting such a threshold are maximal dosing recommendations of 1600 µg per day

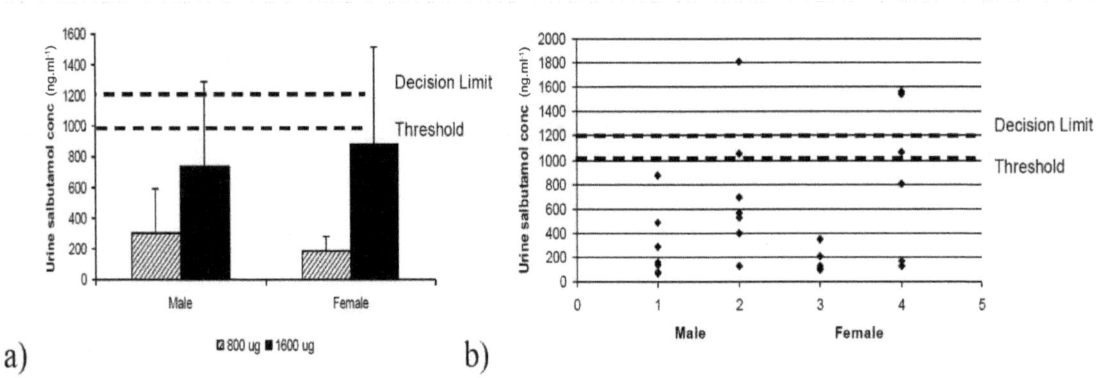

Figure 2: (a) Mean (+ SD) and (b) Individual urine SAL concentration (ng.ml^{-1}) post repeated 17.5 m sprints in temperate (20oC, 40% RH) environment following inhalation of 800 µg or 1600 µg SAL in male and female players.

[3]. However, whilst the recommended dosing regimen is between 100 and 400 µg up to four times daily, salbutamol is typically prescribed pro re nata ('when required'). Individuals encouraged to administer salbutamol pro re nata may inhale doses of salbutamol over and above such recommendations for therapeutic purposes, either intentionally or inadvertently. In such cases athletes are at risk of exceeding the WADA threshold and in doing so, facing possible anti-doping sanctions.

Previous research has attempted to examine the excretion of salbutamol administered by different routes including oral and inhaled [16,17] and across a range of acute doses from 200 µg and 800 µg [18] and repeated doses over several hours [19]. The current study is the first to examine the urinary excretion of an acute, high dose in comparison with an intermediate dose following intermittent running in soccer players. Whilst the findings did not suggest any differences according to gender there was a large variation between individuals at the various doses. This large inter-subject variation confirmed the likelihood that individuals inhaling acute, high doses of salbutamol may exceed the current WADA urinary threshold of 1000 $ng.ml^{-1}$. Indeed the current study also demonstrates that following such a dosing regimen may result in urine salbutamol levels in excess of 1200 $ng.ml^{-1}$. This concentration is significant since it represents a level referred to by WADA as the 'Decision Limit, above which a sample would be classified as an adverse analytical finding (AAF) [9] and warrant further investigation.

The maximal recommended dosing regimen for salbutamol clearly acts as an upper limit for those requiring immediate relief of asthma symptoms. Individuals who regularly use high doses of salbutamol or exceed these recommendations clearly demonstrate poor management of their condition. There lies the problem from an anti-doping regulatory perspective when the evidence to support ergogenic properties is not present and the likelihood of poor control of asthma and EIB are high. From a sports medicine perspective improved care may constitute better diagnosis, management and education amongst athletes. Regardless of whether salbutamol is on or off the WADA list of banned substances team medical officers must follow best practice in the diagnosis of respiratory conditions such as EIB prior to providing inhalers for therapeutic use [20].

Conclusion

Our findings suggest there is no ergogenic benefit, from inhaling up to 1600 µg of salbutamol, on intermittent running performance in soccer players. However, inhalation of 1600 µg may result in a urine concentration above the current WADA upper limit and decision limit leading to a positive test finding. Athletes should ensure they use inhaled salbutamol at therapeutic doses to avoid the risk of breaching the WADA decision limit.

Conflict of Interest

None to declare

Discloser of Funding

This projected was funded by the World Anti-Doping Agency (WADA).

Acknowledgments

The authors would like to thank the technical support of Rob Allan and Andrew Hulton during the data collection phase of this study.

References

1. Dickinson J, Whyte G, McConnell A, Harries M (2005) Impact of change in the IOC-MC asthma criteria: a British perspective. Thorax 60: 629-632.
2. Parsons J, Kaeding C, Phillips G, Jarjoura D, Wadley G, et al. (2007) Prevalence of exercise-induced bronchospasm in a cohort of varsity college athletes. Med Sci Sports Exerc 39: 1487-1492.
3. The World Anti-Doping Agency (2015) The 2015 Prohibited List International Standard.
4. Anderson S, Argyros G, Magnussen H, Holzer K (2001) Provocation by eucapnic voluntary hyperpnoea to identify exercise induced bronchoconstriction. Br J Sports Med 35: 344-347.
5. Drust B, Reilly T, Cable T (2000) Physiological responses to laboratory-based soccer-specific intermittent and continuous exercise. J Sports Sci 18: 885-892.
6. Drust B, Atkinson G, Reilly T (2007) Future perspectives in the evaluation of the physiological demands of soccer. Sports Med 37: 783-805.
7. Draper N, Whyte G (1997) Here's a new running based test of anaerobic performance for which you need only a stopwatch and a calculator. Peak Performance 97: 3-5.
8. Miller M, Hankinson J, Brusasco V, Burgos F, Casaburi R, et al. (2005) Standardisation of spirometry. Eur Respir J 26: 319-338.
9. The World Anti Doping Agency (2010) The International Standards for Laboratories Technical Document 2010: Decision limits for the confirmatory quantification of threshold substances.
10. Pluim B, de Hon O, Staal J, Limpens J, Kuipers H, et al. (2011) β_2-Agonists and physical performance: a systematic review and meta-analysis of randomized controlled trials. Sports Med. 41: 39-57.
11. Dickinson J, Hu J, Chester N, Loosemore M, Whyte G (2014) Acute impact of inhaled short acting b2-agonists on 5 km running performance. J Sports Sci Med 13: 271-279.
12. Elers J, Mørkeberg J, Jansen T, Belhage B, Backer (2012) High-dose inhaled salbutamol has no acute effects on aerobic capacity or oxygen uptake kinetics in healthy trained men. Scand J Med Sci Sports 22: 232-239.
13. Dickinson J, Molphy J, Chester N, Loosemore M, Whyte G (2014) The Ergogenic Effect of Long-Term Use of High Dose Salbutamol. Clin J Sport Med. 24:474-81.
14. Kalsen A, Hostrup M, Bangsbo J, Backer V (2014) Combined inhalation of beta2 -agonists improves swim ergometer sprint performance but not high-intensity swim performance. Scand J Med Sci Sports 24: 814-22.
15. Hostrup M, Kalsen A, Auchenberg M, Bangsbo J, Backer V (2014) Effects of acute and 2-week administration of oral salbutamol on exercise performance and muscle strength in athletes. Scand J Med Sci Sports.
16. Pichon A, Venisse N, Krupka E, Perault-Pochat M, Denjean A (2006) Urinary and blood concentrations of β2-agonists in trained subjects: comparison between routes of use. Int J Sports Med. 27: 187-192.
17. Elers J, Pedersen L, Henninge J, Hemmersbach P, Dalhoff K, et al. (2012) The pharmacokinetic profile of inhaled and oral salbutamol in elite athletes with asthma and nonasthmatic subjects. Clin J sports Med 22: 140-145.
18. Sporer B, Sheel W, McKenzie D (2008) Dose response of inhaled salbutamol on exercise performance and urine concentrations. Med Sci Sports Exerc 40: 149-157.
19. Elers J, Pedersen L, Henninge J, Hemmersbach , Dalhoff K, et al. (2011) Urine concentrations of repetitive doses of inhaled salbutamol. Int J Sports Med 32: 574-579.
20. Parsons J, Hallstrand T, Mastronarde J, Kaminsky D, Rundell K, et al. (2013) An official American Thoracic Society clinical practice guideline: exercise-induced bronchoconstriction. Am J Respir Crit Care Med 187: 1016-1027.

Characteristics of the Japanese National Team of the First Youth Olympic Games

Yoko Tanabe[1,2]*, Shin Asakawa[3], Yuko Arakida[4], Ichiro Kono[5] and Takao Akama[6]

[1]Nihon University, Tokyo, Japan
[2]Graduate School of Sport Sciences, Waseda University, Saitama, Japan
[3]Japan Anti-Doping Agency, Tokyo, Japan
[4]Japanese Olympic Committee Tokyo, Japan
[5]University of Tsukuba, Ibaraki, Japan
[6] Faculty of Sport Sciences, Waseda University, Saitama, Japan

Abstract

Objective: To investigate the change in young elite Japanese athlete's attitudes during the Youth Olympic Games (YOG) in 2010.

Design: Survey study.

Setting: 2010 YOG, Singapore.

Participants: Data were collected from individual surveys completed by 57 athletes selected for the Japanese national team.

Main outcome measures: Main outcome measures were change in athlete's awareness of the equal emphasis on sport, culture, and education and athlete understands of anti-doping education.

Results: A total of 57 athletes agreed to participate in this study, Twenty-five respondents indicated that their main route of entry into their competition sport was family members who played the sport. Thirty-one respondents indicated that fun upon winning the game was their primary motivation for continuing to participate in the sport and 42 respondents stated that a good result in the competition was the main types of satisfaction gained from participation.

Conclusions: The results revealed the influences for taking up sports among young elite athletes on the Japanese national team competing at the Singapore YOG in 2010. The findings indicated that athletes were originally influenced by their parents. Lastly, the attitude of the Japanese athletes was significantly broadened through participation in the YOG.

Keywords: Youth Olympic games; Elite athletes; Anti-doping education; Characteristics; Olympic education

Introduction

The inaugural Youth Olympic Games (YOG) were held in Singapore from August 14 to 26, 2010. The Games accommodated 3,600 athletes aged 14-18 years across 26 sports. The goal of the Olympic Movement is "to contribute to building a peaceful and better world by educating youth people through sport practiced in accordance with Olympism and its values" [1]. The YOG are a realization of that statement, and aims to bring talented young athletes together as part of its greater vision of inspiring young people around the world to participate in sport and to adopt and live within the Olympic values. It is a world-class multi-sport event that integrates various cultural activities through its Culture and Education Program (CEP) in addition to its athletic activities [2,3]. Professor Jigoro Kano, who developed judo from jujutsu, similarly expressed an opinion on the relationship between judo and education. He too, emphasized the importance of education through sports [4-6].

This study focuses on a number of aspects of the YOG and its impact on the members of the Japanese YOG national team. The following topics are covered in this research: the nature of athlete's entry into sport and age at which participation in their competition sport began; their motivation for continuing in the sport and the types of satisfaction gained from participation; the types of positive outcomes experienced from participation in the sport; the existence of role models and their influence; the nature of sacrifices made to compete at the junior elite level; the source, content, and perceived importance of the anti-doping education program; and their reasons for competing at the YOG. The importance of elements of the anti-doping education programs is ethical and health related knowledge and technical knowledge seen as the important impression on anti-doping education program to the elite athletes. Environment is apparent surrounding junior athletes have experienced a Japanese sports and education from the characteristics of the Japanese national team of the first Youth Olympic Games.

Methods

In the 1st YOG, 25 male and 46 female athletes participated as part of the Japanese national team; of them, 23 male and 34 female participants completed a questionnaire (Table 1).

Participants

The protocol was revised and approved by the Ethics Committee on Human Research of Waseda University. The participants included in the study consist of 23 boys (mean age 16.74 years, SD = 0.75) and 34 girls (mean age 16.26 years, SD = 1.11). These 57 young elite athletes were selected from the Japanese national team, which competed at the

***Corresponding author:** Yoko Tanabe, Associate Professor, Nihon University, 2-3-1, Misaki-cho, Chiyoda-ku, Tokyo, 101-8375, Japan
E-mail: yoko@law.nihon-u.ac.jp

	Male		Female		Total	
	n	%	n	%	n	%
Ahtletics	8	34.8	7	20.6	15	26.3
Aquatics	4	17.4	4	11.8	8	14.0
Archery	1	4.3	1	2.9	2	3.5
Badmington	1	4.3	2	5.9	3	5.3
Basketball	0	0.0	4	11.8	4	7.0
Cycling	2	8.7	1	2.2	3	4.3
Gymnastics	2	8.7	6	17.6	8	11.6
Judo	1	4.3	1	2.2	2	2.9
Rowing	0	0.0	1	2.2	1	1.8
Sailing	1	4.3	1	2.2	2	2.9
Table tennis	0	0.0	1	2.2	1	1.4
Tennis	1	4.3	2	4.3	3	4.3
Triathlon	1	4.3	1	2.2	2	2.9
Wrestling	1	4.3	1	2.2	2	2.9
Weightlifting	0	0.0	1	2.2	1	1.4
Total	23	100.0	34	100.0	57	100.0
Sports subjects are categorized based on the sport events featured in the Singapore 2010 Youth Olympic Games						

Table 1: Categorization of sports subjects.

Stage 1	Active Start	Chronological Age	0-6	0-6	- Focus on learning proper movement skills such as running, jumping , wheeling, twisting, kicking, throwing and catching
					- Active movement environment combined with well-structured gymnastics and swimming programs.
Stage 2	Fundamentals	Chronological Age	6-9	6-8	- ABC's of athleticism: agility, balance, coordination and speed
					- ABC's of Athletics: running, jumping, wheeling and throwing
Stage 3	Learning to Train	Chronological/ Developmental Age	9-12	8-11	- Introduction to mental preparation
					- Integrated mental, cognitive and emotional development
Stage 4	Training to Train	Chronological/ Developmental Age	12-16	11-15	- Major fitness development stage: aerobic and strength
					- The onset of Peak Height Velocity (PHV) and PHV are the reference points
					- Peak Strength Velocity (PSV) comes a year or so after PHV (at the age of 13)
					- Develop mental preparation
Stage 5	Training to Compete	Chronological/ Developmental Age	16-23+/-	15-21+/-	- Advanced mental preparation
					- Sport, event, position-specific physical conditioning
					- Sport, event, position-specific tactical preparation
Stage 6	Training to Win	Chronological Age	19+/-	18+/-	- Maintenance or improvement of physical capacities
					- Further development of technical, tactical and playing skills
Stage 7	Active for Life	Enter at any age			- Move from highly competitive sport to lifelong competitive sport through age group competition.
					- Minimum of 60 minutes moderate daily activity or 30 minutes of intense activity for adults.
Long-Term Athlete Development, Canadian Sport for Life center, Resource Paper v2					

Table 2: The seven stages of long-term athlete development.

2010 YOG in Singapore. The surveys were carried out before and after the games, following receipt of an agreement of informed consent from the candidates.

Because the members of the women's volleyball team were not junior national level, they are not included in this study.

Quantitative method

The questionnaire was composed of 12 pre-competition items (12 multiple-choice items, 1 free-response question) and 1 post-competition items (all multiple-choice items). The questionnaire's items addressed motivation and sports, anti-doping, and the significance to participants of participating in the YOG.

Statistical analysis

Boys' and girls' responses were compared using the chi-square test, calculated using IBM SPSS Statistics version 17.0 for Windows. Statistical significance was set at $P<0.05$.

Age categories

The age category at which participation in athlete's competition sports began is discussed on the basis of long-term athlete development (LTAD) which is "based on the physical, mental, emotional, and cognitive development of children and adolescents" (The Canada Sport Centres, 2010: 7). The LTAD focuses on "the general framework of athlete development with special reference to growth, maturation and development, trainability, and sport system alignment and integration". Following a Canadian model of LTAD, which is divided into seven stages in terms of age and gender, the main points of seven stages are described. In terms of the age at which participation in their competition sports began, we can divide three groups: those who began their athlete's lives aged under 6, between the age of 6 and 10, and aged over 10 (Table 2.) [7].

Anti-doping items

The open-ended responses to the themes which were perceived

	Male	Female	Total
	n	n	n
A) Your family was playing the sport	9	16	25
B) Recommended by your family	6	5	11
C) Recommended by your friends	2	6	8
D) Start at school or sports club	3	3	6
E) There were facilities or sports clubs near by	5	8	13
F) Inspired by watching a game	4	5	9
G) Others	0	5	5
Pre Questionnaire 1.-1) What made you start your sports? (Multiple choices allowed)			
The mean difference between boy's and girl's responses was not significant			

Table 3: The nature of the route into sport.

Categorization of sports	Under 6	Form 7-8y	Form 9-10y	Form 11-12y	Form 13-15y	Form 16-18y	Others	Total
Athletics (M)	1	1	2	1	3			8
Athletics (F)	2	1	1		3			7
Aquatics (M)	3	1						4
Aquatics (F)	3	1						4
Archery (M)					1			1
Archery (F)			1					1
Badminton (M)		1						1
Badminton (F)		1	1					2
Basketball (F)		1	2	1				4
Cycling (M)	2							2
Cycling (F)			1					1
Gymnastics (M)	2							2
Gymnastics (F)	4	2						6
Judo (M)	1							1
Judo (F)	1							1
Rowing (F)						1		1
Sailing (M)				1				1
Sailing (F)					1			1
Table tennis (F)		1						1
Tennis (M)		1						1
Tennis (F)	2							2
Triathlon (M)								1
Triathlon (F)			1					1
Wrestling (M)			1					1
Wrestling (F)		1						1
Weightlifting (F)		1						1
	21	16	16	5	10	1		57

Table 4: The age at which participation in their competition sport.

as being important in the anti-doping education session received were analyzed and deemed to fall into one of the following four major categories: ethical and health-related knowledge (side effects, moral principles, reasons to not dope); technical knowledge (how testing is done, how to avoid violation, prohibited substances, attention to contents); implications of failure to comply (sanctions, reasons athletes dope); and the impact of doping on performance.

Results

Nature of athlete's entry into sport

Regarding the nature of the route by which athletes became involved in their sport, 25 respondents indicated that members of their family played the sport and 11 indicated that the sport was recommended to them by their family. In total, 36 of the 57 athletes shared this viewpoint that family was the most influential factor for them in becoming athletes. In the multiple-choice section, 8 athletes indicated that the sport was recommended by their friends and 6 indicated that they started at school or a sports club. Furthermore, 13 athletes said that there were facilities or sports clubs nearby and 9 answered that they were inspired by watching the sport (Table 3).

Age at which athletes began participating in their competition sport

The earliest group of athletes began practicing their sport at below age 6. These athletes were involved in aquatics, cycling, gymnastics, judo, and tennis. The gender and sports of the respondents were as follows: both boys and girls in aquatics; boys in cycling; boys and girls in gymnastics; boys and girls in judo; and girls in tennis. Athletes who began practicing their sport between age 6 and 10 were involved in athletics, archery, badminton, basketball, cycling, table tennis, tennis, triathlon, wrestling, and weightlifting. More specifically, the respondents' gender and sports were as follows: girls in athletics; girls in archery; boys and girls in badminton; girls in basketball; girls in cycling; girls in table tennis; boys in tennis; boys and girls in triathlon; boys and girls in wrestling; and girls in weightlifting. Sports began at over age 10 were athletics, archery, basketball, rowing, and sailing. More specifically, the respondents' gender and sports were as follows: boys

	1st		2nd		Total	
	Male	Female	Male	Female	Male	Female
A) It is fun to win the game	7	15	6	3	13	18
B) Aiming for the best	4	6	1	8	5	14
C) Want to participate in the world championships and the Olympic Games.	9	5	7	9	16	14
D) To get on a scholarship	1	0	0	1	1	1
E) Make friends or to meet variety of people	1	2	6	9	7	11
F) To make people who support me happy	1	4	3	2	4	6
G) Been told by my family/coach to continue	0	0	0	0	0	0
H) Others	0	1	0	1	0	2
Total	23	33	23	33	46	66
Pre Questionnaire 1.-3) Why do you continue playing your sport?						
The mean difference between boy's and girl's responses was not significant						

Table 5: Their motivation for continuing to participate in the sport.

	1st		2nd		Total	
	Male	Female	Male	Female	Male	Female
A) Good result at the game	17	21	2	2	19	23
B) No matter what results are, you performed to your best	2	8	2	5	4	13
C) You performed to the level where your coach expected you to do	0	0	6	3	6	3
D) To beat your rival	2	1	5	2	7	3*
E) To make people around me happy	1	3	5	11	6	14
F) Been able to make friends through competitions	1	0	0	10	1	10*
G) Others	0	0	0	0	0	0
Total	23	33	20	33	43	66
Pre Questionnaire 1.-4) What makes you feel good about yourself as being an athletes?						
n=66 *p<0.05						

Table 6: The types of satisfaction gained from participation.

	1st		2nd		Total
	Male	Female	Male	Female	n
A) Become mentally stronger	11	26	6	2	45
B) Make friends and travel together	6	3	6	21	36
C) Become more polite	6	3	7	8	24
D) More communication with your family	0	0	0	1	1
E) Receive praise from people around you	0	0	1	0	1
F) Become fitter	0	0	2	0	2
G) Others	0	1	0	0	1
Total	23	33	22	32	110
Pre Questionnaire 1.-5) What are the posotive things about playing your sports?					
The mean difference between boy's and girl's responses was not significant					

Table 7: The type of positive outcome experienced from participation in the sport.

and girls in athletics; boys in archery; girls in basketball; girls in rowing; and boys and girls in sailing (Table 4).

Athlete's motivation for continuing in their sport

Regarding their motivation for continuing to participate in the sport, 31 respondents indicated that they participating because they enjoyed competing and winning, 19 that they were aiming to be the best they could, 30 that they wanted to participate in world championships and the Olympic Games, 2 that they wanted to receive a scholarship, 18 that they thought they could make friends and meet a variety of people through sports, and 10 that they wanted to make the people who support them happy (Table 5).

Types of satisfaction gained from participation

The mean difference between boys' and girls' responses was statistically significant at the 0.05 level.

The answer "a good result at the competition" was indicated by 42 respondents, representing a majority of the total. The second-largest number, 20 respondents, chose 'to make people around me happy'. The remaining answers were indicated by a similar number of athletes: 17 respondents indicated "doing one's best, no matter the outcome"; 9 indicated "performing in line with the coach's expectations"; 10 respondents indicated "beating a rival'; and 11 respondents indicated "being able to make friends through competition" (Table 6).

Types of positive outcomes experienced from participation in the sport

The majority of athletes chose "becoming mentally stronger" (45 respondents), "becoming more polite" (24 respondents), and "making friends and traveling together" (36 respondents). Only 2 athletes responded "becoming physically fitter", and only 1 respondent each answered "improving communication with family" and "receiving praise from surrounding people" (Table 7).

Existence of role models

52 of the 56 athletes (92.9%) who participated in the YOG

	Male	Female	Total	%
Yes	22	30	52	92.9
No	1	3	4	71.0
Total	23	33	56	100.0
Pre Questionnaire 2.-2) Do you have a role model athlete?				
The mean difference between boy's and girl's responses was not significant				

Table 8: The existence of role models.

	Male	Female	Total	%
A) Family	4	5	9	15.8
B) Coach	6	9	15	26.3
C) Doctor or trainer	0	1	1	1.8
D) Friends	0	5	5	8.8.
E) Your rival	4	6	10	17.5
F) Role model athlete	8	6	14	24.6
G) Animation or character of TV	0	0	0	0.0
H) Others	1	2	3	5.3
Total	23	34	57	100.0
Pre Questionnaire 2.-1) Who influences you the most when you are playing your sport? (only one)				
The mean difference between boy's and girl's responses was not significant				

Table 9: Their influence when they are playing their sport.

	Male	Female	Total	%
Yes	21	30	51	89.5
No	2	3	5	8.8
N/A	0	1	1	1.8
Total	23	34	57	100.0
Pre Questionnaire 2.-3) Do you have anyting to cut down in your life to become an athlete?				
The mean difference between boy's and girl's responses was not significant				

Table 10: The nature of sacrifices made to be able to compete at the junior elite level.

	1st		2nd		Total	
	Male	Female	Male	Female	Male	Female
A) Meal (Because you have to lose weight for a competition)	3	10	3	0	6	10
B) Play with your friend	13	10	3	10	16	20
C) Fashion or Hairstyle	0	3	6	3	6	6
D) Study hours	1	1	0	1	1	2
E) Spend time with your family	2	4	1	5	3	9
F) Attendance at your school	0	1	3	1	3	2
G) Others	2	0	1	3	3	3
Total	21	29	17	23	38	52
Pre Questionnaire 2.-3-1) Which you have cut down to become an athlete?						
The mean difference between boy's and girl's responses was not significant						

Table 11: The nature of sacrifices made to be able to compete at the junior elite level.

responded that they had an athlete role model and 4 responded that they did not (Table 8).

Influence when playing their sport

Nine athletes (15.8%) answered that family influenced them the most while they were playing their sport, while 5 (8.8%) answered that friends influenced them the most. However, 15 (26.3%) responded that their coaches were the most influencing factor and 1 athlete indicated their doctor or trainer. Other responses were "a rival" (10 athletes, 17.5%), "athlete role models" (14 athletes, 24.6%); and "a television character", (3 athletes, 5.3%) (Table 9).

Nature of sacrifices made to be able to compete at the junior elite level

Table 10 shows that 51 respondents (89.5%) felt they had made sacrifices to compete at the junior elite level and 5 respondents (8.8%) did not. "Playing with friends" was the answer given by the majority (36) of respondents. "Meals (due to the need to lose weight for competition)" was given by 16 respondents, "time with family" was each given by 12 respondents. Furthermore, 12 respondents cited "fashion or hairstyle"; 3 respondents, "study hours" and 5 respondents, "school attendance" (Table 11).

Source, content, and perceived importance of elements of the anti-doping education program

21 respondents stressed ethical and health-related knowledge, 12 stressed technical knowledge, 6 stressed the implications of failure to comply, and no respondents stressed the impact of doping on performance, as shown in (Table 12).

Athlete's main reason for competing in the YOG

Before participating in the YOG, 40 respondents answered that their main purpose was to win the games; 21 respondents, to compete fairly; 36 respondents, as a step toward the Olympic Games; 30 respondents, to meet athletes from all over the world; 22 respondents, to participate in sport and cultural activities simultaneously; and 23 respondents, to enjoy participating in the competition.

After participating in the YOG, 15 respondents answered that their main purpose was to win the competition, 20 respondents, to compete fairly; 42 respondents, as a step toward the Olympic Games; 30 respondents, to meet athletes from all over the world; 31 respondents, to participate in sport and cultural activities simultaneously; 31 respondents, to enjoy participating in the games; and 8 respondents, "other" (Table 13).

	Male	Female	Total
	n	n	n
Impact of doping on performance	0	0	0
Implications of failure comply	2	4	6
Technical knowledge	5	7	12
Ethical and health related knowledge	9	12	21
Total	16	23	39
Pre Questionnair 3.1)-1 What element of the anti-doping session/ lectures left the most important impression?			
The mean difference between boy's and girl's responses was not significant			

Table 12: Source, content, and perceived importance of elements of the anti-doping education program.

	Pre	Post
A) To win the game	40	15
B) To compete fairly	21	20
C) Step towords the the Olympic Games	36	42
D) To meet many athletes from all over the world	30	30
E) To be able to participate in your sport and meny cultural activities at the same time	22	31
F) To enjoy yourself by participating the games	23	31
G) Others	0	8
Post Questionnaire 1. What is your main reason to compete at YOG ? (Multiple choices allowed)		
The mean difference between Pre and Post responses was not significant		

Table 13: What is your main reason to compete at YOG.

Discussion

The surveys were conducted before and after the YOG and a total of 57 young athletes belonging to the national team, in 15 different categories of sports, participated, 23 of whom were male athletes and 34 of whom were female athletes. The questionnaires consisted of 12 questions and were divided into 7 categories as follows.

Nature of athlete's entry into sport and the age at which participation in their competition sport began

Question Pre1-1 "What made you start your sport?" and Question Pre1-2, "When did you start your sport?" will discuss nature of the athlete's entry into sport and the age at which participation in their competition sport began, respectively. Although this implies that athlete's friends and school have some influence, access to facilities is one of the most influential factors for athletes to begin practicing their sport. Therefore, family support and recommendation as well as access to facilities are seen as the most powerful component of athlete's entry into sport [8,9].

The age at which participation in athlete's competition sports began is discussed based on the categories used by the LTAD of Canadian Sport for Life. The earliest age group, those who started their sport at under age 6 years, was reported by 22 athletes. These sports probably require that athletes have agility, balance, coordination, and speed, which are fundamental abilities as defined by the ABCs of Athletics. This categorization also contains running, jumping, wheeled movement (for para sports), and throwing [7].

The second group comprises athletes who began their sports between ages 6 and 10. Most athletes in this group joined team sports, which use equipment. The fact that most athletes who joined team sports that use of equipment usually begin their sports at this age may imply that, this age range between 6 and 10 years is the earliest athletes are normally able to acquire the skills and strategy for understanding how to play such team sports.

The last group comprises athletes who began their sports at over age 10. The athletes practicing these sports probably were expected to possess prerequisite knowledge, such as on water safety, and high skills for utilizing more complicated equipment before they could begin the sport.

Nature of athlete's entry into sport and the age at which participation in their competition sport began is greatly affected by their family and close person and environment around the athletes.

Athlete's motivation for continuing in their sport and the types of satisfaction gained from participation

The second category deals with two factors, the motivation for continuing a sport and the types of satisfaction gained from participation. Question Pre1-3, which asked "Why do you continue playing your sport?" examined motivation for continuing to participate and Question Pre1-4, "What makes you feel good about yourself as an athlete?" examined the relationship with the types of satisfaction gained from participation.

Both questions that the results of athlete's performance can be an important element to make athletes feel good about themselves. Also I think the relationship between the target and the games has a significant impact of Athlete's motivation for continuing in their sport and the types of satisfaction gained from participation.

Types of positive outcomes experienced from participation in the sport

Through Question Pre1-5, which asked "What are the positive aspects of playing your sport?" the young athletes showed their internal development, such as improvement in their personality or attitude toward their competitors, through participation in the event. Athletes tend seeking spiritual growth from participation in the sport.

The existence of role models and their influence

The presence of role models plays an important role for young athletes in establishing themselves and they are strongly influenced by their coaches in terms of playing their sport [10]. The influences has a great impact on children's choices of heroes and role models [11]. This tells us that having a role model strongly motivates and influences young athletes, such as those in this survey. I considered players strong influenced by their coaches and the role model athletes.

Nature of sacrifices made to be able to compete at the junior elite level

In this category, the athletes were asked "Is there anything you had to cut down in your life to become an athlete?" Fifty-one respondents (89.5%) answered "yes", the majority (36) of whom specified that they had to cut down on playing with friends. Athletes in the present study were aged 14-18 years, and youths of this age generally want to play with their friends. Many athletes have cut down to ensure the practice time.

Source, content and perceived importance of the anti-doping education program

Supplements were used for health and well-being by 62.7% of the respondents of the Japanese national YOG team [12]. The use of supplements among athletes is widespread [13,14]. The Japanese national high school curriculum for 2013 includes anti-doping education. Students learn the values of athletics and the basic principles of anti-doping. The curriculum increase the appreciation of athletic values in Japanese society and promote ant-doping activities [15]. The YOG are an opportunity for young athletes to understand for themselves, to discover the social significance of sport, and to learn about fair play through anti-doping education. Of the 39 respondents, 21 stressed ethical and health-related knowledge and 12 identified technical knowledge of anti-doping, for example how testing is done, as being the most significant elements of the anti-doping session. Only 6 respondents stated negative elements as having been emphasized, namely the implications of failure to comply. No respondents responded that the impact of doping on performance had been emphasized. Japan Anti-doping Agency (JADA) opened sports pharmacist system in 2010. Pharmacists are experts in prohibited substance and advice athletes, and to join in the cause against doping [16].

Reasons for competing

This study aimed to identify any change of young athlete's attitude on sport pre- and post-YOG, and there were some changes in young athlete's attitude. Before participating in the YOG, athlete's major aim was to win competitions, while after participating, their aim changed specifically to taking a step closer to the Olympic Games.

Conclusion

This research was aimed at identifying the impact of the YOG on the members of the Japanese national team and contains data from 57 Japanese athletes who participated in the YOG. Concerning the nature of the route into sport and the age at which participation in their competition sport began, friends and school can be influential to the athletes but accessibility to facilities remains a crucial factor. Three groups of respondents implied that the starting age of athletes can be based on the characteristics of the sports being practiced.

The results revealed what athletes experience or learn through sports competitions, the importance of role models to them, and the impact of the role model as a target of the athlete's dream. Even though athletes made sacrifices for the sake of their sports, they perceived themselves as becoming mentally stronger and having more respect for others as a result of taking part in the sports competitions.

Before the YOG, respondents suggested that winning was the most important factor, but their commitments after participating in the YOG was primarily to go forward toward participating in the Olympic Games. This suggests that the attitude of the Japanese athletes was significantly influenced by participation in the YOG, with a greater commitment to future participation in sports at the Olympic level.

Implications for future research

This study suggests that in the future, more systematic and comprehensive investigations on youth athlete education programs, going beyond just the Japanese team, will be needed. This will allow comparison of those athletes participating in different sports, of those who won medals and those who did not, age cohorts, gender and country/continent of origin. It may also allow education of the application of anti-doping regimes to be undertaken across a broader spectrum in different national contexts.

References

1. International Olympic Committee (2011) Olympic Charter in International Olympic Committee.
2. I.O.C.Y.O.G. International Olympic Committee (2010) Youth Olympic Games.
3. International Olympic Committee (2013) Official website of the Olympic Movement.
4. Micheal Jeremy Callan (2008) Elite sport and education support systems: a case study of the team bath judo programme at the university of bath. University of Bath School for Health.
5. Kodokan (2009) Jigoro Kano and the kodokan Editorial Committee. 164-169.
6. Kodokan (1994) Kodokan Judo Jigoro Kano. 20-25.
7. Lund M (2010) Canadian Sport for Life (CS4L), FUNdamental Movement Skills and Paddle Alberta: First Steps.
8. Kirby J (2009) The Importance of Role Models in Making Adolescent Girls More Active. Heriot Watt University.
9. Payne W, Reynolds M, Brown S, Fleming A (2003) Sports role models and their impact on participation in physical activity: a literature review. School of Human Movement and Sport Sciences, University of Ballarat.
10. International Olympic Committee (2012) 8th world conference on sport, education and culture, the amsterdam declaration.
11. Anderson KJ, Cavallaro D (2002) Parents or Pop Culture? Children's Heroes and Role Models. Childhood Education 78,3: 161.
12. Sato A, Kamei A, Kamihigashi E, Dohi MM, Komatsu Y, et al. (2012) Use of Supplements by Young Elite Japanese Athletes Participating in the 2010 Youth Olympic. Games in Singapore. Clin J Sport Med 22: 418-423.
13. Bloodworth A, McNamee M (2010) Clean Olympians? Doping and anti-doping: the views of talented young British athletes. Int J Drug Policy 21: 276-282.
14. Jongkyu Kim, Eung-Joon Kim, Sun-kyung Ki, Jaeryang Yoon, Mi-sook Lee (2011) Anti-doping education and dietary supplementation practice in Korean elite university athletes. Nutrition Research and Practice (Nutr Res Pract) 5: 349-356.
15. Akama T, Abe A (2013) Development and activities of the fight against doping. J Phys Fitness Sports Med 2: 267-274.
16. Ambrose (2011) Educational Opportunities and Anti-Doping Roles and Responsibilities for Pharmacists. Yakugaku Zasshi 131: 1755-1756.

25

Effects of the Menstrual Cycle and Acute Aerobic Exercise on Cytokine Levels

Harumi Hayashida[1,2], Mayura Shimura[3], Kaoru Sugama[2,4], Kazue Kanda[2] and Katsuhiko Suzuki[5*]

[1]*Faculty of Health Promotional Sciences, Tokoha University, Japan*
[2]*Institute for Nanoscience & Nanotechnology, Waseda University, Japan*
[3]*Faculty of Health Sciences, Health Science University, Japan*
[4]*Division of Cell Regeneration and Transplantation, Department of Functional Morphology, Nihon University School of Medicine, Japan*
[5]*Faculty of Sport Sciences, Waseda University, Japan*

Abstract

Objective: The purposes of this study were: 1) to investigate the effects of menstrual cycle on the basal levels of salivary cytokines (interleukin (IL)-6 and IL-8) in young healthy women; 2) to examine the influences of prolonged aerobic exercise at ventilatory threshold (VT) on salivary and circulating IL-6 and IL-8 concentrations during menstrual phase.

Methods: Eight healthy women participated in three visits (saliva sampling during menstrual, follicular and luteal phases) and two trials (exercise and resting trials during a separate menstrual phase). The exercise trial involved a 60- min cycling at VT and the resting trial involved resting for 90 min. Saliva and blood samples were taken at before, immediately after and 30 min post-exercise and equivalent times during the resting trial.

Results: Salivary IL-6 level was higher during the follicular phase than the luteal phase at rest. Salivary IL-8 immediately post-exercise was higher than pre-exercise, and circulating IL-6 was significantly increased from pre-exercise to immediately post-exercise and 30 min post exercise.

Conclusion: The results showed that salivary cytokines are influenced by menstrual cycle and prolonged exercise during menstrual phase. However the levels of IL-6 and IL-8 in saliva do not closely reflect those in plasma, and therefore might reflect a local level of inflammation.

Keywords: Menstrual cycle; Inflammation; Ventilatory threshold; Endurance exercise; Interleukin-6; Interleukin-8

Introduction

It has been shown that physical and psychological stresses are associated with the phases of the menstrual cycle [1,2]. Only few studies have examined the relationship between stress level and inflammation status during different phases of menstrual cycle using biological stress markers and cytokines such as cortisol and interleukin (IL)-6, respectively [1-3]. Cortisol is a well-known biological stress marker whereas IL-6 is a multifunctional cytokine that is secreted by endometrial cells, immune cells and muscle cells [4,5] and is a major factor in the regulation of the inflammatory process, immune response, metabolism and the acute phase response [5,6]. In the previous studies, healthy women with a normal menstrual cycle demonstrated higher serum cortisol levels during luteal phase compared with the follicular phase [1] yet plasma IL-6 levels were higher during the follicular phase compared with the luteal phase [2].

On the other hand, other studies report similar serum IL-6 levels between follicular and luteal phases [3]. To date, no studies have examined markers of inflammation specifically during the menstrual phase of the cycle. This is because the menstrual phase has been considered as a part of the follicular phase [2,3]. Female sex hormones, especially progesterone, influence immune responses by decreasing basal IL-6 levels [2]. Moreover, menstruation, initiated by progesterone withdrawal, is highly inflammatory in nature and involves feedback loops that enhance inflammatory pathways [7]. Therefore, it is important to specifically focus on menstrual phase as a distinct phase.

Recently, saliva sampling has received attention as an alternative to blood sampling to measure stress markers [8-11]. Saliva collection has the advantage over blood sampling in that it is a non-invasive method of sample collection which does not require any specialized training. However, the influence of menstrual cycle on stress markers using saliva has received comparatively little attention. In healthy women with a normal menstrual cycle, saliva samples were taken every evening to compare cortisol levels among menstrual, follicular, ovulatory, luteal and premenstrual phases and the analysis revealed that salivary cortisol level did not differ across the phases [12]. In another study, female participants provided a saliva sample directly after awakening and 30, 45 and 60 min thereafter to measure cortisol levels during the menstrual phase, follicular phase, ovulation and luteal phase. The results showed that there was a significant interaction between time and menstrual cycle and the net increase in cortisol level was larger during the ovulation than during the menstrual, follicular and luteal phases [13,14]. It is well known that saliva cortisol exhibits diurnal variations with concentrations highest in the morning and this may account for the disparities in the apparent influence of menstrual phase on cortisol levels between these studies.

Several studies have examined salivary IL-6 and/or IL-8 concentrations in relation to systemic or local disease conditions including oral cancers [15,16] and Sjögren's syndrome [15], an autoimmune disease that affects mucosal exocrine functions. Other studies have assessed the relationships between salivary IL-6 levels and

***Corresponding author:** Katsuhiko Suzuki, Professor, Faculty of Sport Sciences, Waseda University, #2-579-15 Mikajima, Tokorozawa, Saitama 359-1192, Japan
E-mail: katsu.suzu@waseda.jp

psychosocial factors in middle aged people [17] and in post-menopausal women [18]. Therefore, there is a lack of information regarding salivary IL-6 and IL-8 concentrations on resting healthy women during different phases of menstrual cycle. In addition, previous studies reported that salivary and circulating IL-6 levels do not relate to each other at rest [15,17,18] and at post-exercise [10]. Such findings need to be confirmed in healthy women at different timings of menstrual cycle to demonstrate whether salivary sampling can be employed as an alternative to blood sampling for an examination of inflammation status.

Moderate intensity aerobic exercise is important for maintaining or promoting physical fitness. However, exercise has been shown to induce an inflammatory response and estrogen is associated with an attenuation of the response [19]. Moreover, the secretion of estrogen changes during the menstrual cycle yet reported circulating inflammatory responses to exercise during the different phases of the menstrual cycle are equivocal [20], which may reflect differences in participant fitness, oral contraceptive use and differing exercise protocols used. Considering women's health and safety and the effectiveness of exercise, it is important to assess the influence of exercise or changes in the stress and inflammatory markers during the menstrual cycle [21]. Only one study has examined an influence of prolonged moderate intensity exercise on salivary IL-6 and reported that salivary IL-6 level was higher at 30 min post treadmill running (1 h at 65% VO_2peak) compared to the baseline level during follicular and luteal phases in females [22]. However, the magnitude of increases did not differ between the follicular and the luteal phases. Hence, an influence of exercise on inflammation status during menstrual phase is still unclear.

Therefore, the aims of this study were: 1) to investigate the effects of menstrual cycle on the basal levels of salivary cytokines (IL-6 and IL-8) in young healthy women; 2) to examine the influences of prolonged aerobic exercise at ventilatory threshold (VT) on salivary and circulating IL-6 and IL-8 levels during menstrual phase. It was hypothesised that: 1) basal salivary cytokine levels would be affected by menstrual cycle; and 2) salivary cytokine levels would be affected by acute aerobic exercise at VT.

Materials and Methods

Subjects

Eight healthy young women enrolled in this study (age: 20.5 ± 0.8 years (means ± standard deviation (SD), body mass: 48.3 ± 5.9 kg, height: 155.4 ± 4.9 cm, BMI: 20.0 ± 2.2 kg/m^2, estimated body fat: 23.7 ± 4.0 % and VO_2peak: 1790 ± 281 ml/min). None of them were taking any medications including oral contraceptives or dietary supplements. Their menstrual cycle was regular and there were no menstrual cycle-related disorders (e.g., premenstrual syndrome, dysmenorrhea) for at least one year. All subjects were recreationally active and exercised for less than 1 h/week at moderate intensity (e.g., jogging, recreational volleyball and basketball). Written informed consent was obtained from all participants and they were free to withdraw from the study at any time. The experimental procedure was approved by the Research Ethics Committee at Waseda University.

Experimental design

The subjects attended the laboratory on seven separate occasions for two preliminary trials, three short visits and two main trials. Two preliminary trials were arranged for orientation, to familiarize the subjects with the experimental procedures and to determine their VT, height, body mass, and estimated body fat (OMRON BODY FAT MONITOR HBF-903, Omron Healthcare, Kyoto, Japan). The visits took place during the menstrual phase (day 1-4 from the start of menstrual flow), follicular phase (day 7-11 after the start of menstrual flow) and mid-luteal phase (5-9 days before estimated date of the next menstrual phase) and main trials were conducted during menstrual phase. The subjects refrained from performing any strenuous physical activity and drinking alcohol for at least 24 h prior to the testing trials, and consumed a small meal at 12:00 pm before the trials. To control for diurnal variations in the hormones, all trials were performed at the same time of day from 2:00 to 3:00 pm.

Determination of VT

In a preliminary session, peak oxygen uptake (VO_2peak) was estimated using a continuous incremental exercise test performed on an electromagnetically braked cycle ergometer (AEROBIKE 75XL, Combi, Shinagawa, Tokyo, Japan). Oxygen consumption, ventilation and heart rate were measured during an incremental cycle ergometry test (2 Watts increase every 10 seconds, starting at 20 Watts) with a bicycle ergometer. Ventilation was measured and gas analysis was performed during the test on a breath-by-breath basis (AEROMONITOR AE-300S, Minato, Yodogawa, Osaka, Japan). VT was determined by the modified V-slope method, which is from a plot of VCO_2 as a function of VO_2 [23].

Visits and main trials

For the three visits, the subjects reported to the laboratory in a rested state during the menstrual phase, follicular phase and mid-luteal phase to provide saliva and blood samples. For the main trials, subjects reported to the laboratory at 2:00 pm for the exercise and control trials in a separate menstrual phase. In the exercise trial, subjects cycled for 60 min at the predetermined VT from 2:30 pm and they seated quietly for 30 min after the cycling. Saliva and blood samples were taken at pre-, immediately post- and 30 min post-exercise. Subjects drank water *ad libitum* during each trial to maintain hydration status. Heart rate was measured using a bedside monitor (BSM-2401, Nihonkohden, Shinjuku, Tokyo, Japan). In the control trial, subjects remained seated quietly for 90 min from 2:30 pm and saliva specimens were collected at 0, 60 and 90 min (i.e. at the same times of day as in the exercise trial).

Sample collection and analyses

Each participant was instructed to empty her mouth of pre-existing saliva before sampling. One and a half ml of unstimulated saliva was collected before blood sampling by passive drool for determination of hormone and cytokine levels. Saliva samples were centrifuged at 3,000 rpm for 15 min at room temperature and stored at -30°C until the day of analyses. All salivary samples were centrifuged again on the day of the assay to remove particulate matter.

Capillary blood samples were obtained from the fingertip into at least three heparinized capillary tubes for hematocrit measurement. The capillary tubes were immediately centrifuged at 12,000 rpm for 5 min at room temperature. Hematocrit was measured to confirm changes in plasma volume and hydration status. After the hematocrit measurement, the plasma was put into microtubes and stored at -30°C until the day of assays.

To confirm the menstrual cycle, the hormonal status was determined by measuring salivary 17β-estradiol and progesterone concentrations [24]. The salivary 17β-estradiol, progesterone, cortisol and Dehydroepiandrosterone (DHEA) concentrations were measured using high sensitivity enzyme immunoassay (EIA) kits (Salimetrics LLC, Sate College, PA, USA). The intra-assay coefficients of variation for 17β-estradiol, progesterone, cortisol and DHEA were 8.1%, 6.2%,

3.6 and 5.5%, respectively. The salivary amylase activity was measured using an enzymatic method (AMYLASE MONITOR, Nipro Co., Osaka, Japan) [25]. The saliva concentrations of IL-1β and TNF-α were measured using Quantikine high sensitivity (HS) enzyme-linked immunosorbent assay (ELISA) kits (R&D Systems, Minneapolis, MN, USA). The intra-assay coefficients of variation for IL-1β and TNF-α were 4.4 and 8.5%, respectively. The saliva concentrations of protein were measured by the Bradford method using a protein assay kit purchased from Bio-Rad (Hercules, CA, USA) [26]. Resting and exercise-induced salivary and plasma concentrations of IL-6 were measured using Quantikine HS ELISA kits (R&D Systems, Minneapolis, MN, USA) and IL-8 was measured using OptEIA kits (Becton Dickinson Bioscience, San Diego, CA, USA). The intra-assay coefficients of variation for IL-6 and IL-8 were 7.8 and 5.5%, respectively, and inter-assay coefficients of variation were 14.2 and 10.0%, respectively. These measurements were performed with a microplate reader (VERSAMAX, Molecular Devices Inc. Sunnyvale, CA, USA). Plasma and saliva samples from each individual subject were tested in the same assay run.

Statistical analyses

A one-way analysis of variance with repeated measures was used to assess the differences in basal salivary hormone and cytokine levels among the menstrual, follicular and luteal phases. A two-way (trial x time) analysis of variance with repeated measures was used to examine the differences in cytokine levels. When a main effect was observed, *post hoc* tests using Bonferroni adjustment was employed for multiple comparisons. Normality plots with tests (Shapiro-Wilks) were performed and log transformed before statistical analysis when data were not normally distributed. After log transformation, data were investigated again and considered to be normally distributed. Effect sizes (η^2) were calculated using guidelines of Cohen [27], and were considered as follows: 0.01 = small effect; 0.06 = moderate effect; and 0.14 = large effect. Data are presented as mean ± SD. Spearman's correlation coefficients were employed to assess the relationships between the salivary and plasma values. Statistical significance was set at $P<0.05$. Statistical analyses were performed using PASW Statistics 18 software (SPSS, Chicago, IL, USA).

Results

Menstrual cycle effects

The descriptive data for resting salivary hormones and plasma cytokines during each menstrual phase are presented in Table 1. Salivary 17β-estradiol concentration was not different between menstrual and follicular phases, however, the concentration increased by 41% from follicular phase to luteal phase (Table 1). Salivary progesterone concentration was increased by 156% from menstrual phase to luteal phase, and 177% from follicular phase to luteal phase (Table 1).

Salivary IL-6 concentration significantly differed between different phases of menstrual cycle ($P = 0.023$, $\eta^2 = 0.42$). When Bonferroni adjustment was conducted, salivary IL-6 concentration was significantly higher during the follicular phase compared with the luteal phase ($P = 0.036$) (Figure 1). Salivary TNF-α, IL-1β and IL-8 concentrations tended to decrease from the menstrual phase to the luteal phase but the concentrations were not significantly affected by menstrual cycle (TNF-α: $P = 0.059$, $\eta^2 = 0.33$, IL-1β: $P = 0.474$, $\eta^2 = 0.10$, IL-8: $P = 0.256$, $\eta^2 = 0.18$) (Figure 1).

Similarly, plasma IL-6 and IL-8 concentrations tended to decrease from the menstrual phase to the other phases but these were not significantly affected by menstrual cycle (IL-6: $P = 0.153$, $\eta^2 = 0.18$, IL-8: $P = 0.180$, $\eta^2 = 0.16$) (Table 1). There were no significant relationships between saliva and plasma IL-6 concentrations and between saliva and plasma IL-8 concentrations.

Salivary cortisol, DHEA concentrations and salivary amylase activity at rest were unaffected by the menstrual cycle (Table 1).

	Menstrual	Follicular	Luteal	
Salivary hormone				
17β-estradiol (pg/ml)	2.43 ± 0.70	2.51 ± 0.60	3.53 ± 1.18	*
Progesterone (pg/ml)	105.21 ± 49.21	97.23 ± 37.30	269.56 ± 145.35	*#
Salivary stress marker				
Cortisol (pg/ml)	0.19 ± 0.13	0.23 ± 0.14	0.20 ± 0.11	
DHEA (pg/ml)	174.60 ± 115.99	258.68 ± 282.79	149.19 ± 55.29	
Amylase activity (KIU/L)	67.50 ± 52.37	60.50 ± 33.95	60.13 ± 61.33	
Plasma cytokine				
IL-6 (pg/ml)	1.23 ± 0.90	0.59 ± 0.34	0.65 ± 0.45	
IL-8 (pg/ml)	5.38 ± 2.65	3.35 ± 2.10	3.89 ± 1.86	

Table 1: Salivary hormone, stress marker and plasma cytokine data at baseline with regard to menstrual cycle phases. Data are presented as means ± SD (n = 8). *DHEA*: Dehydroepiandrosterone, *IL-6*: Interleukin-6, *IL-8*: Interleukin-8. * $P < 0.05$ follicular versus luteal phase; # $P < 0.05$ menstrual versus luteal phase

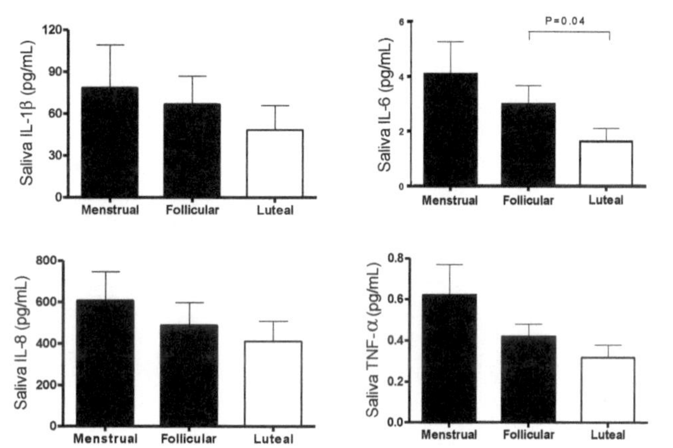

Figure 1: Salivary inflammatory cytokine data at baseline with regard to menstrual cycle phases. Data are presented as means ± SE (n = 8). *IL-1β*: Interleukin-1β, *IL-6*: Interleukin-6, *IL-8*: Interleukin-8, *TNF-α*: Tumor necrosis factor-α

Exercise effects

During the 60-min cycling at VT, subjects cycled at 63.3 ± 9.3 Watts, corresponding to 78.5 ± 15.4% HRmax (using Karvonen formula). The changes in salivary and plasma IL-6 and IL-8 concentrations during the exercise and control trials are presented in Figure 2. A significant interaction (trial by time) was found in plasma IL-6 ($P = 0.001$). Immediately and 30-min post-exercise plasma IL-6 concentrations were significantly higher than that of pre-exercise (pre: 0.92 ± 1.03 pg/mL, immediately post-exercise: 1.85 ± 1.23 pg/mL, $P = 0.013$, 30 min post-exercise: 2.38 ± 2.43 pg/mL, $P = 0.001$) (Figure 2). No significant time and trial effects were found in plasma IL-8, salivary IL-6 and protein. However, a significant interaction (trial by time) was found in salivary IL-8 ($P = 0.004$). Immediately post-exercise salivary IL-8 concentration was significantly higher than that of pre-exercise (P =

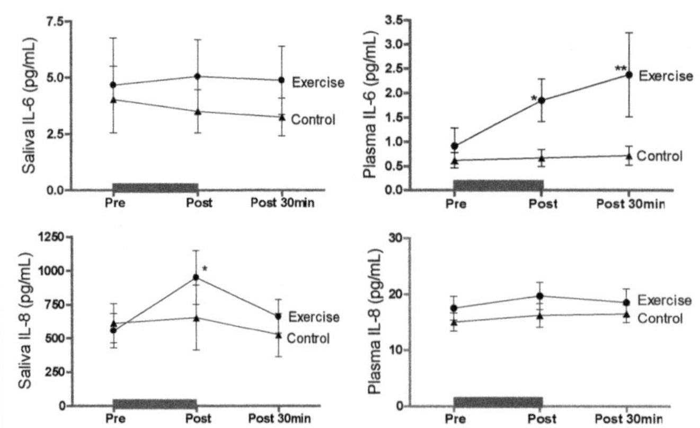

Figure 2: Changes in IL-6 and IL-8 levels in saliva and plasma during cycling at ventilator threshold (VT) and the control trial (n = 8). The data given refer to exercise during the menstrual period, since, as shown in Figure 1, interleukin levels vary throughout the menstrual cycle. Data are presented as means ± SE. *IL-6*: Interleukin-6, *IL-8*: Interleukin-8. * $P < 0.05$ versus pre-exercise, ** $P < 0.001$ versus pre-exercise

0.019) (Figure 2). No significant relationships were found between the concentrations of saliva and plasma IL-6 and IL-8 (IL-6: $r = 0.366$, $P = 0.08$, IL-8: $r = 0.312$, $P = 0.14$).

Discussion

The current study investigated the effects of the menstrual cycle on basal salivary stress hormone and cytokine levels, and the influences of aerobic exercise at VT on cytokine levels in healthy recreationally active women. The main findings of this study were; (1) resting salivary IL-6 concentration was significantly higher during the follicular phase compared with the luteal phase; (2) immediately post-exercise salivary IL-8 concentration was significantly higher than that of pre-exercise; (3) salivary and plasma cytokines were influenced differently by menstrual cycle and exercise.

Menstrual cycle effects

In the present study, salivary IL-6 concentration was significantly affected by menstrual cycle, whereas plasma IL-6 concentrations were unaffected by menstrual cycle in young healthy women at rest. Our findings in plasma are in contrast to a previous study that reported menstrual cycle influences on circulating IL-6 concentrations [2].

In the current study, plasma IL-6 level showed small (1.9 fold) insignificant decreases from menstrual phase to luteal phase, but no differences were observed between the follicular phase and luteal phase. However, Angstwurm et al. [2] reported that plasma IL-6 decreased from follicular phase to luteal phase. This may be related to the timing of sample correction during the menstrual cycle. This conflicting result could be attributable to the current study having used three phases of the menstrual cycle (menstrual, follicular and luteal) as opposed to two phases (follicular and luteal) used in the study by Angstwurm et al. [2].

However, no significant relationships were found between saliva and circulating IL-6 (and IL-8) concentrations in recreationally active healthy women at rest in the current study. Previous studies agree with the current study as they reported that salivary IL-6 level was not related to circulating IL-6 at rest and post-exercise conditions in patients and mixed gender athletes [10,15,17,18]. Moreover, it has been discovered that IL-6 mRNA are up regulated in salivary glands of mouse models [28] and in humans [29]. Furthermore, salivary IL-6 (and IL-8) has been used to assess immunological patterns relevant to systemic or local disease conditions and its levels were altered in patients with oral health problems [15,16,30]. Therefore, salivary IL-6 is possibly reflecting a local level of inflammation and as such it is understandable that saliva IL-6 concentrations are not a good refection of circulating values.

In the present study, salivary IL-6 level was the lowest when concentrations of female sex hormones (17β-estradiol and progesterone) were the highest (luteal phase). This is possibly because female sex hormones reduce inflammations as previous studies reported that estradiol showed an anti-inflammatory action and down regulated IL-6 *in vitro* [31,32].

All other salivary and plasma cytokines were not significantly affected by menstrual cycle. However, salivary levels of TNF-α, IL-1β and IL-8 tended to decrease between the menstrual and luteal phases. Although a significant difference was not found, moderate or large effect sizes were demonstrated for these relationships, perhaps suggesting that these markers are also worthy of future attention.

In the present study, cortisol and DHEA in saliva and salivary amylase activity did not significantly differ among the menstrual cycle phases. Generally, these hormones have been used as stress markers [11,25,33]. Bernstein et al. [34] investigated an association between sympathetic responsiveness and the serum concentration of IL-6 in young women. However, changes in salivary amylase activity, an index of sympathetic tone according to menstrual cycle was not observed in the current study. Therefore, salivary IL-6 concentration at rest seems to reflect the inflammatory conditions which is influenced by menstrual cycle, but not influenced by sympathetic tone.

Exercise effects

In the present study, there were no differences in salivary IL-6 concentration among before, immediately after and 30-min post cycling at VT during menstrual phase in recreationally active women with a normal menstrual cycle. However, a previous study reported that salivary IL-6 concentration increased after a prolonged moderate intensity exercise in sedentary women [22]. In the previous study, salivary IL-6 concentration increased significantly from baseline to 30 min post 1 h treadmill running at 65% VO_2peak during follicular and luteal phases. Potential rationales for the different outcomes are an employment of different exercise intensity and conducting the studies during different phases of menstrual cycle. In general, 65% VO_2peak is higher than VT and ventilation rates increase at higher exercise intensities which may lead to increased airway inflammation. Hence, higher exercise intensities may be linked with a greater local inflammation which is reflected in an increased concentration of salivary IL-6. Moreover, resting salivary IL-6 concentration is the highest during menstrual phase compared to the other phases as observed in the current study; this may limit further elevations in saliva IL-6 concentration in response to exercise during menstrual phase.

In the current study, salivary IL-8 concentration significantly increased from pre- to post-exercise. In contrast to the salivary IL-8 concentration, circulating IL-8 concentration did not change throughout the trial. IL-8 is a neutrophil chemotactic factor, released by immune cells and endothelial cells to recruit neutrophils to sites of tissue damage (i.e. inflammation) [35-37]. Hence, the increase in salivary IL-8 observed in the present study after exercise may also simply reflect local inflammation due to increased ventilatory rates with exercise. Currently, there are no other studies which examined an influence of exercise on cytokine levels during menstrual phase using both salivary and circulating IL-8 concentrations. Therefore, further research is required to confirm the findings from the present study.

In conclusion, salivary cytokines (IL-6) is influenced by menstrual cycle at rest in recreationally active healthy women. Moreover, salivary IL-6 and IL-8 responded differently to both the menstrual cycle and to exercise compared with their counterparts in plasma. Therefore saliva sampling should not be considered as a non-invasive alternative to blood sampling for examining the inflammation status in women as it may simply reflect local inflammatory events related to increased ventilatory rates.

Acknowledgements

This study was supported by a Grant-in-Aid for the Global COE "Sport Sciences for the Promotion of Active Life", Scientific Research (A) 15H0183, and the Strategic Research Foundation at Private Universities, 2015-2020 from the Ministry of Education, Culture, Sports, Science and Technology (S1511017) of Japan.

The authors would like to thank Dr. Nicolette Bishop for her help with preparing this manuscript.

References

1. Tersman Z, Collins A, Eneroth P (1991) Cardiovascular responses to psychological and physiological stressors during the menstrual cycle. Psychosom Med 53: 185-197.
2. Angstwurm MW, Gärtner R, Ziegler-Heitbrock HW (1997) Cyclic plasma IL-6 levels during normal menstrual cycle. Cytokine 9: 370-374.
3. Chiu KM, Arnaud CD, Ju J, Mayes D, Bacchetti P, et al. (2000) Correlation of estradiol, parathyroid hormone, interleukin-6, and soluble interleukin-6 receptor during the normal menstrual cycle. Bone 26: 79-85.
4. Ray P, Ghosh SK, Zhang DH, Ray A (1997) Repression of interleukin-6 gene expression by 17 beta-estradiol: inhibition of the DNA-binding activity of the transcription factors NF-IL6 and NF-kappa B by the estrogen receptor. FEBS Lett 409: 79-85.
5. Pedersen BK, Febbraio MA (2008) Muscle as an endocrine organ: focus on muscle-derived interleukin-6. Physiol Rev 88: 1379-1406.
6. Pedersen BK (2011) Muscles and their myokines. J Exp Biol 214: 337-346.
7. Evans J, Salamonsen LA (2012) Inflammation, leukocytes and menstruation. Rev Endocr Metab Disord 13: 277-288.
8. Kirschbaum C, Kudielka BM, Gaab J, Schommer NC, Hellhammer DH (1999) Impact of gender, menstrual cycle phase, and oral contraceptives on the activity of the hypothalamus-pituitary-adrenal axis. Psychosom Med 61: 154-162.
9. Minetto M, Rainoldi A, Gazzoni M, Terzolo M, Borrione P, et al. (2005) Differential responses of serum and salivary interleukin-6 to acute strenuous exercise. Eur J Appl Physiol 93: 679-686.
10. Minetto MA, Gazzoni M, Lanfranco F, Baldi M, Saba L, et al. (2007) Influence of the sample collection method on salivary interleukin-6 levels in resting and post-exercise conditions. Eur J Appl Physiol 101: 249-256.
11. Thomasson R, Baillot A, Jollin L, Lecoq AM, Amiot V, et al. (2010) Correlation between plasma and saliva adrenocortical hormones in response to submaximal exercise. J Physiol Sci 60: 435-439.
12. Brown SG, Morrison LA, Calibuso MJ, Christiansen TM (2008) The menstrual cycle and sexual behavior: relationship to eating, exercise, sleep, and health patterns. Women Health 48: 429-444.
13. Kudielka BM, Kirschbaum C (2003) Awakening cortisol responses are influenced by health status and awakening time but not by menstrual cycle phase. Psychoneuroendocrinology 28: 35-47.
14. Wolfram M, Bellingrath S, Kudielka BM (2011) The cortisol awakening response (CAR) across the female menstrual cycle. Psychoneuroendocrinology 36: 905-912.
15. Tishler M, Yaron I, Shirazi I, Yossipov Y, Yaron M (1999) Increased salivary interleukin-6 levels in patients with primary Sjögren's syndrome. Rheumatol Int 18: 125-127.
16. St John MA, Li Y, Zhou X, Denny P, Ho CM, et al. (2004) Interleukin 6 and interleukin 8 as potential biomarkers for oral cavity and oropharyngeal squamous cell carcinoma. Arch Otolaryngol Head Neck Surg 130: 929-935.
17. Sjögren E, Leanderson P, Kristenson M, Ernerudh J (2006) Interleukin-6 levels in relation to psychosocial factors: studies on serum, saliva, and in vitro production by blood mononuclear cells. Brain Behav Immun 20: 270-278.
18. Fernandez-Botran R, Miller JJ, Burns VE, Newton TL (2011) Correlations among inflammatory markers in plasma, saliva and oral mucosal transudate in post-menopausal women with past intimate partner violence. Brain Behav Immun 25: 314-321.
19. Kendall B, Eston R (2002) Exercise-induced muscle damage and the potential protective role of estrogen. Sports Med 32: 103-123.
20. Gillum TL, Kuennen MR, Schneider S, Moseley P (2011) A review of sex differences in immune function after aerobic exercise. Exerc Immunol Rev 17: 104-121.
21. Northoff H, Symons S, Zieker D, Schaible EV, Schäfer K, et al. (2008) Gender- and menstrual phase dependent regulation of inflammatory gene expression in response to aerobic exercise. Exerc Immunol Rev 14: 86-103.
22. Ives SJ, Blegen M, Coughlin MA, Redmond J, Matthews T, et al. (2011) Salivary estradiol, interleukin-6 production, and the relationship to substrate metabolism during exercise in females. Eur J Appl Physiol 111: 1649-1658.
23. Sue DY, Wasserman K, Moricca RB, Casaburi R (1988) Metabolic acidosis during exercise in patients with chronic obstructive pulmonary disease. Use of the V-slope method for anaerobic threshold determination. Chest 94: 931-938.
24. Gandara BK, Leresche L, Mancl L (2007) Patterns of salivary estradiol and progesterone across the menstrual cycle. Ann N Y Acad Sci 1098: 446-450.
25. Yamaguchi M, Kanemaru M, Kanemori T, Mizuno Y (2003) Flow-injection-type biosensor system for salivary amylase activity. Biosens Bioelectron 18: 835-840.
26. Bradford MM (1976) A rapid and sensitive method for the quantitation of microgram quantities of protein utilizing the principle of protein-dye binding. Anal Biochem 72: 248-254.
27. Cohen JW (1988) Statistical power analysis for the behavioral sciences. Lawrence Erlbaum, Hillsdale, NJ: pp 380-403.
28. Tanda N, Ohyama H, Yamakawa M, Ericsson M, Tsuji T, et al. (1998) IL-1 beta and IL-6 in mouse parotid acinar cells: characterization of synthesis, storage, and release. Am J Physiol 274: G147-156.
29. Boumba D, Skopouli FN, Moutsopoulos HM (1995) Cytokine mRNA expression in the labial salivary gland tissues from patients with primary Sjögren's syndrome. Br J Rheumatol 34: 326-333.
30. Korostoff A, Reder L, Masood R, Sinha UK (2011) The role of salivary cytokine biomarkers in tongue cancer invasion and mortality. Oral Oncol 47: 282-287.
31. Pottratz ST, Bellido T, Mocharla H, Crabb D, Manolagas SC (1994) 17 beta-Estradiol inhibits expression of human interleukin-6 promoter-reporter constructs by a receptor-dependent mechanism. J Clin Invest 93: 944-950.
32. Kovacs EJ, Plackett TP, Witte PL (2004) Estrogen replacement, aging, and cell-mediated immunity after injury. J Leukoc Biol 76: 36-41.
33. Cadore E, Lhullier F, Brentano M, Silva E, Ambrosini M, et al. (2008) Correlations between serum and salivary hormonal concentrations in response to resistance exercise. J Sports Sci 26: 1067-1072.
34. Bernstein IM, Damron D, Schonberg AL, Shapiro R (2009) The relationship of plasma volume, sympathetic tone, and proinflammatory cytokines in young healthy nonpregnant women. Reprod Sci 16: 980-985.
35. Suzuki K, Totsuka M, Nakaji S, Yamada M, Kudoh S, Liu Q (1999) Endurance exercise causes interaction among stress hormones, cytokines, neutrophil dynamics, and muscle damage. J Appl Physiol 87: 1360-1367.
36. Suzuki K, Nakaji S, Yamada M, Totsuka M, Sato K, Sugawara K (2002) Systemic inflammatory response to exhaustive exercise: cytokine kinetics. Exer Immunol Rev 8: 6-48.
37. Suzuki K, Nakaji S, Yamada M, Liu Q, Kurakake S, et al. (2003) Impact of a competitive marathon race on systemic cytokine and neutrophil responses. Med Sci Sports Exer 35: 348-355.

Brief Exercise Enhances Blood Hypocretin-1 in Sedentary Men

Giovanni Messina, Giovanni Di Bernardo, Antonietta Messina, Carmine Dalia, Sergio Chieffi, Umberto Galderisi and Marcellino Monda*

Department of Experimental Medicine, Section of Human Physiology and Clinical Unit of Dietetics and Sports Medicine, Second University of Naples, Naples, Italy

Abstract

The aim of this experiment was to test the effect of brief exercise on the concentration of plasma hypocretin-1, a peptide that regulates many physiological variables. Blood samples were collected from participants (men, n=6) before (time 0 min) and after (times 15 and 30 min) a cycle ergo meter exercise at 75 W for 15 min. The physical exertion was monitored by heart rate registration. The exercise causes a significant increase in plasmatic hypocretin-1, in association with an increase of hearth rate. These results are the first demonstration, which indicates that plasma hypocretin-1 is involved in the reactions induced by physical activity.

Keywords: Hypocretin-1; Exercisel; Heart rate

Introduction

The hypothalamic neuropeptide "hypocretin-1" [1] is also named orexin-A for its influence on food intake [2,3]. An intracerebroventricular injection of hypocretin-1 does not merely affects food intake, but it also causes an increase in heart rate (HR) [4], blood pressure [5], and metabolic rate [6]. These autonomic modifications indicate that this neuropeptide plays a role in the control of vegetative functions. Hypocretin-1 also affects thermoregulation, including changes in "core" temperature and temperature of interscapular brown adipose tissue (IBAT) [7,8].

The presence of hypocretin receptors in many cerebral areas indicates that several functions are played by hypocretin-1 [9]. Some antipsychotic drugs, as haloperidol, clozapine, risperidone, and quetiapine, modify the sympathetic and hyperthermic reactions due to hypocretin-1 [10-13]. A role for the hypocretin-1 in sleep regulation has been demonstrated [14]. Deficiency in hypocretin-1 causes narcolepsy in mice, cats, dogs, and humans [15-18]. Studies in rodents have indicated that hypocretin-1 crucial for the regulation of respiration [19-22].

Since there are few studies concerning the modification of plasmatic hypocretin-1 in humans and, in particular, there is no study during exercise, the aim of the present research was to investigate the effect of exercise on the concentration of plasma hypocretin-1. This experiment could reveal a role for hypocretin-1 in the reactions induced by physical activity.

Methods

Subjects

Six male sedentary were enrolled among those who contacted the Clinical Unit of Dietetics and Sports Medicine of the Second University of Naples. Age and anthropometric values, expressed as mean ± standard error (SE) are reported in Table 1.

Ethics statement

The experimental procedures followed the rule approved by Ethic Committee of the Second University of Naples. Patients were informed on the research and permission for the use of plasma samples was obtained. All procedures were conforming to the directives of the Declaration of Helsinki.

Age (Years)	23.7 ± 3.12
BMI (Kg/m^2)	20.09 ± 1.9

Table 1: Age, Body mass index (BMI) of subjects.

Study protocol

The study protocol consisted of one day of testing in which each participant was asked to continue his normal work and leisure activities. The subjects were instructed to consume food and beverages as usual and to sleep a sufficient amount of hours. The period of experiment was divided in 3 times: resting time (0 min), exercise time (1-15 min) and recovery time (16-30 min). Three blood samples were collected in all periods of experiment. One sample at resting time, one sample at last min of exercise, and one sample at recovery time. The physical activity consisted in a cycle ergometer exercise at 75 W for 15 min, performed at 1-15 min period. All tests were performed in laboratory environment with a normal ambient climate.

Measurement of HR

After standard adjustments of seat and handlebar, the participants cycled on a calibrated mechanically braked cycle ergometer (Kettler ergometer E7) at 75 W, with no stop for 15 minutes. HR data were recorded during all period of experiment. Each participant wore a chest belt hard-wired to a digital R-R recorder (BTL08 SD ECG), where the QRS-signal wave-form R-R signal was sampled at the resolution of 1 ms. The HR (beats min-1) was calculated according to the following formula: HR = 60 R-R interval-1; where, R-R interval was converted into seconds.

Plasma hypocretin-1 detection

Blood samples were collected from all participants in the study. Blood samples were drawn from forearm vein at 8:00 a.m. after overnight fast into Vacutainer tubes (BD, Franklin Lakes, NJ) containing EDTA and 0.45 TIU/ml of aprotinin. Samples were gently mixed and then immediately centrifuged at 3000 rpm for 12 min at 4 °C. Plasma was stored at – 80°C until analysis. Plasma hypocretin-1 levels were measured using commercially available enzyme-linked immunoassay (ELISA) kits. Hypocretin-1 ELISA kit was purchased from Phoenix Pharmaceuticals. Before measurement, plasma hypocretin-1 was extracted using Sep-Pak C18 columns (Waters, Milford, MA). The columns were activated using

***Corresponding author:** Marcellino Monda, Professor, Department of Experimental Medicine, Second University of Naples, via Costantinopoli, 16, I-80138 Naples, Italy, E-mail: marcellino.monda@unina2.it

10 ml of methanol and 20 ml of H2O. 1-2 ml of sample was applied to the column and washed with 20 ml of water. Samples were eluted slowly with 80% acetonitrile and resulting volume was reduced to 400 µl under nitrogen flow. Aliquot was further evaporated into dryness using Speedvac (Savant Instruments, Holbrook, NY). The dry residue was dissolved in water and used for ELISA. There was no crossreactivity of the antibody for hypocretin-1(16–33), hypocretin-2, agouti-related protein(83–132)-amide. The minimal detectable concentration was 0.37 ng/ml, the intra-assay error < 5% and the inter-assay error < 14%.

Statistical analysis

The values are presented as means ± SE, Statistical analysis was performed using analysis of variance. Multiple comparisons were performed by the Newman-Keuls post hoc test. All data were analyzed with GraphPad Prism-version 5.01 statistical software package (GraphPad, CA, USA).

Control group

Three subjects without any exercise were used as controls. HR and hypocretin-1 were monitored as exercising subjects.

Results

Figure 1 illustrates the modification of the HR. Exercise induced an increase in HR. The analysis of variance showed significant effects [$F(2, 15) = 87.42$, $p<0.01$]. The post-hoc test showed a difference between pre-exercise and post-exercise values.

Figure 2 shows changes in blood concentration of hypocretin-1.

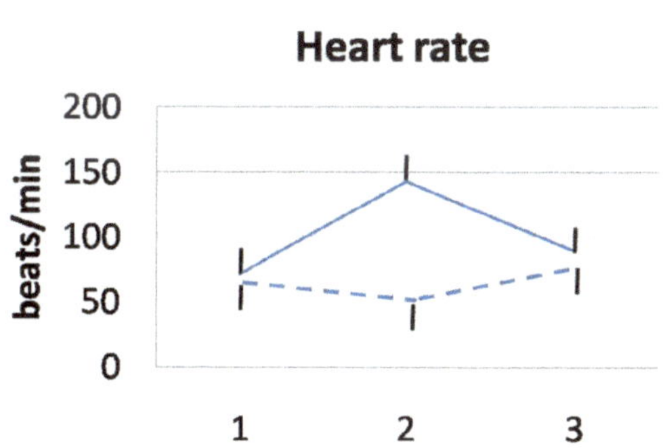

Figure 1: Changes in heart rate during resting (time 1), exercise (time 2), and recovery (time 3).

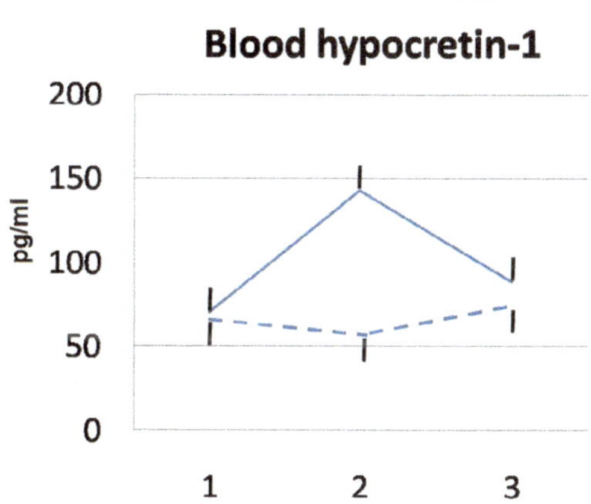

Figure 2: Changes in hypocretin-1 during resting (time 1), exercise (time 2), and recovery (time 3).

The physical activity caused an increase in hypocretin-1. The analysis of variance showed significant effects [$F (2, 15) = 22.24$, $p<0.01$]. The post-hoc test showed a difference between pre-exercise and post exercise values.

In the control group, HR and hypocretin-1 level did not modify during the times of the experiment. The data are not reported in the figures.

Discussion

This experiment is the first demonstration showing an increase of plasmatic hypocretin-1 during exercise in humans. The values of hypocretin-1 concentration are plausible with published reports. The peripheral origin of hypocretin-1 is not well known. The pancreatic beta-cells are retained secretor cells of hypocretin-1. Double immunohistochemical staining, using a polyclonal anti-insulin antibody, showed that hypocretin-1 is co-expressed with insulin [23]. In our experiment, the increase of plasmatic hypocretin-1 probably is due to an increase in the secretion of hypocretin-1 by pancreatic beta-cells. Since the sympathetic nervous system is involved in the regulation of pancreatic hormonal secretion [24], an enhancement of the sympathetic discharge of nerves to pancreas could increase the secretion of hypocretin-1.

Exercise is associated to the sympathetic activation, as demonstrated by increase in HR. Exercise elicits adaptive responses to sustain muscle engagement. Physical activity induces not only the sympathetic activation, but also hormonal changes [25,26]. The increase in plasmatic hypocretin-1 could be included among hormonal adaptations due to exercise. Plasmatic hypocretin-1 could be involved in the control of cortisol secretion. Indeed, relationship between hypocretin-1 and cortisol has been described. Since hypocretin-1 increases the expression of steroidogenic enzymes in human adrenocortical cells [27], an influence of hypocretin-1 on cortisol secretion (enhanced during physical activity) is conceivable. In further studies, determination of plasma insulin and cortisol levels will be measured using the present experimental design.

In the present experiment, the sympathetic discharge is positively associated with level of plasmatic hypocretin-1. Muscle exercise induces an increase in HR, controlled by the sympathetic nervous system, which is accompanied by an increase in plasmatic hypocretin-1, as demonstrated by the findings of the present experiment. Although it is well established that cerebral hypocretin-1 is related to the sympathetic discharge, the results of our research are the first ones showing an association between the plasmatic hypocretin-1 and HR, as expression of the sympathetic activity. An intracerebral injection of hypocretin-1 causes a generalized increase in the sympathetic discharge with augmented firing rate of sympathetic fibers innervating interscapular brown adipose tissue [28,29] heart [30], kidneys [31], etc. Studies in rodents have concluded that hypocretin neurons have a major role in the regulation of HR. Intracisternal hypocretin administration increases HR and blood pressure [32-34] and microinjections into the nucleus of the solitary tract elicit dose dependent changes in HR and blood pressure.

These evidences suggest that cerebral hypocretinergic pathway controls the sympathetic nervous system with possible relationship of "cause-effect" between hypocretin-1 and sympathetic activation. Although the findings of the present experiment do not indicate a secure "cause-effect" relationship, but only an association, it is very possible that hypocretin-1 could influence the sympathetic activity and/or vice-versa. Since hypocretin-1 rapidly enters brain from blood by simple diffusion [35], it is possible that increased plasmatic hypocretin-1during exercise time could induce cerebral stimulation of areas that, in turn, control the sympathetic reactions.

In a broader vision of the physiological role of hypocretin-1, the benefits of physical activity [36] in the control of body weight could include an increased peripheral secretion of this peptide. Since hypocretin-1 is involved in the regulation of body weight [37,38], and in the patho-physiology of obesity, an increased secretion of plasmatic hypocretin-1during physical activity, as showed in this experiment, could influence body weight probably through an activation of energy expenditure [39]. The findings of this experiment shed further light on the positive effects of exercise, including hypothetic positive effect exerted by plasmatic hypocretin-1.

In conclusion, our study represents the first demonstration that the exercise induces an increase in plasmatic hypocretin-1 and this peptide could play an important role in the peripheral adaptations to physical activity.

Acknowledgements

The present work received financial support from the Postgraduate School in Sports Medicine of the Second University of Naples (process numbers 2013/13-0).

Competing Interest

The authors declare that they have no competing interests.

References

1. de Lecea L1, Kilduff TS, Peyron C, Gao X, Foye PE, et al. (1998) The hypocretins: hypothalamus-specific peptides with neuroexcitatory activity. Proc Natl Acad Sci U S A 95: 322-327.
2. Sakurai T, Amemiya A, Ishii M, Matsuzaki I, Chemelli RM, et al. (1998) Orexins and orexin receptors: a family of hypothalamic neuropeptides and G protein-coupled receptors that regulate feeding behavior. Cell 92: 573-585.
3. Monda M1, Viggiano A, De Luca V (2003) Paradoxical [correction of parodoxical] effect of orexin A: hypophagia induced by hyperthermia. Brain Res 961: 220-228.
4. Monda M1, Viggiano AN, Viggiano A, Viggiano E, Lanza A, et al. (2005) Hyperthermic reactions induced by orexin A: role of the ventromedial hypothalamus. Eur J Neurosci 22: 1169-1175.
5. Shirasaka T1, Nakazato M, Matsukura S, Takasaki M, Kannan H (1999) Sympathetic and cardiovascular actions of orexins in conscious rats. Am J Physiol 277: R1780-1785.
6. Lubkin M1, Stricker-Krongrad A (1998) Independent feeding and metabolic actions of orexins in mice. Biochem Biophys Res Commun 253: 241-245.
7. Monda M1, Viggiano A, Mondola P, De Luca V (2001) Inhibition of prostaglandin synthesis reduces hyperthermic reactions induced by hypocretin-1/orexin A. Brain Res 909: 68-74.
8. Monda M1, Viggiano A, Viggiano A, Fuccio F, De Luca V (2004) Injection of orexin A into the diagonal band of Broca induces sympathetic and hyperthermic reactions. Brain Res 1018: 265-271.
9. Kukkonen JP1, Holmqvist T, Ammoun S, Akerman KE (2002) Functions of the orexinergic/hypocretinergic system. Am J Physiol Cell Physiol 283: C1567-1591.
10. Monda M, Viggiano A, De Luca V (2003) Haloperidol reduces the sympathetic and thermogenic activation induced by orexin A. Neurosci Res 45: 17-23.
11. Monda M1, Viggiano A, Viggiano A, Fuccio F, De Luca V (2004) Clozapine blocks sympathetic and thermogenic reactions induced by orexin A in rat. Physiol Res 53: 507-513.
12. Monda M1, Viggiano A, Viggiano A, Viggiano E, Messina G, et al. (2006) Quetiapine lowers sympathetic and hyperthermic reactions due to cerebral injection of orexin A. Neuropeptides 40: 357-363.
13. Monda M1, Viggiano A, Viggiano A, Viggiano E, De Luca V (2006) Risperidone potentiates the sympathetic and hyperthermic reactions induced by orexin A in the rat. Physiol Res 55: 73-78.
14. Beuckmann CT1, Yanagisawa M (2002) Orexins: from neuropeptides to energy homeostasis and sleep/wake regulation. J Mol Med (Berl) 80: 329-342.
15. Kiyashchenko LI1, Mileykovskiy BY, Maidment N, Lam HA, Wu MF, et al. (2002) Release of hypocretin (orexin) during waking and sleep states. J Neurosci 22: 5282-5286.
16. Taheri S1, Zeitzer JM, Mignot E (2002) The role of hypocretins (orexins) in sleep regulation and narcolepsy. Annu Rev Neurosci 25: 283-313.
17. Wu MF1, John J, Maidment N, Lam HA, Siegel JM (2002) Hypocretin release in normal and narcoleptic dogs after food and sleep deprivation, eating, and movement. Am J Physiol Regul Integr Comp Physiol 283: R1079-1086.
18. Zhang S1, Lin L, Kaur S, Thankachan S, Blanco-Centurion C, et al. (2007) The development of hypocretin (orexin) deficiency in hypocretin/ataxin-3 transgenic rats. Neuroscience 148: 34-43.
19. Zhang W1, Fukuda Y, Kuwaki T (2005) Respiratory and cardiovascular actions of orexin-A in mice. Neurosci Lett 385: 131-136.
20. Zhang W, Zhang N, Sakurai T, Kuwaki T (2009) Orexin neurons in the hypothalamus mediate cardiorespiratory responses induced by disinhibition of the amygdala and bed nucleus of the stria terminalis. Brain Res 1262: 25-37.
21. Corcoran A1, Richerson G, Harris M (2010) Modulation of respiratory activity by hypocretin-1 (orexin A) in situ and in vitro. Adv Exp Med Biol 669: 109-113.
22. Terada J1, Nakamura A, Zhang W, Yanagisawa M, Kuriyama T, et al. (2008) Ventilatory long-term facilitation in mice can be observed during both sleep and wake periods and depends on orexin. J Appl Physiol (1985) 104: 499-507.
23. Dall'Aglio C1, Pedini V, Scocco P, Boiti C, Ceccarelli P (2010) Immunohistochemical evidence of Orexin-A in the pancreatic beta cells of domestic animals. Res Vet Sci 89: 147-149.
24. Thorens B (2010) Central control of glucose homeostasis: the brain--endocrine pancreas axis. Diabetes Metab 36 Suppl 3: S45-49.
25. Messina G, Vicidomini C, Viggiano A, Tafuri D, Cozza V, et al. (2012) Enhanced parasympathetic activity of sportive women is paradoxically associated to enhanced resting energy expenditure. Auton Neurosci 169: 102-106.
26. Viggiano A, Vicidomini C, Monda M, Carleo D, Carleo R, et al. (2009) Fast and low-cost analysis of heart rate variability reveals vegetative alterations in noncomplicated diabetic patients. J Diabetes Complications 23: 119-123.
27. Wenzel J1, Grabinski N, Knopp CA, Dendorfer A, Ramanjaneya M, et al. (2009) Hypocretin/orexin increases the expression of steroidogenic enzymes in human adrenocortical NCI H295R cells. Am J Physiol Regul Integr Comp Physiol 297: R1601-1609.
28. Monda M1, Viggiano A, Viggiano A, Viggiano E, Messina G, et al. (2007) Sympathetic and hyperthermic reactions by orexin A: role of cerebral catecholaminergic neurons. Regul Pept 139: 39-44.
29. Monda M1, Sullo A, De Luca E, Pellicano MP (1996) Lysine acetylsalicylate modifies aphagia and thermogenic changes induced by lateral hypothalamic lesion. Am J Physiol 271: R1638-1642.
30. Shahid IZ1, Rahman AA, Pilowsky PM (2012) Orexin and central regulation of cardiorespiratory system. Vitam Horm 89: 159-184.
31. Tanida M1, Niijima A, Shen J, Yamada S, Sawai H, et al. (2006) Dose-different effects of orexin-A on the renal sympathetic nerve and blood pressure in urethane-anesthetized rats. Exp Biol Med (Maywood) 231: 1616-1625.
32. Hirota K1, Kushikata T, Kudo M, Kudo T, Smart D, et al. (2003) Effects of central hypocretin-1 administration on hemodynamic responses in young-adult and middle-aged rats. Brain Res 981: 143-150.
33. Jochem J1, Zwirska-Korczala K, Zabielski R, Kato I, Kuwahara A (2006) Cardiovascular effects of centrally acting orexin A in haemorrhage-shocked rats. J Physiol Pharmacol 57 Suppl 11: 115-124.
34. Huang SC, Dai YW, Lee YH, Chiou LC, Hwang LL (2010) Orexins depolarize rostral ventrolateral medulla neurons and increase arterial pressure and heart rate in rats mainly via orexin 2 receptors. J Pharmacol Exp Ther 334: 522-529.
35. Kastin AJ1, Akerstrom V (1999) Orexin A but not orexin B rapidly enters brain from blood by simple diffusion. J Pharmacol Exp Ther 289: 219-223.

36. Garland TJr, Schutz H, Chappell MA, Keeney BK, Meek TH et al. (2011) The biological control of voluntary exercise, spontaneous physical activity and daily energy expenditure in relation to obesity: human and rodent perspectives. J Exp Biol 15: 206-229.

37. Boughton CK1, Murphy KG (2013) Can neuropeptides treat obesity? A review of neuropeptides and their potential role in the treatment of obesity. Br J Pharmacol 170: 1333-1348.

38. Perez-Leighton CE, Boland K, Teske JA, Billington C, Kotz CM (2012) Behavioral responses to orexin, orexin receptor gene expression, and spontaneous physical activity contribute to individual sensitivity to obesity. Am J Physiol 303: E865-E874.

39. Panossian LA1, Veasey SC (2012) Daytime sleepiness in obesity: mechanisms beyond obstructive sleep apnea--a review. Sleep 35: 605-615.

Physiological Implications of Two versus Three Sets in the Development of Quadriceps Muscle Strength in Untrained Men

Baker JS[1]*, Buchan DS[1], Wong DP[2], Davies B[3], Cooper SM[4], Davies M[3] and Kilgore L[1]

[1]*Institute for Clinical Exercise & Health Science, University of the West of Scotland, Hamilton, ML3 0JB, Scotland, UK*
[2]*Human Performance Laboratory, Technological and Higher Education Institute of Hong Kong, Hong Kong, P.R. China*
[3]*Health and Exercise Science Research Unit, School of Applied Sciences, University of South Wales, Pontypridd, CF37 1DL, Wales, UK*
[4]*Cardiff School of Sport, Cardiff Metropolitan University, Cardiff CF23 6XD, Wales, UK*

Abstract

Background: The purpose of this study was to determine if differences in strength gain are apparent following resistance training at two different exercise volumes (2-sets versus 3-sets).

Methods: Seven men (age=21.6 ± 1.5) completed the study. Each subject trained one leg in the leg extension exercise using two sets and trained the other using three sets. Subjects were randomly assigned to two groups then treatments were randomly assigned to groups to minimize bias: one group assigned two sets right leg and three sets left leg (3L 2R; n = 3), one group assigned three sets right leg and two sets left leg (3R 2L; n=4). One repetition maximum (1RM) was determined for each leg of each participant for the leg extension prior to the three sessions per week and six week duration training program. Each set included in training consisted of six repetitions at a workload of 80% 1RM during each session. 1RM was tested after 2 and 4 weeks allowing for training workloads to be adjusted to 80% of current 1RM to apply the principle of progression.

Results: Significant differences were apparent when comparing pre- and post-training absolute 1RM measures for both the two set and three set legs ($p<0.05$). There was a significant difference in magnitude of change between the two set and three set legs, 12.6 kg versus 19.4 kg respectively ($p=0.02$).

Conclusion: While six weeks of either two or three sets of the leg extension exercise training both significantly increase quadriceps strength, the three set configuration creates a significantly larger magnitude of change compared to two sets.

Keywords: Strength training; Muscle adaptation; 1RM

Introduction

Resistance training has been well established as a highly effective method for improving muscular strength for more than half a century [1-4]. Resistance training is beneficial to the development of musculoskeletal fitness and is known to decrease the risk of injury and disease to the individual, both cardiovascular and orthopaedic in the elderly [5-7]. There is further evidence that low muscle strength significantly compromises mobility and function in the elderly increases the prevalence of obesity and is associated with increased all-cause mortality in both the elderly and young [8-11].

The manner in which strength training programs should be structured to increase strength and reap functional benefits continues to be a source of practitioner and scientific debate. Resistance training and its effects are dependent on several factors, including the intensity and frequency of training, rest interval duration and exercise volume. In relation to volume of training, although the number of sets and repetitions prescribed for strength gain is not precisely known [3,12,13]. The prevailing consensus, derived from studies generally examining programs using 1-set or 3-sets, is that execution of multiple sets of an exercise is required to elicit optimal increases in muscular strength [2,14-16]. Typically this is the general information included in coaching and fitness professional instructional materials. The validity of this one-size-fits-all prescription can be questioned as several studies are present in the literature suggesting that single set programs may be as efficient as multiple sets in the development of muscular strength [13,17-22].

The concept that single set training is as strong of a stimulus for strength gain as multiple sets was presented in the paper by Carpinelli and Otto [2]. They suggested, based on the literature they reviewed, if three sets does not succeed in bringing about significantly greater increases in strength than a single set then it seems plausible that considerable time and effort could be spared by weight trainees by simply performing a single set per exercise per training session. It must be noted that numerous professionals and scientists claimed the review was biased in papers included [23]. Further, a meta-analysis by Krieger suggests that multiple sets produce 40% greater hypertrophy than single sets in both untrained and trained subjects [24]. Although hypertrophy is a different training goal than strength gain, the findings suggest that there is an authentic difference in anatomical and physiological adaptations between single and multiple set programs.

A number of training studies report similarity in results after single and multiple set programs undertaken for the short term (7-10 weeks in duration) [17,19-21]. These findings have come under criticism for being too short in duration to elicit statistically significant changes. The short term nature of these studies seemingly provides some of an explanation as to why single sets, in many authors' work, indicate similar strength improvements with one or multiple sets. Galvao and Taaffe agree with this, stating that many programs do not exceed a 14 week time course, which may limit the potential for strength gain [12]. To address this concern De Hoyos et al. and Vincent et al. conducted studies that took place over a period of 25 weeks, and produced similar conclusions to the shorter tem studies – that both single and

***Corresponding author:** Julien Baker, Institute for Clinical Exercise & Health Science, University of the West of Scotland, Hamilton, ML3 0JB, Scotland, UK
E-mail: julien.baker@uws.ac.uk

multiple set groups improved strength to a significant degree, but that any differences noted between the groups were not large enough to be statistically significant [18,22].

It has been suggested by Fleck and Kraemer that resistance training consisting of single sets may well be suitable for beginning trainees commencing a strength training program and that multiple sets will be most advantageous in terms of producing physiological adaptations once an initial fitness level has been reached through the initial single set regime [3]. This concept was refined and linked to Selye's general adaptation syndrome by Rippetoe and Kilgore through a definition of training progression (novice, intermediate, advanced and elite) who respond to general training parameters at different rates and with differing magnitudes of strength gain [25,26]. Essentially, exposure to strength training of previously untrained subjects will produce similar rates and magnitudes to strength gain across all resistance training procedures. Beginning trainees respond to all programs as a general stimulus for adaptation thus the similarity of response. More advanced trainees require more specific sources of stress (i.e., multiple sets) to produce fitness gains. A paper by Silvester et al. analysed single set versus multiple set programs and are in agreement with this concept, finding that single set protocols result in similar strength increases as multiple sets over short durations of training in untrained subjects, but that as the individual's strength was enhanced multiple set resistance training protocols were more advisable and effective [19]. This finding is suggestive that beyond the short term nature of studies proposing that single set training is as effective as those using multiple sets another concern is the training progression status of the subjects. It is often the case that untrained subjects are the focal point of the investigations thus providing another factor needing attention and description in experimentation. Studies using novice trainees as subjects are quite valid and informative, however their findings must be restricted to similar populations, those with no or limited training experience.

There has been a large degree in dissimilarity in the repetition ranges and set numbers used in the one versus multiple set investigations to date. Kraemer et al. [27] illustrated that significantly greater increases in 1RM squat ability were acquired by subjects undertaking a multiple set program (3×10 repetitions) in comparison to those performing a single set protocol (1×12 repetitions), where both groups trained three times a week for a 14 week period. Schlumberger et al. [28] also presented evidence that superior strength gains were associated with those that trained with 3 sets in comparison to those using a single set resistance training program, with a study focused on leg extension strength improvements. Conflicting evidence to this was provided by Ostrowski et al. [29], whose study on recreational weightlifters it was concluded after a 10 week program that three sets per exercise was as effective as 6 or 12 sets for inducing strength gains. Hass et al. [13] supplied further support for single set training being sufficient for strength increases in recreational weightlifters, with a study involving two groups, one of which performed 1 set of 8-12 repetitions and the other 3 sets of 8-12 repetitions both at 70% of 1RM. The results obtained indicated that leg extension strength increased significantly in both groups from pre-training to midpoint measures and from midpoint to post-training measures, but also that at no time during the program did the differences in leg extension 1RM between the groups differ significantly. Conclusions regarding multi-set versus single set training that are based on differing volumes (repetitions and sets) and intensities is problematic as they have been shown to be linked to differential physiological adaptations in muscle [30].

Due to the variance in approaches to constructing experimental training programs, there has been contrasting evidence to date concerning single versus multiple set resistance training. The strength

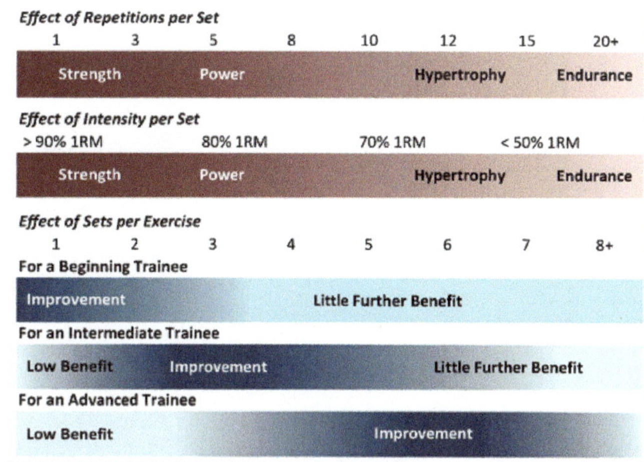

Figure 1: Box-whisker-plot of the ratio testosterone (T) to epitestosterone (E) at baseline (V2) and end of trial after 12 weeks (V4) for both treatment groups. Shown are the median (small line within the box) with interquartile range ICR (upper and lower quartile), 5th and 95th percentiles and minimum and maximum values (+).

continuum that is an operational construct in professional strength training practice has been supported in the literature (Figure 1) [30]. However a complete and systematic exploration of repetition and set schemes need to be undertaken to more fully establish its accuracy. The most complete analysis of the effects of different set numbers was that of Berger [1]. Given the limited literature in existence regarding discriminating between the differences in the amount of strength two and three set program organizations induce, this set range was compared, as it has received the least attention but may have a profound utility in lower volume training programmes. The present small-scale study proposed to examine strength changes in the quadriceps after four weeks of training in beginning weight trainees. A within subjects method was used (right and left legs receiving differing training) to control for inter-individual variance.

The most common repetition per set recommendations for beginners currently in use are for five repetitions and 6-12 repetitions [26,31,32]. The present study examined a 6 repetition per set organization, similar to popular and exercise authority recommendations. The experimental hypothesis was that three sets of exercise would produce a larger change in strength than two sets of exercise (Figure 1).

Materials and Methods

Subjects

Ten male subjects volunteered for this study, ranging from 19-24 years of age. All 10 subjects were apparently healthy and were beginners and not involved in any other type of training for strength development, in order to ensure that no muscle strength gains were due to any means other than those set out in this investigation. In addition to this, no other leg exercises or leg training (other than normal ambulation) was performed by the participants either within the study or outside of it throughout the entire program duration. The descriptive data of the subjects are presented in Table 1. Prior to the commencement of the study the participants were fully instructed of what was required of them and they each gave written informed consent, with the knowledge that at any time they could voluntarily withdraw from the investigation.

Experimental design

This investigation centred on the increases in quadriceps strength

Group	Age (y)	Height (cm)	Weight (kg)
3R 2L (n=4)	21.8 (2.1)	177.1 (3.7)	74.6 (5.3)
3L 2R (n=3)	21.3 (0.6)	181.6 (6.5)	73.4 (2.0)

Table 1: Subject descriptive data presented as means (standard deviation).

1RM strength	Pre-Training	2-week	4-week	6-week	% change	Effect size between pre- and post-test
2-set leg	52.0 (11.1)	57.1 (10.3)	61.1 (10.8)	64.6 (9.1)*	24.2	1.24
3-set leg	51.4 (12.9)	58.9 (13.0)	65.7 (14.8)	70.9 (15.6)*	37.9	1.36

*Denotes significant differences of pre- to post-training 1RM values within legs ($P < 0.05$). **Table 2:** Changes in mean 1RM over the experimental period. All results in kg (SD).

Subject	2-set leg	3-set leg
1	20	40
2	12	16
3	16	24
4	8	20
5	8	8
6	16	16
7	8	12
Mean (SD)	12.6 (4.9)	19.4 (10.4)*

Table 3: Comparison of magnitude of strength gain in legs trained with 2 sets and 3 sets of the leg extension exercise using 80% 1RM for six weeks. Results in kg (SD).*indicates statistically different value from 2-set training protocol ($p<0.05$).

obtained through different protocols of resistance training. As part of the experiment, each subject was required to train both their right and left leg quadriceps muscles, but in a dissimilar fashion. One leg was trained with two sets of six repetitions in the leg extension exercise and the other with three sets of six repetitions per training session. The 10 subjects were randomly assigned into two groups: (1) five subjects trained using three sets with the right leg and two sets with the left (3R 2L) and (2) five subjects trained using two sets with the right leg and three sets with the left leg (3L 2R). This orientation was selected to reduce bias in the test regarding right or left leg dominance in subjects. The program lasted for a period of six weeks with three sessions being performed each week (Monday-Wednesday-Friday at the same time of day), with at least 48 hours between sessions. The six weeks of training were consecutive to ensure that no reversible effects to training could occur during the program and that the subjects were training at an identical frequency. The training sessions were undertaken on a standard leg extension exercise machine (Power sports International Ltd., UK) adjusted according to tibial length so that the machine pad rested at a level just above the level of the lateral malleolus of each subject. Subjects sat on the machine seat in a position where their gastrocnemius was approximately 1-2 cm in advance of the forward edge of the seat. Each repetition began with the tibia perpendicular to the floor, went through complete extension (180 degrees) of the knee, and ended with return of the tibia to a perpendicular position.

One repetition maximum (1RM) for leg extension of each leg of each subject was tested prior to the commencement of training as a baseline for the later comparison of strength gains. Two further 1RM tests were conducted as strength re-tests after the second and fourth weeks of training and again at the end of the program (sixth week).

During each training session both legs were separately exercised at a workload of 80% of each subject's 1RM, as calculated from their pre-program 1RM measurements for each respective leg. Following re-test measurements after two and four weeks the workload of the training sessions was increased to 80% of the new 1RM result to account for any increases in strength occurring in that time period. Each set consisted of six repetitions with a standardized two minute rest interval observed between sets. Before any training session, a standard warm-up was undertaken by all participants consisting of 10-12 repetitions on the leg extension machine at a low weight appropriate to each individual, or approximately 50% 1RM.

Statistical analysis

As the research hypothesis assumed directionality in strength gain, as a consequence critical values were established using one-tailed tests (i.e., strength gain). Two sets of data (pre-experimental 1RM versus post-experimental 1RM; magnitude of 1RM change) were analysed using paired t-tests to determine if any significant differences existed between the two. Level of significance was set *a priori* at $p<0.05$. Mean improvements in strength for both the two set and three set legs were calculated from initial and end 1RM values.

Results

Of the ten original subjects recruited for this study, only seven successfully completed the entire six week training period. Two subjects voluntarily withdrew from the study for personal reasons and one withdrew due to an injury sustained outside of the investigation. As only complete data sets could be used, data from seven subjects was included in the final analysis. Of the remaining seven participants, three were part of the 3L 2R group, and the other four were in the 3R 2L group.

Table 2 illustrates the mean and standard deviations (SD) 1RM for two sets versus three sets of unilateral leg extension training for the seven subjects. The results are presented in 1RM means (SD) for pre-training, following two weeks, four weeks, and at the end of the six week training program. Intermediate 1RM values (second and fourth weeks) were only used for program modification and not included in statistical analysis of the efficacy of the two or three set training organizations.

Both the two set and three set trained legs experienced large increases in 1RM of 24.2% and 37.9% respectively. Both findings are statistically significant when comparing pre-training and post-training data ($p<0.05$). Comparison of these pre-training and post-training 1RM values between resulted in a $p=0.14$, a value that was not statistically significant.

However, as the intent of the project was to detect any differences between 2 or 3 set groups in the magnitude of change in 1RM following training (Table 3). The magnitude of change elicited was calculated, five (71.4%) of the seven subjects increased their 1RM differentially between legs, favouring the three set intervention. Two subjects (28.6%) experienced similar results between exercise treatments. The average difference in strength gain between two set trained and three set trained legs was 6.9 kg (± 7.2) in favour of three set trained legs. This differential in magnitude of 1RM gain was statistically significant ($p=0.02$) suggesting that there is an authentic difference in the effect of increased training volume (2 sets versus 3 sets) on strength gain.

Discussion

When comparing pre- and post-training strength increases following the 6 week resistance training program, it can be statistically shown that both training with 2 sets and 3 sets per session elicit significant strength gains in the quadriceps muscles of untrained men ($p<0.05$). This finding was expected when considering work of other authors having presented similar conclusions [2,13,18,22]. There have been mixed findings in the literature supporting higher volumes (3 set) being superior to lower volumes (1 set) of training [1,14,33]. Alternatively there is data suggesting that single set training is just as efficient in eliciting strength gain as multiple sets of exercise [13,20]. Most available studies have focused upon comparison of single set exercise organizations and three or more sets of exercise. This small scale study attempted to explore the controversial proposition that that exercise volume (number of sets completed) is directly related to magnitude of strength gain and to examine an intermediary number of sets of exercise, two versus three sets, thus adding further information on the validity of the frequently proposed strength continuum.

The variability in previous findings may have been induced by lack of attention to protocol design. Methods for ensuring equity and accuracy included adjusting the exercise machine relative to specific anatomical landmarks on the individual, employing identical exercise postures between subjects, and ensuring that the range of motion was identical between subjects. Some studies have come under criticism as their results may have been affected by confounding variables such as inappropriate or irregular rest intervals. In this study rest intervals between sets were restricted to two minutes [13,14,20,27,33].

The premise of modern strength training programs is largely based on the general adaptation syndrome theory forwarded by Selye [25]. In Selye's original synthesis, exhaustive exercise was considered a noxious stress, thus the theory's application in modern exercise prescription has to be carefully considered and modified. The crux of the general adaptation syndrome, in application to exercise, is that exercise must induce a non-lethal disruption of homeostasis in a target cell, tissue, organ or system and then the organism must be allowed sufficient opportunity to recover and adapt. This adaption enhances survivability and carries with it improved fitness. The magnitude of loading (sets of exercise at 80% 1RM here) is the external stress that requires adaptation. The very similar nature of the load used in this project, one set versus two sets, and the resulting findings indicate that the body is very capable of an exquisitely sensitive detection of loading magnitudes and adaptive variation.

While the present study found significant differences in elicited strength gain between two and three sets, the examination of differences between immediately sequential ordinal numbers of sets is not common in the literature. Few papers have tested for differences in strength gain between one and two sets and two and three sets. The primary rationale for this exclusion is that in Berger's seminal work comparing one, two, and three sets of exercise it was concluded that one and two sets of exercise is not as effective as three sets [1]. So it is common that single sets are compared to larger multiples of sets [34,35]. Our study is similar to that of Berger in that our findings were that three sets are superior to two sets. In the paper by Limke et al. a discernibly different strength adaption was not seen in trainees following single or two set training protocols [36]. Combined, the present data and that of Limke support the findings presented by Berger. It could be suggested, based on these observations, that a single set and two sets of weighted exercise does not disrupt muscle homeostasis as effectively as three sets as evidenced by the larger magnitude of 1RM increase after three-set training.

There is a limitation in this study that must be considered, the attrition of subjects resulted in a very low final *n*. Despite the low subject numbers, the results are paired and genetically matched. The right and left legs of the subjects each received different training interventions and reduced intra-subject variability between treatments. This is the same genetic pairing approach that enabled elucidation of the mechanism of hypertrophy by Gollnick et al. in 1981 [37]. This pairing enables a more robust comparison of data and strengthens the ability to make relevant conclusions regarding the two treatments.

The magnitude of increase in 1RM was significantly larger for the three set intervention compared to two sets (mean of 19.4 kg compared to 12.6 kg). These increases may be specific to machine exercise in magnitude and time course. Free weights represent a potentially larger homeostatic disruption than possible with machine weights, as machines have pre-determined movement patterns not requiring contributions from synergists active in coordinated movement of free weights or in the maintenance of balance. The use of machine weights may also have affected both 1RM testing and training progression. The leg extension machine used was designed to allow resistance increases in 4 kg increments. This placed a limitation in sensitivity of 1RM testing as any strength gain of less than 4 kg would have been undetectable. This could have resulted in an under-representation of 1RM. The limitation in increment to 4 kg may also have affected loading and resulted in lower weights being used in training than potentially supported by subject adaptive capacity. Neither of these issues could have been avoided given the equipment available. Future studies should consider using free weight exercises as weight addition increments can be accommodated down to 0.25 kg.

Conclusions and Practical Implications

This study demonstrated that a three times per week and six week duration machine resistance training program, using six repetitions and either two sets or three sets of leg extension exercise with 80% 1RM will elicit significant increases in quadriceps muscle strength. However, three sets of exercise increased the magnitude of strength gain by an additional 53.9% over two sets of exercise. These findings suggest that practitioners can indeed produce significant strength gains using two sets, which may be of value to trainers and coaches working with time limited individuals. However, three sets were clearly more effective in producing a change in strength. Given that the additional time to do a third set is two additional minutes for recovery and less than a minute for conduct of the third exercise set, this may mitigate against the rationale of not doing a third set in the interest of saving time.

References

1. Berger RA (1962) Effect of varied weight training programs on strength. Research Quarterly 33: 168-181.
2. Carpinelli RN, Otto RM (1998) Strength training. Single versus multiple sets Sports Med 26: 73-84.
3. Fleck S, Kraemer W (1997) Designing resistance-training programs. (2nd edn), Human Kinetics, Champaign, USA.

4. McDonagh MJ, Davies CT (1984) Adaptive response of mammalian skeletal muscle to exercise with high loads. Eur J Appl Physiol Occup Physiol 52: 139-155.

5. Pollock ML, Wilmore JH (1990) Exercise in health and disease. (2nd Edn), W.B. Saunders, Philadelphia, USA.

6. Artero EG, Lee DC, Lavie CJ, España-Romero V, Sui X, et al. (2012) Effects of muscular strength on cardiovascular risk factors and prognosis. J Cardiopulm Rehabil Prev 32: 351-358.

7. Fiatarone MA, O'Neill EF, Ryan ND, Clements KM, Solares GR, et al. (1994) Exercise training and nutritional supplementation for physical frailty in very elderly people. N Engl J Med 330: 1769-1775.

8. Marsh AP, Rejeski WJ, Espeland MA, Miller ME, Church TS, et al. (2011) Muscle strength and BMI as predictors of major mobility disability in the Lifestyle Interventions and Independence for Elders pilot (LIFE-P). J Gerontol A Biol Sci Med Sci 66: 1376-1383.

9. Jackson AW, Lee DC, Sui X, Morrow JR Jr, Church TS, et al. (2010) Muscular strength is inversely related to prevalence and incidence of obesity in adult men. Obesity (Silver Spring) 18: 1988-1995.

10. Ruiz JR, Sui X, Lobelo F, Morrow JR Jr, Jackson AW, et al. (2008) Association between muscular strength and mortality in men: prospective cohort study. BMJ 337: a439.

11. Ortega FB, Silventoinen K, Tynelius P, Rasmussen F (2012) Muscular strength in male adolescents and premature death: cohort study of one million participants. BMJ 345: e7279.

12. Galvão DA, Taaffe DR (2004) Single- vs. multiple-set resistance training: recent developments in the controversy. J Strength Cond Res 18: 660-667.

13. Hass CJ, Garzarella L, de Hoyos D, Pollock ML (2000) Single versus multiple sets in long-term recreational weightlifters. Med Sci Sports Exerc 32: 235-242.

14. Kraemer WJ (1997) A series of studies: The physiological basis for strength training in American football: Facto over philosophy. J Strength Cond Res. 11: 131-142

15. Kraemer WJ, Ratamess N, Fry AC, Triplett-McBride T, Koziris LP, et al. (2000) Influence of resistance training volume and periodization on physiological and performance adaptations in collegiate women tennis players. Am J Sports Med 28: 626-633.

16. Marx JO, Ratamess NA, Nindl BC, Gotshalk LA, Volek JS, et al. (2001) Low-volume circuit versus high-volume periodized resistance training in women. Med Sci Sports Exerc 33: 635-643.

17. De Hoyos DV, Herring D, Garzarella L, Weber G, et al. (1997) Effect of strength training volume on the development of strength and power in adolescent tennis players. Med Sci Sports Exerc 29: 164.

18. De Hoyos DV, Herring D, Abe T, Garzarella L (1998) Effect of 6 months of high- or low-volume resistance training on muscular strength and endurance. Med Sci Sports Exerc 30: 165.

19. Silvester LJ, Stiggins C, McGown C, Bryce R (1982) Effect of variable resistance and free-weight training programs on strength and vertical jump. Natl Str Cond Assoc J 3: 30-33.

20. Stadler Jr VL, Stubbs NB, Vokovich M D (1997) A comparison of a 2-day and 3-day per week resistance training program on strength gain in older adults. Med Sci Sports Exerc. 29: 254

21. Tim Stowers, Jim McMillan, Dwight Scala, Voris Davis, Dennis Wilson, et al. (1983) The short term effects of three different strength-power training modes. Natl Str Cond Assoc J 5: 24-27.

22. Vincent K, DeHoyos D, Garzarella L, Hass C, Nordman M, et al. (1998) Relationship between indices of knee extension strength before and after resistance training. Med Sci Sports Exerc 30: 163.

23. Byrd R, Chandler TJ, Conley MS, Fry AC, Haff GG, et al. (1999) Strength training: single versus multiple sets. Sports Med 27: 409-416.

24. Krieger JW (2010) Single vs. multiple sets of resistance exercise for muscle hypertrophy: a meta-analysis. J Strength Cond Res 24: 1150-1159.

25. Selye H (1936) A syndrome produced by diverse nocuous agents. Nature 138: 32.

26. Rippetoe M, Kilgore L (2009) Practical Programming for Strength Training (2nd Edn), Aasgaard Company, Wichita Falls TX, USA.

27. Kramer JB, Stone MH, O'Bryant HS, Conley MS, Robert L Johnson, et al. (1997) Effects of single vs. multiple-sets of weight training: impact of volume, Intensity, and variation. J Strength Cond Res. 11: 143-147.

28. Schlumberger A, Stec J, Schmidtbleicher D (2001) Single- vs. multiple-set strength training in women. J Strength Cond Res 15: 284-289.

29. Ostrowski K, Wilson G, Weatherby R, Murphy P, Andrew D Lyttle (1997) The effects of weight training volume on hormonal output and muscular size and function. J Strength Cond Res 11: 154.

30. Campos GE, Luecke TJ, Wendeln HK, Toma K, Hagerman FC, et al. (2002) Muscular adaptations in response to three different resistance-training regimens: specificity of repetition maximum training zones. Eur J Appl Physiol 88: 50-60.

31. Starr B (2007) Strongest Shall Survive: Strength training for football. Five Starr Productions, Baltimore MD, USA.

32. American College of Sports Medicine (2009) American College of Sports Medicine position stand. Progression models in resistance training for healthy adults. Med Sci Sports Exerc 41: 687-708.

33. Rhea MR, Alvar BA, Ball SD, Burkett LN (2002) Three sets of weight training superior to 1 set with equal intensity for eliciting strength. J Strength Cond Res 16: 525-529.

34. Kelly SB, Brown LE, Coburn JW, Zinder SM, Gardner LM, et al. (2007) The effect of single versus multiple sets on strength. J Strength Cond Res 21: 1003-1006.

35. Munn J, Herbert RD, Hancock MJ, Gandevia SC (2005) Resistance training for strength: effect of number of sets and contraction speed. Med Sci Sports Exerc 37: 1622-1626.

36. Limke JC, Rainville J, Peña E, Childs L (2008) Randomized trial comparing the effects of one set vs two sets of resistance exercises for outpatients with chronic low back pain and leg pain. Eur J Phys Rehabil Med 44: 399-405.

37. Gollnick PD, Timson BF, Moore RL, Riedy M (1981) Muscular enlargement and number of fibers in skeletal muscles of rats. J Appl Physiol Respir Environ Exerc Physiol 50: 936-943.

The Eurycoma Longifolia Freeze-Dried Water Extract-Physta® Does not Change Normal Ratios of Testosterone to Epitestosterone in Healthy Males

George A[1]*, Liske E[2], Chen CK[3] and Ismail SB[4]

[1]*Biotropics Malaysia Berhad, Lot 21, Jalan U1/19, Section U1, Hicom-Glenmarie Industrial Park, 40150 Shah Alam, Selangor, Malaysia*
[2]*Departments of Life Sciences, Technical University of Braunschweig, Germany*
[3]*Sports Science Unit, School of Medical Sciences, Universiti Sains Malaysia, Malaysia*
[4]*Department of Family Medicine, School of Medical Sciences, Universiti Sains Malaysia, Malaysia*

Abstract

Eurycoma longifolia is traditionally known for its adaptogenic properties and often used for the general well-being and increased performance in daily life.

Methods: In a randomized, double blind, placebo-controlled clinical trial, 40 Malaysian men aged 30-55 years performed a battery of physical testings during which the ratio of Testosterone (T) to Epitestosterone (E) was analyzed. The daily intake was 300 mg of the freeze-dried water extract of Eurycoma longifolia root (Physta®, Biotropics Malaysia) or placebo for a period of 12 weeks.

Results: At the end of the study the T/E-ratio in the herbal group ranged from 0.03 to 2.95 and was not significantly different from values at baseline (p=0.49). Further, the ratio-values for E. longifolia compared to placebo did not change over time. The weight lifting force which measures muscular strength using back & leg strength test, increased significantly from baseline to end of the study in the herbal group by approximately 14 kg (p=0.0166).

Conclusion: The ratios of testosterone to epitestosterone did not change during a 12-weeks E. longifolia intake. The data suggest that this herb does not exhibit "doping"- like effects. Instead, muscular strength improved significantly in the back and leg with E. longifolia supplementation rendering this herb good for physical performance minus the doping effects.

Keywords: Eurycoma longifolia; Strength; Quality of life; Doping; Testosterone; Epitestosterone

Introduction

It is a common human attitude to want to perform better, particularly in sports and tournaments/competitions. The desire to be better with the use of banned performance-enhancing drugs is considered to be "doping". Anti-doping rules and testing have been established as an independent and globally accepted standard by the World Anti-Doping Agency (WADA) [1]. Biochemical measurements for the ratio of Testosterone ("T") to Epitestosterone ("E") are often used in the fight against doping. The hormones are endogenously built in the body and T increases protein-synthesis resulting in growth of cellular tissue, especially in muscles ("anabolic steroids"), whereas E is an inactive isomer of testosterone. In general, the normal ratio of T to E in urine samples is found similar to be 1:1.

Due to the intake of anabolic steroids or products with similar function, testosterone levels increases while E levels remain stable, resulting in a change in T/E-ratio from normal levels. In 2005, a threshold of T/E-ratio higher than 4:1 (>4) was considered by the WADA as a proof of exogenous intake of anabolic substances [2]. The significance of these measures as well as factors which may influence and possibly facilitate false-positive results have been discussed controversially, e.g., non-steroidal products capable of changing T/E-ratio, specified/non-specified stimulants, pathological androgen metabolism, individual genetic variations and enzyme polymorphism [1-4].

Adaptogenic substances, including many herbal medicines have been used traditionally with the goal of increasing physical performance. The history of herbs in sports can be traced back to ancient Greek [5]. Famous examples of herbs for sports purposes are among others Panax ginseng, caffeine, and ephedrine and Eurycoma longifolia E. longifolia, also known as "Tongkat ali" or "Malaysian ginseng", is well-known in Southeast Asian countries and used traditionally for the general well-being and better performance in daily living [5-9]. In a randomized, double-blind placebo controlled trial, healthy male subjects on E. longifolia experienced significant improvement in physical functioning, one of the 9 domains found in the SF-36 Quality of Life questionnaire [9]. The question items in this domain were on moderate and vigorous activities, climbing, bending and kneeling, walking, and bathing/dressing, role physical, and vitality. The supplementation with E. longifolia improved strength in physically active male and female seniors between 57 and 72 years of age in an open pilot study and additionally increased muscle mass and fat free mass in men, in another study [10,11]. The ergogenic properties of the herb appear prevalent in these studies. The proandrogenic effect on the laevator ani muscle by an increase in its weight was also seen in rats [12]. It was shown that E. longifolia contains the presence of a 4.3 kDa peptide which increases testosterone levels in rat leydig cells [13]. However, a few clinical data on the effects of E. longifolia in exercise performance are available, such as endurance bicycling and running which still render non-conclusive the effect of E. longifolia in sports performance [6].

***Corresponding author:** Annie George, Biotropics Malaysia Berhad, Lot 21, Jalan U1/19, Section U1, Hicom-Glenmarie Industrial Park, 40150 Shah Alam, Selangor, Malaysia, E-mail: annvalu@yahoo.com

Here we report the non-doping effects and the benefits in sport performance during a 12-weeks treatment of Eurycoma longifolia. These data were obtained as an addendum from a randomized, placebo-controlled trial on the quality of life and sexual well-being in men [9].

Methods

Study design and subjects

The randomized, double-blind, placebo-controlled and parallel group study was performed at the Clinical Trial Unit (CTU), Hospital Universiti Sains Malaysia (HUSM), Kubang Kerian, Malaysia. It was conducted in accordance with the Guideline for Good Clinical Practice (ICH-6), Declaration of Helsinki and approved by the Human Research and Ethics Committee for Clinical Studies at HUSM (approval date 24 Dec 2008). An addendum to approve additional endpoints was approved by the Ethics Committee for Clinical Studies at HUSM on 23 Dec 2009 (Ref. USM/PPP/Ethics Com./2009(146)).

One hundred and nine healthy Malaysian men aged between 30 years to 55 years were included. The inclusion/exclusion criteria, randomization and intervention, primary and secondary endpoints as well as sample size estimation and statistical analyses for the study are described in detail in Ismail et al. [9]. Forty subjects agreed for an additional doping test (verum: n=21; placebo: n=19). The subjects were randomly selected and were from the tail end of the ongoing (larger population) study. The additional doping test was added to the protocol at mid-way of the study (larger population) to address possible doping effects upon suggestions by the local Sports Council. The investigators, subjects and study coordinators were double blinded and the products were randomized prior to shipment to the Investigators. The information of the product whether placebo or treatment were sealed in an envelope labeled with the corresponding randomization number and could only be broken upon occurrence of serious adverse event or at the completion of the trial, during data analysis. The envelope containing information of the subjects was checked to ensure there was no breaking of seal.

The subjects were non-athletes and were instructed not to participate in any form of physical training during the study period. A total of four interval visits were scheduled for the entire study: screening (visit 1, week -1 to week-2), measurements taken at baseline (visit 2, day 0: randomisation), at week-6 (visit 3, day 42 ± 3 days) and end-of-study at week-12 (visit 4, day 84 ± 3 days) followed by a follow-up visit (visit 5 at week-14, via telephone or face to face). At screening (visit 1), clinical examinations and interviews were conducted to select subjects who fulfilled the study criteria. Blood samples were collected from the subjects for routine health check (hematological, renal and liver parameters) and Prostatic Specific Antigen (PSA). At each other visit (V2, V3, V4) Physical Fitness Testings were performed (see Methods 2.3). The primary endpoints for the ratio of hormonal values for Testosterone (T) to Epitestosterone (E) were taken at baseline (V2) and end of the study (V4). The safety was assessed based on documented Adverse Events, physical examinations, clinical and laboratory measures as published [9].

Study medication

Each subject consumed four capsules per day containing either herbal extract or placebo. One capsule contained 75 mg of freeze-dried water extract of Eurycoma longifolia root (Physta®, Biotropics Malaysia Berhad, Kuala Lumpur, Malaysia) as active ingredients, manufactured under Good Manufacturing Process requirements (GMP) with continuous quality control (DER 20:1). Consumption of 500 to 1000 mg root extracts has been reported traditionally, and clinical data show safe consumption of the water soluble extract between 200 to 600 mg [7,14]. Since the present investigation was the first randomized, placebo controlled clinical trial in a large population, a middle range of 300 mg/day extract was selected. The total daily intake was therefore 300 mg/day herbal extract. The placebo medication (containing maltodextrin) was identical to the active medication however without the herbal extract.

Procedures for the physical fitness tests

Tests for physical fitness were performed: each session of the physical fitness tests contained a battery of different types of tests so that various physiological and muscular parameters could be activated/stimulated, finally leading to an improvement of these fitness activities: flexibility-(type of test: Sit & Reach), muscular strength (Hand grip; Back & Leg), muscular endurance (Sit-up & Push up) and body composition (Bioelectrical Impedance Analysis). All these tests were carried out on the same day for each participants and the duration took approximately two hours for each session of five to eight subjects.

Sit and reach: The subjects sat on the floor with legs stretched out straight ahead. They were bare-footed and the soles of the feet are placed flat against the sit and reach box. Both knees were locked and pressed flat to the floor. With the palms facing downwards, and the hands on top of each other, the subjects were told to reach forward along the measuring line as far as possible. Then, the subjects hold that position for at least two seconds while the distance was recorded. The subjects were given three trials and the longest distance to the nearest centimeter reached was noted.

Hand grip: The subjects held the hydraulic hand dynamometer (Jamar, United Kingdom) in the hand to be tested, with the arm at right angles and the elbow by the side of the body. The handle of the dynamometer was adjusted if required and the base was rested on the first metacarpal (heel of palm), while the handle rested on the middle of four fingers. Then, the subjects squeezed the dynamometer with maximum isometric effort, which was maintained for about 5 seconds. No other body movement was allowed. The subjects were strongly encouraged to give a maximum effort. The best result in kilograms from three trials for the dominant hand was recorded, with at least 15 seconds recovery between each effort.

Back and leg strength: The subjects stood upright on the base of the back and leg dynamometer (VacuMed, USA: http://www.vacumed.com/images/12-0403.JPG) with their feet shoulder width apart. They were instructed to hang their arms straight down to hold the centre of the bar with both hands, and with the palms facing toward the body. The chain was adjusted so that the knees are bent at approximately 110 degrees. In this position the subjects' back are bent slightly forward at the hips, their heads held upright and looking look straight ahead. Then without bending their backs, they pulled as hard as possible on the chain and try to straighten their legs while keeping their arms straight. Additionally, they were told to pull against the weight steadily whilst keeping the feet flat on the base of the dynamometer. The subjects were reminded that maximum performance will result when their legs are almost straight at the end of the lift. The best result in kilograms from three trials was recorded, with at least 15 seconds recovery between each effort.

Sit-up: The subjects lay on a carpeted floor with their knees bent at approximately right angles, with feet flat on the ground. They were instructed to rest their hands on their thighs. Then, they pushed their backs flat and raised high enough for their hands to slide along their thighs to touch the tops of their knees. They were also reminded not to pull with their necks or heads and to keep their lower backs on the floor. They were required to do as many sit-ups as possible in one minute. The number of sit-ups performed in one minute was recorded.

Push-up: The subjects were instructed to use the standard "military style" push-up position with only the hands and the toes touching the floor in the starting position. They were told to lower the chest down towards the floor, always to the same level each time, either till their elbows was at right angles or their chests touch the ground. They were required to do as many push-ups as possible in one minute. The number of push-ups performed in one minute was recorded.

Body composition: A body fat analyzer (Omron HBF 306, Japan) was used to analyze the percent body fat of the subjects. Personal information such as age, gender, weight and height were keyed into the analyzer. Then the subjects were told to grip the device handles and held arms straight out at a 90° angle to the body. Percent body fat, fat mass content and Body Mass Index was calculated automatically in seconds.

Analysis of testosterone T/epitestosterone E

The analysis of urine samples was performed by the Doping Control Centre, Penang, a NATA -accredited laboratory (National Association of Testing Authorities, Australia). The quantification of T/E ratio was determined by Gas Chromatography–Mass Spectrometry (GC-MS). The free and conjugated T and E were extracted by solid phase extraction using the Nexus (Varian) column combined with liquid-liquid extraction using tert-Butyl methyl ether, followed by hydrolysis using enzyme β-glucuronidase from Esherichia Coli K12 (Roche Diagnostics Mannheim, Germany); extracts were then derivatized with activated N-methyl-N-(trimethylsilyl)-trifluoroacetamide (MSTFA). The calibration of T was performed using concentration levels of between 2 ng/mL and 80 ng/mL while the values for E were between 2 ng/mL to 20 ng/mL. Selected ion monitoring mode with electron ionization on the GC-MS was used for identification and quantification of both T and E.

Statistical analyses

Detailed description on the statistical evaluation was already published elsewhere [9]. Data was explored and descriptive statistical analysis was conducted to measure changes in the parameters between E. longifolia and placebo groups at baseline, week 6 and/or end of treatment. Mean (SEM, standard error of the mean) were used for continuous variables of normality distributed data and median (IQR, inter quartile range) for non-normal distribution. The ratio T/E is visualized by Box-Whisker-Plots, showing the spread of the set of data without any assumption of the underlying data distribution. Independent t-test and non-parametric test (as appropriate, Mann-Whitney) were used for comparison of the two randomized groups. Significant changes in the parameters are referred to a p-value of ≤ 0.05.

Results

Forty males agreed for the additional testings: Verum n=21, age (mean ± SD) 45.19 ± 5.37 years (range 30-54 years); Placebo n=19, age 44.63 ± 7.05 years (30-52 years). The flowchart of the study design, bibliographic as well as clinical baseline data of these subjects is listed elsewhere [9].

Hormones

During treatment, hormonal values for Total Testosterone (TT), Free Testosterone (FT), Dehydroepiandrosterone-SO4 (DHEA), the metabolic intermediate in biosynthesis of androgens and Sexual Hormone Binding Globulin (SHBG), the testosterone carrier protein were analyzed for the two treatment groups and are shown in Table 1. There were slight increasing trends in almost all of the values during E. longifolia intake from baseline (V2) to end of study (V4), however, none reached significance: TT median V2-V4: 15.3-16.5 nmol/L (p=0.34), FT 31.4-34.9 pmol/L (p=0.24), SHBG 22.6-25.2 nmol/L (p=0.86). The hormone DHEA increased by 13.6% from baseline (4.2 μmol/L) after 6 weeks (p=0.25), however, at the end of treatment, the value dropped back to the basic value (4.23 μmol/L, p=0.87).

In the placebo-group, FT and DHEA showed increasing values compared to baseline, at the end of trial, (after 12 weeks) (V2-V4: 32.4-36.5 pmol/L; p=0.58) and 3.6-4.5 μmol/L; p=0.62) respectively. Comparisons between groups demonstrated no significant deviations over time for all the hormonal values except for SHBG, which already had a significantly higher starting value in the placebo group at baseline (V2: p=0.03).

Ratio Testosterone to Epitestosterone

After 12 weeks, the T/E-ratio values in the E. longifolia group ranged from 0.03 to 2.95 with a median of 0.2 (n=21) compared to a median (V2) of 0.16 (n=3) at baseline as shown in Figure 1. This would mean no changes occurred in the hormonal relationship during herbal treatment (p= 0.49). At the end of the study, approximately 91%

Hormones	*Eurycoma longifolia*			Placebo		
	Baseline V2 (n=21) Median IQR Mean (SEM)	**6 weeks V3** (n=21) Median IQR Mean (SEM)	**12 weeks V4** (n=21) Median IQR Mean (SEM)	**Baseline V2** (n=19) Median IQR Mean (SEM)	**6 weeks V3** (n=18) Median IQR Mean (SEM)	**12 weeks V4** (n=17) Median IQR Mean (SEM)
Total Testosterone (nmol/L)	15.3 11.4-19.15 15.89 (1.15)	12.6 10.35-18.35 14.40 (1.12)	16.5 12.35-20.35 16.77 (1.25)	19.8 14.0-21.3 18.72 (1.16)	21.05 16.5-22.25 19.93 (1.41)	19.4 13.55-24.05 18.79 (1.49)
Free Testosterone (pmol/L)	31.4 25.35-40.55 32.53 (2.16)	33.7 22.75-40.4 31.84 (2.17)	34.9 29.5-40.05 35.41 (2.88)	32.4 27.0-40.5 35.01 (2.61)	33.85 26.9-43.4 34.48 (2.81)	36.5 30.4-45.65 37.37 (2.88)
DHEA (μmol/L)	4.1 3.2- 5.4 4.4 (0.4)	3.9 2.9-5.9 4.86 (0.75)	4.0 3.05-5.8 4.23 (0.37)	3.6 2.9-5.3 4.15 (0.31)	4.0 2.85-5.13 4.14 (0.37)	4.5 3.15-5.5 4.36 (0.34)
SHBG (nmol/L)	22.6 17.95-29.45 25.44 (2.4)	22.9 17.85-32.6 24.27 (1.98)	25.2 15.3-30.0 25.27 (2.39)	30.8 26.5-33.3 32.03 (1.87)	30.1 26.1-37.13 33.59 (2.8)	29 26.15-38.35 33.41 (3.02)

Table 1: Testosterone (free and total), Dehydroepiandrosterone (DHEA) and the Sexual Hormone Binding Globulin (SHBG) for the two treatment groups over time.

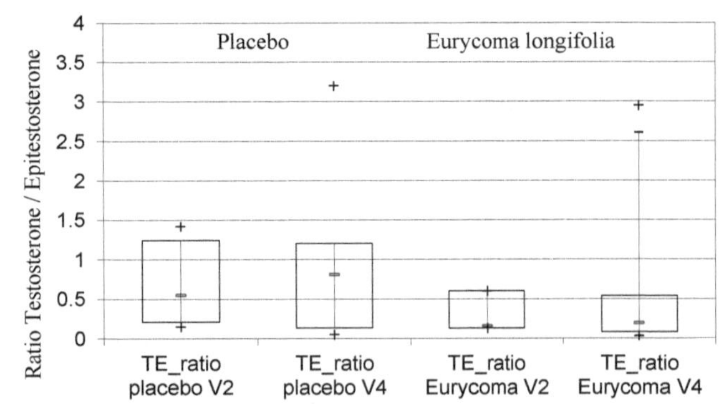

Figure 1: Box-whisker-plot of the ratio testosterone (T) to epitestosterone (E) at baseline (V2) and end of trial after 12 weeks (V4) for both treatment groups. Shown are the median (small line within the box) with interquartile range ICR (upper and lower quartile), 5th and 95th percentiles and minimum and maximum values (+).

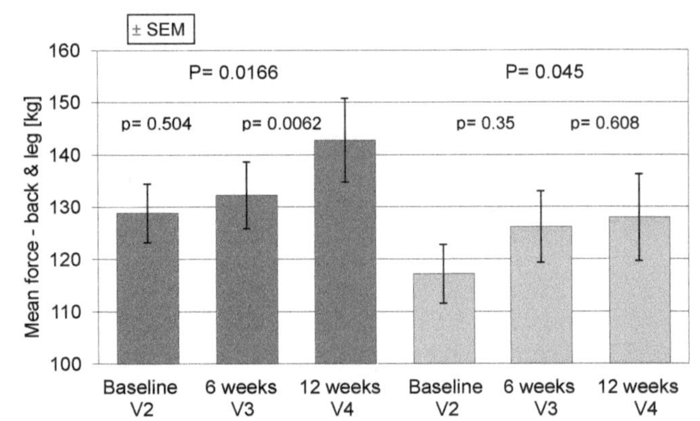

Figure 2: Mean amount of weight lifting force (kg) for one repetition at muscular strength training during treatment of Eurycoma longifolia (black bars) and placebo (grey bars).

of the subjects had T/E-ratios of up to 1, which is considered to be a "normal" ratio. Similar data were obtained in the placebo group: after 12 weeks, the T/E-ratio values ranged from 0.05 to 3.3 with a median of 0.81 (n=18). Roughly 72% of the subjects had T/E-ratios of up to 1. At baseline, the median value was 0.55 (n=4), demonstrating no changes during treatment (p= 0.82). Between group comparisons showed no statistical differences in the ratios of testosterone to epitestosterone: V2 -EL/placebo: p=0.33; V4 -EL/Placebo: p=0.11). Almost all single values measured in both treatment groups fall within the interquartile range IQR (lower quartile: 25% value and upper: 75% value), except for the minimum and maximum values as well as the 95th percentile value of the T/E ratio in the E. longifolia group (Figure 1).

Physical fitness tests

Flexibility (sit & reach), muscular strength testing: back & leg (kg), hand grip (kg), muscular endurance: sit-up and push-up (times/min) as well as body composition: percent body fat (%) were measured at screening (V1), 6 weeks (V3) and end of treatment visits (V4).

In all the fitness settings no noticeable changes and significant beneficial effects were observed either within treatment groups or between group comparisons, except for back and leg muscular strengths.

The amount of strength the subjects can exert for one repetition during treatment is shown in Figure 2. At baseline (V2), subjects in the E. longifolia group who started with mean ± SEM strength of 128.81 kg ± 5.63 kg (range: 75 kg-196 kg, n=21), increased to 132.26 kg ± 6.39 kg (82 kg-195 kg, n=19) at 6 weeks (V3) and finally reached mean values of 142.78 kg ± 7.95 kg (70 kg-205 kg, n=18) after 12 weeks of treatment (V4). This increase with an approximately 14 kg strength from baseline to end of the study was highly significant with p=0.0166 and from V3 (6 weeks) to V4 (12 weeks) with p=0.0062. In contrast, subjects in the placebo group had a moderate gain (approx. 10.8 kg) in back and leg strength with mean values of 128 kg ± 8.31 kg, n=13 at the end of the trial compared to baseline mean values (117.21 kg ± 5.62 kg, n=19), barely reaching significance (p=0.045).

Discussion

The supplementation of 300 mg per day of Eurycoma longifolia root water extract in healthy middle-aged men, for a period of 12 weeks, was evaluated here for the ratio of Testosterone (T) to Epitestosterone (E) and physical fitness. To the best of our knowledge, this anti-doping measurement, established by the WADA, was applied for the first time in a controlled clinical trial with E. longifolia intake.

In none of the analyzed subjects were the T/E-ratios greater than 4 observed: a threshold which is considered by WADA as an adverse analytical finding requiring further investigations of the individuals. The maximum T/E-ratio of 2.95 was observed after daily intake of 300 mg of E. longifolia water extract. The majority of subjects (>90%) had T/E-ratios of up to 1, in the treatment group. The highest ratio for subjects on placebo was 3.3 and more than 72% of the subjects had values of up to 1. Since between-group comparisons showed no noteworthy and statistical significance, the results show that a 12 weeks treatment with 300 mg daily of E. longifolia water extract did not interfere with the normal ratio of testosterone to epitestosterone in middle-aged active and healthy men.

Several other hormones involved in the androgenic metabolism were analyzed in this study: total (TT) and Free Testosterone (FT), Dehydroepiandrosterone (-Sulfate) (DHEA) and sex-hormone binding globulin (SHBG). Although increasing values of these parameters ranging from 7% to 11% could be observed during E. longifolia extract intake, it did not reach significance when compared to baseline or when comparing with the placebo-group. However, literature on E. longifolia states conflicting results on its' influence in androgenic hormones. It is reported in animal studies that the anabolic action of this herb is in increasing levels of testosterone and human studies suggested that this herb facilitates the production of testosterone by reducing SHBG, thus releasing free circulating testosterone [15,16]. The study, randomized to various doses of standardized E. longifolia extract (200-600 mg daily), showed testosterone and DHEAS at "high normal levels" compared to baseline, in middle aged subjects, after an 8-weeks treatment (statistics were not mentioned in the reference) [17]. In another placebo controlled study, thirty male endurance cyclist, received either 100 mg E. longifolia–water extract (n=15) or placebo (n=15); approximately 30 minutes before and after each of a four 14.91 miles laps, in a high-intensity 24-hrs bicycling program [18]. Supplementation of E. longifolia resulted in testosterone levels 16.4% higher while cortisol levels were 32% lower when compared to placebo (p<0.05). The biochemical profile of the cyclists appeared to be in an anabolic hormonal state. In hypogonadic men who have low serum testosterone levels, E. longifolia supplementation was able to significantly increase testosterone levels to normal levels as well [19].

While the role of testosterone is known to affect muscles [20], the role of E. longifolia may not only be limited to testosterone enhancing. In this study, the muscle strengthening effect did not appear to be related to a significant increase in testosterone hormones. This is probably due to E. longifolia purportedly being a natural adaptogenic energizer in the maintenance and healthy ageing in men, suggesting E. longifolia's role in optimizing testosterone levels only when sup-optimal [21]. It can be suggested that E. longifolia supplementation does not indiscriminately increase testosterone levels as do exogenous testosterone supplementation but modulates to optimal levels according to ones' current hormonal levels. Furthermore, the standardized water extract of E. longifolia (Physta®) contains >22% protein and peptides possibly adding to the ergogenic benefit despite non-significant elevation of testosterone [13,22]. Hence, future studies on the role of the active ingredients in E. longifolia on the contractile properties of the muscles are warranted.

According to recently published reviews on herbs/botanicals including E. longifolia, dietary supplements and herbal medicines, only little conclusive clinical evidence is available to justify the herb's effects on exercise and sports performance [5,6]. Nevertheless, in this study, the test for muscular strength resulted in significant effects after 12-weeks of Eurycoma-extract intake. There was a highly significant 14 kg improvement (approx. 10% increase) in back and leg strength after 12 weeks (142.78 kg) of E. longifolia intake compared to baseline (128.81 kg; $p=0.0166$). Placebo-group only reached values of up to 10.8 kg (approx. 8% increase) with a borderline significance of $p=0.045$. No significant changes in hand grip strength was observed in this study although in physically active male and female seniors aged between 57-72 years of age, increased muscle strength (measured similarly with a hand grip dynamometer) accompanied with significant testosterone elevation, was observed with E. longifolia supplementation of 5 weeks [10]. The ages of the subjects in this study was below 55 years hence the effect of E. longifolia may be more intense in older subjects where sub optimal levels of testosterone normally occurs. An elevation of testosterone in the older subjects may have therefore contributed to the significant improvement of handgrip strength. The precise mechanism attributing to increase in muscular strength is currently inconclusive since in some studies it is accompanied by testosterone elevation and in others, it either did not increase or was not tested. This is particularly important as strength training can provide functional benefits (ergogenic properties): improve general health and well-being as seen in both groups of this study, however, with an enhanced effect present in the E. longifolia group.

There were also other studies demonstrating possible ergogenic properties of E. longifolia. In one randomized placebo-controlled trial, both groups on either 100 mg E. longifolia-extract or placebo, demonstrated a significant increase in muscle strength after 5 weeks of intensive strength training program. However the increase was larger in the treatment (herbal) group compared to the placebo: 6.78% ($p=0.006$) vs. 2.77% ($p=0.011$) respectively [11]. Subjects on E. longifolia extract had improved significantly in fat-free mass, fat mass, maximal strength (1-RM) and arm circumference when compared to the placebo group. This data corresponds with data from our study where a similar increase of muscle strength (approximately 10% compared to 6.78%) demonstrated by the back and leg strength test during E. longifolia intake, was observed. This study however did not measure testosterone levels.

The supplementation with E. longifolia did not significantly affect flexibility of the subjects evaluated through the 'sit and reach' activity. The mechanism of action for this herb is likely to be proandrogenic whereby testosterone is unlikely to affect the flexibility of subjects [13].

Other studies evaluating endurance were unable to demonstrate the effect of E. longifolia [23,24]. In a previous trial, 12 male athletes (mean age 23.3 years) who received 2 capsules of 75 mg E. longifolia-extract or placebo for 7 days, 1 hour before a 60 min run on the treadmill, showed no changes in running distance and physical responses compared to placebo [23]. In addition, in a separate study, six male cyclists who received a low-dose of E. longifolia medication (0.67 mg), showed no improvement in cycling performance and physical parameters [24]. In this current study, no significant changes were observed in muscular endurance evaluated through Sit-up and Push-ups. In these three situations, it is possible that supplementation of E. longifolia could not affect sports endurance of the subjects which is also dependent on aerobic fitness levels. Furthermore, a short supplementation period (7 days) and low dosage (0.67 mg) of E.longifolia may have also contributed to the lackluster performance of the subjects. In a trial of endurance cyclists supplemented with 100 mg of E. longifolia in a 24-hr mountain biking event, cortisol levels were 32% lower and testosterone levels were 16% higher in supplemented subjects compared to placebo, indicating a biochemical profile that promotes an "anabolic" hormonal state during the intense endurance exercise [18]. The type of exercise which engage different muscle group, anaerobic or aerobic exercise may play a role in the effectiveness of E. longifolia. In the exercise that engaged the larger muscle group such as quadriceps in intense cycling and back muscles in back and leg strength exercises, a beneficial effect of E. longifolia was invoked. Both strength training and intense cycling are primarily anaerobic. Anabolic activity is primarily during anaerobic respiration and was observed in the intense cycling [18]. Hence, it is possible that E. longifolia affects muscle strength in an anaerobic state than endurance which is influenced by aerobic fitness levels such as running and moderate cycling [24,25].

The body fat composition remained unchanged in this study. This was also the case in the larger population [9]. Only in men with BMB>25 kg/m^2 was fat loss observed. Overall, the size of the population may be too small to reach statistical significance in other parameters within the physical fitness test and hormonal profiles especially the androgenic hormones. The subjects were also non athletes hence may not actually be physically motivated to be evaluated in physical fitness, leading to poorer performance overall in the fitness test. A population of athletes or recreational athletes could be evaluated in the future to gauge E. longifolia as an effective supplement for sports performance. Additionally, it could be that the study duration of 12 weeks may have been too short and the given daily dose of E. longifolia was not optimal for the desired effect in all physical tests.

Besides ergogenic benefits, the supplementation with E. longifolia may have other beneficial effects, e.g. increase in physical performance, vigor and calmer mood [10,25-28]. An overall clarity of mind and mood elevation accompanied by vigor and muscle strength could be an additional useful attribute in a supplement for sports enthusiast in the future.

Conclusion

The ratio of testosterone to epitestosterone was measured for the first time in healthy males during a 12 weeks intake of 300 mg/day Eurycoma longifolia-extract (Physta®), in a randomized, double-blind and placebo-controlled trial. In both treatment groups, the T/E ratio was normal and below 4. A significant increase in muscle strength was observed for the herbal group compared to placebo in the back and leg strength test though muscular endurance, flexibility and body fat composition remained unchanged with 300 mg daily dose of Eurycoma longifolia over 12 weeks.

Acknowledgements

We would like to thank the phyto-pharmaceutical company Biotropics Malaysia Berhad, Kuala Lumpur, Malaysia, for financial support of the clinical trial.

References

1. World Anti-Doping Agency (WADA) February 19, 2013.
2. Wood RI, Stanton SJ (2012) Testosterone and sport: current perspectives. Horm Behav 61: 147-155.
3. Mareck U, Geyer H, Fusshöller G, Schwenke A, Haenelt N, et al. (2010) Reporting and managing elevated testosterone/epitestosterone ratios--novel aspects after five years' experience. Drug Test Anal 2: 637-642.
4. Anielski P, Simmchen J, Wassill L, Ganghofner D, Thieme D (2011) Epidemiological investigation of the UGT2B17 polymorphism in doping control urine samples and its correlation to T/E ratios. Drug Test Anal 3: 645-651.
5. Stafford ML (2012) Dietary supplements and botanicals in sports: evidence, regulation, and doping controversies. HerbalGram 96: 55-63.
6. Chen CK, Muhamad AS, Ooi FK (2012) Herbs in exercise and sports. J Physiol Anthropol 31: 4.
7. Goreja WG (2004) Tongkat Ali: The Tree That Cures A Hundred Diseases. Amazing Herbs Press.
8. Burkill IH, William Birtwistle; Frederick William Foxworthy; John Brooke Scrivenor; James Gilbert Watson (1966) A Dictionary of the Economic Products of the Malay Peninsula. (2nd Edn) Kuala Lumpur: The Ministry of Agriculture and Cooperatives, Malaysia.
9. Ismail SB, Wan Mohammad WM, George A, Nik Hussain NH, Musthapa Kamal ZM, et al. (2012) Randomized Clinical Trial on the Use of PHYSTA Freeze-Dried Water Extract of Eurycoma longifolia for the Improvement of Quality of Life and Sexual Well-Being in Men. Evid Based Complement Alternat Med 2012: 429268.
10. Henkel RR, Wang R, Bassett SH, Chen T, Liu N, et al. (2013) Tongkat Ali as a Potential Herbal Supplement for Physically Active Male and Female Seniors-A Pilot Study. Phytother Res.
11. Hamzah S, Yusof A (2003) The ergogenic effects of Tongkat ali (Eurycoma longifolia): A pilot study. Br J Sports Med 37: 464-470.
12. Ang HH, Cheang HS (2001) Effects of Eurycoma longifolia jack on laevator ani muscle in both uncastrated and testosterone-stimulated castrated intact male rats. Arch Pharm Res 24: 437-440.
13. Sambandan TG, Rha CK, Kadir AA, Aminudim N, Saad J, Mohammed M: Bioactive fraction of Eurycoma longifolia. United States.
14. Tambi MIM (2005) Standardized water soluble extract of Eurycoma longifolia (LJ100) on men's health. Int of J Androl 28: 25-44.
15. Zanoli P, Zavatti M, Montanari C, Baraldi M (2009) Influence of Eurycoma longifolia on the copulatory activity of sexually sluggish and impotent male rats. J Ethnopharmacol 126: 308-313.
16. Tambi MI, Kadir AA (2006) Eurycoma longifolia jack: a potent adaptogen in the form of water-soluble extract (LJ100) with the effect of maintaining men's health Asian J Androl 8: 49-50.
17. Tambi MI (2009) Nutrients and botanicals for optimizing men's health. Examining the evidence for Eurycoma longifolia Jack, the Malaysian Ginseng in men's health. Asian Journal of Andrology 11: 37-38
18. Talbott S, Talbott J, Negrete J, Jones M, Nichols M, et al. (2006) Effect of LJ100 on anabolic balance during endurance exercise. Journal of International Society of Sports Nutrition 3: S32
19. Tambi MI, Imran MK, Henkel RR (2012) Standardised water-soluble extract of Eurycoma longifolia, Tongkat ali, as testosterone booster for managing men with late-onset hypogonadism? Andrologia 44 Suppl 1: 226-230.
20. Herbst KL, Bhasin S (2004) Testosterone action on skeletal muscle. Curr Opin Clin Nutr Metab Care 7: 271-277.
21. Tambi MI (2005) Standardized water soluble extract of Eurycoma longifolia on men's health In abstracts of 8th International Congress of Andrology, 12–16 June, Seoul, Korea. Int J Androl 28: 27.
22. Certificate of Analysis (2008) Freeze dried water extract of Eurycoma longifolia (Physta®). Biotropics Malaysia Bhd.
23. Muhamad AS, Keong CC, Kiew OF, Abdullah MR, Lam CT (2010) Effects of Eurycoma longifolia Jack supplementation on recreational athletes' endurance running capacity and physiological responses in the heat. Int J Appl Sports Sci 22: 1-19.
24. Ooi FK, Singh R, Sirisinghe RG, Ang B, Jamalullail S (2001) Effects of a herbal ergogenic drink on cycling performance in young cyclists. Malays J Nutr 7: 33-40.
25. Talbott S, Talbott J, George A, Pugh M (2013) Effect of Tongkat Ali on stress hormones and psychological mood state in moderately stressed subjects. J Int Soc Sports Nutr 10: 28.
26. Ang HH, Cheang HS (1999) Studies on the anxiolytic activity of Eurycoma longifolia Jack roots in mice. Jpn J Pharmacol 79: 497-500.
27. Ang HH, Ngai TH, Tan TH (2003) Effects of Eurycoma longifolia Jack on sexual qualities in middle aged male rats. Phytomedicine 10: 590-593.
28. Ang HH, Lee KL, Kiyoshi M (2004) Sexual arousal in sexually sluggish old male rats after oral administration of Eurycoma longifolia Jack. J Basic Clin Physiol Pharmacol 15: 303-309.

Modelling Effects of Drug Testing Procedures on Performance Trends in the Shot Put

Leon I Foster[1]*, Steve J Haake[1], Dave M James[1] and Alan M Nevill[2]

[1] *The Centre for Sports Engineering Research, Faculty of Health and Wellbeing, Sheffield Hallam University, UK*
[2] *Faculty of Education, Health and Wellbeing, University of Wolverhampton, UK*

Abstract

Objectives: The effect of performance enhancing drugs on historic performance records in sport is open to interpretation and needs empirical support. Here we addressed this contentious issue by assessing whether a double sigmoidal model could detect decrements in sporting performance attributed to introduction of drug testing protocols.

Methods: Distances thrown by the top 25 male and female shot putters since the end of the 19th century were modelled using a double sigmoid.

Results: First-phase peak acceleration in the men's and women's shot put was reached in 1981 and 1986 respectively coinciding with advent of systematic doping programs. Shot put performance of men and women underwent a second-phase decline of 5.3 m and 8.9 m, in 1991 and 1994, respectively. Performance decrements in women's shot put were nearly double that for men, but much of this difference resulted from the reduced mass of their shot. Controlling for changes in mass, women's shot put performance appears to decline to a greater extent than men's, based on raw energy calculations.

Conclusions: The double sigmoidal model detected a second-phase decline in shot put performances. We attribute this data feature to onset of improved drug testing protocols and a consequential reduction of doping. The assumption is that drug testing programs of shot putters has been successful and reduced the prevalence of drug taking in that sport. The application of a double sigmoidal model to historic performance statistics can be used to detect unknown interventions in analyses of sports performance.

Keywords: Double logistic curves; Nonlinear regression; Drug testing interventions; Performance modelling; Shot put performance; Doping

Introduction

It has been well documented that athletic performance has increased since the start of the modern Olympic Games in 1896, and many factors have been attributed to this improvement, including changes in population [1,2], globalization [3], technological interventions [4,5] and use of performance enhancing drugs [6]. Performance trends in various sports have been modelled through the implementing various growth functions with the aim of quantifying these influential factors [5,7,8], and predicting limits of human ability [9,10].

One notable, but thus far challenging, intervention to gauge is the influence of performance enhancing drugs, mainly because of uncertainty due to their secretive use in elite-level sport programs. Evidence suggests that from the 1950s to 1980s systematic doping programs were implemented by Eastern bloc countries, as well as the USA, in various "power" events [11,12]. Athletes were, putatively, surreptitiously prescribed different drugs (often without their knowledge), such as anabolic steroids and hormones, to increase muscle mass and, ultimately, their performance [11,12]. Results of these programs can be observed in specific events, where performance curves display an unanticipated trend and peak in the 1980s, before dropping to the present day. Here we implement a model to interpret whether this observed performance decrement might be attributed to the introduction of more effective drugs testing programs during that decade.

One method of investigating effects of drugs testing programs, proposed by Haake and Foster [7,8] to gauge the influence of performance enhancing drugs, was through the modelling of step interventions in 1989 and 2000 using [0,1] indicator variables. These step changes accounted for instantaneous reductions in running performance, presumed to be related to the introduction of improved drug testing protocols. The disadvantages of this method are: (1) the introduction of drug testing procedures might not follow an instantaneous discrete step change profile; and (2), choosing specific dates in which to apply a step change is a subjective process, and date selection might influence reported effects.

An alternative approach is adapted from the methods proposed by Balmer et al. [5] who originally used a double sigmoidal model to identify specific technological interventions in jumping events (e.g. to separate the effect of the Fosbury flop from the evolutionary growth in high-jump performances). In this study, we sought to ascertain whether the model could be used to overcome disadvantages of our original method. We sought to separate the development of drug testing procedures and consequential performance declines, from evolutionary growth in shot put performance. Specifically, we focused on understanding whether the double sigmoidal method could be used to model the effects on shot put performance statistics of improved drug testing procedures.

Recent research [7,8,13] has made use of established online databases [14] that contain all performance statistics since modern competitive records began. Application of a double sigmoidal model

***Corresponding author:** Leon Foster, Research Associate, Centre for Sports Engineering Research, Sheffield Hallam University, A129 Collegiate Hall, Collegiate Crescent, Sheffield, S. Yorks S10 2BP, UK
E-mail: l.i.foster@shu.ac.uk

to this type of data would facilitate modelling of an underlying evolutionary improvement curve (phase one growth), in addition to curves predicated an external intervention events (phase two growth).

To achieve our aims we chose the shot put event for men and women as a task vehicle for analysis. Performance in such athletic field events is predominantly related to the power an athlete can produce. The shot put event has a competitive aim of "putting" a shot the greatest distance over a number of rounds. Unlike other field events, like the high jump, a single dominant shot putting technique has not emerged, with athletes favoring either the "Glide" or the "Spin" actions. This feature suggests that putting technique is not a dominant factor and that historic technical changes are assumed not to have significantly influenced trends in overall shot put performance. This suggestion makes it an ideal event to examine the evolutionary development of athletic performance over the past century, since few outside interventions, other than possibly drug taking and drug testing, are likely to have influenced performance over time. The shot put is also an old event in which performance data are found in the earliest records of international competitions, signifying that entire historic trends in shot put performance can be examined.

In this study our aim was to utilise the double sigmoidal model originally proposed by Balmer et al. [5] to model the top 25 best performances in each year in male and female shot put competitions recorded over the past century. Model fitting would enable us to quantify the evolutionary development in shot put performances in the past century, in addition to the influence of drug testing procedures, and consequential performance declines, in more recent years. This information will assist in providing potential estimates of current doping levels in elite shot put and whether implemented drug testing procedures have been successful.

Methods

With institutional ethics approval, data on the top 25 performances were collected from open-source, performance statistics websites [14,15] for the men's and women's shot put event between 1891 and 2012 (women's data from 1921 onwards). Performances were collated such that each athlete appeared only once in the annual list. Figure 1a shows the top 25 performances for the men's shot put event from the 1890s onwards and Figure 1b shows the same data for the women's event from the 1920s onwards.

Inspection of the raw data indicates the following:

1. Performance in the men's shot put appears to initially evolve slowly, whereas the women's event appears to improve at a greater rate;
2. Performances for both men and women appear to peak during the 1980s before declining and leveling off;
3. The peak in the women's event appears more pronounced than the men's event;
4. There are performance declines emerging during the years of the 1st and 2nd World Wars.

There are many limitations in the modelling of athletic performance data using linear and polynomial models [1,7,8]. These types of models become unsuitable for extrapolation beyond an observed range, contain no asymptotes, and some model parameters lack biological meaning. Therefore, it is preferential to use logistic and exponential growth functions when seeking to model the evolution of athletic performance [5,8,9].

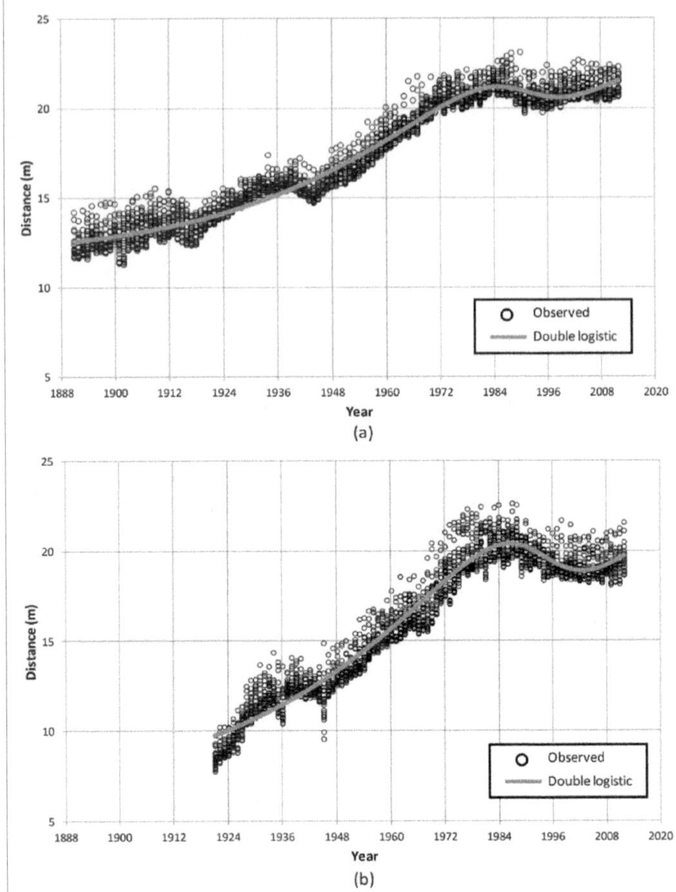

Figure 1: Double sigmoidal models of the shot put performance over time plotted alongside observed performance values (yearly top 25) for (a) men and (b) women.

In cases where there are two acceleration phases in athletic performance, a double logistic model is preferable because it can detect both the underlying evolutionary global improvement in performances (phase 1), as well as further accelerations in performance as a result of a technological or other interventions (phase 2) [5]. For example, the double logistic model could also be employed to model a second phase performance decline due to implementation of improved drug testing procedures. Equation (1) shows the adapted double logistic model employed by Balmer et al. [5] to search for technological interventions within the jumping category of field events.

$$f(t) = P_0 + \frac{a_1}{1+e^{-a_2(t-t_1)}} + \frac{b_1}{1+e^{-b_2(t-t_2)}} \qquad [1]$$

The model sums two logistic functions, where P_0, is the baseline performance at the beginning of the model. $P_0 + a_1$ is the upper limit of performance which would have been obtained if an intervention had not occurred. a_1 is the modelled contribution from the underlying evolutional improvement or global improvement of that particular event; a_2 reflects the rate of this global improvement trend and is symmetrical about $t = t_1$, the point of inflection. b_1 is the contribution to performance of the second phase or the level of effect from the intervention being modelled. b_2 reflects the rate of change of the second phase and is symmetrical about $t = t_2$. Where there is a negative second phase growth (where the product of b_1 and b_2 is negative) performance peaks at $P_0 + a_1 - |b_1|$ as time tends towards infinity.

	Men			Women		
Parameter	Estimate	Standard error	95% CI	Estimate	Standard error	95% CI
P_0	6.53	1.24	2.43	6.66	0.53	1.04
a_1	19.77	3.18	6.23	30.46	7.76	15.21
a_2	0.04	0.00	0.00	0.03	0.00	0.01
t_1	1980.68	7.29	14.30	1985.55	11.74	23.01
b_1	5.28	1.16	2.27	-8.93	2.16	4.23
b_2	-0.18	0.03	0.05	0.18	0.03	0.05
t_2	1991.39	0.62	1.22	1994.23	0.72	1.40
Peak after phase 1		26.29			37.12	
Peak after phase 2		21.01			28.18	
R^2		0.9603			0.9472	
R^2 adjusted		0.9602			0.9471	

Table 1: Non-linear regression output for the double logistic models of the men's and women's shot put by year.

All performance data available, both for the men's and women's shot put events, were modelled using a double logistic model. The double logistic model was fitted to each data set using non-linear least squares estimation [16] both in SPSS and manually using the solver function in EXCEL to confirm model parameters (see Supplemental Digital Content 1 for the adopted SPSS syntax text).

Results

(Table 1) shows non-linear regression outputs for the double logistic model when applied to all annual shot put performance data in both the men's and women's events. Fitted and observed data are shown in Figure 1a for the men's event and (Figure 1b) for the women's event. Examining (Table 1), the double logistic model in both the men's and women's shot put have similar baseline values, 6.53 m and 6.66 m respectively. The expected growth in the first phase in the men's shot put event is 19.77 m, resulting in an estimated peak of this phase at 26.29 m. This first phase growth is centred around 1981 (Figure 2a). The women's event demonstrated a very large expected growth in the first phase at 30.46 m resulting in a peak of 37.12 m. The women's first phase growth centred around 1986, slightly later than the male event (Figure 2b). The second phase decline in shot put performance, attributed to the uptake of better drug testing procedures in the men's event, is 5.28 m, with a point of inflection around 1991. In the women's event this modelled decline is 8.93 m, with a point of inflection around 1994 (Figure 2a).

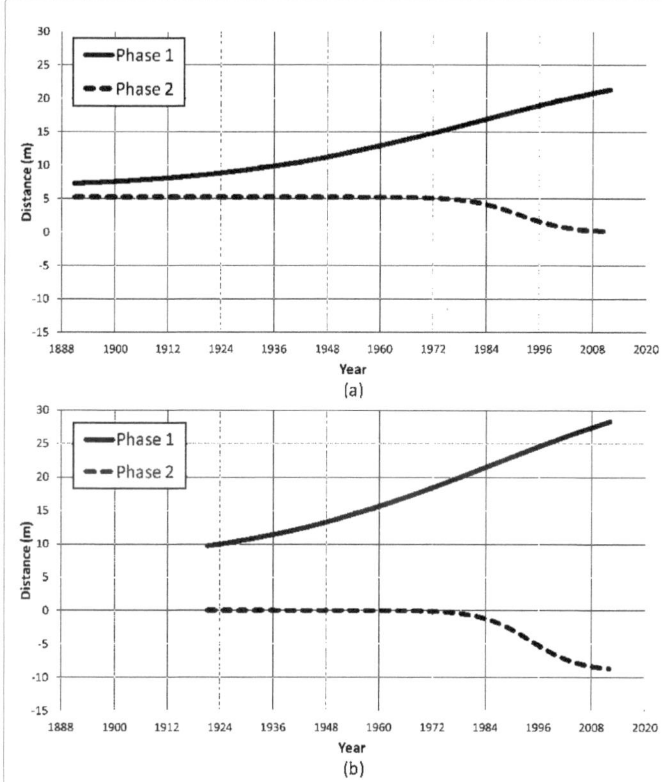

Figure 2: The first and second phase of growth in the (a) men's and (b) women's shot put, the second phase is attributed to the improvements in drug testing procedures.

Discussion

As hypothesised, performance trends in both the men's and women's shot put event showed evidence of two phases: the first phase being positive and the second being negative. All model parameters were significant (i.e., parameter estimates greater than 2*SE, see Table 1) and the magnitude of these estimates, together with the explained R^2 and R^2 adjusted, demonstrated that the double sigmoidal model was a good fit to the two data sets.

The estimates associated with the first phase suggested a general evolutionary growth over the whole of the 20th century in both the men and women's shot put performances. The minimum shot put distance value estimates for men and women are very similar at 6.5 m and 6.7 m respectively, and the year of maximum acceleration in shot put performance also occurred at approximately 1981 for men and 1986 for women athletes. This maximum acceleration in performance coincides with the prevalence of early systematic steroid doping programs [11,12].

The maximum second phase decline in performance in the women's event is predicted to be 8.93 m, 70 % more than the predicted men's second phase decline at 5.28 m. One reason for this large variation is the difference in mass between the men's and women's shot put. The mass of the women's competition shot (4 kg) is almost half that of the men's (7.26 kg). According to Newton's second law of motion, if the athlete can produce an increase in propulsive impulse, the acceleration of a heavier shot will be proportionally smaller, and the increase in distance projected will be smaller. (Table 2) within the supplemental material shows the approximate peak launch velocities and impulse values for men and women shot putters. These values have been calculated by taking the peak throw distances in the 1st and 2nd phase growth functions, and applying them to a simple projectile model [17]. The launch angle of the shot was taken to be 38° and the launch height was assumed to be 2.20 m for men and 2.07 m for women, because these parameters are typical values observed in elite shot put performance [16]. It can be seen that the predicted drop in women's performance, due to the onset of

		Men	Women
	Shot mass (kg)	7.26	4
	Launch angle of shot (°)	37	37
	Launch height (m)	2.22	2.07
Phase 1 growth peak	Throw distance (m)	26.29	37.12
	Launch velocity (ms^{-1})	15.53	18.78
	Impulse (Ns)	112.77	75.12
Phase 2 growth peak	Throw distance (m)	21.01	28.183
	Launch velocity (ms^{-1})	13.71	16.19
	Impulse (Ns)	104.22	64.75
	Impulse drop (Ns)	8.55	10.37
	Impulse drop (%)	7.58%	13.80%

Table 2: Launch velocities and impulse values for the men's and women's doped and un-doped peak performances.

better drug testing protocols, is about 10.37 Ns, or 13.80%. This figure is still higher when compared to the men's drop in performance of 8.55 Ns, or 7.58%. This comparison indicated that, based on impulse values, women shot putters were influenced more by the onset of better drug testing protocols. Findings suggest that anti-doping measures have had a greater effect on women's performance than men's. Female physiology with artificially elevated testosterone levels may account for this [18]; the normal levels of testosterone present in females are generally several times lower than males [19]. The artificial administration of this type of hormone could have pushed women's performance close to values for men's performance levels in the absence of doping interventions.

Contemporary female shot putters are predicted to produce about 62% of the propulsive impulse, compared to male counterparts, whereas a doped women shot putter could have been as close as 72% to an un-doped male counterpart.

Both the modelled second phase reductions in performances appear to be ongoing with both the men's and women's shot put reaching 99.9 % of the maximum decline in 2030 and 2033 respectively. It is assumed that within 0.1 % of the asymptotic limit, the decline has practically reached this limit. In 2012 the modelled decline in performance in the men's and women's event is at 97.6% and 96.1% of the maximum respectively. These data may indicate that anti-doping measures have been successful and that the majority of performance gains seen by doping have almost been eradicated.

(Figure 2) represents the two separate phases of the double logistic model. Phase two begins to have an influence on both events in 1970s with maximum rate (deceleration) of decline in performance in 1991 and 1994 for the men's and women's event respectively. The start of this second phase decline coincides with the first introduction of testing procedures for anabolic steroids at the 1976 Montreal Olympic Games [20]. Eight athletes tested positive for anabolic steroids in those Olympic Games. The peak rate of decline in the men's and women's shot put also occurs slightly after the introduction of out-of-season random drug testing around the late 1980s, the reunification of Germany in 1990, and the fall of the Soviet Union in 1991.

Examining (Figure 2) further, it is apparent that there are two different types of second phase reduction in the men's and women's shot put. The men's event appears to have an underlying positive influence of 5.23 m from the second phase throughout historic performance data. The positive influence starts to drop to zero with the advent of drug testing in the 1970s. In contrast the women's event experiences zero influence from the second phase function throughout the 20th century and then experiences a negative influence with the onset of drug testing. This statistical evidence suggests that the influence of women's drug taking was a gradual occurrence that was incorporated as part of the evolutionary growth of phase one. In contrast, the men's shot put event may have been influenced by doping measures throughout its more recent history. The development and isolation of steroids like testosterone did not occur until 1930s. However, this does not rule out the historic use of other performance enhancing drugs such as stimulants which may have underlined historic performance, and which are now prohibited and tested as part of anti-doping measures. In the women's event there is no underlying influence from the second phase function, but a negative effect can be seen with the onset of drug testing. One reason for this observation could be that the model finds it difficult to distinguish between the positive effects from doping and the general evolution of the women's shot put event. Therefore, any influence seen from an underlying second phase is hidden within the global evolution from the phase one growth function.

The model parameters show that, if phase two of the double logistic model were omitted, maximum performance in 2012 would reach 26.68 m in the men's shot put event and 37.12 m in the women's event. The underlying global progression of athletic performance modelled in the first phase of the double logistic model appears to show that performances are still improving and will not reach 99.9% of the predict limit until 2167 in the men's and 2183 in the women's shot put event. At first glance, the women's upper limit in shot put performance appears to be unrealistic. Nonetheless, based solely upon Newton's second law of motion, a lighter shot will travel further if propelled at the same force. In theory, and ignoring air resistance, a shot putter who threw a 7.26 kg shot 26.68 m will throw a 4 kg shot 48.42 m. Therefore, a maximum value of 37.12 m in the women's event does not seem an unreasonable expectation. However, it must be noted that there is a high degree of uncertainty when extrapolating limits from any model that is based solely on historic performance data. This is because it is impossible to account for any future factors and events that may influence performance.

Conclusion

Up until now, the evidence for any advantage gain of performance enhancing drugs has been mainly anecdotal and subjective. Based on statistical evidence of performance evaluated in this paper it seems apparent that anti-doping measures initially employed in the last two decades of the 20th century have been effective. The result has been a reduction in the men's and women's shot put performances that are likely to now reflect the true limits in shot put performance in the absence of illegal drug assistance.

There will be some uncertainty as to the true effect of performance enhancing drugs on the shot put and other elite sports, as well as uncertainty as to whether their use is still on-going within elite performance programs. However, evidence presented here suggests that performances have declined on top of underlying global performance improvement since the introduction of anti-doping measures in the late 1960s. Therefore, it seems likely that current athletic performances have been influenced to a lesser extent by doping than before drugs testing programs were introduced.

The methods developed in this study reveal that application of a double sigmoidal model to historic performance statistics can be used to objectively detect an intervention, in this case, the effect of anti-doping testing measures on shot put performance. These methods could, also be used to gauge other unknown interventions in sports performance statistics, and potentially be a new method used in sports performance analysis.

Acknowledgements

No funding was received for this study.

The authors have no conflict of interest to declare and all authors meet the uniform requirements of the Journal of Sports Medicine & Doping Studies criteria for authorship.

References

1. Denny MW (2008) Limits to running speed in dogs, horses and humans. J Exp Biol 2213836-3849.
2. Foster L, James D, Haake SJ (2010) Understanding the influence of population size on athletic performance. Procedia Eng 2: 3183-3189.
3. Lippi G, Banfi G, Favaloro EJ, Rittweger J, Maffulli N (2008) Updates on improvement of human athletic performance: focus on world records in athletics. Br Med Bull 87: 7-15.
4. Haake SJ (2009) The impact of technology on sporting performance in Olympic sports. J Sports Sci 27: 1421-1431.
5. Balmer N, Pleasence P, Nevill A (2012) Evolution and revolution: Gauging the impact of technological and technical innovation on Olympic performance. J Sports Sci 30: 1075-1083.
6. Ernst S, Simon P (2012) A quantitative approach for assessing significant improvements in elite sprint performance: Has IGF-1 entered the arena? Drug Test Anal 5: 384-389.
7. Haake SJ, Foster L, James D (2014) An improvement index to quantify the evolution of performance in running. J Sports Sci 32: 610-622.
8. Foster L (2012) Modelling the effect of technology on elite sport [PhD Thesis]. Sheffield Hallam University 343.
9. Nevill AM, Whyte G (2005) Are there limits to running World Records? Med Sci Sports Exerc 37: 1785-1788.
10. Morton RH (1983) The Supreme Runner: What Evidence Now? Aust J Sports Sci 3: 7-10.
11. Kammerer RC (2001) What Is Doping and How Is It Detected? In: Wilson W, Derse E, editors. Doping in elite sport: the politics of drugs in the Olympic movement. JHK 3-28.
12. Franke WW, Berendonk B (1997) Hormonal doping and androgenization of athletes: a secret program of the German Democratic Republic government. Clin Chem 43: 1262-1279.
13. Berthelot G, Tafflet M, El Helou N, Len S, Escolano S, et al. (2010) Athlete atypicity on the edge of human achievement: performances stagnate after the last peak, in 1988. PLoS One 5: e8800.
14. Rabinovich M (2013) Track and Field Statistics.
15. IAAF (2013) International Association of Athletics Federations, records.
16. Seber GAF, Wild CJ (2003) Nonlinear regression. Hoboken (NJ): Wiley-Interscience.
17. Linthorne NP (2001) Optimum release angle in the shot put. J Sports Sci 19: 359-372.
18. Seiler, S, De Koning, JJ, Foster C (2007) The Fall and Rise of the Gender Difference in Elite Anaerobic Performance 1952-2006. Med Sci Sports Exerc 39: 534-540.
19. Weiss LW, Cureton KJ, Thompson FN (1983) Comparison of serum testosterone and androstenedione responses to weight lifting in men and women. Eur J Appl Physiol 50: 413-419.
20. World anti-doping agency (2013) About WADA website [Internet]. Montreal (Canada): World anti-doping agency.

The Epo Fable in Professional Cycling: Facts, Fallacies and Fabrications

Hein FM Lodewijkx*

Faculty of Psychology and Educational Sciences, Open University of The Netherlands, Heerlen, The Netherlands

Abstract

The massive doping schemes that surfaced in professional cycling suggest that riders' performances, realized in the controversial 'epo era' (>1990), are a cut above achievements delivered by their forerunners. We examined this superior performances assumption (SPA) by conducting six historic studies, which all scrutinized archival records of winning riders' stage race and time trial performances demonstrated in the three European Grand Tours (Tour de France, Giro d'Italia, and Vuelta a España; 1903–2013), including Lance Armstrong's wins. Findings revealed that all riders' wins in the epo years are no exception to the variability in speed progress observed in the three races over time and none of their achievements proved to be outliers. This also holds true for Armstrong's performances. These findings agree with results of a meta–analysis of epo studies we conducted, indicating that the ergogenic effects of epo and blood doping on riders' aerobic performances and associated cycling speeds are overrated. In conclusion, we argue that our observations render the SPA doubtful. They also made us realize that arguments used in contemporary discussions about effects of doping in cycling often involve psychological biases, false reasoning and fabrications. They are presented in the closing sections of this contribution.

The Epo Fable in Professional Cycling: Facts, Fallacies and Fabrications

The recent history of doping affairs in professional cycling placed the sport into grim light and left individual riders with a tainted image [1-6]. Reckoning the proposed, powerful performance–enhancing (or ergogenic) effects of epo and blood doping used by riders in the 'epo era' (>1990), it is often argued that riders' sportive achievements in these years are therefore superior to accomplishments delivered by riders in prior years [7,8] (USADA, 2012a, b). The current paper examines the soundness of this superior performances assumption (SPA) in two different ways. First, at a physiological level, the SPA presupposes strong ergogenic effects of, for instance, epo doping on aerobic performances of endurance athletes such as cyclists, resulting in strong increases in cycling speed. However, as will be shown, findings of a meta–analysis of epo studies we carried out indicated that these effects are far less powerful than generally presumed. These results constitute a first, yet indirect, indication that the SPA may be invalid. Second, to directly evaluate the SPA, we conducted six historic studies which all scrutinized annals of the three main European cycling races: Tour de France, Giro d'Italia, and Vuelta a España (1903–2013). With these records we not only assessed riders' winning performances in stage races, but in time trials as well. The studies were guided by the doping hypothesis model (DHM) that permits a critical appraisal of the SPA because it takes account of the variation in riders' sportive achievements in actual races over time. Alternatively, the same historic performance variation also enables us to examine whether riders' feats in the epo years can be explicated by various historic measures from the past which are unrelated to doping, such as the distances of the races or the years in which riders competed.

In the next sections, we will first elaborate on the DHM. We will then present a short theoretical outline of the physiological reasons why cyclists are tempted to manipulate their blood with doping agents that augment the volume of red blood cells (RBCs), i.e., epo and blood doping. We will then summarize main findings of the meta–analysis and the archival studies. As noted, findings of the meta–analysis evoked our reservations against the SPA. All historic studies confirmed these initial reservations, making the SPA doubtful. Little by little, our empirical facts made us aware that arguments put forward in present–day discussions about effects of doping in professional road racing too often involve psycho–logical fallacies and fabrications. They will be discussed at length in the concluding sections of this paper.

The Doping Hypothesis Model

For many fans the doping affairs that plagued the cycling world in recent years put great pressure on their enthusiasm for the sport. The scandal that struck the final blow involved American, ex–professional racer Lance Armstrong. He was the only rider ever to win seven consecutive Tours de France. The doping agents used by Armstrong and eleven of his team mates at the U.S. Postal and Discovery Channel teams predominantly involved epo, blood transfusions (doping with own blood, or with blood harvested from a compatible donor), and anabolic steroids such as testosterone [8] (USADA, 2012b). Worldwide, the Armstrong affair aroused strong punitive, moral outrage and cleansing responses [9-12] that appear to be fueled by popular beliefs about the potent ergogenic effects of aforementioned doping agents. Intriguingly, these beliefs are questioned by Kuipers [13] in a paper with the compelling title: "Putative effects of doping in cycling." He doubts whether said doping agents indeed improve performances of endurance athletes such as cyclists. Given his conclusions, he further plausibly contends that the doping problem in the sport is therefore partly "due to superstition, hearsay, and insufficient knowledge among the athletes' support personnel, which frequently leads to medical malpractice in sport" (ibid., p. 2645).

One cannot imagine a bigger contrast: The downfall of Lance Armstrong versus Kuipers' arguments that the ergogenic effects of many of the modern doping agents used by cyclists are overestimated and conceivably might even rest on mountebankery and deception. However, Kuipers is not the only dissenting voice. Other scholars arrived at similar conclusions and their arguments will be presented in the pages to follow. When taking the findings and arguments of these

***Corresponding author:** Hein Lodewijkx, Faculty of Psychology and Educational Sciences, Open University of The Netherlands, Stationsweg 3A, 4811 AX, Breda, The Netherlands
E-mail: Hein.Lodewijkx@ou.nl, lodex@ziggo.nl

scholars seriously, it would be better to speak of a *doping hypothesis* which is still in search of empirical support.

Clearly, many riders in recent years were involved in epo and / or blood doping affairs or acknowledged afterward that they used these aids during their active career [2,14]. So, the pivotal question we sought to answer is not about whether cyclists give in to doping use. In all likelihood they do. While its prevalence is estimated in some studies to be 3-7% [15-18], solid figures, however, are still not available. Rather, reckoning the opposing voices, the essential question of the study became: "To what extent did the use of RBC–augmenting doping aids enhance riders' performances in actual races?" As is the case with the unknown pervasiveness of doping use in the cycling world, research also demonstrates an impressive lack of independent, verifiable and conclusive empirical evidence concerning the effects of doping on riders' sportive achievements in real competitions over the years [1,3,19]. To fill this gap and to resolve our uncertainty concerning the status of the doping hypothesis, we conducted a series of empirical studies that were guided by the doping hypothesis model (DHM). As can be seen in Figure 1, it only consists of question marks.

Lack of Research

Some scholars attempted to fill the lacunae in the model [1,3-6] leading to very interesting, yet undependable insights into the customs and traditions pertaining to doping use in the cycling world. Furthermore, some ex–professional cyclists wrote about their own personal experiences with doping use during their sportive career [20-27]. There are also sketchy accounts about these relationships written by members of the support staff of different cycling teams, such as Willy Voet [28], former 'soigneur' of the much disputed French Festina team, and Jef D'Hont [29], who worked with the controversial German Telekom team. Medical doctors also wrote personal accounts about these subjects, such as Eric Ryckaert [30] who was involved in the 1998 Festina doping affair, and Gérard Porte [31] who served as a physician in the Tour de France for nearly forty years. Finally, you have the journalists and writers, who attempted to uncover the 'omerta' or unwritten code of silence concerning doping use in the professional group of riders [32-35].

Although these sources yield an understanding of the mores in professional cycling, they still mainly concern anecdotic attempts to clarify the historic, sociological, psychological, and physiological reasons as to why riders resort to doping use. As Brewer [1] observed, this is due to the lack of systematic research into actual cycling contests,

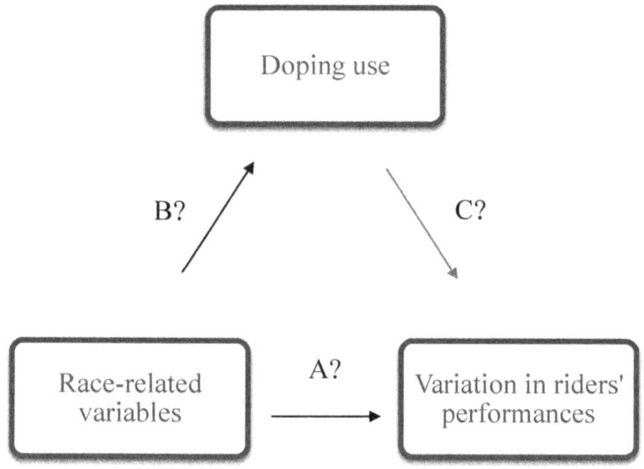

Figure 1: The Doping Hypothesis Model (DHM).

which is why scholars often built on their own experiences as fans of, and participants in, cycle races. Consequently, much of the writings about the cycling world necessarily had to fall back on the 'grey' literature, i.e., publications that appeared in magazines, on websites, and in popular books, to some of which we referred to previously. This also means that research that methodically attempted to investigate the relationships between the variables presented in the DHM is practically absent. Our own studies leave the relationships presented in path B unrequited, but they do permit to give direct answers to the relationships presented in path A and some indirect answers to the relationships presented in path C. The latter replies can only be indirect, since there are simply no studies available that unequivocally assessed the statistical relationships between these variables in actual cycle races over time and our studies also failed to do so. Then again, we argue that our answers constitute a rather inconvenient truth concerning the SPA. A first, indirect indication of the unsoundness of the SPA relates to findings of a meta–analysis we conducted [36]. It evaluated results of laboratory studies that all assessed effects of epo administration on aerobic performance and extrapolated the estimated epo–stimulated improvements in performance to cycling speeds in actual races. Main findings are summarized in the next section, preceded by a short outline of the physiological reasons why endurance athletes are tempted to manipulate their blood with RBC–augmenting doping aids.

RBC-augmentation: Physiology and Estimations of its Effects on Performance Physiology

Building on the cardiovascular/anaerobic model [37,38], the proposed, causal chain between epo/blood doping and aerobic performance runs as follows:

Epo / blood doping → RBCs↑ →Ht↑ → O_2-transport capacity↑ → VO_{2max}↑→ W_{map}↑ → Cycling speed↑

The key variable in the chain constitutes VO_{2max}, described as an estimate of cardio–respiratory, circulatory and muscular fitness that measures the fastest rate at which oxygen (O_2) can be delivered and consumed by the body during strenuous exercise. The model assumes that high levels of VO_{2max} are a prerequisite for top–level accomplishments in endurance sports such as cycling [39]. Through the process of erythropoiesis, the hormone erythropoietin (or epo) stimulates the bone marrow to produce newly formed red blood cells (RBCs), or reticulocytes. After one to two days, they grow into mature cells, or erythrocytes, which for 99% make up the population of blood cells. Hemoglobin (Hb) is a protein in RBCs which carries oxygen and, hence, it is essential in the chain of oxygen transport from the lungs to O_2–consumers such as the muscles. A single RBC contains ~250 million Hb–molecules which each can bind four O_2–molecules. This is the reason why it is proposed that the oxygen–transport capacity of blood can be improved by augmenting the volume of RBCs in the blood (RBCV) and thereby the blood's Hb mass. Hematocrit (Ht) is commonly used to assess the concentration of RBCs in the blood, or the thickness (viscosity) of the blood. It constitutes the ratio of RBCV vs. PV (blood plasma volume, the liquid part of the blood). For instance, a value of Ht=45% means that one litre blood contains 450 ml RBCV and 550 ml PV. Further note that only mature, but not immature RBCs can bind oxygen. This means that, in contrast to blood transfusions that immediately supply the blood with mature RBCs, administration of artificial epo does not have this instant effect. Accordingly, the physiological grounds why cyclists are inclined to boost their performances through RBC–augmenting doping aids is because it is proposed that this augmentation elevates the Ht level in the blood, thereby increasing the corresponding oxygen–carrying capacity.

This increase subsequently improves athletes' aerobic performance capacity (VO_{2max}) and the associated maximal aerobic power output, expressed in watts (W_{map}). These improvements are presumed to result in increased speeds in races and, ultimately, even in victories [22,40].

According to Catlin et al. [41] and Joyner [42] the use of artificial epo as an ergogenic aid became rampant in endurance sports such as cycling in the early 1990s. Verbruggen [82], former chairman of the International Cycling Union (UCI), the sport's governing body, labeled the 1990-2000 period in professional cycling as an "epo epidemic", maintaining that epo improved athletes' endurance capacity by as much as 20%. In 2013, Vandeweghe — president of the Flanders Cycling Federation (WBV, Wielerbond Vlaanderen) — arrives at a similar conclusion concerning the estimated, cumulative effects of epo in actual competitions. Lundby and Olsen [43] reviewed findings of laboratory studies which examined the relationship between epo administration and aerobic performance in normal, healthy humans. They concluded that —if Ht is artificially increased by epo treatment from pre-test baseline values to around Ht=50% posttest— VO_{2max} is estimated to improve by 8-12%. For blood doping the estimates are 5-10% improvement [44]. Descriptively, Ninot et al. [45] concluded that the ergogenic effects of, for example, synthetic epo are "dramatic", whilst effects of blood transfusions are labeled "gigantic" in a study by Lundby et al. [46].

Estimations of Effects

Seemingly, the use of descriptive terms such as 'dramatic' and 'gigantic' may lead to the impression that the SPA is indeed valid. However, notice that these are rather suggestive terms that do not have any statistical meaning. To reach some solid, yet preliminary answers concerning the validity of the SPA, we therefore decided to statistically estimate the ergogenic effects of RBC-augmenting doping agents on riders' aerobic performances and the corresponding improvements in cycling speeds by conducting a meta-analysis of epo studies [36]. Kuipers [13] already contended that effects of RBC-doping aids on cyclists' maximal aerobic power output (W_{map}) are overestimated, while Heuberger et al. [58] even maintain that the epo doping - aerobic performance hypothesis is not supported by empirical evidence. In our meta-analysis, we evaluated findings of seventeen laboratory studies and assessed effect sizes (unbiased d, r and r^2) of the epo-stimulated increases in VO_{2max} and W_{map}. The Forest plot in Figure 2 summarizes effect sizes of pre vs. posttest comparisons on these measures, relating to all epo treatments of the studies. The average effect size amounted to d=0.54. Figure 2 additionally shows that 31 (77.5%) of the forty d values did not surpass the bandwidth of the 95%-confidence interval. This means that many of the epo-induced improvements in performance yielded by the studies did not exceed chance level. Note, however, that negative and small d's may have inflated these findings. Additional results revealed that these values could either be attributed to submaximal performances measured in distinct studies, or to specific experimental treatments manipulated in the studies, such as performances assessed at moderate altitudes (hypoxia) or at sea level (normoxia). Of the nine values that did surpass the 95%-bandwidth, five could be traced to two studies, which mainly concern large positive d's obtained on W_{map} [47,48]. After refining analyses to maximal performances demonstrated by participants at sea level in double-blind, placebo-controlled studies the fixed, pooled effect sizes were moderate: d=0.41-0.49. These values slightly deviate from the overall d=0.54 described previously. According to Cohen [49] an effect size of roughly half SD (d=0.50) indicates that in 67% of the observations the epo studies are not able to discriminate between maximal performances demonstrated by participants that were administered epo or not. The observed amounts of explained

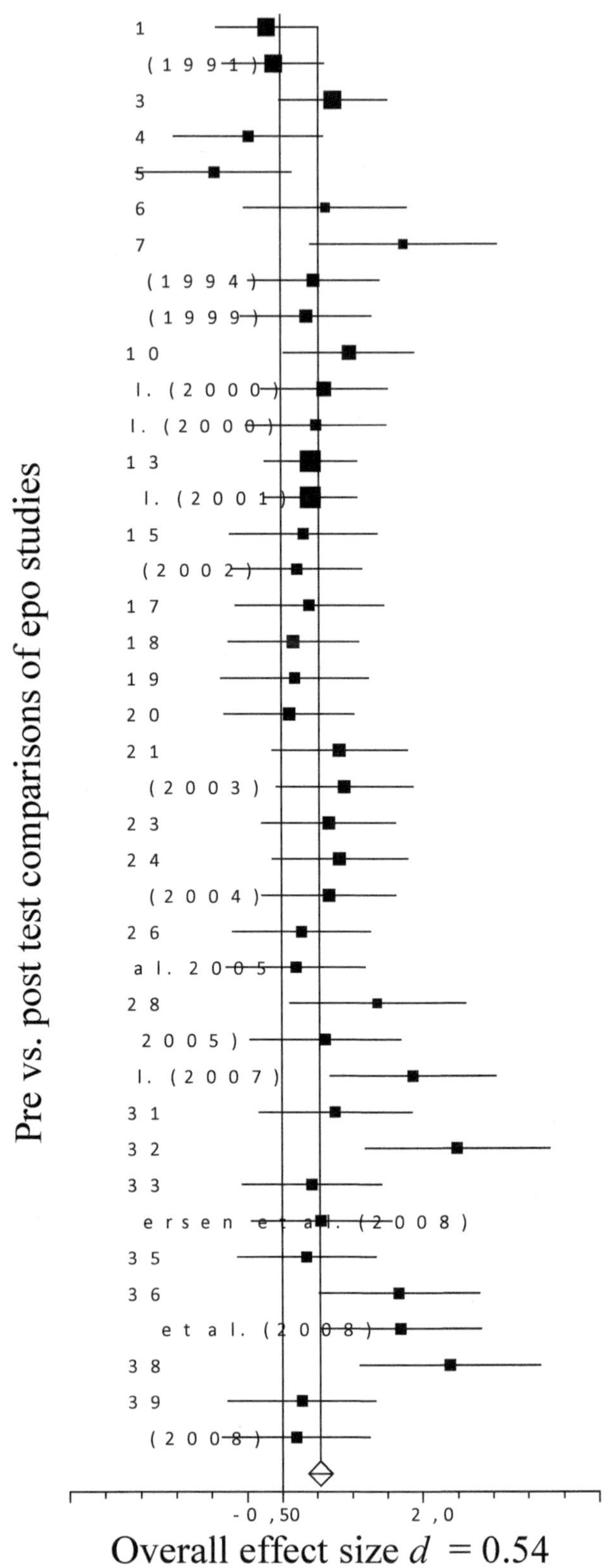

Figure 2: Forest plot of effect sizes (unbiased d) of pre vs. post test comparisons on VO_{2max} and W_{map} within epo treatments of seventeen epo studies included in the meta-analysis (N = 40 strata). The size of the solid black squares represents the weight the corresponding study exerts in the analysis. The 95%–confidence interval of the estimates is displayed as a horizontal line through the black square. The unfilled diamond presents the pooled estimate. (Source: Lodewijkx et al., 2013).

variation in epo-stimulated performance improvement of 4–19% mean that a considerable 81–96% of these improvements cannot be attributed to the effects of experimental conditions. Percentages improvement from pre to post tests ranged between M=6–7% (VO_{2max}) and M=7-8% (W_{map}). Important for the SPA, based on Nevill et al. [50], we estimated that the largest improvement in VO_{2max} of $M_{post - pre}$=0.29 l/min yielded by the analysis corresponded to an increase in velocity of about one kilometer per hour (km/h). Perneger [51] reports a similar increase in speed. However, Hopkins et al. [52] strongly warn against directly generalizing this increase to actual races. Additionally, Heuberger et al. [53] and Lodewijkx et al. [36] argue that the epo/blood doping-aerobic performance relationship suffers from external, ecological, and predictive validity problems. For instance, the relationship becomes very limited if we consider the well-known fact that elite athletes, such as professional cyclists, are estimated to be able to exercise at peak VO_{2max} levels for approximately ten minutes before reaching the different stages in the lactate threshold [54]. So, after this period cyclists' exercise capacity will be greatly reduced. Hence, the influence of epo doping on cyclists' performances in actual races is also strongly constrained by time limits.

All these observations suggest that the effects of RBC-augmenting doping aids might indeed be strongly overvalued in actual competitions, including the races that were scheduled during the epo era. Yet, the meta- analysis mainly evaluated achievements of non-athletes who delivered their performances in laboratory situations. It did not examine achievements demonstrated by professional riders in real races. Only a critical appraisal of these performances may provide some conclusive answers concerning the validity of the SPA. In our six archival studies we therefore evaluated these performances.

Historic Studies: Performances in the Three European Grand Tours

Findings of two studies which examined the annals of the three major European stage races appear to agree with the SPA. Perneger [51] investigated mean km/h performances of riders who ranked fifth in the overall standings of the three tours in the period 1990-2009. He reported that between 1990 and 2004, riders' speed increased by 0.16 km/h per year and further observed a decrease in speed of 0.22 km/h per year since 2004. El Helou et al. [21] analyzed mean km/h performances of riders who reached the first ten places in the final standings of eleven European races from 1892 to 2008, which included all famous one-day classic races as well as the three main stage races. They found that, relative to the pre-epo years (1946-1992), riders' performances in the epo years (1993–2008) showed a significant improvement in km/h of 6.38%.

We also decided to scrutinize archival records [55] of the three main stage races and to assess winning riders' km/h and time performances. However, consistent with Perneger [51] and Vandeweghe [14], we realized that riders' first-ranking achievements, demonstrated after three weeks of competition, could bias conclusions relating to the SPA. In the end, selecting riders' final rankings as the measure to evaluate the SPA may be false, since the very same performances also result from the joint and coordinated labors in the total group of cyclists participating in the races. Hence, these group labors can be considered contaminating variables which may strongly impede a sound evaluation of individual riders' final achievements. Conversely, in time trials riders in person race against the clock and compete for the fastest time. Since they cannot benefit from the efforts of other riders in these races through drafting, time trialing requires the maximum of individual riders' stamina and aerobic exercise capacity [56]. To validly evaluate the SPA, we therefore followed Vandeweghe's [14] recommendation and decided to gather data concerning individual riders' time trial accomplishments as well.

Table 1 presents an overview of the studies and the descriptive statistics of the variables we assessed. Riders' mean km/h and time performances served as the dependent variables. Column five shows that we used seven DHM measures from the past to account for the historic variation in riders' wins. Regarding stage races, we measured the years in which cyclists competed (Y), the distances of the races (D) as well as the number of stages in the races (N_{ST}), which inclined with advancing years. We further developed the brutality rate (B), measuring the harshness of the races. In the early years of the tours sometimes only 30% of the riders managed to finish the race, while in 2011 more than 80% succeeded to do so. Findings revealed that lower distances and brutality rates and increases in the number of stages facilitated riders' speed to a lesser or greater extent over the years. We additionally took

Study	*N*	Wins	Years	DHM variables[1]	R^2_{adj} (%) explained by DHM variables[2]		Main explanatory variable (*r*)				Outliers (1990–2013)
							Km/h		Time		
					Km/h	Time	Y	D	Y	D	-
1 (Lodewijkx & Brouwer, 2011)	181	Stage race	1947–2008	Y, D, B, N_{ST}, SR	84***	98***	.79***	-.42***	-.60***	.92***	None
2 (Lodewijkx & Brouwer, 2012)	256	Stage race	1903–2011	Y, D, B, N_{ST}, SR	94***	90***	.92***	-.31***	-.68***	.85***	None
3 (Lodewijkx & Verboon, 2013)[3]	62	Time trial (50–61 km)	1934–2010	Y, D, A	58***	56***	.77***	-.16	-.71***	.41**	None
4 (Lodewijkx & Bos, 2014)[3]	100	Time trial (multiple winners)	1949–2013	Y, D, A	55***	98***	.73***	-.24*	-.21*	.98***	Indurain (Tour, 1992)
5 (Lodewijkx, 2013)[4]	19	Time trial (mountain)	1958–2004	Y, CL_I, A	93***	88***	.48*	.83***	.14	.94***	Berzin (Tour, 1996)
6 (Lodewijkx & Verboon, 2014)[5]	324	Time trial (all)	1933–2013	Y, D, SR	60***	98***	.71***	-.28***	-.34***	.97***	Plaza (Vuelta, 2005)

Notes:
[1] Y = Competition year. D = Distance of stage race / trial. B = Brutality rate. N_{ST} = Number of stages in the race. SR = Stage race (Tour vs. Giro vs. Vuelta). A = Comparisons of Armstrong vs. other riders. CL_I = Climbing index. Findings concern observations across the Tour, Giro, and Vuelta.
[2] % Performance differences (R^2_{adj}) explained by DHM variables. R^2_{adj} are rounded off.
[3] These studies compared Armstrong's (A) time trial victories to other riders, demonstrated on flat and rolling terrain, excluded are mountain time trials.
[4] We only examined mountain trials in the Tour de France.
[5] Included in this study are all trials on flat and rolling terrain, excluded are prologues, mountain trials, and team time trials.
* $p \leq .05$; ** $p \leq .01$; *** $p \leq .001$

Table 1: Main Findings of Historic Studies.

account of the influence the three different stage races (SR) exerted on riders' achievements over time.

As to time trials, Table 1 shows that the years of competition (Y) and the distances (D) of the trials again served as predictor variables. Study 6 investigated all victories realized by riders on flat and rolling terrain in the three tours over the years (1933–2013). The remaining studies all compared Armstrong's (A) achievements to other riders. Study 3 evaluated his wins against other riders who, from 1934 to 2010, won trials in the three major races and all faced distances comparable to Armstrong's (50–61 km) in the seven Tours he won. Study 4 relates to comparisons of Armstrong's victories with wins of all other famous multiple Grand Tour winners (Coppi, Anquetil, Merckx, Hinault, and Indurain) as well as victories of riders who either were, or were not, involved in doping affairs in the years following Armstrong's domination in professional road racing (2006-2013). Study 5 evaluated Armstrong's 2001 and 2004 wins in mountain time trials (racing uphill). We developed a climbing index (CL_I) to capture the demanding nature of these trials, operationalized as the rise (the corrected altitude of the climbs in km) over the run (the total distance of the trial in km). Higher values of the Cl_I designate more demanding trials in terms of riders' instant climbing efforts.

In the sections to follow, we will first discuss the total amounts of variation (R^2_{adj}) the various DHM variables conjointly explained in riders' performances in the different studies as well as the single variables that explained the largest amounts of variation in these achievements. We will then proceed with a comprehensive appraisal of the SPA relating to different findings in different studies: (1) stage race wins; (2) time trial wins; (3) outlying performances; and (4) Armstrong's achievements. The appraisal additionally involves an alternative assessment of riders' performance progress over time, since km/h and time performances *per sé* do not permit valid estimates of this progress. The differencing method, used in time–series analysis [57], enables one to appraise the proportional progress (%) in riders' performances per year. We therefore also employed this method to examine the SPA. Last, as can be seen in the figures and tables, we partitioned the years of competition into periods of approximately ten years, using El Helou et al.'s critical year 1993 as the standard to classify the ten–year periods after WW II. Because our main objective is to examine the validity of the SPA, we will restrict the presentation and discussion of our findings to three bordering time periods: the epo era (1993–2002) vs. the immediate preceding years (1983-1992) vs. the following years (2003-2011/2013). A thorough elaboration of developments in the remaining time periods and associated differences between races is beyond the scope of the present thesis. We refer to the separate studies for information concerning these developments.

Main Findings

The sixth column in Table 1 presents the total amounts of variation (R^2_{adj}) the various DHM measures together explained in riders' achievements. As to km/h performances, the amounts range between 55– 94%. For time performances they vary between 56–98%. The lowest amounts are found in the first Armstrong time–trial study (Study 3; R^2_{adj}=56-58%). In this study, distance did not significantly contribute to the R^2_{adj}, because it examined a restricted range in the distances of the trials (50–61 km), thereby decreasing the overall R^2_{adj}. The correlations presented in the seventh column show that two variables account for most of the differences in riders' achievements over time. Competition year constitutes the main explanatory variable of riders' km/h performances (r=0.48-0.92). As the years proceed, riders race faster. The exception is the mountain time trial study (Study 5) in which the positive influence of distance (r=0.83) was stronger than the influence of competition year (r=0.48). Distance turned out to be the main explanatory variable of riders' mean time performances. Larger distances are associated with slower performances. Except for Study 3, which evaluated restricted trial distances (r=0.41), the remaining studies yielded robust correlations ($r_=$0.85-0.98). Table 1 additionally reveals that, as far as time trials are concerned, competition year has a relatively minor and inconsistent influence on riders' time performances (r=-0.34-0.14). We will deal with these relationships in the sections on the psycho–logical fallacies, because they have consequences for the SPA.

Speed Progress in Stage Races

The six panels in Figure 3 graphically present the relationships between competition year and the two performance measures, providing some first answers to the soundness of the SPA. We confined the plots to findings of the study with the largest number of observations (Study 2; N=256). The correlations in Panel A and B reveal a linear progress in speed over the years, which is stronger for km/h than for time performances. Notice, first, that the negative competition year–time performance relationship in Panel B also indicates faster time performances over the years. Second, both panels reveal a steady improvement in performance from the epo era up to 2011, designating that riders in the '90s did not outperform riders in succeeding years. This observation constitutes a first indication of the invalidity of the SPA.

A second indication concerns the annual proportional changes in performance we computed. The relationships are illustrated in Panel C and D of Figure 3. Positive numbers on km/h performances denote an incline in performance per year, 0% indicates no progress, and negative numbers indicate a decline. The reverse relationships hold for time performances. The original linear relationships, depicted in Panel A en B, are illustrated by the mean proportional changes in Panel C and D: $M_{km/h}$=0.52%; M_{time}=0.42%. These percentages indicate, for instance, that riders increased their km/h with approximately 52% within a time span of 100 years, i.e., from the 1900s (M=26 km/h) to the 2010s (M=39.5 km/h; excluding the years of the two world wars).

Furthermore, in disagreement with the SPA the mean proportional changes in both panels reveal no striking increase in the epo years. As to km/h performances, the analysis yielded r=-.05 (b=-0.007%; p=.41) and the individual 95%–prediction interval varies between -7.8-8.9%. For time performances, the correlation amounts to r=- .10 (b=-0.04%; p=.10; 95%–prediction interval: -21.9-22.9%). The same panels additionally designate that the prediction intervals apply to all time periods and, hence, to riders' disputed wins in the epo era as well.

A third indication concerning the unsoundness of the SPA involves the distribution of the mean annual changes that can be seen in Panel E and F of Figure 3. The changes concerning km/h performances are normally distributed, while this is not true for the changes involving time performances, which show kurtosis. This can be explained by the relatively large number of observations that revolve around zero. Importantly, both distributions indicate a symmetrical dispersion of inclines and declines in riders' performances over time. Accordingly, there is no evidence at all for the existence of extraordinary 'superior' developments in riders' first–ranking achievements in the three stage races over the years.

A final indication relates to the evaluation of the predicted, proportional progress in performance realized in the epo era compared to the directly adjacent time periods. Using regression analyses, we assessed the influence of stage races and competition year on the

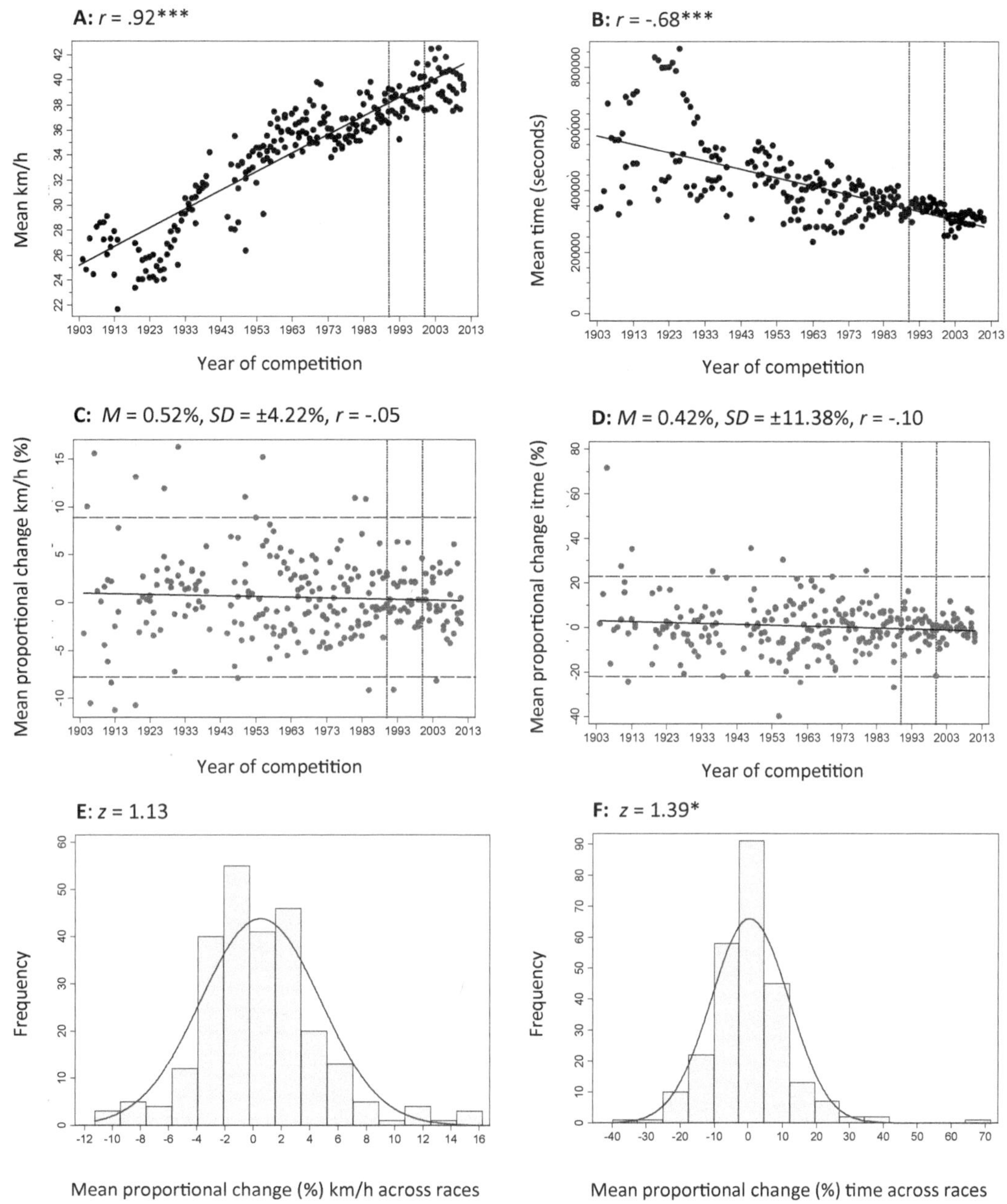

* $p \leq .05$; *** $p \leq .001$

Figure 3: Panel A and B present Pearson correlation coefficients between competition year and winning riders' mean km/h and time performances across stage races. Panel C and D show the Pearson correlation coefficients between competition year and the mean proportional changes (%) per year for both performance measures, averaged across races. Panel E and F present the distribution of the latter performance measures. Vertical dotted lines mark the epo era (1990–2000), horizontal dashed lines present the individual 95%–prediction interval.

percents change per year in which we controlled for the influence of the corresponding annual changes in the three covariates alluded to above (distance, number of stages, and the brutality rate). We will restrict the presentation of the regression findings solely to km/h performances, since time performances yielded virtually identical results. Main findings are summarized in Table 2 and Figure 4. First, relative to Panel C in Figure 3, Figure 4 shows a strong reduction in the variability of the changes that can be attributed to the influence of the variables included in the analyses. Second, Table 2 reveals that, within the epo era, none of the predicted, mean changes differ significantly from zero. Likewise, the changes in the epo years do no differ significantly from the changes in the immediate bordering years (or from all the other time periods we distinguished). These conclusions hold within and across races. The findings additionally indicate that the relationships between competition year and the mean changes across and within races are small and negative: in speed progress Across races, r=-0.13, b=-0.007% per year, R^2_{adj}=1.2%, ($p \leq 0.05$); Tour: r=-0.15, b=-0.008% per year, R^2_{adj}=1.3%, (p=0.14); Giro: r=-0.14, b=-0.008% per year, R^2_{adj}=1%, (p =0.18); Vuelta: r=-0.11, b=-0.01% per year, R^2_{adj}=1%, (p=0.39). The relationships reveal a minor, gradual decline over time in the three

	Stage Races[1]				Time Trials[2]			
	Year	*N*	*M* (*SE*)[3]	95%-CI	Year	*N*	*M* (*SE*)[3]	95%-CI
Across Races	1903-1914	16	0.21 (0.47)$_a$	-0.72–1.14	-	-	-	-
	1919-1929	22	1.48 (0.37)*$_a$	0.75–2.22	-	-	-	-
	1930-1940	22	1.18 (0.64)$_a$	-0.08–2.43	1933-1942	9	1.46 (0.19)*$_b$	1.07–1.86
	1946-1952	18	0.93 (0.42)*$_a$	0.11–1.75	1946-1952	15	1.10 (0.13)*$_b$	0.85–1.35
	1953-1962	28	0.26 (0.33)$_a$	-0.40–0.91	1953-1962	24	0.73 (0.10)*$_b$	0.52–0.93
	1963-1972	30	0.49 (0.32)$_a$	-0.14–1.12	1963-1972	28	0.56 (0.09)*$_b$	0.38–0.74
	1973-1982	30	0.27 (0.32)$_a$	-0.36–0.90	1973-1982	29	0.34 (0.09)*$_a$	0.17–0.52
	1983-1992	30	0.26 (0.32)$_a$	-0.37–0.89	1983-1992	30	0.33 (0.09)*$_a$	0.15–0.50
	1993-2002	**30**	**0.48 (0.32)$_a$**	**-0.15–1.11**	**1993-2002**	**30**	0.15 (0.09)$_a$	-0.02–0.33
	2003-2011	27	0.27 (0.34)$_a$	-0.39–0.94	2003-2013	33	-0.11 (0.08)$_a$	-0.27–0.06
Tour	1983-1992	10	-0.14 (0.55)$_a$	-1.23–0.95	1983-1992	10	0.32 (0.15)*$_a$	0.01–0.62
	1993-2002	**10**	**0.52 (0.55)$_a$**	**-0.57–1.61**	**1993-2002**	**10**	0.20 (0.15)$_a$	-0.10–0.51
	2003-2011	9	0.19 (0.58)$_a$	-0.96–1.34	2003-2013	10	-0.01 (0.15)$_a$	-0.29–0.28
Giro	1983-1992	10	0.40 (0.55)$_a$	-0.69–1.49	1983-1992	10	0.39 (0.15)*$_a$	0.09–0.70
	1993-2002	**10**	**0.41 (0.55)$_a$**	**-0.68–1.50**	**1993-2002**	**10**	0.13 (0.15)$_a$	-0.18–0.43
	2003-2011	9	0.19 (0.58)$_a$	-0.97–1.33	2003-2013	10	-0.16 (0.15)$_a$	-0.45–0.13
Vuelta	1983-1992	10	0.52 (0.55)$_a$	-0.57–1.61	1983-1992	11	0.27 (0.15)$_a$	-0.04–0.57
	1993-2002	**10**	**0.50 (0.55)$_a$**	**-0.59–1.59**	**1993-2002**	**11**	0.13 (0.15)$_a$	-0.17–0.43
	2003-2011	9	0.46 (0.58)$_a$	-0.69–1.60	2003-2013	11	-0.16 (0.15)$_a$	-0.44–0.13

Notes:

[1] Number of stage race wins between time periods vary due to WW I and II and the Spanish civil war. The years of the epo era are in bold type face. Predicted mean proportional changes are based regression analyses in which we used competition year, stage races, distances of the stage races, number of stages in the races, and the brutality rate of the races as predictor variables. *N* = 253 because proportional changes cannot be computed for the intial races.

[2] The first time trial ever in professional cycling was scheduled in the 1933 Giro, followed by the Tour in 1934, and in 1941 by the Vuelta. Predicted mean proportional changes are based regression analyses in which we used competition year, stage races, and the distances of the time trials as predictor variables. We aggregated the time trials per year (*N* = 198).

[3] Means without a common subscript differ significantly, $p \leq .05$. Across stage races, we contrasted the epo period against all other periods. For separate stage races, contrasts compared the epo years to immediate adjacent time periods. To prevent Type I-errors, we adjusted the 95%-CI using the Bonferroni procedure.

* Within time periods mean proportional changes differ significantly from zero, $p \leq .05$.

Table 2. Descriptive Statistics of Predicted Mean Proportional Changes (%) in Winning Riders' Km/h Performances per Time Period in Stage Races and Time Trials.

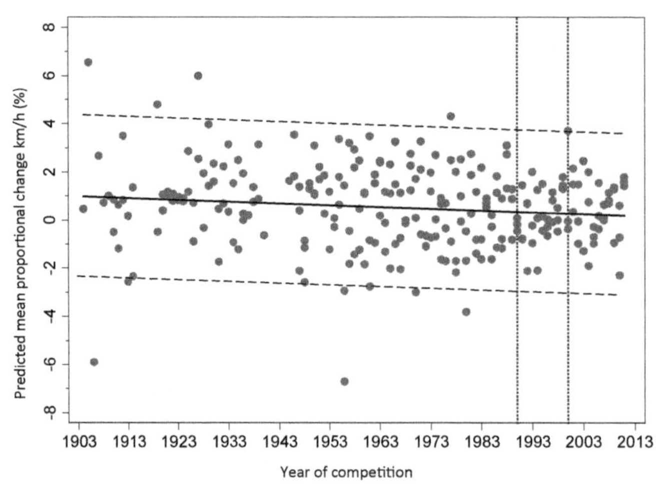

Figure 4: Relationship between predicted mean proportional changes (%) in winning riders' km/h performances and competition year, aggregated across stage races. Changes are based on the regression analyses of the stage race data in Table 2. Vertical dotted lines mark the epo era (1990–2000), dashed lines the individual 95%-prediction interval.

races and competition year explains 1–1.3% of the differences in these developments.

To sum up, all these observations invalidate the SPA as well as conclusions drawn by El Helou and colleagues [16] and Perneger [51]. They indicate that riders perform progressively faster over time, but this progress gradually levels off with advancing years. However, the progress in the epo period is not superior compared to the progress observed in immediate bordering periods and, most importantly, does not constitute an exception to the overall, historic variability in speed progress observed in the three main stage races.

Speed Progress in Time Trials

Findings concerning riders' time trial achievements are presented in an identical way as the stage race data. Panel A en B in Figure 5 present the zero-order correlations between competition year and the two performance measures for the study with the largest number of observations (Study 6; *N*=324). In regard to km/h performances, Panel A shows a linear progress in speed, indicating that riders perform faster with advancing years. Again the panel shows that riders in the epo era did not perform faster than riders in succeeding years. Besides, Panel B reveals that for mean time performances the relationship is not linear, but resembles a significant M-curve, or quartic relationship. Riders raced slower in the '40s, faster in the post-WW II years up till the mid-'70s, slower in the '80s and '90s, and faster again after 2003. By itself, this M-curve again disproves the SPA, because riders in the epo era

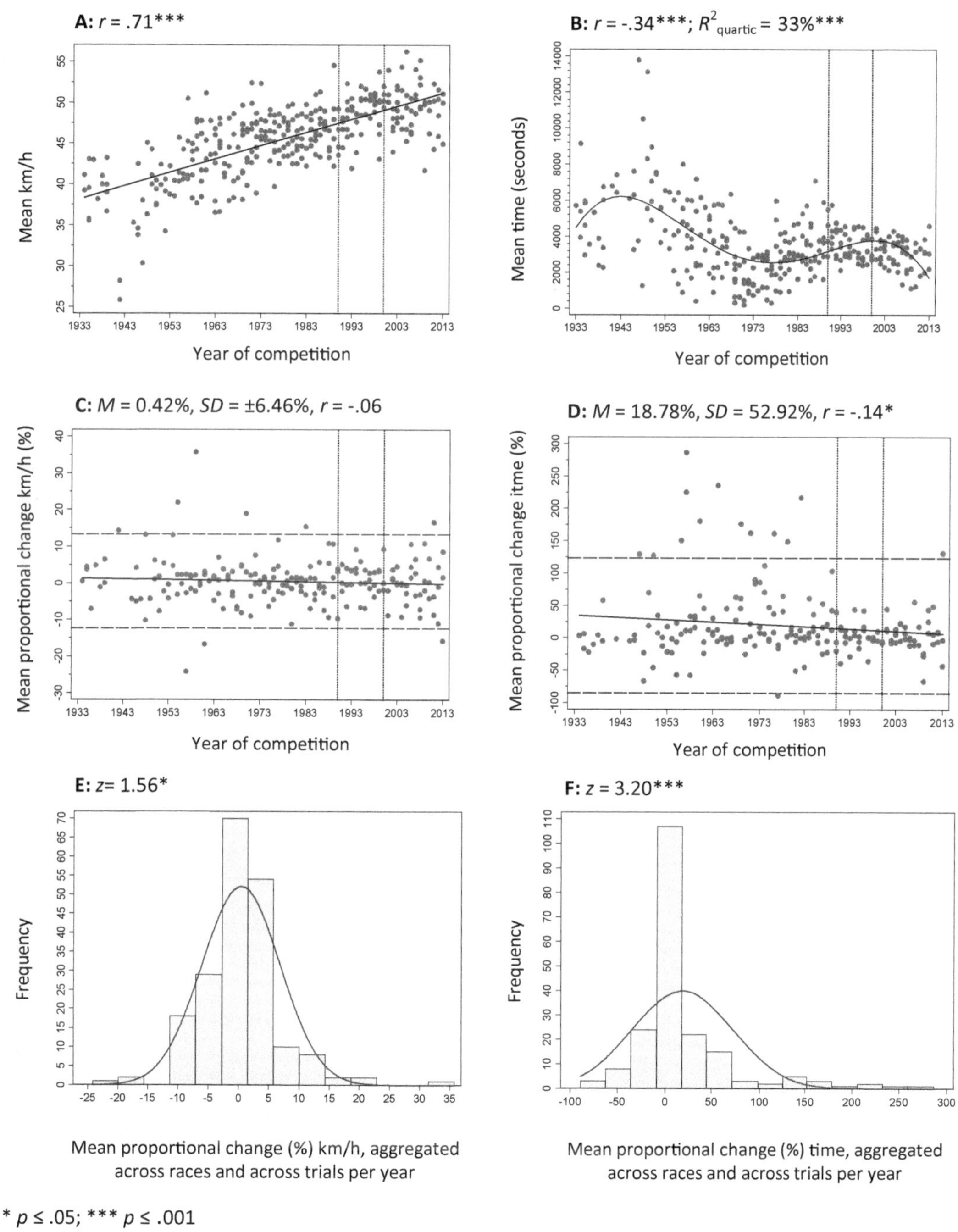

Figure 5: Panel A and B present the Pearson correlation coefficients between competition year and winning riders' mean km/h and time performances in time trials across stage races. Panel C and D show the Pearson correlation coefficients between competition year and the mean proportional changes (%) per year on both performance measures, averaged across races and across trials per year. Panel E and F show the distribution of the latter performance measures. Vertical dotted lines mark the epo era (1990–2000), dashed lines the individual 95%–prediction interval.

delivered comparatively slower not faster time performances compared to riders' achievements in the 2000s. Additional analyses indicated that this M-curve can be explained by the distances of the time trials. This variable shows a robust correlation with time performances (r=0. 97) and, hence, a development over the years which is similar to the M-curve obtained on the time performance measure. Accordingly, the variation in riders' mean time performance over the years is due to the closely matching variation in trial distances. These observations imply that we should control for the influence of distance on riders' performances.

Panel C and D in Figure 5 illustrate the relationships between the estimated proportional changes and competition year for both dependent variables. To estimate these changes we transformed the data by aggregating the time trials per year. The reason is that the public in the '50s, '60s and '70s wanted to see the performances of the legendary and renowned time trialists Fausto Coppi, Jacques Anquetil, and Eddy Merckx. To satisfy the interest of the public in these riders they therefore faced many trials in their stage races, the distances of which sometimes varied extremely (between 8 and 137 km). These large differences led to huge bandwidths on both performance measures. To circumvent this problem we therefore averaged the time trial performances per year. Consistent with the stage race data, findings of the regression analyses reject the SPA. Regarding the mean proportional changes in km/h, the analyses produced r=-0.06 (b=-0.019%; p=0.39) and the individual 95%-prediction interval varies between -12.4–13.3%. For time performances, the correlation is r=-.14 (b=-.35%; p=.051) with the individual 95%-prediction interval ranging between -85.1–123.2%. Notice again that for time performances, positive numbers indicate a decrease and negative numbers an increase in performance. Thus, the negative correlation found for time performances designates a progress in these performances that lessens with proceeding years. As to these performances, we stress that Panel D still reveals a huge variation, despite the data transformation we applied.

Panel E and F in Figure 5 present the distributions of the aggregated, annual changes for the two performance measures, revealing deviations from normality. Similar to the stage race data, the deviations cannot be attributed to a relatively large number of observations that involve extreme forms of fast progress, but rather to a comparatively large number of observations that hover around zero. Once more, both distributions show no evidence for the existence of extraordinary 'superior' developments in riders' time trial performances over the years.

Last, we evaluated the proportional progress in performance in the epo era vs. the directly bordering time periods in which we controlled for the associated yearly changes in trial distances and differences between stage races. Again, the presentation of the regression results will be confined to km/h performances. Findings are presented in Table 2 and Figure 6. Relative to Panel C in Figure 5, Figure 6 shows a strong reduction in the variability of the changes owing to the variables we entered into the regression equation. Additionally, Table 2 reveals that the predicted mean changes in the epo years do not differ significantly from zero. Examination of differences between the three time periods also produced no significant effects across and within races. However, inconsistent with findings relating to the stage races, the regression results revealed strong, significant decreases in the predicted speed progress over time: Across races, r=-.64, b=-.019% per year, R^2_{adj}=41%; Tour: r=-.62, b=-.017% per year, R^2_{adj}=37.8%; Giro: r=-.82, b=-.022% per year, R^2_{adj}=67.3%; Vuelta: r=-.50, b=-.017% per year, R^2_{adj}=23.5% (all $p \leq$ .001). All relationships indicate a strong downturn in predicted speed progress per year within and across races. Inconsistent with the SPA,

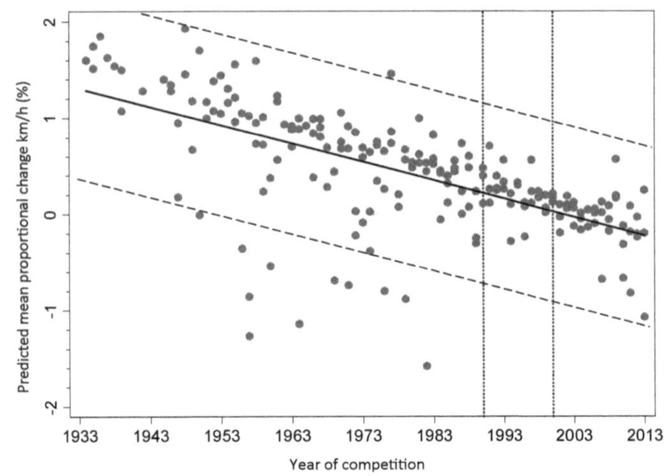

Figure 6: Relationship between predicted mean proportional changes (%) in winning riders' km/h performances in time trials and competition year, aggregated across races. Changes are averaged across trials per year and based on the regression analyses of the time trial data in Table 2. Vertical dotted lines mark the epo era (1990–2000), dashed lines the individual 95%-prediction interval.

however, Table 2 and Figure 6 show that riders' progress in the epo era does not constitute an exception to these developments. The observed decrease in progress can be explained by the fact that, over time, riders deliver faster performances in time trials. However, the more enhanced the speed the more difficult it becomes to make a difference. Hence, the diminishing annual progress in speed demonstrated by riders in these individual races against the clock over the years.

On the whole, we conclude that the time trial data corroborate findings relating to the stage races. Neither the SPA, nor conclusions drawn by El Helou et al. [16] and Perneger [51] are supported.

Outliers

An assessment of outlying (very fast) performances perhaps makes up the most valid way to test the SPA. To determine outliers, we applied the rigorous criterion of ≥ ± 2SD from the sample mean (the individual 95%-confidence and prediction intervals), while conventionally the criterion of ≥ ± 3SD is used (or z ≥ ± 3.30 with N <1000; [58]). As to the mean proportional changes, the 95%-prediction intervals and the normal distributions depicted in Figure 3 to 6 already indicate that outliers are very rare indeed. In all analyses, the one and only rider that slightly surpassed the bandwidth in the epo era involved the victory of Spanish rider Roberto Heras in the 2000 Vuelta (z=2.01). However, when considering achievements within the Spanish race itself, his performance did not went beyond the criterion anymore.

The last column of Table 1 presents findings of the separate studies. They are based on regression analyses in which riders' observed mean km/h and time performances served as the dependent variables. The table shows that none of the performances of the stage-race winners in the epo era or thereafter fell outside the 95%-bandwidth. This conclusion does not change much after the evaluation of riders' time trial accomplishments. Only three riders surpassed the 95% band width: Spanish rider Miguel Indurain, Russian rider Yevgeny Berzin, and Spanish rider Ruben Plaza. Indurain's performance failed to be an outlier after having taken account of all time trial performances realized by winning riders over the years in the three tours (Study 6). Besides, it can be doubted whether Plaza's achievement in the 2005 Vuelta can be regarded an outlier as well, because the conditions during his race must have been very good. Closer scrutiny of the overall standings of the trial showed that the rider who reached the 100th position (Alberto Ongarato) already achieved a speed of nearly 50 km/h [55]. Of all riders we investigated, perhaps only Berzin realized a striking performance in his race uphill. Then again, even his achievement did not surpass the bandwidth of ± 3*SD*.

Once more, these results disprove the SPA. Reckoning the historic variation in riders' achievements in stage races and time trials, all riders' performances in the epo era fell within the range of expected variability. Evidently, many of these performances are outstanding. However, this does not mean to say that, therefore, they are 'abnormal.' Our findings persuasively suggest that this is not the case.

Armstrong's Wins

Study 3 evaluated whether Armstrong's seven time trial wins on flat and rolling courses, demonstrated in the Tour de France from 1999 to 2005, were faster compared to wins of riders who faced similar trial distances (50–61 km) in the three tours from 1934 to 2010. Findings of the study indicated that the American racer initially did realize significantly faster performances relative to the other riders (M=4.70 km/h, R^2=6.4%). However, after statistically controlling for the significant influence of competition year, he ultimately raced somewhat slower (M=-0.43 km/h, R^2=0.1%). Only one of his wins exceeded the bounds of the 68%–bandwidth (i.e., ± 1*SD* from the sample mean), while all his remaining six achievements fell within the bandwidth of this very stringent criterion. Thus, when considering the historic performance variation in these trials of limited distance, all individual accomplishments of the controversial American were not superior.

Study 4 evaluated his time trial–wins against victories of all other multiple Grand Tour winners and against riders who were, or were not, involved in doping affairs in the 2006–2013 periods. It yielded virtually identical results as Study 3. Ultimately, analyses revealed a non–significant difference of M=142 seconds (M=0.33 km/h) between Armstrong vs. all the aggregated other riders, which explained a trivial 0.1% of the variation in riders' performances. Only two of Armstrong's wins surpassed the bandwidth of the 68%–CI and none went beyond the 95%–CI. The study further revealed that riders who were involved in doping affairs (including Armstrong) raced somewhat slower than riders who were not (M=-68 s; M=-1.17 km/h). Yet, these differences were far from significant and explained an inconsequential 0.1–3.2% of the performance differences between riders.

Findings of the mountain time trial study (Study 5) confirmed the findings of the two other studies. The climbing index (CL_l) had a robust influence on riders' speed (r=-.97; R^2=94%), indicating that riders raced b=2.302 km/h slower per unit of the index. The significant mediating influence of the index subsequently reduced riders' yearly progress in speed to a non–significant b=26 m per year (R^2=0.3%). Besides, Armstrong's wins did not prove to be outliers, but came out comparatively slow. As to the results of the remaining studies, they all substantiate the foregoing conclusions: None of his performances were extraordinary, including his controversial seven victories in the Tour de France.

As a final conclusion, we maintain that all our empirical facts convincingly invalidate the SPA. Implications of this conclusion for contemporary discussions about the effects of doping in the cycling world will be addressed in the next sections.

Implications: Fallacies and Fabrications

Logical fallacies

As our body of evidence against the SPA accumulated, we came to realize that arguments used in these discussions often involve logical fallacies and psychological biases. We will first discuss the logical fabrications. An often heard argument refers to the appeal to ignorance (*argumentum ad ignorantiam*), which poses that "something is true only because it has not been proved false, or that something is false only because it has not been proved true" [59]. Evidently, this logic again exemplifies the SPA, because it illustrates the assumed, strong positive association between the year in which riders competed with the concomitant doping use (i.e., in the epo era) and their performances. Our stage race and time trial data reject this logic. Findings relating to the predicted, mean proportional changes in stage races indicated that competition year explained a minor 1–1.3% of the differences in winning riders' progress in speed over time. The small, negative relationships we found indicate that this progress slowly levels off up till the present. We emphasize that riders do perform increasingly faster over the years, but the speed progress in the epo era is consistent with the progress observed in the other time periods we distinguished. The negative relationships we found for riders' predicted progress in time trials were more substantial, explaining 23.5%-67.3% of the performance differences between riders over time. Yet, they do not alter our main conclusion. Again, our findings revealed that the speed progress in the epo period was not superior compared to the progress observed in immediate bordering time periods and did not constitute an exception to the overall, historic variability in speed progress in time trials in the three main stage races. Besides, the assessment of the magnitude of the competition year– performance relationship is also contingent upon whether or not research examines the powerful influence of distance on riders' achievements. For instance, the last three time trial studies in Table 1 indicate that the impact of this variable on riders' time performances (r=.94–.98) is far more substantial and consistent than the influence of competition year (r=-0.34–0.14). All these observations render the reasoning underlying the appeal to ignorance implausible.

Study 5 illustrates the *post hoc ergo propter hoc fallacy* (translation: after this, therefore because of this). It reflects the erroneous belief that, because there is a temporal sequence in events, one event is the cause of the other. For example, Armstrong's winning achievements in mountain time trials in 2001 and 2004 ('after this') are assumed to be caused by his doping use ('because of this'). However, Study 5 revealed that the main determinant of riders' wins in these trials appeared to be the climbing index rather than the year in which riders won their trial and the doping use associated with it. Thus, when taking race–related variables into consideration that are essential for mountain time trialing, Armstrong's victories did not prove to be superior to achievements realized by famous climbers such as Charly Gaul in 1958 or Frederico Bahamontes in 1959 or 1962. These findings invalidate the logic used in the post hoc fallacy in addition to the reasoning presented in the argument from ignorance. They further entail that we tend to underestimate the athletic achievements demonstrated by the very gifted riders in the early days of the races and to overestimate riders' performances in the modern era.

Study 6 elucidates the *Texas sharpshooter fallacy.* If research is based on selective or limited data or uses an invalid dependent variable, this may result in biased conclusions concerning riders' evolution in speed over time. This fallacy applies to the two archival studies [16,51], described previously, that both supported the SPA. However, the 6.38% performance progress in the epo era, reported by El Helou and co-workers, can be attributed to the selective way this increase was statistically tested [16]. The researchers aggregated all riders' performances demonstrated in the pre–epo years (1946–1992) and compared the resulting mean performances to the aggregated mean performances of riders in the epo years (1993–2008). Because they also found a strong linear increase in speed over time, the observed difference might thus have been inflated by the relatively slower speeds demonstrated by riders in the years following WW II (see also Panel A in Figure 3). In a similar vein, Perneger based his conclusions on limited data. He restricted his analyses to performances delivered by riders between 1990 and 2009, but did not include performances demonstrated by riders in 1980s in his sample. However, the choice of an alternative way to measure developments in performance (annual proportional changes), the decision to include confounding variables (the control variables) in our studies and to examine all stage race and time trial wins as well as performance differences between the epo era and directly bordering time periods proved them wrong.

All in all, the logical fallacies suggest that discussions about the (reputed) effects of doping in cycling may often involve false reasoning and fabrications. According to Carroll [59], the use of these errors becomes more tempting among 'believers'. Thus, for people who believe in the effects of doping, the lack of opposing empirical evidence may be germane to sustaining their belief.

Psychological fallacies

Psychological research shows that some very powerful social-cognitive biases may reinforce these beliefs, offering partial explanations for the naming, blaming, and shaming of cyclists. Our judgments may be guided by the availability heuristic [60], a rule of thumb whereby people base a judgment on the ease with which they can bring something to mind. Regretfully, winning cyclists who are accused of cheating can be brought to mind all too easily. This heuristic is further associated with some other biases that may well clarify stereotypic reactions towards cyclists. The base rate fallacy leads us to overestimate the number of (winning) riders that used doping substances. We also may engage into biased sampling and illusory correlations [61]. Both involve making sweeping statements based on selective samples of information that are atypical, i.e., on the basis of a few selected observations we come to the conclusion that, because some performances were associated with doping use, all endeavors of cyclists probably have to do with cheating.

These biases may have an influence on people's attribution of blameworthiness. In his culpable control model, Alicke [62] argues that such attributions or often guided by automatic, heuristic processes, not by rational arguments. If we apply his arguments to the doping problem in cycling they mean that, whenever we are confronted with a rider that by hook or by crook is associated with doping use, we implicitly tend to "exaggerate his volitional or causal control, lower evidential standards for blame, or seek information that supports our blame attribution" (ibid., p. 558).

This blaming may be directed by the fundamental attribution error [63], which refers to the tendency to strongly overestimate the extent to which people's behavior is caused by internal, dispositional factors and to underestimate the role of external, situational factors that may plausibly account for the same behavior. So, if we are confronted with an outstanding achievement of a cyclist in a mountain stage, the heuristic tendency will be to attribute this performance to some internal factors (athletic capability, training, doping/cheating?) and to underestimate the role of external, race-related circumstances (favorable wind, competition between teams, distance, relatively easy stage) that may have strongly affected the very same achievement. Three factors facilitate the operation of this bias. It occurs if performances are evaluated as being highly distinctive ("I've never seen a rider race so fast"), if we all agree that this is indeed the case (high consensus), and if there is low consistency in the performance ("He has never climbed like that before"). According to Hilton and Slugoski's [64] abnormal conditions focus model, the combination of high distinctiveness, high consensus and low consistency will result in the conclusion that riders' performances are 'abnormal'. Combined with the culpable control processes and the other biases we described this will lead us to implicitly construe that these 'abnormal' winning achievements probably involve the use of banned substances and their attributed ergogenic effects. To his regret, Christopher Froome, winner of the 2013 Tour de France, faced this kind of reasoning throughout the entire race.

Conclusions

In the Introduction of this contribution we argued that the findings yielded by our studies would constitute a rather inconvenient truth concerning the validity of the SPA. We additionally put forward that our studies would permit to give direct answers to the relationships presented in path A of the DHM (Figure 1) and some indirect answers to the relationships presented in path C. Our findings indicated that the race-related variables we distinguished in path A explained considerable amounts of 90–94% (Study 2, all stage races) and 60–98% (Study 6, all time trials) of the performance differences between riders over time. These percentages imply that 6–10% (stage races) or 2–40% (time trials) of these differences are not explained by our DHM variables. The rather high 40% of unexplained differences, obtained on km/h performances in Study 6, can be attributed to the weak influence of distance (r=-0.28) on these particular performances, while the influence of the same variable on cyclists' time performances is robust (r=0.97). Therefore it seems fair to discard this 40%. This means that, ultimately, 2–10% of the differences in riders' achievements over the years in stage races and time trials can be attributed to other, unknown and perhaps confounding variables which we did not include in our studies. Doping use is but one of the variables to account for these differences next to other performance-enhancing variables, many of which relate to the circumstances under which cyclists practiced their sport over the years [1,3-6,14,33,34,56]. They all facilitated riders' achievements with advancing years, such as more favorable road, terrain, and race conditions; less demanding racing programs; growing insights from exercise physiology with associated sophisticated and effective training regimes; improved technology of bikes and racing gear; increased specialization of riders; and improvements in nutrition and hydration, leading to an enhanced maintenance of riders' energy balance during stage events [13]. In addition, in his socio-historical analysis of the cycling sport, Brewer [1] describes other facilitative factors relating to changes in team organization and inter-team dynamics, sponsorship, financial incentives, and a progressively deepening commercialization of the sport, which led to increased speed in races from the mid-1980s onward. We emphasize that this list of expediting variables is by no means exhaustive. They can all be regarded variables which, apart from doping use, may plausibly account for the unexplained performance differences between riders we obtained.

Importantly for the present thesis, the indirect relationships we found for path C render the superior performances assumption doubtful. Our empirical facts yielded no proof that riders in the epo era raced strikingly faster than riders in immediate adjoining years. Moreover, their first-ranking performances in stage races and time trials did not constitute outliers and the progress in performance they demonstrated did not depart from the variation in progress observed in the three major European stage races over time. These null results are consistent with findings of the meta-analysis we carried out, from which we concluded that the ergogenic effects of RBC-augmenting doping agents on riders' aerobic performances and associated cycling speeds are overestimated. However, despite the clear uniformity in our findings, we stress that conclusions from the historic studies can only be tentative. The studies lack essential base lines and control conditions and the findings may have been influenced by an inestimable, systematic error: We have no idea how riders would have performed over the years, had they abstained from taking banned substances.

Nevertheless, we argue that awareness of our empirical observations and their implications would greatly contribute to the exchange of evidence-based pros and cons in the sometimes frenzied, societal discussions about the effects of doping in the cycling world, set in motion by the Armstrong affair. Moreover, Kuipers [13] and Heuberger et al. [53] might not be mistaken in their final conclusion that the doping problem in professional cycling indeed rests on superstition, hearsay, insufficient knowledge, medical malpractice, and lack of (opposing) empirical evidence. On balance, the sportive feats demonstrated by riders in the years of the 'epo epidemic' were not exceptional at all, despite their doping use.

References

1. Brewer BF (2002) Commercialization in professional cycling 1950–2001: Institutional transformations and the rationalization of doping. SSJ 19: 276-301.
2. Dilger A, Frick B, Tolsdorf F (2007) Are athletes doped? Some theoretical arguments and empirical evidence. Contemporary Economic Policy 25: 604-615.
3. Dimeo P (2007) A history of drug use in sport 1876–1976. New York: Routledge / Taylor & Francis Group.
4. Hoberman J (1992) Mortal engines: The science of performance and the dehumanization of sport. The Free Press, New York.
5. Hoberman JM (2005) Testosterone dreams: Rejuvenation, aphrodisia, doping. University of California Press, Berkeley/Los Angeles.
6. Lodewijkx HFM (2011) Reasoned decision of the United States Anti–Doping Agency on disqualification and ineligibility. Rotterdam: 2010 Uitgevers.
7. USADA (2012a) Statement from USADA CEO Travis T. Tygart regarding the U.S. Postal Service Pro Cycling Team doping conspiracy.
8. USADA (2012b) Reasoned decision of the United States Anti–Doping Agency on disqualification and ineligibility.
9. Lodewijkx HFM, Brouwer B (2011) Some empirical notes on the 'epo epidemic' in professional cycling. Res Q Exerc Sport 82: 740-754.
10. Lodewijkx HFM, Verboon P (2013) Lance Armstrong's era of performance – Part I: Are his time trial performances much different from other winners? Journal of Athletic Enhancement 2:1.
11. Tetlock PE (2003) Thinking the unthinkable: Sacred values and taboo cognitions. Trends in Cognitive Sciences 7: 320-324.
12. Tetlock PE (2003) Thinking the unthinkable: sacred values and taboo cognitions. Trends Cogn Sci 7: 320-324.
13. Tetlock PE1, Kristel OV, Elson SB, Green MC, Lerner JS (2000) The psychology of the unthinkable: taboo trade-offs, forbidden base rates, and heretical counterfactuals. J Pers Soc Psychol 78: 853-870.
14. Kuipers H (2006) [Putative effects of doping in cycling]. Ned Tijdschr Geneeskd 150: 2643-2645.
15. Diamanti-Kandarakis E1, Konstantinopoulos PA, Papailiou J, Kandarakis SA, Andreopoulos A, et al. (2005) Erythropoietin abuse and erythropoietin gene doping: detection strategies in the genomic era. Sports Med 35: 831-840.
16. El Helou N1, Berthelot G, Thibault V, Tafflet M, Nassif H, et al. (2010) Tour de France, Giro, Vuelta, and classic European races show a unique progression of road cycling speed in the last 20 years. J Sports Sci 28: 789-796.
17. Gaudard A1, Varlet-Marie E, Bressolle F, Audran M (2003) Drugs for increasing oxygen and their potential use in doping: a review. Sports Med 33: 187-212.
18. Juhn M (2003) Popular sports supplements and ergogenic aids. Sports Med 33: 921-939.
19. Joyner MJ1, Coyle EF (2008) Endurance exercise performance: the physiology of champions. J Physiol 586: 35-44.
20. Bobet J (2008) Tomorrow, we ride. Norwich (UK), Mousehold Press/Hampstead (UK), Sport and Publicity.
21. Fignon L, Ducoin JE (2009) We were young and carefree [In French: Nous étions jeunes et insouciants]. Editions Grasset & Fasquelle, Paris.
22. Hamilton T, Coyle D (2012) The secret race. Bantam Books, New York.
23. Kimmage P (2007) Rough ride: Behind the wheel with a pro cyclist. Yellow Jersey Press / Random House, London.
24. Krijgsman E, Dekker Th (2011) Clean enough [In Dutch: Schoon genoeg]. Amsterdam, Arbeiderspers.
25. Millar D, Whittle J (2011) Racing through the dark. Orion Books, London.
26. Vanwalleghem R, Museeuw J (2009) Museeuw speaks [In Dutch: Museeuw spreekt]. Tielt (Belgium): Lannoo.
27. Winnen P (2000) From Santander to Santander. [In Dutch: Van Santander naar Santander]. Thomas Rap, Amsterdam.
28. Voet W (2001) Breaking the chain. Yellow Jersey Press / Random House, London.
29. D'Hont J (2007) Recollections of a 'soigneur' [In Dutch: Mémoires van een wielerverzorger]. Halewyck, Leuven, Belgium.
30. Rijckaert E (2000) The Festina affair [In Dutch: De zaak Festina]. Tielt (Belgium): Lannoo.
31. Porte G (2011) Physician in the Tour [In French: Médécin du Tour]. Editions Albin Michel, Paris.
32. Ballester P, Walsh D (2009) L.A. Confidentiel: Les secrets de Lance Armstrong [In Dutch: Vuil spel: het systeem Armstrong]. No Monkey Books, Westmalle, Belgium.
33. Fotheringham W (2009) Fallen angel: The passion of Fausto Coppi. Yellow Jersey Press, London.
34. Maso B (2005) The sweat of the Gods. Mousehold Press, Norwich, (UK).
35. Whittle J (2008) Bad blood. The secret life of the Tour de France. Yellow Jersey Press / Random House, London.
36. Lodewijkx HFM, Brouwer B, Kuipers H, Van Hezewijk R (2013) Overestimated effect of epo administration on aerobic exercise capacity: A meta–analysis. American Journal of Sports Science and Medicine 1: 17-27.
37. Noakes TD (2000) Physiological models to understand exercise fatigue and the adaptations that predict or enhance athletic performances. Scandinavian Journal of Medicine & Science in Sports 10:123-145.
38. Noakes TD (2008) Testing for maximum oxygen consumption has produced a brainless model of human exercise performance. Br J Sports Med 42: 551-555.
39. Varlet–Marie E, Gaudard E, Audran M, Bressolle F (2003) Pharmacokinetics / pharmacodynamics of recombinant human erythropoietins in doping control. Sports Medicine 33: 301-315.
40. Joyner MJ (2003) VO2MAX, blood doping, and erythropoietin. Br J Sports Med 37: 190-191.
41. Catlin DH, Hatton CK, Lasne F (2006) Abuse of recombinant erythropoietins by athletes. In Moulineux G, Foote MA, Elliott SG (Eds.) Erythropoietins and erythropoiesis. Basel, Birkhäuser Verlag, 205-228.
42. Verbruggen H (2001) The EPO epidemic in sport. Bloodline Reviews 1: 3-4.
43. Lundby C1, Olsen NV (2011) Effects of recombinant human erythropoietin in normal humans. J Physiol 589: 1265-1271.
44. Bytomski JR, Moorman III CT, MacAuley D (2010) Oxford American handbook of sports medicine. Oxford University Press, Oxford.
45. Ninot G1, Connes P, Caillaud C (2006) Effects of recombinant human erythropoietin injections on physical self in endurance athletes. J Sports Sci 24: 383-391.
46. Lundby C1, Robach P, Saltin B (2012) The evolving science of detection of 'blood doping'. Br J Pharmacol 165: 1306-1315.
47. Lundby C1, Robach P, Boushel R, Thomsen JJ, Rasmussen P, et al. (2008) Does recombinant human Epo increase exercise capacity by means other than augmenting oxygen transport? J Appl Physiol (1985) 105: 581-587.
48. Thomsen JJ, Rentsch RL, Robach P, Calbet JAL, Boushel R, et al. (2007) Prolonged administration of recombinant human erythropoietin increases submaximal performance more than maximal aerobic capacity. European Journal of Applied Physiology 101: 481-486.

49. Cohen J (1988) Statistical power analysis for the behavioral sciences (2nd Edn.). Lawrence Earlbaum Associates, Hillsdale.

50. Nevill AM1, Jobson SA, Palmer GS, Olds TS (2005) Scaling maximal oxygen uptake to predict cycling time-trial performance in the field: a non-linear approach. Eur J Appl Physiol 94: 705-710.

51. Perneger TV (2010) Speed trends of major cycling races: does slower mean cleaner? Int J Sports Med 31: 261-264.

52. Hopkins WG1, Hawley JA, Burke LM (1999) Design and analysis of research on sport performance enhancement. Med Sci Sports Exerc 31: 472-485.

53. Heuberger JA1, Cohen Tervaert JM, Schepers FM, Vliegenthart AD, Rotmans JI, et al. (2013) Erythropoietin doping in cycling: lack of evidence for efficacy and a negative risk-benefit. Br J Clin Pharmacol 75: 1406-1421.

54. Johnson AT (2007) Biomechanics and exercise physiology: Quantitative modeling. Taylor and Francis Group, CRC Press, New York.

55. Magnier D, Picq P, Debreilly M, Zingoni P, Haffreingue H , et al. (2014) Cycling remembered. [In French: Mémoires du cyclisme].

56. Lucia A1, Earnest C, Arribas C (2003) The Tour de France: a physiological review. Scand J Med Sci Sports 13: 275-283.

57. Koop G (2000) Analysis of economic data. John Wiley & Sons, New York.

58. Tabachnick BG, Fidell LS (2001) Using multivariate statistics (4th Edn.). Allyn and Bacon / Pearson Education Company, Boston.

59. Carroll RT (2003) The skeptic's dictionary: A collection of strange beliefs, amusing deceptions, and dangerous delusions. John Wiley & Sons, Hoboken (NJ).

60. Tversky A, Kahneman D (1973) Availability: A heuristic for judging frequency and probability. Cognitive Psychology 5: 207-232.

61. Hilbert M (2012) Toward a synthesis of cognitive biases: how noisy information processing can bias human decision making. Psychol Bull 138: 211-237.

62. Alicke MD (2000) Culpable control and the psychology of blame. Psychological Bulletin, 126: 556-574.

63. Ross L (1977) The intuitive psychologist and his shortcomings: Distortions in the attribution process. In Berkowitz L (Ed.), Advances in experimental social psychology Academic Press, New York 10: 174-221.

64. Hilton DJ, Slugoski BR (1986) Knowledge–based causal attribution: The abnormal conditions focus model. Psychological Review 93: 75-88.

Time Lost from Play in Foot and Ankle Injuries of Professional Soccer Players

Haluk H. Oztekin* and Bulent Zeren

Orthopaedic Surgeons, Private Clinic for Sports Traumatology and Orthopaedics, 1738 Sokak, No: 10, Karsiyaka, Izmir, Turkey

Abstract

Objective: Ankle and foot injuries are common in professional soccer players, but the relation between injury severity and time lost from play is not well known. The aim of this study is to investigate the relationship between diagnosis, injury severity and time lost to play of professional soccer players with severe ankle and foot injuries with reviewing the recent literature.

Design: Prospective evaluation of retrospectively collected data and review of the literature.

Setting: Primary private practice.

Patients: The medical records of two hundred lower extremity injuries of professional soccer players who admitted to our private clinic during the 2003-2004 professional national soccer league season were reviewed. Collected data of sixty-six players with severe ankle and foot injuries were included in the study. Type of injury, diagnosis, treatment, injury severity and finally, time lost from play were evaluated from the medical records. Injury severity ('severe' if >28 days, 'moderate' if between 8-28 days) and time lost from play were calculated from medical records and by telephone interviews with the players.

Results: Most injuries (n=20, 32%) occurred during player-to-player contact. The most common diagnosis was ankle sprain (30.3%) with anterior talofibular ligament injury. Most (55%) hindfoot injuries were Achilles tendinopathy with or without rupture. Treatment was surgical in 23 patients (35%). The mean time lost from play for players with severe foot and ankle injuries was 61days (range 21-240 days); after Achilles tendon ruptures, the mean time lost was 180 days. Injury severity was severe (>28 days lost from play) in 64% patients and moderate (8-28 days lost from play) in 36% patients.

Conclusion: Time lost to play can dramatically increase by the presence of severe ankle and foot injuries. Serious ankle and foot injuries in this study resulted in players being out of professional competition for about two months.

Introduction

Soccer carries a certain risk of injury for its participants, from 13 to 35 injuries per 1000 player-hours of competition [1]. However, less is known about the risk factors, mechanisms, injury severity of soccer-related injuries and their resulting time lost to play while players recover [2,3]. In addition, no consensus exists about study design, data collection, and injury definitions in the epidemiological studies of soccer injuries to date [3].

After the thigh, the feet and ankles are the most common locations for injury (19% and 7% of match injuries) in professional players during competition, with an incidence of 39 injuries per thousand hours of competition [4]. Soccer players with 'footballer's ankle' develop ankle osteoarthritis at a much higher rate than the general population [5,6]. Identifying the causes, type of injury and injury severity of foot and ankle injuries in soccer players may influence efforts for preventive strategies [7].

Some studies have explored the mechanism and type of injury in soccer related ankle and foot injuries with or without video-based analyses, however much less is known about the real diagnosis, treatment and true time loss [7-13]. The aim of this study was to investigate the relationship between diagnosis, injury severity and time lost to play of professional soccer players with severe ankle and foot injuries.

Methods

Retrospectively, records of 200 professional soccer players with a primary complaint of having injured their lower extremity during practice or competition were reviewed. All players presented for care to our private sports/orthopaedic clinic during the 2003-2004 professional national outdoor soccer league season and were cared for by one orthopaedic surgeon. Sixty-six were found to have had severe ankle and/or foot injuries according to Chomiak [10] criteria and included in the study. Injury severity was categorized as minor (1–7 days absence), moderate (8–28 days), and severe (>28days) [11]. The primary mechanism and type of injury were determined by patient history.

Injuries were classified anatomically as being in the ankle, midfoot, or hindfoot. Achilles tendinopathy and ruptures were classified as hindfoot injuries. The Orava [14] modification [3] of injury classification was used. After clinical examination, conventional radiographs were obtained as per the Ottawa [15] criteria. Ultrasonography (USG) with a high-resolution probe with or without dynamic scanning was performed when needed by a musculoskeletal ultrasonographer experienced in sports trauma scanning. Magnetic resonance imaging (MRI) was performed if chronic overuse syndrome, impingement syndrome, bone bruise or ankle joint instability was

***Corresponding author:** Haluk H. Oztekin, MD, Orthopaedic Surgeon, 6345 Sokak, No: 6/11 35540, Karsiyaka, Izmir, Turkey
E-mail: hhoztekin@isbank.net.tr

suspected clinically and radiographically. The same surgeon performed all surgical treatments and prescribed rehabilitation treatments to be performed by one sports physiotherapist. The "return to play" decision was made after completing rehabilitation, a final clinical examination, and a field test.

The time lost from participation was calculated from our own medical records and confirmed by telephone interviews with the each player. After returning to the field, follow-up examinations were performed over the course of two months to determine if reinjury had occurred. Results were analysed and discussed with recent literature.

Results

Of 200 patients with lower extremity soccer-related injuries, 66 had severe ankle and foot problems (33%). Sixty-one patients of 66 were male and the mean age was 23 years old (range 17 and 31 years old). Patient demographics are summarized in Table 1. The majority (61%) injured themselves during a competition. No ankle bracing, taping, bandages or orthoses were used in any patient, but all of them had worn shin guards at the time of injury. All matches were played on natural grass. The injury mechanism was direct player-to-player contact (32%), overuse (26%), tripping on the grass (10,5%), landing (7,5%), jumping and jumping/landing (7,5%), tackling (4,5%), being tackled (4,5%), shooting (3%), kicking and kicking/shooting (3%), sprinting (1,5%). Most (59%) had injuries of the right foot/ankle, and 79% were in the dominant extremity.

The anatomical sites of injury were the ankle in 56%, hindfoot in 30% and midfoot in 14%. The majority of injuries were ankle sprains and anterior talofibular ligament (ATFL) lesions (n=20); others were overuse impingement syndromes (n=10), Achilles overuse with strain (n=11; tendinopathy in 6 hindfeet of 5 players, and 5 ruptures), metatarsal fractures (n=7), ankle contusions (n=3), malleolus fractures (n=3), symptomatic os trigonum (n=3), osteochondral talar lesions (n=2), fracture dislocation of the ankle (n=1), tibial shaft fracture (N=1) and plantar fasciitis (n=1). Achilles tendon ruptures happened during jumping and jumping/landing in three of five players during training.

Twenty-seven players with ankle sprains had X-rays and musculoskeletal USG performed. Eleven players had X-rays only. Tendinopathies were confirmed by USG only in nine players. Nineteen players needed MRI (Table 1). No scintigraphy (bone scan) was performed.

Treatment was surgical in 23 patients (35%); in four of these, ankle arthroscopy was performed, followed by early rehabilitation. Others were treated with only an aggressive sports rehabilitation program. "Return-to-play" decisions were made after an on-field observational test (eg. plyometric exercises). All players were contacted by telephone and confirmed the "return-to-play" date.

The mean time lost to play was 61 days (range 21-240 days). The mean time lost to play after an Achilles tendon rupture was 180 days. When Achilles tendinopathy and ruptures were excluded from the study, the overall mean time lost to play was 48 days. In 21 "player-to-player contact" injuries, the mean time lost to play was 56 days and the injury severity 'major', in 17 players with 'overuse injuries', a similar mean time lost to play was found (56 days). Injury severity was severe (>28 days lost to play) in 64% of patients and moderate (8-28 days lost to play) in 36%. No player experienced a reinjury in the two-month follow-up period.

Discussion

The most common injury mechanisms for foot and ankle injuries in soccer are direct contact in 58% of our patients, and in 59% in a study among professional English football players [12]. As found in similar studies, the dominant foot is most commonly injured and the majority of injuries happen during competition rather than during training [16,17]. Wong and Hong [13] described this as "the higher the speed of play, the higher the rate of injury".

According to Woods et al. [12], ankle sprains occurred most often during tackles (54%). Biomechanical studies have shown that the ATFL is the first ligament to be tensed and rupture when forced inversion of the ankle occurs [7]. Our findings correlate with the other studies [1,4,7,12,13] suggesting that the typical responsible mechanism is inversion. Because our results relied on the player's recollection of the event, the position of the foot as the injury occurred was not as clear as it might have been on a video replay. (Table 1)

Achilles tendinopathy and ruptures are sometimes classified as 'lower leg injuries' rather than foot and ankle injuries, but in a recently published review, Achilles tendinopathies and ruptures were categorized as hindfoot problems [18]. Hindfoot injuries occurred frequently (30% of all ankle-foot injuries) in the players in our series, with most (55%) being Achilles tendinopathy and ruptures. Although these injuries caused a time lost to play of 180 days in our study, few studies mention Achilles tendinopathy and rupture among professional soccer players [10,11,19,20,21]. The frequency of Achilles tendon ruptures varies considerably from country to country, perhaps due to the variation in sports traditions and popularity [21], which may explain the small number of studies in the literature.

Although we have classified Achilles ruptures in "strain" group, we believe that they must be categorized as both overuse injuries and strains. Achilles tendinopathy could be a main risk factor in Achilles ruptures. In a recent study, Mahieu et al. [22] described intrinsic risk factors that play an important role in Achilles tendon overuse injuries. Other well known risk factors are hard ground, resumption of training after a break, poor footwear and increased intensity of training and running [23]. Therefore, paying attention to the player's plantar flexor strength and amount of dorsiflexion excursion [an intrinsic risk factor mentioned by Mahieu [22]], minimising overtraining in the pre- or mid-season, wearing better shoes and playing on suitable ground may prevent such injuries.

While few studies [10,11,24] describe the mechanism and type of injury in soccer-related ankle and foot injuries, even fewer elaborate on the true diagnosis and real time loss. Hoy et al. [24] reported a very low "average duration of lost work time" as five days in 715 soccer injuries in their epidemiological study, while Chomiak et al. [10] reported a mean 57 day duration of absence. However, both of these studies were focused on general trauma in soccer players rather than ankle/foot-related injuries. Our injury severity was higher than in other published studies [10,17,24].

Video-based investigations or baseline forms [3] may be suitable for recording the mechanism and type of injuries, but not for the final diagnosis and time lost to play. Recording the true diagnosis and time lost to play are also problematic though: recovering original on-field injury records, harmonising original injury records with the final diagnosis, following-up a player who has changed physicians, and crude estimations of the period away from play may result in inaccurate data. In most studies to date, the diagnoses, time lost to play and injury severity calculations were made by estimations [1,4,7-9,24] rather than from medical and on-field playing records [3].

The populations surveyed and the definitions of injury severity and time lost to play vary between studies, making comparisons difficult [9]. For example, most epidemiological studies report general soccer trauma [10,17,20,24] with a few exceptions reporting specific anatomical sites [4,6,7,21]. We preferred using the UEFA model for interpreting the time lost to play and injury severity [3]. We agree with Ekstrand [25] that the real time loss must be "an injury that occurred during a scheduled training session or match that caused absence from the next training session or match". Time lost to play was dramatically increased by the presence of an Achilles rupture or fracture, and was especially lengthy in player-to-player contact and overuse injuries. One survey among professional, adolescent, adult and child soccer players found most ankle and foot injuries to be minor [13]. Our patients were likely self-selected, most not seeking care at our sports medicine clinic for more minor injuries.

The limitations of this present study were its retrospective design and the lack of video recordings for determining the exact mechanism of injury. Although we calculated the time lost to play from our medical records and by telephone interviews, calculations from the attendance records of the teams would be more accurate. Patient based questionnaires, clinician based evaluation using objective criteria must

Case	Age	Gender	Dom. Ext.	Injury during	Injury Mechanism	Ankle	Midfoot	Hindoot	Type of Injury	Diagnostic Tool	Diagnosis	Treatment	Time loss in days
1	27	M	R	T	Sprinting			R	Strain	USG/ MRI	Achilles rupture	Surg	240
2	31	M	L	M	Tripping			L	Strain	USG/ MRI	Achilles rupture	Surg	180
3	25	M	L	M	Overuse	L			Other	x ray	Lat.mall. pseudoarthrosis	Surg/Greft	200
4	27	M	R	M	Overuse	R			Overuse	x ray	Footballer's ankle/Imp.	Arth/Surg	45
5	21	M	L	M	P/P		L		Fx	x ray	1st Tarso/metatarsal fx.	Surg	105
6	26	M	R	M	P/P	R			Fx	x ray	Tibial shaft fx.	Surg	240
7	22	M	R	M	P/P	L			Fx	x ray	Maisonneuve fx.	Surg	150
8	29	M	R	M	Jumping			R	Strain	USG/ MRI	Achilles rupture	Surg	150
9	27	M	L	T	Overuse			L	Strain	x ray/USG	Ach.Tendinopathy/O. Trigonum	Surg	150
10	25	M	L	T	J/Landing			L	Strain	USG/ MRI	Achilles rupture	Surg	180
11	22	M	L	M	Tackling		L		Fx	x ray	5th metartarsal fx.	Surg	90
12	19	M	L	T	Overuse			L	Fx	MRI	Sympt. os trigonum	Surg	45
13	21	M	R	M	b/Tck?		L		Fx	x ray	5th metartarsal fx.	Surg	150
14	19	M	R	M	Overuse	R			Overuse	MRI	A/L impingement	Surg	90
15	25	M	L	T	Landing	R			Strain	x ray/USG	Peroneal tendon luxation	Surg	60
16	26	M	L	T	Overuse	L			Overuse	MRI	A/M impingement	Arth	60
17	28	M	L	M	Overuse	L			Overuse	MRI	Ant. impingement	Arth	30
18	27	M	L	T	Tripping	L			Overuse	x ray/USG	ATFL sprain	Sport.Rehab.	30
19	30	M	R	M	Overuse			R	Overuse	USG	Achilles tendinopathy	Sport.Rehab.	30
20	19	M	L	T	K/S	L			Contusion	MRI	Bone bruise/Lat.mall.	Sport.Rehab.	60
21	23	M	L	T	Tripping	L			Sprain	x ray/USG	Deltoid lig. Sprain	Sport.Rehab.	30
22	20	M	L	M	P/P	L			Sprain	x ray/USG	ATFL sprain	Sport.Rehab.	90
23	27	M	R	M	Tripping	R			Fx/Sprain	x ray/USG	Lat.mall.fx/Delt.lig. rupture	Surg	150
24	24	M	R	M	P/P		R		Strain	x ray/USG	Peroneal Tendon strain	Sport.Rehab.	60
25	27	M	L	M	Overuse			L	Overuse	MRI	Post. Impingement	Art/Surg	30
26	21	M	R	M	Overuse			R	Overuse	MRI	Post. Impingement	Local Inj. Sp.Rehab	30
27	22	M	R	M	Landing	R			Sprain	x ray/USG	ATFL Sprain	Sport.Rehab.	45
28	26	M	L	T	Overuse			L	Overuse	USG/ MRI	Achilles tendinopathy	Surg	45
29	17	M	R	T	P/P		R		Fx	x ray	5th metartarsal fx.	Cast	90
30	19	M	L	M	Overuse			L	Overuse	USG	Achilles tendinopathy	Sport.Rehab.	21
31	25	M	R	M	P/P	R			Sprain	x ray/USG	ATFL Sprain	Sport.Rehab.	21
32	33	M	R	T	P/P	R			Sprain	x ray/USG	ATFL Sprain	Sport.Rehab.	21
33	32	M	R	M	P/P	R			Sprain	x ray/USG	ATFL Sprain	Sport.Rehab.	30
34	25	M	R	M	Tripping	R			Sprain	x ray/USG	ATFL Sprain	Sport.Rehab.	21
35	19	M	R	T	Tackling?	L			Overuse	USG	Ganglion of peroneal Tendon	Surg	30
36	17	M	R	M	b/Tck	R			Contusion	x ray/USG	Contusion/Post. tibial tendon	Sport.Rehab.	21
37	16	M	R	M	Overuse	R			Overuse	MRI	Post.Imping./O. Trigonum	Loc.Inj/Rehab.	21
38	27	M	R/L	T	Overuse			R/L	Overuse	USG	Achilles tendinopathy	Sport.Rehab.	30
39	26	M	R	M	Shooting?	R			Sprain	x ray/USG	C/F Lig. Sprain	Sport.Rehab.	30

Case	Age	Gender	Dom. Ext.	Injury during	Injury Mechanism	Ankle	Midfoot	Hindoot	Type of Injury	Diagnostic Tool	Diagnosis	Treatment	Time loss in days
40	26	M	R	T	Tripping			R	Overuse	MRI	P/M impingement	Sport.Rehab.	21
41	18	M	R	M	P/P			R	Overuse	MRI	P/L impingement	Sport.Rehab.	21
42	18	M	R	T	Tackling			R	Contusion	MRI	Bone bruise(talus)	Sport.Rehab.	21
43	22	M	L	M	b/Tck	L			Sprain	x ray/USG	ATFL Sprain	Sport.Rehab.	21
44	20	M	R	T	P/P	R			Strain	x ray/USG	Syndesmotic Injury	Sport.Rehab.	30
45	28	M	L	M	P/P	L			Sprain	x ray/USG	ATFL sprain	Sport.Rehab.	21
46	24	M	R	T	Tripping			R	Overuse	MRI	Posterior impingement	Surg	60
47	25	M	L	T	P/P	L			Sprain	x ray/USG	ATFL Sprain	Sport.Rehab.	21
48	25	M	L	M	Kicking	L			Sprain	x ray/USG	ATFL Sprain	Sport.Rehab.	21
49	20	M	R	M	P/P	R			Sprain	x ray/USG	ATFL rupture	Sport.Rehab.	30
50	17	M	R	M	P/P		R		Fx	x ray	3rd metatarsal stress fx.	Sport.Rehab.	75
51	29	M	R	T	Shooting			R	Fx	USG	Achilles tendinopathy	Sport.Rehab.	30
52	17	M	R	T	Overuse?		R		Fx	x ray	4th metatarsal stress fx.	Cast	90
53	25	M	R	T	P/P		R		Fx	x ray	3rd metatarsal stress fx.	Sport.Rehab.	75
54	29	M	R	M	P/P	R			Sprain	x ray/USG	ATFL Sprain	Sport.Rehab.	21
55	21	M	L	M	P/P	L			Sprain	x ray/USG	ATFL Sprain	Sport.Rehab.	21
56	24	M	L	T	Overuse			L	Overuse	USG	Achilles tendinopathy	Sport.Rehab.	21
57	23	M	L	M	Landing	L			Sprain	USG	ATFL Sprain	Sport.Rehab.	15
58	25	M	R	T	P/P	R			Sprain	x ray/USG	ATFL Sprain	Sport.Rehab.	21
59	27	M	R	M	Landing	R			Sprain	x ray/USG	ATFL Sprain	Sport.Rehab.	21
60	20	M	L	M	P/P	L			Sprain	USG	ATFL Sprain	Sport.Rehab.	15
61	22	M	R	M	P/P	R			Strain	x ray/USG	Syndesmotic Injury	Sport.Rehab.	21
62	25	F	R	M	Jumping			R	Overuse	USG/ MRI	Achilles rupture	Surg	150
63	22	F	R	M	Landing		R		Contusion	x ray/MRI	Contusion/ Cuboid	Sport.Rehab.	15
64	33	F	R	M	Jumping	R			Sprain	x ray/USG	ATFL Sprain	Sport.Rehab.	30
65	17	F	R	T	Jumping	R			Sprain	x ray/USG	ATFL Sprain	Sport.Rehab.	21
66	27	F	R	T	Overuse			R	Overuse	USG	Plantar fasciitis	Sport.Rehab.	15

Table 1: Patients demographics and characteristics. (Dom. Ext.= Dominant extremity, M=Male, F=Female, R=Right, L=Left, T=Training, M=Match, P/P=Player-to-player contact, J=Jumping, Tck=Being tackled, K/S=Kicking and shooting, A=Anterior, P=Posterior, M=Medial, L=Lateral, Fx=Fracture, Surg=Surgery, Arth=Arthroscopy).

be the gold standard in a future scientific research in determination of return to play after ankle injury. The other weakest point of the study is the decision to return the athlete to play was made by one single clinician using subjective criteria.

Prevention of these serious ankle/foot injuries in professional soccer players should receive considerable attention, given the almost 2 months time away from the field that results. The development of effective prevention programs first involves collecting detailed information on the injury mechanism [3,7,12]. A soccer-specific injury reporting system with uniform diagnostic and return-to-play criteria should be developed and widely implemented [3,26]. Video-based studies are ideal for documenting injury mechanisms, but not for establishing the final diagnosis or time lost to play. The Orchard OSIFC model [27], the Oslo group's model, the ICD-10 coding system and the UEFA model can be used for establishing uniform diagnostic criteria [3].

Take Home Message

We feel that the UEFA model is the best of these for reporting injuries in epidemiological studies. Even with optimal operative and rehabilitative therapy, foot and ankle injuries among professional soccer players result in a lengthy time away from the field, a loss to their team. Efforts to minimise these injuries and time away from play needs to begin with a comprehensive plan for prospectively collecting data for long-term comparison studies.

References

1. Junge A, Dvorak J, Graf-Baumann T (2004) Football injuries during the World Cup 2002. Am J Sports Med 32: 23S-27S.
2. Dvorak J, Junge A (2000) Football injuries and physical symptoms. A review of the literature. Am J Sports Med 28: S3-S9.
3. Hagglund M, Walden M, Bahr R, Ekstrand J (2005) Methods for epidemiological study of injuries to professional football players: developing the UEFA model. Br J Sports Med 39: 340–346.
4. Giza E, Fuller C, Junge A, Dvorak J (2003) Mechanisms of foot and ankle injuries in soccer. Am J Sports Med 31: 550-554.
5. Injuryupdate.com.
6. Larsen E, Jensen PK, Jensen PR (1990) Long-term outcome of knee and ankle injuries in elite football. Scan J Med Sci Sports 9: 285-289.
7. Andersen TE, Floerenes TW, Arnason A, Bahr R (2004) Video analysis of the mechanisms for ankle injuries in football. Am J Sports Med 32: 69-79.
8. Andersen TE, Tenga A, Engebretsen L, Bahr R (2004) Video analysis of injuries and incidents in Norwegian professional football. Br J Sports Med 38: 626–631.
9. Arnason A, Tenga A, Engebretsen L, Bahr R (2004) A prospective video-based analysis of injury situations in elite male football. Am J Sports Med 32: 1459-1465.
10. Chomiak J, Junge A, Peterson L, Dvorak J (2000) Severe injuries in football players: influencing factors. Am J Sports Med 28: S58-S68.
11. Hawkins RD, Hulse MA, Wilkinson C, Hodson A, Gibson M (2001) The

association football medical research programme: an audit of injuries in professional football. Br J Sports Med 35: 43–47.

12. Woods C, Hawkins RD, Hulse M, Hodson A (2003) The Football Association Medical Research Programme: An audit of injuries in professional football: An analysis of ankle sprains. Br J Sports Med 37: 233–238.

13. Wong P, Hong Y (2005) Soccer injuries in the lower extremities. Br J Sports Med 39: 473-482.

14. Orava S (1980) Exertion injuries due to sports and physical exercise. A clinical and statistical study of nontraumatic overuse injuries of the musculoskeletal system of athletes and keep-fit athletes. Thesis: University of Oulu, Finland.

15. Stiell IG, McKnight RD, Greenberg GH, McDowell I, Nair RC, et al. (1994) Implementation of the Ottawa ankle rules. JAMA 271: 827-832.

16. Hawkins RD, Fuller CW (1999) A prospective epidemiological study of injuries in four English professional football clubs. Br J Sports Med 33: 196-203.

17. Ekstrand J, Gillquist J (1983) Soccer injuries and their mechanisms: a prospective study. Med Sci Sports Exerc 15: 267–270.

18. Miller RA, DeCoster TA, Mizel MS (2005) What's new in foot and ankle surgery? J Bone Joint Surg Am 87: 909-917.

19. Cretnik A, Frank A (2004) Incidence and outcome of rupture of the Achilles tendon. Wien Klin Wochenschr 116: 33-38.

20. Orchard J (2003) Management of muscle and tendon injuries in footballers. Aust Fam Physician 32: 489-493.

21. Kannus P and Natri A (1997) Etiology and pathophysiology of tendon ruptures in sports. Scand J Med Sci Sports 7: 107-112.

22. Mahieu NN, Witvrouw E, Stevens V, Van Tiggelen D, Roget P (2006) Intrinsic risk factors for the development of Achilles tendon overuse injury. A prospective study. Am J Sports Med 34: 226-235.

23. Woods C, Hawkins RD, Hulse M, Hodson A (2002) The Football Association Medical Research Programme: an audit of injuries in professional football: analysis of preseason injuries. Br J Sports Med 36: 436–441.

24. Hoy K, Lindblad BE, Terkelsen CJ, Helleland HE, Terkelsen CJ (1992) European soccer injuries. A prospective epidemiologic and socioeconomic study. Am J Sports Med 20: 318-322.

25. Ekstrand J (1982) Soccer injuries and their prevention. Linköping: Department of Surgery, Linköping University.

26. Ekstrand J, Karlsson J (2003) The risk for injury in football. There is a need for a consensus about definition of injury and the design of studies. Scand J Med Sci Sports 13: 147–149.

27. Orchard J (1993) Orchard Sports Injury Classification System (OSICS). Sports Health 11: 39–41.

Temporomandibular Joint Disorders and Preventive Methods in Boxing Athletes

Elif Ozcan[1] and Guhan Dergin[2]*

[1]Marmara University Faculty of Dentistry Department of Oral and Maxillofacial Surgery, Turkey
[2]Associate Professor, Marmara University Faculty of Dentistry Department of Oral and Maxillofacial Surgery, Turkey

Abstract

Oral and maxillofacial injuries are common in sporting activities, especially in contact combat sports. It has been stated by a number of researchers that obligatory dental and orofacial protection for all athletes have major effects in preventing injuries and associated life-long discomfort, as well as reducing the treatment costs. Boxing exposes athletes to severe head impacts and risk of brain injury, as well as disorders resulting from chronic recurrent traumas. The purpose of this report is to state the causes of temporomandibular joint disorders in boxing athletes and emphasize the importance of preventive measures and routine screening by a TMJ specialist maxillofacial surgeon.

Keywords: Temporomandibular joint disorder; Trauma; Boxing

Introduction

As a contact combat sport, boxing is an universally exercised discipline since earliest periods of history. Boxing exposes athletes to repetitive, occasionally severe head impacts. As a result, boxing athletes are among high-risk group for encountering maxillofacial and brain injuries [1].

Maxillofacial injuries and temporomandibular disorders are very common and comprises the results of various types of sporting activities such as soccer, skiing, basketball, cycling, hockey, snowboarding, boxing and other contact combat sports [2-4]. Contact sports are reported to be cause of about 19% of maxillofacial and 33% of dental injuries [5,6]. Retrospective analyses by Tanaka et al., and Mourouzis and Koumoura reported the incidence of boxing-related maxillofacial fractures as 2% and 1.6%, respectively [3,4].

Boxing-related injuries are considered more serious among other sports due to repetitive and direct traumas to head and face region, which are prohibited in other disciplines [7]. Kumamoto and Maeda reported that 33-72% of boxing athletes have encountered dental injuries in their career [8]. According to study examining the epidemiology of boxing injuries in the U.S. within a 19-year study period by Potter et al., the most common diagnosis was fracture (27.5%). Most frequently injuried body region was the hand (33.0%), followed by head and neck (22.5%). Lacerations in this region involved face, mouth and eyes (87%) [6]. As reported by Jerolimov, all orofacial injuries comprised soft tissue injuries (50%), dental injuries (40%), jaw fractures and temporomandibular joint injuries (10%). Among these, injuries of TMJ and related structures consist of about 2-6% of cases, but there is lack of reliable data on this subject [9-12].

Anatomy and Biomechanics of the Temporomandibular Joint

The Temporomandibular Joint (TMJ) is a true synovial joint and composed of the temporal bone and the mandible, and a specialized dense fibrous structure, the distinct fibrocartilaginous articular disk, articular ligaments, and surrounding muscles. Anatomically the TMJ is a diarthrodial joint, which is formed by mandibular condyle and the glenoid fossa of the temporal bone. Movement of TMJ is adjusted by muscles of mastication, and limited by ligaments. Certain movements of mandible and opening against resistance requires the activation of suprahyoid and infrahyoid muscle groups, digastic and mylohyoid muscles [13,14].

Functionally the TMJ is a compound ginglymoarthrodial joint. The lower compartment provides hinge motion and is termed as ginglymoid. The superior compartment conducts translatory movements and hence termed as arthroidal. Pure hinge motion of 2.5 cm measured at the interincisal opening is possible, further movements of the mandible involves translatory and involves a gliding motion between disk and the temporal fossa. Complex free movements of the mandible are made possible by the relation of four articulating compartments bilaterally [15].

Temporomandibular Joint Trauma in Boxing Discipline

Most of orofacial and temporomandibular injuries in boxing, are predictable and preventable. There are three main types of appliances exist as extraoral, intraoral (mouthguards) and combined ones. Intraoral appliances (mouthguards) can be stock, mouth-formed orcustom-made [16]. A continuing education should be followed on the importance of prevention methods for boxing injuries for sports physicians, coaches and athletes, thus making the role of the maxillofacial surgeon in this sport persistent [17].

Types of boxing injuries depends on impact areas on the maxillofacial region and mechanism of transmitted force. Magnitude and vector of the force, as well as absorbing mechanisms and transmitting patterns should be taken into account.

Traumatic effect of the force can be absorbed by surrounding musculatory, articular and extraarticular ligaments, articular disc and the teeth [9].

There are two essential mechanisms of boxing injuries and related TMJ disorders as microtraumas and macrotraumas in direct and indirect routes (Figure 1). Repeated trauma to the mandible can lead to inflammatory responses in the masticatory muscles, laxity of the ligaments, and TMJ internal derangements [14]. Microtraumas generated

***Corresponding author:** Guhan Dergi, Marmara University Faculty of Dentistry Department of Oral and Maxillofacial Surgery, Turkey
E-mail: guhandergin@yahoo.com

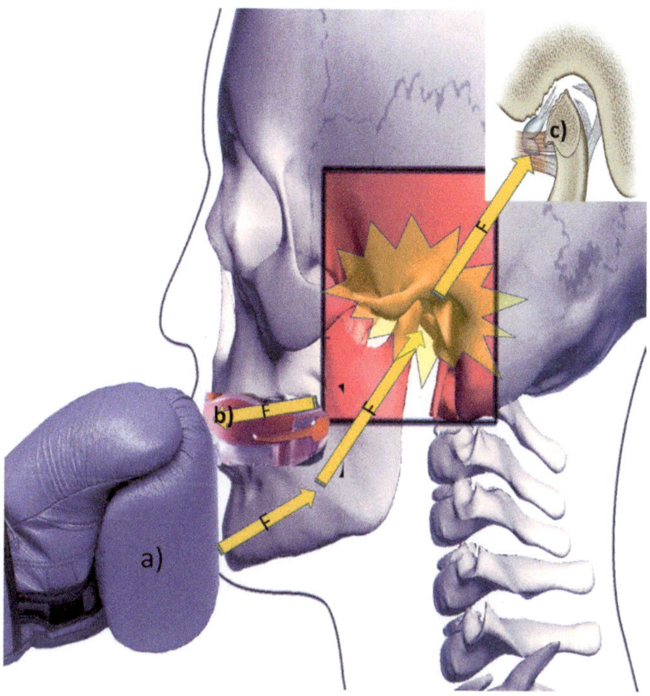

Figure 1: a) Direct or indirect blow trauma to the mandible which is conducted to the TMJ.

b) Mouthguard which fixates maxilla and mandible, so the condyle at a certain position, which decreased the transmitted forces to the condyle and articular structures.

c) Degenerated disk and articular surface of the temporomandibular joint with chronic macro and micro trauma.

by internal factors, such as chronic overloads and parafunctional habits such as bruxism and clenching. Constant clenching and lateral pterygoid muscle spasm during practice leads to disc deplacements in long term. Chronic microtraumas to the temporomandibular joint can result in synovitis, capsulitis, tendinitis, reducing and non- reducing disc deplacements, osteoarthritis, subluxation and condylar dislocation as well as periodontal disorders and luxation of the teeth [18-23].

Consistent microtrauma causes releasing of certain inflammatory mediators, such as NO, arachidonic acid and prostaglandin E2. These cytokines starts a cascade that leads decomposing of cross collagen content of the articular surfaces, which leads to degeneration of articular disc, retrodiscal tissues and eventually reducing and non-reducing disc deplacement [24]. Clinical symptoms of internal derangements include limited mandubular range of motion, deviation of the mandible to the affected side, joint sounds and pain, generally associated with painful sensation of muscular tissues [15].

Repetitive loading of articulation system may result in osteoarthrosis. Bruxism and clenching habits may mimic excessive load forces. Internal derangement of the temporomandibular joint leads to alteration of forces transmitted to condyle-glenoid fossa complex, thus weakening of the functional areas of join elements. These changes often results cartilage tissue proteoglicans to undergo destruction with decreasing lubricative and protective properties of the cartilage. Eventually, osteoarthrosis may lead to perforation of articular disc and/or remodeling of bony structures of the joint such as flattening of the condyle. Macrotraumas are external factors such as acute, high magnitude blows. These traumas likely will result in maxillo-mandibular and condylar fractures, condylar dislocations, dental traumas, fibrous or bony ankylosis, cranial base fractures and concussions. Bechor and Zadik reported a case of maxillary incisor being laterally luxated due to long term boxing practice without protection [18].

Traumatic arthritis represents the acute intraarticular response to temporomandibular joint trauma. The resulting inflammation effusion and occasional hemarthrosis causes limited range of mandibular movement, pain on the affected side. Direct blows to the mandible may result in anterior dislocation, capitular fractures, contusions of the condylar head and condylar neck fractures. Direct trauma to the sympyhseal area is likely to cause bilateral condylar fractures upon transmission of force, whereas blows to the parasympyseal area will likely cause fracture of contralateral condyle due to indirect conducting of trauma and rotational forces [25].

Besides taking medical history and clinical examination of the patient, diagnostic measures include plain panoramic radiographs, CT scans and MRIs [26]. It should be emphasized that, microtraumas are easily overlooked in diagnostic procedure, since their chronic and occasionally non subjectively-symphtomatic nature. Microtroumas has a cumulative effect on TMJ and it is the serious causative factor of TMJD. Besides athletes may not refer to microtraumas in their medical history, which can result in wrong diagnosis.

Depending on the type of disorder and/or injury, treatment modalities include, anti-inflammatory medications, analgesic drugs, myorelaxants, anestethics, soft diet regimen, passive opening excersises, heat applications, cold applications, arthrocentesis and surgical procedures under general anesthesia. Masticatory muscle disorder and disc derangement may lead to each other and frequently appear simultaneously, therefore it is essential to determine the primary disorder so that effective treatment may be executed. As a general rule, non-invasive and reversible forms of treatment should be initially performed for management and unnecessary surgical approaches should be avoided. According to the results, the need for more aggressive or irreversible forms of treatment may be determined. Since misdiagnosis is the most common reason for failure of the treatment, meticulous examination of underlying mechanism is mandatory for executing especially surgical treatment modalities [15].

Since such injuries, symptoms and their treatment process result in interruption of athlete's professional activities, risk of acute or chronic injuries should be limited or completely eliminated [21-23,27].

Prevention of Maxillofacial and Temporomandibular Injuries

Most of athletic injuries are predictable, therefore preventable. Protection and education of athletes are essential for reducing boxing related injuries and disorders. World Dental Federation (FDI) classified sporting activities into two risk groups in 1990, according to the risk level of orofacial injuries in which the protection is recommended [28]. Prevention of maxillofacial injuries in sports can be achieved by appliances such as helmets, face shields and mouthguards.

Many reports have demonstrated that using mouthguards can reduce the incidence of maxillofacial injuries significantly [29,30]. By absorbing, limiting, and distributing the power of impact that tends to be transferred along osseous structures of the skull to the central nervous system, mouthguards reduce the risk of cerebral concussion and subarachnoid hemorrhage [16]. Use of mouthguards are vital in preventing TMJ injury in any high risk sports and even became obligatory in certain disciplines such as skiing, hockey and boxing [31].

Mouthguards can be classified as three groups:

- Extraoral mouthguards are attached to head or helmet and in the form of a wire cage.
- Intraoral mouthguards rest within dental arches, usually fits to maxillary teeth and shaped accordingly.
- Combined mouthguards have an extraoral part for soft tissues and intraoral part for protection of the teeth.

Intraoral mouthguards are superior appliances in various aspects, and have significant roles in mitigating trauma to the maxillofacial region [19,31].

- Reducing the risk of fractures and luxations in anterior dentition by direct blows and posterior dentition from sudden impacts
- Distributing the force and creating a recoil space allows the interface between condyle and glenoid fossa, hence preventing condylar dislocations towards the cranial base [32]
- Protection of soft tissues from being lacerated by edges of the teeth
- Reducing the possibility of maxillary and mandibular fractures by absorbing the impact force
- Increasing the athlete's ability to focus on performance by increased comfort
- By activation and contraction of head and neck muscles, providing increased resistance to rotational forces upon impact, and reducing injuries to cervical spine and possibility of concussions [33-36].

There have been three types of intraoral mouthguards have been used:

- Stock mouthguards are available commercially in varying sizes, composed of rubber or polyvinyl chloride. These type of mouthguards are not recommended by TMJ professionals although being most widely used.
- Mouth-formed mouthguards are preferred for their price and quick fabrication, but their retention decreases over time. These type of appliances can be manufactured by heating and shaping according to arch shape, or they can be prepared on cast models.

As presented by Shimoyama et al., boil and bite type of mouthguards considered to be limitedly effective against injuries due to unfitness. Lack of occlusion in mouthguards especially in intercanine area would instead increase the probability of injury, and cause mandibular and condylar fractures [37-39].

Custom-made mouthguards are fitted to dental arch, show higher retention and offer more effective absorption and distribution of forces. These appliances can also ensure the proper positioning of condyle in the fossa. Custom made mouthguards can be manufactured as monomaxillary and bimaxillary. Monomaxillary appliances mostly fit onto maxilla, except in cases of mandibular prognathism.

Bimaxillary appliances should have air openings for maintaining adequate breathing and stabilizes the mandible in order to reduce the risk of fractures as well as injuries to TMJ [2,19].

Thickness of the material usually adjusted to 3-4 mm in general, which provides a adequate absorption of forces. Although being more difficult to use, vertical thicknesses up to 6 mm are used for high risk occasions.

Inappropriately manufactured mouthguards lead clenching habits

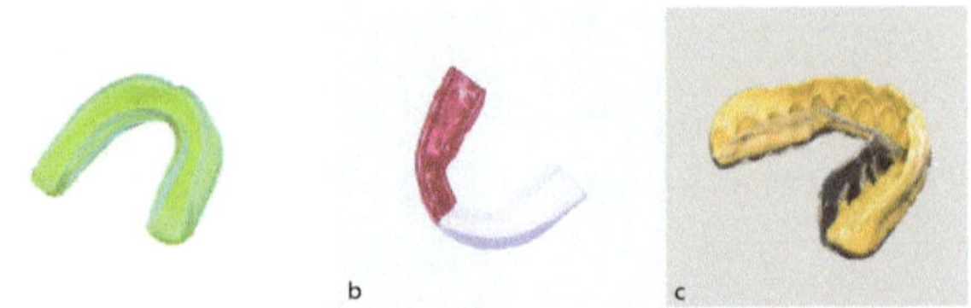

Figure 2: a) Stock-type mouthguard
b) Mouth-formed mouthguard
c) Custom-made mouthguard

by its own, and have insufficient protective properties by means of force tranmission to cranium and mandibular condyle. Therefore, these appliances should be produced under the supervision of TMJ specialists [34]. It has been reported that custom made mouthguards with adequate occlusal and labial thickness provides significant protection against maxillomandibular injuries by their resilient nature [16]. However, there is insufficient evidence confirming that usage of appliances prevent brain concussions [8,33,40].

Several authors have tested the mechanical properties of mouthguards based on standards established by American Society of the Testing Materials (ASTM) [41,42]. Also, response of human mandible to the impact loading of the chin and relationship between joint dynamics and mouthguards have been studied on cadaver, fabricated hybrid dummy models and finite element models. Though there is no established standard test method exist for biomechanical evaluation of mouthguards [29,32,43,44] (Figure 2).

Conclusion

To prevent TMJ complications of boxing sport and early diagnosis of clinical signs of TMJ micro-macro trauma, boxers should be routinely examined by TMJ specialist maxillofacial surgeons and neurocognitive tests must be performed on a regular basis. Athletes should not wear mouthguards which is not approved and adjusted by TMJ specialist. Custom made mouthguards should be preferred for a better protection of temporomandibular joint structures and dental arch. In some cases, TMJ MRIs, clinical signs and TMJ sounds should be evaluated to identify the severity of the problem. After these, pharmacological, physical or surgical therapy should be executed. The profession should make efforts to promote the use of mouthguards by informing athletes of the possibilities of active prevention against injuries to dental/oral regions in order to reduce their incidence.

References

1. Gartland S, Malik MH, Lovell ME (2001) Injury and injury rates in Muay Thai kick boxing. Br J Sports Med 35: 308-313.
2. Badel T, Jerolimov V, Panduric J (2007) Dental/Orofacial trauma in contact sports and intraoral mouthguard programmes. Kinesiology 39: 97-105.
3. Tanaka N, Hayashi S, Amagasa T, Kohama G (1996) Maxillofacial fractures sustained during sports. J Oral Maxillofac Surg 54: 715-719.
4. Mourouzis C, Koumoura F (2005) Sports-related maxillofacial fractures: a retrospective study of 125 patients. Int J Oral Maxillofac Surg 34: 635-638.
5. Glendor U (2009) Has the education of professional caregivers and lay people in dental trauma care failed? Dent Traumatol 25: 12-18.
6. Potter MR, Snyder AJ, Smith GA (2011) Boxing injuries presenting to U.S. emergency departments, 1990-2008. Am J Prev Med 40: 462-467.
7. Emerich K, Nadolska-Gazda E (2013) Dental trauma, prevention and knowledge concerning dental first-aid among Polish amateur boxers. J Sci Med Sport 16: 297-301.
8. Kumamoto DP, Maeda Y (2004) A literature review of sports-related orofacial trauma. Gen Dent 52: 270-280.

9. Jerolimov V (2010) Temporomandibular injuries and disorders in sport. Medical Sciences 34: 149-165.

10. Jerolimov V, Seifert D, Carek V (2000) Injuries to the orofacial structure in a selected sample of handball players. Kinesiology 32: 93-98.

11. Lombardi S, Sheller B, Williams BJ (1998) Diagnosis and treatment of dental trauma in a children's hospital. Pediatr Dent 20: 112-120.

12. Flanders RA, Bhat M (1995) The incidence of orofacial injuries in sports: a pilot study in Illinois. J Am Dent Assoc 126: 491-496.

13. Du Brul EL (1980) Sicher's oral anatomy. (7thedn.), C.V. Mosby, St. Louis (MO), 146-61, 174-209.

14. Sailors ME (1996) Evaluation of sports-related temporomandibular dysfunctions. J Athl Train 31: 346-350.

15. Okeson JP (1989) Management of temporomandibular disorders and occlusions. (2nd Edn.), CV Mosby St. Louis (MO) 3-26.

16. Gawlak D, Mierzwińska-Nastalska E, Mańka-Malara K, Kamiński T (2013) Comparison of usability properties of custom-made and standard self-adapted mouthguards. Dent Traumatol .

17. Federation Dentaire Internationale (1990) Guidelines for dental protection during sporting activities; Drugs and Sports, London.

18. Bechor R, Zadik Y (2008) An unusual lateral luxation of an upper incisor owing to long-term boxing without protection. Dent Traumatol 24: 550-552.

19. Ranalli DN (2000) Advances in sports dentistry. Dent Clin North Amer 44: 1-235.

20. Yildirim D, Dergin G, Tamam C, Moroglu S, Gurses B (2011) Indirect measurement of the temporomandibular joint disc elasticity with magnetic resonance imaging. Dentomaxillofac Radiol 40: 422-428.

21. Tippett SR (1990) Coaches guide to sport rehabilitation. Leisure Press, Champaign (Illinois).

22. Torg JS (1991) Athletic injuries to the head, neck, and face. (2ndedn), Lea & Febiger, USA.

23. Mellion MB, Michael WW, Shelton GL (2002) The Team physician's handbook. (3rd edn), Hanley & Belfus, USA.

24. Fonseca (2000) Temporomandibular joint disorders, oral and maxillofacial surgery. WB Saunders Company, Philadelphia, Pennsylvania, USA.

25. Mafee MF, Valvassori GE, Becker M (2005) Imaging of the Head and Neck. (2nd Edn.) Thieme Medical Publishers, Stuttgart, Germany.

26. Dergin G, Kilic C, Gozneli R, Yildirim D, Garip H, et al (2012) Evaluating the correlation between the lateral pterygoid muscle attachment type and internal derangement of the temporomandibular joint with an emphasis on MR imaging findings. Journal of Cranio-Maxillo-Facial Surgery 40: 459-463.

27. Jerolimov V (2009) Temporomandibular disorders and orofacial pain. Medical Sciences 33: 53-77.

28. World Dental Federation (FDI) Guidelines for dental protection during sporting activities. London.

29. Takeda T, Ishigami K, Hoshina S, Ogawa T, Handa J, et al. (2005) Can mouthguards prevent mandibular bone fractures and concussions? A laboratory study with an artificial skull model. Dent Traumatol 21: 134-140.

30. Lieger O, von Arx T (2006) Orofacial/cerebral injuries and the use of mouthguards by professional athletes in Switzerland. Dent Traumatol 22: 1-6.

31. Ranalli DN (2002) Sports dentistry and dental traumatology. Dent Traumatol 18: 231-236.

32. Walilko T, Bir C, Godwin W, King A (2004) Relationship between temporomandibular joint dynamics and mouthguards: feasibility of a test method. Dent Traumatol 20: 255-260.

33. Labella CR, Smith BW, Sigurdsson A (2002) Effect of mouthguards on dental injuries and concussions in college basketball. Med Sci Sports Exerc 34: 41-44.

34. Winters JE Sr (2001) Commentary: Role of Properly Fitted Mouthguards in Prevention of Sport-Related Concussion. J Athl Train 36: 339-341.

35. Seals RR Jr, Dorrough BC (1984) Custom mouth protectors: a review of their applications. J Prosthet Dent 51: 238-242.

36. Patrick DG, van Noort R, Found MS (2005) Scale of protection and the various types of sports mouthguard. Br J Sports Med 39: 278-281.

37. Chalmers DJ (1998) Mouthguards. Protection for the mouth in rugby union. Sports Med 25: 339-349.

38. Takeda T, Ishigami K, Ogawa T, Nakajima K, Shibusawa M, et al. (2004) Are all mouthguards the same and safe to use? The influence of occlusal supporting mouthguards in decreasing bone distortion and fractures. Dent Traumatol 20: 150-156.

39. Shimoyama T, Masuda I, Numa T, Horie N (2009) Mandibular fracture with a mouth formed mouthguard in kickboxing. Dent Traumatol 25: 242-244.

40. Knapik JJ, Marshall SW, Lee RB, Darakjy SS, Jones SB, et al. (2007) Mouthguards in sport activities : history, physical properties and injury prevention effectiveness. Sports Med 37: 117-144.

41. Westerman B, Stringfellow PM, Eccleston JA, Harbrow DJ (2002) Effect of ethylene vinyl acetate (EVA) closed cell foam on transmitted forces in mouthguard material. Br J Sports Med 36: 205-208.

42. Tran D, Cooke MS, Newsome PR (2001) Laboratory evaluation of mouthguard material. Dent Traumatol 17: 260-265.

43. Craig M, Bir C, Viano D, Tashman S (2008) Biomechanical response of the human mandible to impacts of the chin. J Biomech 41: 2972-2980.

44. Walilko TJ, Viano DC, Bir CA (2005) Biomechanics of the head for Olympic boxer punches to the face. Br J Sports Med 39: 710-719.

Deep Oscillation® Therapy in the Treatment of Lateral Epicondylalgia: A Pilot Randomized Control Trial

O'Brien CP[1] and Watson A[2*]

[1]*Sports Surgery Clinic, Santry Demesne, Dublin, Ireland*
[2]*Raglan Sports Medicine, 4 Fitzwilliam Square East, Dublin, Ireland*

Abstract

Introduction: DEEP OSCILLATION® therapy has been shown to improve wound healing, inflammation, pain and most prominently its effect on lymphoedema. It has been indicated for use in musculoskeletal injuries but few studies on its effectiveness exist. Therefore, the purpose of this study was to measure the effect DEEP OSCILLATION® (DOT) had on patients with lateral epicondylalgia (LE).

Methods: Twenty subjects aged between 18-55 years who had a diagnosis of LE took part in this trial. Group A (Control) underwent the protocol of injection therapy with 5 mg of Adcortyl and Lignocaine, topical Diclofenac anti-inflammatory gel applied three times per day and supervised rest over a two week period. Patients were then referred for physiotherapy where they completed a baseline PRTEE and were instructed on a home exercise program (HEP) for 4 weeks. Group B, test, received the same protocol from the physician as Group A and referred for physiotherapy where they completed a baseline PRTEE and received the same HEP as Group A. Group B also received DOT consisting of two-25 minute sessions per week for 4 weeks, eight treatment sessions in total. Outcome measures were the PRTEE and VAS to measure pain at baseline and end of treatment at 6 weeks. Further follow-up was performed at 6 months post treatment.

Results: The baseline mean of pain for Group A was 18.9 (SD 4.5) and at 6 weeks the mean was 13(3.09). The baseline mean of pain in Group B was 18.4 (4.5) and at 6 weeks it was 10.3(3.8). Repeated measure ANOVA on Pain showed significant difference between measurement from baseline to 6 weeks ($F(1,18)=530.52$, $p \le 0.001$). Results for the Time x Group interaction effect was not significant ($F(1,18)=1.76$, $p=0.20$), indicating that the changes in Pain measurements from baseline to 6 weeks were not significantly different for Control and Test groups. The mean function baseline for Group A was recorded as 13 (3.09) and 12.95 (2.76) at 6 weeks. The mean function for Group B was recorded as 22.5 (3.9) and 11.35 (4.10) at 6 weeks. Repeated measure ANOVA on Function showed significant difference between measurement from baseline to 6 weeks ($F(1,18)=98.82$, $p \le 0.001$). Time x Group interaction effect were found significant ($F(1,18)=10.59$, $p=0.004$), indicating that the changes in measurement from baseline to 6 weeks was significantly different for Control and Test groups.

Conclusion: A significant improvement in patients function at 6 weeks post treatment was found with 70% of the treatment group requiring no further treatment from 6 weeks to 6 months post treatment. DOT is beneficial in the treatment of TE and may further enhance the benefit from local steroid injection. Further research on the use of DOT in musculoskeletal injury and relevant protocols are needed.

Keywords: Lateral epicondylalgia; Tennis elbow; Physiotherapy; Deep oscillation therapy; Sports medicine; Rehabilitation

Introduction

Lateral Epicondylalgia (LE), commonly known as "Tennis Elbow", is a frequent complaint in primary healthcare settings with an occurrence rate of 4-7 per 1000 patients seen per year in general practice [1]. It is one of the most common upper extremity conditions [2] affecting 1-3% of the population with both sexes between 40-60yrs of age being equally susceptible [3]. It is caused by tendinosis of the common extensor tendon complex, primarily the extensor carpi radialis brevis (ECRB) at the lateral humeral epicondyle [4]. As over-use is a common causative factor, approximately 70% of cases are work-related leading to a significant loss of revenue due to sick leave [5].

Various treatment methods have been proposed in the management of lateral epicondylalgia. Labelle and colleagues [6] found evidence for approximately 40 treatment modalities with no one specific treatment proving to be superior. In 1936, Cyriax suggested that lateral epicondylalgia would spontaneously resolve in 8-12 months [7], a statement that has yet to be disproven. In many review papers, long-term follow up of 12 months or more, show little difference between placebo groups and intervention [8] with "wait and see" groups performing as good as groups that received physiotherapy or other treatment methods at 12 months follow-up.

Three treatment methods in particular have become the most common intervention for the management of lateral epicondylalgia. Local steroid injection has been shown to reduce pain and increase function in the acute stages of the pathology, particularly at 4 week follow up [9-13]. Work by Burnham et al., [14] showed topical diclofenac to be beneficial in reducing pain when applied directly to the site of pain for one week in patients with lateral epicondylalgia. The influence of exercise therapy has also been shown to give long-term improvement with a combination of stretching and strengthening helping to improve outcome measures of pain and function [15]. DEEP OSCILLATION® therapy has been shown to improve wound healing, [16] inflammation, pain [17] and most prominently its effect on lymphoedema [18]. The mechanism by which the therapy is achieving results is due to the

***Corresponding author:** Mr. Andrew Watson, Head Athletic Therapist and Chartered Physiotherapist, Raglan Sports Medicine, 4 Fitzwilliam Square East, Dublin, E-mail: info@raglansportsmedicine.com

mobilisation of interstitial fluids therefore enhancing the body's natural lymphatic drainage reducing inflammation [19] and activation of mechanoreceptor cells causing a reduction in pain sensitivity. It has been indicated for use in musculoskeletal injuries but few studies on its effectiveness exist.

Therefore, the purpose of this study was to measure the effect DEEP OSCILLATION® (DOT) had on patients with lateral epicondylalgia (LE).

Materials and Methods

Twenty subjects aged between 18-55 years took part in this trial from patients whom attended a sports medicine physician at the Sports Surgery Clinic, Dublin for the treatment of lateral elbow pain over the course of 12 months. A consultant physician with over 25 years of expertise in the area made the diagnosis of LE. The diagnostic criteria included an appropriate subjective history of the injury and an objective physical examination. To make a diagnosis of LE a positive Stoddard's test, pain on palpation of the origin of ECRB at the lateral epicondyle and pain at the lateral epicondyle with resisted wrist extension were all required. Exclusion criteria included patients whom had a negative Stoddard Test and did not have pain from either palpation or resisted wrist extension or had a pathology that was causing lateral elbow pain that was not related to tendinosis of the common extensor origin. Any subject with an underlying pathology that DOT treatment was contraindicated was also excluded. Ethical approval was granted through the ethics board at the Sports Surgery Clinic, Dublin and written consent was received from all participants.

Subjects individually completed a Patient Rated Functional Tennis Elbow Evaluation (PRTEE) [20] to assess their baseline perceived pain and function levels using a ten point Visual Analogue Scale (VAS) with 0 indicating no pain and 10 indicating the worst pain possible.

A baseline measure of grip strength was also collected by all subjects using a Baseline Hydraulic Hand Dynamometer (Fabrication Enterprises Inc, New York). This was recorded with the subject standing, elbow flexed to 90 degrees and wrist in a neutral position. Subjects were then randomised into two groups, Group A, control and Group B, intervention. Randomization was performed using random order allocation using SPSS software with subjects stratified for age and sex.

Group A (Control) underwent the protocol of injection therapy with 5 mg of Adcortyl and Lignocaine, patients were advised to apply approximately 1inch of topical Diclofenac anti-inflammatory gel themselves three times per day and undergo supervised rest over a two week period. Patients were then referred for physiotherapy where they completed a baseline PRTEE and were instructed on a home exercise program (HEP) for 4 weeks. The HEP consisted of stretching of the forearm extensors with the elbow extended, holding for 30 seconds for 2 sets twice per day. Wrist extension and radial deviation strength exercises performed with resistance band were performed for 3 sets of 10 repetitions each.

Group B (Test) received the same protocol from the physician as Group A and referred for physiotherapy where they completed a baseline PRTEE and received the same HEP as Group A. Group B also received DOT consisting of two-25minutes session per week for 4 weeks, eight treatment sessions in total. All subjects received one-to-one treatment and therefore had no interaction with other subjects.

The extensor tendon and the extensor muscle mass were both treated with two applicator heads using a custom protocol stored on the Evident Clinical Unit, designed and supplied by Physiomed Elektromedizin AG, Germany.

Protocol

The DOT treatment protocol consisted of 10minutes @ 200Hz-250Hz, 5minutes @ 40Hz-65Hz and a final 10minutes @ 85Hz. Intensity was set as close to 100% manually based on patients' response and sensitivity. Application was performed using two 5 cm diameter treatment heads using effleurage strokes treating the extensor mass of the affected forearm from distal to proximal with a proximal end point of 3 cm proximal to the lateral epicondyle. The mode was set to 2:1. Protocol design was customized by the authors and was based on parameters stored within the Evident unit and literature provided by manufacturers on effects of varying frequency ranges. High frequency oscillations for pain reduction, low frequency for reduction of scar tissue due to the deeper oscillations and medium frequency to reduce inflammation by mobilizing interstitial fluid. Do date; no current evidence is available on specific protocols for specific soft tissue injuries.

Follow-up

After the four week protocol and 6 weeks from the start of the treatment with the consultant physician, both groups returned for follow up PRTEE, grip strength and further assessment. At 6 months, information on any further treatment was recorded through telephone and email correspondence. The purpose of this was to ascertain if the subjects still had symptoms and did they seek further treatment since the 6 week follow up.

Statistical analysis

Data recorded on the PRTEE was collected from the groups. Pain scores were added to give a figure out of a maximum of 50 and the sum of the function scores were divided by 2 to also give a figure out of 50. Grip strength scores were recorded from baseline and at 6 weeks post treatment to analyze for comparison. Statistical analysis was performed using SPSS version 20 software for Windows. Data was tested for normality and analysis was performed using a repeated measure ANOVA to assess the significant difference between groups' pain and function from baseline to 6 weeks. Significance levels report at $p < 0.05$ with a confidence interval of 95%.

Results

Twenty subjects, 14 females and 6 males, between the age of 18 and 55 years with a mean age of 38.8 yrs (± 12.02) took part in the study and met the criteria. The remaining subjects were randomized into control and intervention groups with equal number of males and females per group. Descriptive statistics for the groups are displayed in Table 1.

Due to insufficient grip strength data at 6 weeks being recorded, there was no benefit in analyzing the collected results. This was due to a number of subjects being unable return to the test center at the allocated time therefore PRTEE data was recorded via email and telephone correspondence.

Descriptive statistics above show mean age to be 38.8 yrs with a SD of 12.02. Sex has a mean of 0.3 indicating 30% of the subjects were male. A mean of 0.5 indicates equal numbers in each group. The baseline mean of pain for Group A was 18.9 (SD 4.5) and at 6 weeks the mean was 13 (3.09). The baseline mean of pain in Group B was 18.4 (4.5) and at 6 weeks it was 10.3 (3.8). The results of the repeated measure ANOVA on Pain showed significant difference between measurement from baseline to 6 weeks ($F(1,18)=530.52$, $p \leq 0.001$). However, Results for the Time x Group interaction effect was not significant ($F(1,18)=1.76$, $p=0.20$),

	N	Minimum	Maximum	Mean	Std. Deviation
Age:	20	18	55	38.8	12.016
Sex:	20	Female	Male	0.3	0.47
Group:	20	Group A	Group B	0.5	0.513
Subject:	20	1	20	10.5	5.916
Valid N (list wise)	20				

Table 1: Descriptive statistics.

indicating that the changes in Pain measurements from baseline to 6 weeks were not significantly different for Control and Test groups. This is also shown in the Figure 1.

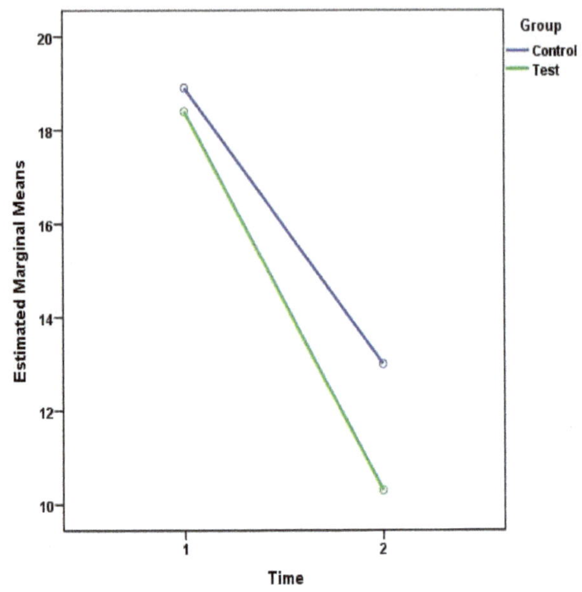

Figure 1: Results of pain difference between groups.

The figure above shows the Mean difference between 1 (baseline) and 2 (6-weeks post) for each group. The mean function baseline for Group A was recorded as 13 (3.09) and 12.95 (2.76) at 6 weeks. The mean function for Group B was recorded as 22.5 (3.9) and 11.35 (4.10) at 6 weeks. The results of the repeated measure ANOVA on Function showed significant difference between measurement from baseline to 6 weeks ($F(1,18)=98.82$, $p \leq 0.001$). Furthermore, the results for the Time x Group interaction effect were found significant ($F(1,18)=10.59$, $p=0.004$), indicating that the changes in measurement from baseline to 6 weeks was significantly different for Control and Test groups. This is also shown in the Figure 2.

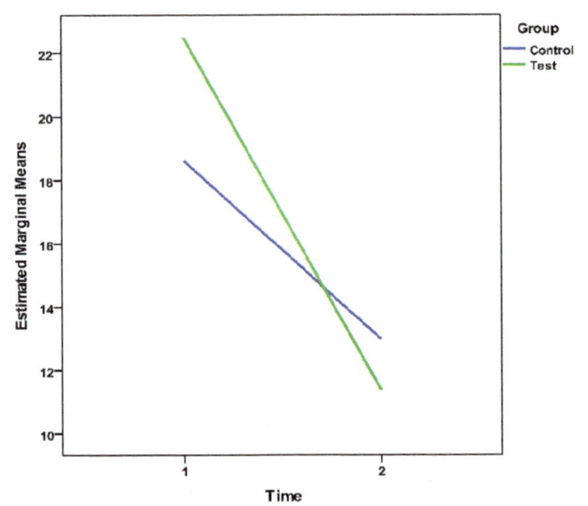

Figure 2: Results of function difference between groups.

The figure above indicates the mean scores for both groups for function at 1. (baseline) and at 2. (6 weeks post). On follow up at 6 months, 7 of the 10 subjects in Group A required further treatment between 6 weeks and the 6 month period. Only 3 subjects from Group B required further treatment within the same period. The methods of further treatment was not considered in the study design but data collected ranged from further physiotherapy, injection therapy and continued topical ketoprofen gel use.

Discussion

The results of this pilot study show the benefit both groups received from the treatment intervention given but that Group B reported better outcomes on follow-up. Both groups pain significantly reduced in the 6 week period which is supported by research by Bisset et al. [9]. They compared mobilization techniques, injection therapy and "wait and see" in 65 patients with TE. Corticosteroid injection was found to give the best results at 6 weeks compared to the other modalities. They also found a high regression rate with 47 out of the 65 patients' symptoms regressing between 6 and 52 weeks post injection. Work by Ozturan et al., [10], Verhar et al., [12] and Price et al., [13]; all found corticosteroid injection therapy to give the most benefit in the treatment of TE from baseline to 6 weeks but they also found approx 50% of these patients symptoms would regress in the weeks following. This finding was similar in this current study with 7 of the 10 patients in Group A requiring further treatment between 6 week and 6 months.

The current study did not show a statistically significant difference in pain of Group A compared to Group B on 6 week follow-up. However, the significant improvement of Group B's function over Group A may have been the deciding factor in patient's recovery. Only 3 out of the 10 subjects (30%) in Group B required further treatment from 6 weeks to 6 months compared to 7 out of the 10 (70%) in Group A. As both groups received the same protocol except for the eight DOT treatment sessions, it can be hypothesized that the improvement in function and in pain scores was due to the treatment effect. Similar effects were found in research by Jahr et al. [18] in which DOT was also found to reduce pain and increase function when used in conjunction with lymphatic drainage massage to patients with secondary lymphoedema following breast surgery. Twenty one subjects were used in total with the treatment group of 11 subjects receiving 12 treatments of DOT lymphatic drainage massage. The control group received lymphatic massage without the aid of DOT. The treatment group received 45min sessions 2-3 times per week performed at 100Hz for 30mins and 30Hz for 15mins. As the control group did not receive any placebo or sham DOT, the benefit in the treatment group of this study may be due to the placebo effect in having a new treatment. This was also a limitation of this current study.

As the mean function difference of Group B was larger than

Group A, the difference can be assumed to be the impact DOT had on the corticosteroid injection therapy each patient received. We have hypothesised that the oscillation of the tissue increases permeability of the target tissue increasing the therapeutic effect of the corticosteroid and lignocain solution. There is no literature to the authors' knowledge that supports this claim other than comparing the therapy to iontophoresis which it is not. DOT has been shown to mobilise interstitial fluid which may help to disperse the corticosteroid throughout the target tissue. In this current study, it was found that patients whom received DOT closer to their time of injection described a greater reduction of pain post treatment session. This observation may be a consideration in further study designs.

The Patient Rated Tennis Elbow Evaluation (PRTEE) as designed by MacDiarmuid et al. [20] was used to assess pain and function in this trial. Martinez-Silvestrini et al., [21] indicated in their work that as the PRTEE specifically focuses on the forearms pain and function it is therefore the best tool for studying lateral epicondylitis. Poltawski and Watson [22] showed in their work using the PRTEE that what may indicate a statistical difference may not yield a compelling clinic difference. They set the minimal clinical importance difference (MCID) at 11/100 on the PRTEE, defined as "much better" or "completely recovered". Taking this information into account, when the pain and function results are combined in order to mark the score out of 100, Group A improved by 11.55/100 and Group B improved by 19.25/100. This would indicate that both groups showed a clinical difference with Group B showing a greater clinical improvement overall. However, it was the intention to also measure grip strength to further correlate subject improvement of symptoms as Nilsson et al., [15] among others have done, but as enough follow-up data could not be collected, the small amount of collected data was not presented in this work.

There are some limitations with this work. Low subject numbers do not give the ability to make any substantial claims about the effectiveness of DOT in the treatment of TE. The significant improvement in such a small number does however give strong indication that the therapautic benefit could be even more significant on a larger test group. As the trial was not a double blind design, the impact of placebo effect of the test group receiving DOT over the control must be taken into consideration. As very little research on DOT and particularly effective protocols for different pathologies exist, the possibility that the protocol used in this current research may not be optimal for TE. The protocol was based on set protocols stored in the Evident Clinical Unit and practitioner experience of the therapy and not on published results.

Conclusion

This pilot study indicates the potential benefit DOT has in musculoskeletal pathologies such as TE and how it can be used in conjunction with injection therapy to improve on results already gained. A significant improvement in patients function at 6 weeks post treatment was found with 70% of the treatment group requiring no further treatment from 6 weeks to 6 months post treatment. DOT is beneficial in the treatment of TE and may further enhance the benefit from local steriod injection. Further research on the use of DOT in musculoskeletal injury and relevant protocols are needed.

Ethical Approval

Ethical approval was granted through the ethic committee of the Sports Surgery Clinic, Santry Demesne, Dublin 9, Ireland.

Funding

The research paper was funded by the authors.

Sponsors

Equipment was provided on loan for the duration of the testing in the trial by Physiomed Elektromedizin AG, Germany.

References

1. Hamilton PG (1986) The prevalence of humeral epicondylitis: a survey in general practice. J R Coll Gen Pract 36: 464-465.
2. Allander E (1974) Prevalence, incidence, and remission rates of some common rheumatic diseases or syndromes. Scand J Rheumatol 3: 145-153.
3. Putnam MD, Cohen M (1999) Painful conditions around the elbow. Orthop Clin North Am 30: 109-118.
4. Nirschl RP1 (1992) Elbow tendinosis/tennis elbow. Clin Sports Med 11: 851-870.
5. Kivi P (1983) The etiology and conservative treatment of humeral epicondylitis. Scand J Rehabil Med 15: 37-41.
6. Labelle H, Guibert R, Joncas J, Newman N, Fallaha M, et al. (1992) Lack of scientific evidence for the treatment of lateral epicondylitis of the elbow. An attempted meta-analysis. J Bone Joint Surg Br 74: 646-651.
7. Cyriax JH (1936) The pathology and treatment of tennis elbow. J Bone Joint Surg Am 4: 921-940.
8. Hong QN, Durand MJ, Loisel P (2004) Treatment of lateral epicondylitis: where is the evidence? Joint Bone Spine 71: 369-373.
9. Bisset L, Beller E, Jull G, Brooks P, Darnell R, et al. (2006) Mobilisation with movement and exercise, corticosteroid injection, or wait and see for tennis elbow: randomised trial. BMJ 333: 939.
10. Ozturan KE, Yucel I, Cakici H, Guven M, Sungur I (2010) Autologous blood and corticosteroid injection and extracoporeal shock wave therapy in the treatment of lateral epicondylitis. Orthopedics 33: 84-91.
11. Newcomer KL, Laskowski ER, Idank DM, McLean TJ, Egan KS (2001) Corticosteroid injection in early treatment of lateral epicondylitis. Clin J Sport Med 11: 214-222.
12. Verhaar JA, Walenkamp GH, van Mameren H, Kester AD, van der Linden AJ (1996) Local corticosteroid injection versus Cyriax-type physiotherapy for tennis elbow. J Bone Joint Surg Br 78: 128-132.
13. Price R, Sinclair H, Heindrich I, Gibson T (1991) Local injection treatment of Tennis Elbow-hydrocortisone, triamcinolone and lignocaine compared. Br J Rheumatol 30: 39-44.
14. Burnham R, Gregg R, Healy P, Steadward R (1998) The effectiveness of topical diclofenac for lateral epicondylitis. Clin J Sport Med 8: 78-81.
15. Nilsson P, Thom E, Baigi A, Marklund B, Månsson J (2007) A prospective pilot study of a multidisciplinary home training programme for lateral epicondylitis. Musculoskeletal Care 5: 36-50.
16. Mikhalchik E, Titkova S, Anurov M, et al. (2005) Wound healing effects of DEEP OSCILLATION. 1st International Conference on Skin and Environment, Moscow, St Petersburg, Russia.
17. Janik H et al. (2010) Treatment of patients with fibromyalgia syndrome with vibration massage by deep oscillations. Eur J Phys Rehabil Med 46: 42.
18. Jahr S, Schoppe B, Reisshauer A (2008) Effect of treatment with low-intensity and extremely low-frequency electrostatic fields (Deep Oscillation) on breast tissue and pain in patients with secondary breast lymphoedema. J Rehabil Med 40: 645-650.
19. Gasbarro V, Bartoletti R, Tsolaki E, Sileno S, Agnati M, et al. (2006) Role of Hivamat (Deep Oscillation®) in the treatment for the lymphedema of the limbs. Eur J Lymphol 16: 13-15.
20. Macdermid J (2005) Update: The Patient-rated Forearm Evaluation Questionnaire is now the Patient-rated Tennis Elbow Evaluation. J Hand Ther 18: 407-410.
21. Martinez-Silvestrini JA, Newcomer KL, Gay RE, Schaefer MP, Kortebein P et al., (2005) Chronic Lateral Epicondylitis: Comparative effectiveness of a home exercise program including stretching alone versus stretching supplemented with eccentric or concentric strengthening. J Hand Ther 18: 411-420.
22. Poltawski L and Watson T (2011) Measuring clinically important change with the Patient-rated Tennis Elbow Evaluation. J Hand Ther 16: 52-57.

Oxygen Consumption during Different Exercise Protocols in the Aged

Mark R McKean*, Timothy B Stockwell and Brendan J Burkett

Faculty of Science, Health, Education and Engineering, University of Sunshine Coast, Queensland, Australia

Abstract

Objectives: The objective of this study was to compare response; specifically oxygen consumption; of a single bout of exercise using two different (constant and interval) intensity protocols in an aged population.

Design: Ten males (68.8 ± 3.7 years) and six females (66.2 ± 3.5 years) were recruited for this study. All participants were actively involved in three hours of physical activity per week and were able to use a cycle ergometer unaided.

Methods: Participants completed two randomised 20 min exercise protocols on a cycle ergometer, each with equal work output. The constant intensity session was at 50% of Vo_{2max}, and the 1 min interval session varied from 70% to 30% Vo_{2max}. Oxygen consumption was measured during the following phases; resting, warm-up, exercise, cool-down and 20 mins post-exercise.

Results: Similar values were found when comparing the overall oxygen consumption for the constant and interval protocols respectively. However, significant differences ($p<0.05$) were found between the two different intensities during the exercise phase.

Conclusions: The interval training protocol consumed higher levels of oxygen during the exercise phase when compared to the constant intensity protocol, despite the participants reporting similar RPE. These age-specific differences should be considered for future exercise prescription for this at-risk population.

Keywords: Aged; Exercise test; Energy expenditure; EPOC

Introduction

Regular physical activity has been linked to reductions in the risk factors for chronic disease and disability [1]. The aging process, however, tends to decrease the intensity and duration of spontaneous physical activity [2] and also the decline in functional capacity [3]. These factors have been linked to the reduction in the quality of life from the second to the seventh decade of life [4] as well as a decrease in muscle mass every year from the fourth decade of life [5].

Traditionally, exercise protocols of intensity and duration have been determined for a broad and general population, and from this information the protocols are extrapolated and assumed to be suitable for other populations, such as the at-risk aged population. Health practitioners have previously avoided using interval training in the past due to concerns over increased heart rates and stress which are held at an even level during constant cardiovascular training sessions in comparison. With recent research supporting the use of interval training for increased cardiovascular effect [6,7], patients with COPD [8,9], and fat oxidation [10] health practitioners may need to reconsider the use of interval training methods in other low risk populations. The aging population is one such group of people who are looking for ways to maintain good health and participate in a range of fitness activities and evidence suggests these leisure-time activities are an important promoter of health [11]. The mode of exercise can influence oxygen consumption, with differences in the physiological responses found between a single continuous exercise protocol and three different intermittent exercise protocols [12]. The three intermittent training protocols, at both 50% and at 70% Vo_{2Peak}, showed significantly lower heart rate, minute ventilation and Vo_2 when compared to a similar amount of work done within the constant load protocols. This finding suggests that intermittent training is more efficient than constant load training. However, there were no significant differences found between the 15, 30, and 60 second intermittent protocols, when compared to each other. Furthermore, heart rate, minute ventilation and Vo_2 were only taken at the mid-point of each stage of exercise, which meant that the total expired gas and energy expenditure for the entire duration of exercise were not examined. A similar finding was made when comparing constant walking or high-intensity interval walking, with high-intensity interval walking resulting in greater increases in Vo_{2Peak} [13]. If high-intensity interval walking helps to protect older persons against some of the age-related reductions in muscle strength and Vo_{2Peak}, exercise prescription should encourage a high-intensity component during walking. For the sedentary aged population the problems of joint degeneration and the associated high ground force impact from walking may inhibit this mode of physical activity. Consequently the low impact and simple nature of cycle ergometers are often preferred by people with orthopaedic disabilities of the lower extremities, which are more prevalent in elderly people than younger populations. To date, there is little literature which specifically examines the differences in total oxygen consumption during exercise between constant load and interval training in the elderly (65 years and older). This lack of knowledge for what is an important aspect of exercise, particularly in such a crucial population as the elderly, has left many questions unanswered, especially in regards to exercise efficiency and the short-term physiological responses of exercise[14]. This knowledge will facilitate the global aging process [15] and will help to maintain improved health and wellbeing. Reductions in Vo_{2max} in non-endurance-trained individuals are thought to be justified by the loss of muscle mass, which is observed with advancing age [16]. Regular activity is known to reduce the risk factors of chronic disease and disability, and the aging process is known to correlate with a reduction in physical activity, further reinforcing the need for exercise protocols for the elderly that are not only efficient but also beneficial.

***Corresponding author:** Mark McKean, Faculty of Science, Health, Education and Engineering, University of Sunshine Coast, Queensland, Australia
E-mail: mmckean@usc.edu.au

Therefore, the objectives of this study were to directly examine the differences in oxygen consumption, perceived effort and efficiency in the elderly using cycle ergometers across two different protocols, constant and interval. The authors hypothesized there will be little or no difference for oxygen consumption and perceived effort for the interval protocol compared with the constant protocol.

Materials and Methods

Ten males (aged 68.8 ± 3.7 y, height 173.7 ± 7.5 cm, weight 85.2 ± 17.6 kg and predicted Vo_{2max} 36.4 ± 5.2 ml.kg-1.min-1) and six females (aged 66.2 ± 3.5 y, height 163.4 ± 6.9 cm,weight 69.3 ± 8.6 kg and predicted Vo_{2max} 32.8 ± 5.5 ml.kg-1.min-1) were recruited to participate in this study. Participants were informed of the research risks and ll signed University ethics committee approved consent forms before data were collected.

All participants were active, currently participating in a minimum of three hours of physical activity per week, and able to use a cycle ergometer unaided. Additionally, participants were not on any medication that would inhibit any physical activity, and were classified in the 'moderate' category through the risk stratification process [17].

Participants were tested on three separate mornings, having fasted overnight. Participants were also requested to refrain from strenuous exercise and activity on the preceding day to testing. The first session involved a pre-exercise screening questionnaire [17], a 20 min supine resting 12-lead echocardiogram (ECG) and a sub-maximal fitness assessment. All participants were classified as 'moderate risk' due to their age; however they did not require medical clearance due to the relative sub-maximal nature of the exercise being performed. The 12-lead ECG placement was as per standard protocol [18]. Participants were required to rest in a supine position for 20 min, after which time a sample heart trace was taken and assessed for any abnormalities.

Participants then undertook a sub-maximal Vo_2 test to predict their Vo_{2max}. The test was performed on a cycle ergometer (Jaeger ER800, Bitz, Germany). The test commenced with participants cycling at 60 revolutions per minute (rpm) for 3 mins at 20 W. The resistance was then increased to 50 W for 2 mins, and then a further 25 W every subsequent 2 mins until participant's heart rate reached 75% of their age-predicted maximal heart rate, using the formula; 208 – [0.7 × age] [19], or until they were unable to continue to pedal at 60 rpm. Vo_{2max} was calculated by extrapolation using the Multi-stage Model [20]. These values were used to base the percent effort protocol of the two 'exercise' sessions. Heart rate was measured and rating of perceived exertion (RPE) was taken during the last 5 s of each stage for safety and comfort reasons. The second and third morning exercise sessions consisted of either the constant or interval exercise protocol, which was randomised to eliminate any bias from protocol order. Subsequent to each of the two 'exercise' sessions, participants completed another resting 12-lead ECG to ensure consistency and accuracy of initial readings.

Expired gas samples were collected in 15 s averages through a one-way non re-breather mask (Hans-Rudolph 7930 breathing valve, Kansas City, MO, USA) and analysed using a calibrated TrueMax 2400 metabolic measurement system (Parvo Medics, Sandy, UT, USA) as per existing protocol. The gas collection in each session was broken up into five different phases; (i) resting baseline, (ii) warm-up, (iii) exercise, (iv) cool-down, and (v) post-exercise resting. Baseline values were collected with participants seated on the cycle ergometer at rest. This was followed by the warm-up, which consisted of 2 mins of 60 rpm pedalling at 20 W. The exercise phase involved 20 mins of pedalling at 50% of extrapolated Vo_{2max} for the constant session, or 20 mins alternating 70% Vo_{2max} for 1 min followed by 1 min of 30% Vo_{2max} in the interval session. Participants were asked to indicate their (RPE) using the 6-20 Borg [21] scale after each minute of exercise in the exercise phase. The cool-down involved 2 mins at 20 W, and the post-exercise collection phase was 20 mins of supine resting. All protocols for the two exercise sessions, pre and post-exercise, were identical with the exception of the 'exercise' phase of the session. Data was analysed using two-way analysis of variations (ANOVA) and is reported as means with 95% confidence intervals, upper and lower bounds where applicable. Changes in effect statistics are presented in raw and percentage changes.

Results

Total oxygen consumption and heart rate, broken up into the five phases, for both protocols are shown in table 1. Mean values for oxygen consumption were found to be similar between the two protocols for all subjects. Table 2 presents the effect changes expressed as raw and percentage differences between oxygen consumption and heart rate across the two protocols. Whilst there were no significant differences here, it was shown that the EPOC phase of gas analysis was 11.8% greater in the interval session when compared to the constant session. Figure 1 illustrates the total oxygen consumption comparisons between the two protocols. The means of the two oxygen consumptions for the entire sessions did not show any significant differences ($p=0.627$). However, when the 15 s averages were compared between the two sessions, significant differences ($p<0.001$) were seen relating to constant (28.3 L) and interval (30.0 L) data. Males and females showed similar values across most of the other data, except for heart rates during the exercise ($p=0.029$) and cool-down ($p=0.021$) phases in the constant

Period	O_2 Consumption (Litres)				Heart Rate (bpm)			
	Constant (50%)		**Interval (70%:30%)**		**Constant (50%)**		**Interval (70%:30%)**	
Pre (0-2 min)	**0.31**	(0.24–0.38)	**0.30**	(0.22-0.38)	**63.61**	(58.17-69.05)	**66.29**	(60.81-71.77)
Warm Up (2-4 min)	**0.81**	(0.68-0.95)	**0.84**	(0.68-0.99)	**73.19**	(68.69-77.68)	**74.97**	(70.26-79.69)
Exercise (4-24 min)	**21.46**	(17.26-25.65)	**22.67**	(18.93-26.42)	**104.65**	(100.25-109.05)	**105.56**	(100.89-110.23)
Cool Down (24-26 min)	**1.60**	(1.30-1.89)	**1.52**	(1.20-1.76)	**98.78**	(94.16-103.40)	**96.97**	(91.04-102.91)
Post (26-46 min)	**4.15**	(3.26-5.04)	**4.64**	(3.62-5.66)	**73.75**	(68.47-79.03)	**74.21**	(69.11-79.31)

Table 1: Oxygen consumption and heart rate during the five phases of gas collection for constant and interval protocols presented as means (95% CI).

	Difference (Litres)		**% Difference**		**Difference (bpm)**		**% Difference**	
Pre (0-2 min)	**-0.01**	(-0.07-0.04)	**-3.2%**	(-37.1-18.6)	**2.68**	(0.45-4.90)	**4.2%**	(0.5-8.2)
Warm Up (2-4 min)	**0.03**	(-0.11-0.16)	**3.7%**	(-15.0-30.0)	**1.78**	(0.17-3.40)	**2.4%**	(0.1-4.7)
Exercise (4-24 min)	**1.22**	(-0.63-3.06)	**5.7%**	(-12.5-54.9)	**0.91**	(-1.18-2.99)	**0.9%**	(-1.1-2.8)
Cool Down (24-26 min)	**-0.08**	(-0.26-0.10)	**-5.0%**	(-24.6-50.9)	**-1.81**	(-4.75- 1.13)	**-1.8%**	(-5.1-1.0)
Post (26-46 min)	**0.49**	(-0.58-1.56)	**11.8%**	(-16.3-47.6)	**0.46**	(-1.51-2.43)	**0.6%**	(-1.9-3.3)

Table 2: Comparison of interval to constant protocols for oxygen consumption and heart rate presented as absolute and percentage differences (95% CI).

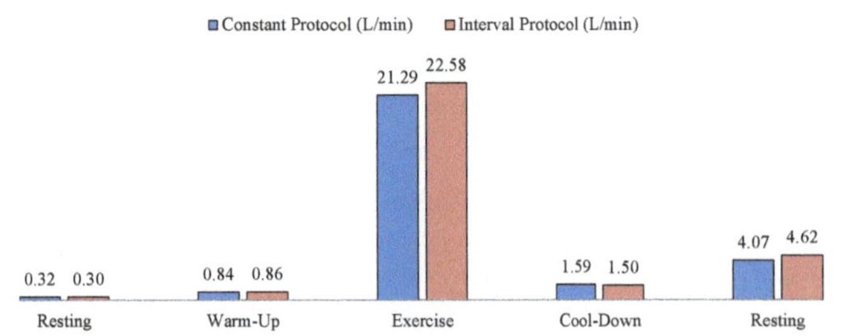

Comparison of Oxygen Consumption per Section

Figure 1: Oxygen consumption (L/min) during the five phases of gas collection for constant and interval protocols presented as means.

protocol, and the warm-up (p=0.013), exercise (p=0.009) and cool-down (p=0.050) phases of the interval protocol.

Most of the participants (10 of the 16 in the constant protocol, and 11 of the 16 in the interval protocol) returned to within 1 standard deviation (SD) of mean pre-exercise oxygen consumption levels within the 20 mins of post-exercise gas collection. Three more returned to within 2 SD in both protocols, with only a small minority (<18%) not returning to within either of these ranges of their baseline levels during the 20 min post-exercise data collection phase.

The mean magnitude of the constant protocol EPOC was found to be 13.6% of the total oxygen consumption for the session and the exercise component of this same session was found to be 71.1% of the total oxygen consumption. This resulted in the ratio of EPOC to exercise oxygen consumption for the constant session being 1:5.2 (19.1%). Similarly, the mean magnitude of the interval protocol EPOC was found to be 15.2%, the exercise component was found to be 75.6%, and the resultant ratio of EPOC to exercise oxygen consumption for the interval session was 1:4.9 (20.5%).

Average RPE's for both exercise phases of the different protocols were almost identical with the exercise phase of constant session being 11.4, and the interval session being 11.3. This average is consistent with an RPE just above the 'light' level of exertion in both protocols.

Discussion

The objective of this study was to directly examine the differences in oxygen consumption, perceived effort and efficiency in the elderly using cycle ergometers across two different protocols, constant and interval. The mean oxygen consumption was found to be slightly higher for the interval protocol when compared to the constant intensity of identical work output, with mean consumption readings of 30.0 and 28.3 L respectively, although these differences were not statistically significant. However, significant differences (p<0.05) were found in the 15 sec oxygen consumption samples between the two different intensities during the exercise phase, with the interval protocol eliciting higher oxygen consumption. No comparable studies were found that assessed elderly male and female participants with a similar mean age of around 67, however past research conducted on 12 physically active 30 year-old males concluded the interval exercise session generated significantly higher oxygen consumption during exercise [22]. Whilst this other study had protocols that involved slightly higher intensities and longer durations, it does not explain the lack of significant differences in oxygen consumption found in this current study. This leads the authors to believe that age has a potential influence in the differences of oxygen consumption in relation to exercise. The similar values of EPOC across both genders, and both protocols of similar work output found in the current study, highlight the conflict in previous research into this area. These results are supported by earlier studies where similar EPOC values were found [22], but in conflict with another study [23] which found that both duration and magnitude of EPOC are significantly greater for interval exercise when compared to constant protocols. This study indicated that, in a younger male population, interval exercise would be more advantageous in regards to exercise energy expenditure and oxygen consumption. This suggests that the EPOC response may be specific to the participants with respect to age, along with the intensity and duration of exercise.

This current study found similar gender-based values in the analysis performed on oxygen consumption, implying that males and females in an aged population will both use the same amount of oxygen during exercise, and therefore gain similar relative physiological benefits from either constant or interval-based exercise protocols. The effect of gender on oxygen consumption has not yet been fully clarified [24] and the authors were unable to find any other studies that found similar results comparing oxygen consumption in males and females within a similar age group.

The similar values from this current study are contradicted by an earlier study [25] on younger participants (males 21.1 ± 3.6 years and females 20.4 ± 3.1 years) which showed a significantly higher amount of oxygen consumption in males when compared to the women for 40% (16.3 to 12.1L), 50% (22.1 to 21.8L) and 70% (28.1 to 24.3L) protocols respectively. In all three protocols, steady-state energy expenditure, and therefore oxygen consumption, was significantly higher in the males than the females. These results imply that a combination of age and gender result in a leveling out, or balancing, effect of oxygen consumption seen with advancing age.

The males and females in this current study had similar ages and also presented similar Vo_{2max} scores (p=0.11), which indicates no difference in physical performance due to gender. The current study exercise phase was 20 min, which would be classified as aerobic or endurance type activity. A similar finding of no difference between genders in an aged population was reported when comparing the endurance swimming performance across genders [25]. Differences however were found in the short sprint swimming events. This indicates that the declines which are associated with age in the physiological influences of sprinting and endurance performance may occur at different rates and at different ages in men and women. A relative rate of the decline in maximal oxygen consumption, which is a key determinant of endurance performance, is similar in both men and women, and therefore further supports the findings of the current study.

This study examined EPOC as a percentage of total oxygen consumption during the two exercise session, with outputs of 14.7% and 15.5% during the constant and interval sessions respectively. These values are within previously reported study which found EPOC of nine healthy participants' percentages to be between 7% and 21% during cycling [26]. These results support the current studies results in regards to the percentage of EPOC to overall total oxygen consumption.

This current study also examined EPOC as a percentage of exercise phase oxygen consumption, and participants achieved values of 19.3% during constant exercise and 20.5% during interval exercise. The previous study found that EPOC in six healthy males was proportional to exercise duration and equalled around 5.1% after 20 min of exercise [27]. These results are not similar to the results of the current study and suggest that healthy males either consume a much smaller amount of oxygen during EPOC, or they consume a much higher amount of oxygen during exercise.

Conclusion

Increased life expectancy within the global aging process, combined with the degrading and potentially debilitating effects associated with aging make exercise of any description a priority later on in life. Associated with this at-risk population is the need to develop age-specific protocols. Furthermore, to overcome the de-motivation to exercise necessitates the development of efficient protocols with 'high benefit' versus 'low effort' exercise need to be developed. There has been conflicting results from previous research as to which type of exercise, constant or interval shows the greater benefits in regards to either aerobic capacity or immediate physiological effects. Similar mean values were found in this study's oxygen consumption measures, however a significant increase in 15 s average oxygen consumption was found for the variable intensity exercise protocol. The similar perceived effort for either exercise protocol suggests the aged population will benefit more by engaging in variable intensity exercise. The author's research hypothesis was proven to hold true in that there was little difference between constant and interval protocols for the elderly.

Acknowledgements

The authors would like to thank Dr. Christopher Askew and Dr. Dale Lovell for their expertise and assistance in this project.

References

1. Warburton DE, Nicol CW, Bredin SS (2006) Prescribing exercise as preventive therapy. CMAJ 174: 961-974.
2. Prentice AM (1992) Energy expenditure in the elderly. Eur J Clin Nutr 46: S21-28.
3. Chatard J, Denis C (1994) Physical fitness of elderly = Physical fitness of elder people. Ann Phys Rehabil Med 37: 423-429.
4. Vaughan L, Zurlo F, Ravussin E, (1991) Aging and energy expenditure. Am J Clin Nutr 53: 821-825.
5. Seguin R, Nelson ME (2003) The benefits of strength training for older adults. Am J Prev Med 25: 141-149.
6. Wisloff U, Stoylen A, Loennechen JP, Bruvold M, Rognmo O, et al. (2007) Superior cardiovascular effect of aerobic interval training versus moderate continuous training in heart failure patients: a randomized study. Circulation 115: 3086-3094.
7. Helgerud J, Hoydal K, Wang E, Karlsen T, Berg P, et al. (2007) Aerobic high-intensity intervals improve VO2max more than moderate training. Med Sci Sports Exerc 39: 665-671.
8. Arnardóttir RH, Boman G, Larsson K, Hedenstrom H, Emtner M (2007) Interval training compared with continuous training in patients with COPD. Respir Med 101: 1196-1204.
9. Vogiatzis I, Nanas S, Roussos C (2002) Interval training as an alternative modality to continuous exercise in patients with COPD. Eur Respir J 20: 12-19.
10. Talanian JL, Galloway SD, Heigenhauser GJ, Bonen A, Spriet LL (2007) Two weeks of high-intensity aerobic interval training increases the capacity for fat oxidation during exercise in women. J Appl Physiol 102: 1439-1447.
11. Paganini-Hill A, Kawas CH, Corrada MM (2011) Activities and mortality in the elderly: The Leisure World cohort study. J Gerontol A Biol Sci 66: 559-567.
12. Morris N, Gass G, Thompson M, Conforti D (2003) Physiological responses to intermittent and continuous exercise at the same relative intensity in older men. Eur J Appl Physiol 90: 620-625.
13. Nemoto K, Gen-no H, Masuki S, Okazaki K, Nose H (2007) Effects of high-intensity interval walking training on physical fitness and blood pressure in middle-aged and older people. Mayo Clin Proc 82: 803-811.
14. Janz KF (2006) Physical activity in epidemiology: moving from questionnaire to objective measurement. Br J Sports Med 40: 191-192.
15. Anderson GF, Hussey PS (2000) Population aging: a comparison among industrialized countries. Health Aff (Millwood) 19: 191-203.
16. Fleg JL, Lakatta EG (1988) Role of muscle loss in the age-associated reduction in VO2 max. J Appl Physiol 65: 1147-1151.
17. Norton K, Olds T, Bowes D, Van Ly S, Gore C (1998) Applying the Sports Medicine Australia pre-exercise screening procedures: who will be excluded? J Sci Med Sport 1: 38-51.
18. Phibbs BP, Buckels LJ (1975) Comparative yield of ECG leads in multistage stress testing. Am Heart J 90: 275-276.
19. Tanaka H, Monahan KD, Seals DR (2001) Age-predicted maximal heart rate revisited. J Am Coll Cardiol 37: 153-156.
20. Thompson WR, Gordon NF, Pescatello LS, American college of sports medicine, et al. (2010) ACSM's guidelines for exercise testing and prescription: Wolters Kluwer/Lippincott Williams & Wilkins.
21. Borg G (1970) Perceived exertion as an indicator of somatic stress. Scand J Rehabil Med 2: 92-98.
22. McGarvey W, Jones R, Petersen S (2005) Excess post-exercise oxygen consumption following continuous and interval cycling exercise. Int J Sport Nutr Exerc Metab 15: 28-37.
23. Ziegendfuss TN, Sedlock DA (1992) Excess post-exercise oxygen consumption following continuous and interval cycling exercise. Medicine & Science in Sports & Exercise 24: S97.
24. Borsheim E, Bahr R (2003) Effect of exercise intensity, duration and mode on post- exercise oxygen consumption. Sports Med 33: 1037-1060.
25. Smith J, Mc Naughton L (1993) The effects of intensity of exercise on excess postexercise oxygen consumption and energy expenditure in moderately trained men and women. Eur J Appl Physiol Occup Physiol. 67: 420-425.
26. Elliot DL, Goldberg L, Kuehl KS (1992) Effect of resistance training on excess post- exercise oxygen consumption. The Journal of Strength & Conditioning Research 6: 77.
27. Bahr R, Ingnes I, Vaage O, Sejersted OM, Newsholme EA (1987) Effect of duration of exercise on excess postexercise O2 consumption. J Appl Physiol 62: 485-490.

Physical Activity, Physical Fitness and Overweight in Early Schoolchildren

Paschaleri Z, Arabatzi F*, Papitsa A, Giagazoglou P and Kellis E

Aristotle University of Thessaloniki, Serres, Greece

Abstract

Purpose: The aim of this study was to evaluate physical activity and physical fitness levels in children 7-8 years old with different body mass index (BMI).

Methods: Eighty nine children (age 7.6 ± 0.4) participated in this study. BMI was used as obesity indicator and children were categorized in normal-weight and overweight/obese groups. Daily physical activity was assessed by RT3 accelerometer (Stayhealthy Inc, Monrovia, CA) and physical fitness was assessed using the European physical fitness test battery (Eurofit).

Results: Analysis of variance (ANOVA) indicated no significant differences in the average daily total counts of physical activity and in scores of four fitness tests between the overweight/obese and normal-weight group ($p>0.05$). However, boys were significantly more physically active than girls ($p<0.05$) and the level of physical activity was higher on weekdays than on weekend for both BMI groups ($p<0.05$).

Conclusion: The results indicate that physical activity is not the main contributing factor for childhood overweight at this age. Sufficient levels of daily physical activity were also shown to lead in good physical performance.

Keywords: Childhood obesity; Accelerometer; Physical performance

Introduction

The prevalence of obesity in children (from 6 to12 years old) has been increasing worldwide in the last decades. From 1980 to 2013, prevalence in developing countries has increased in children and adolescents, from 8.1% to 12.9% for boys and from 8.4% to 13.4% in girls [1]. Excess body weight in childhood and adolescence is associated with a higher risk of premature death and disability in adulthood, but overweight children and adolescents are also more likely to develop non-communicable diseases such as diabetes at a younger age [2]. A recent Greek national study which assessed BMI and prevalence of obesity/overweight in a representative sample of 8130 Greek children [3] showed overall 73.7% of the 7-year-olds children retain their classification of weight status at 18 years and a cross-national comparison in the same study confirmed higher levels of overweight youth at 7 years in Greece, compared to England.

The specific causes of overweight and obesity in childhood is complex, but despite the consideration of genetic and physiologic aspects, a reduction in physical activity (PA), an increased amount of time devoted to sedentary lifestyle and increased caloric intake due to environmental changes seem to be important factors for weight gain [4]. While PA levels of adolescents have been studied more frequently because it seems that the decline in PA begins near the onset of puberty, it is unclear whether PA affects weight status at earlier ages. A recent review of cross-sectional studies conducted over the last ten years reported a negative relationship between PA and child weight status in some studies and no association in others [5].

Except PA, a decrease in physical fitness (PF) has been associated with childhood obesity. It has been shown that regular PA in children improves PF, which helps in the management of childhood obesity [6]. The health-related components of PF are cardiorespiratory endurance, muscular strength and endurance, balance and flexibility. Of all these components, only cardiorespiratory fitness has been frequently studied and associated with childhood obesity [7-9]. This may be because of the possible interaction of obesity and cardiorespiratory fitness with cardiovascular disease risks. However in order to design successful interventions and policies to promote PA, PF and reduce childhood obesity, there is a need to better understand how PA and different parameters of PF affect body composition even from a very young age.

To guide the development and implementation of such programs objective measures of PA must be used. Self-report methods that are widely used in many studies for the assessment of PA have the major limitation of inability to accurately recall daily physical activities, especially by young children [10]. Accelerometry provides a unique way to examine associations between body fatness and amount of time spent in activities of varying intensities [11]. Triaxial accelerometers have been developed to detect body acceleration in all three planes and provide more accurate results than uniaxial accelerometers, when assessing PA in children [12-14].

Comparison of habitual PA, assessed with heart rate monitors, between boys and girls has led to conflicting results in the literature. Some studies have reported that boys were more active than girls, whereas others did not find any gender differences [15]. Additionally previous studies using accelerometers for measuring PA have suggested that boys are more active than girls [16] but these findings refer mainly to older children [5,8,10,17]. The patterns of children's PA across days have not been thoroughly examined in younger children [16] despite that weekdays and weekend are likely to provide different opportunities for children to be active [18]. Previous research studies showed controversial results on this subject because of the different habits of children in different age, in different countries [11,15,19]. Hence there is a need of more research on the timing and magnitude of these trends in Greece.

Thus the purpose of this study was to evaluate the association between weight status, PA and PF, in children 7-8 years old with special focus on gender and between days PA differences.

***Corresponding author:** Fotini Arabatzi, Assistant Professor, Aristotle University of Thessaloniki, Serres, Greece
E-mail: farabaji@phed-sr. auth.gr

Material and Methods

Participants

Eighty-nine healthy children (47 boys, 42 girls; mean age 7.6 years, s=0.4) volunteered to participate in this study. BMI was used as an obesity indicator. Using the international cutoff points for BMI, proposed by Cole et al. [20] subjects were classified as normal-weight (NW) (BMI<17.34 kg/m^2) and overweight/obese (OV/OB) (BMI ≥17.34 kg/m^2) groups, according to the age-adapted values. Written informed consent was obtained from parents/guardians of the children. Participants were recruited from a primary school in Serres, Greece. This study was approved by the ministry of education Athens, Greece and by the Research Ethics Board, Aristotle University of physical education, Serres, Greece.

Measures

Height was measured to the nearest centimeter without shoes and body mass was measured to the nearest 0.1 kg with the participants dressed in light-weight clothing. Waist circumference (WC) was also measured and BMI (kg/m^2) was calculated. BMI and WC correlate with cardiovascular (CV) risk factors in children which track into adulthood. WC provides a measure of central obesity, which has been specifically associated with CV risk factors [21].

Accelerometry: Accelerometry was determined using the RT3 accelerometer (Stayhealthy Inc., Monrovia, CA, USA), which measures PA in three individual planes (vertical, X; anteroposterior, Y; mediolateral, Z) and integrates acceleration to yield the "vector magnitude" (VM) calculated as $VM= (X^2+Y^2+Z^2)^{0.5}$. The epoch interval of data collection was set at 1 min. Children were instructed to wear the device to the right side of the anterior torso at the level of the waist. The device was placed into a small bag and on a belt round the waist for safety. Parents were given both verbal and written instructions on how to use the accelerometer and were instructed to put it on the child each morning of the study when the child woke and to remove it during sleeping, bathing, or swimming. Measurements were made for four consecutive days, two school days and a weekend. At least 3 days of recording, with a minimum of 8 hours registration per day, was set as an inclusion criterion. Accelerometry data were downloaded using manufacturers' software. Total PA (TPA) was expressed as total counts recorded divided by total daily registered time (counts/min). The time engaged in moderate PA (MPA) and vigorous PA (VPA) was calculated and presented as the average time per day. The activity counts thresholds for MPA/min was set from 970-2333 counts (3.0 to 5.99 METS) and for VPA/min >2333 counts (>6.00 METS) [22]. All minutes above 970 counts during a day were summarized and expressed as time spent in moderate to vigorous PA (MVPA). Overall mean PA was also compared among weekdays and weekends and among two different genders for two BMI groups.

Assessment of fitness parameters: All participants underwent four fitness tests from Eurofit physical fitness test battery [23]. These included flamingo balance test, sit-and-reach (flexibility), standing long jump (explosive muscular strength) and 10X5m shuttle run (agility). Brief descriptions of the tests follow below.

Flamingo balance test (FBT): This test assesses the strength of the leg, pelvic, and trunk muscle as well as dynamic balance. While balancing on the preferred leg, the free leg is flexed at the knee and the foot of this leg held close to the buttocks. We count the number of falls in 60 seconds of balancing. If there are more than 15 falls in the first 30 seconds, the test is terminated and a score of zero is given.

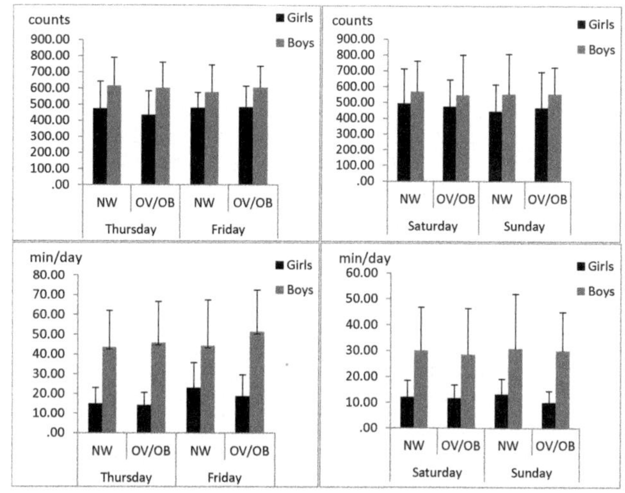

Figure 1: (a) Total physical activity (counts/day) between boys and girls for both BMI groups (b) Vigorous physical activity (min/day) between boys and girls for both BMI groups

Sit and reach (SAR): This test measures the flexibility of the hamstring, buttocks and lower back. It involves sitting on the floor with legs stretched out straight ahead. The soles of the feet are placed flat against a box. With the palms facing downwards, the subject reaches forward along a long ruler, fixed on the box, as far as possible. Indication of 15 cm is at the level of the feet.

Standing long jump (SLJ): Jumping for distance from a standing start. This test measures explosive strength. Children stands behind a line marked on the ground with feet slightly apart. A two foot take-off and landing is used, with swinging of the arms and bending of the knees to provide forward drive. The subject attempts to jump as far as possible, landing on both feet without falling backwards. Two attempts are allowed and the best counts in cm.

10 × 5 meters agility shuttle run (ASR): This test measures speed and agility of lower limb movement. Children stand behind a line and run a distance of 5 meters and back five times (covering 50 meters total). We record the total time taken to complete the 50 m course.

Statistical analysis

All analyses were performed using the Statistical Package for the Social Sciences (SPSS VERSION 17.0) and the level of significance was set as $p< 0.05$. Descriptive statistics for participant characteristics are displayed as means and SD. Pearson correlation was performed to examine the association between BMI and WC. For each of the four days, a Two-way ANOVA was used to examine the differences in TPA, MPA and VPA between the two BMI groups and two genders as independent factors. ANOVA with a repeated measures design was used to examine the differences in mean score of TPA, MPA and VPA of weekdays and weekend between the two BMI groups and two genders (2X2X2). Two-way ANOVA was used to examine the differences between the two BMI groups and two genders in four fitness performances tests.

Percentage frequency analysis was used to evaluate the percentage of the two groups who met the 60-minutes/day MVPA recommendation.

Results

Subjects Participant characteristics are provided in Table 1. Pearson correlation analysis showed a high correlation between BMI and WC (r =0.91, df=87, p<.001).

	Combined	Girls		Boys	
		NW	OV/OB	NW	OV/OB
	n=89	n=20	n=22	n=25	n=22
AGE (years)	7.6 ± 0.4	7.6 ± 0.5	7.5 ± 0.5	7.8 ± 0.4	7.4 ± 0.5
MASS(kg)	30.3 ± 7.0	24.8 ± 3.4	33.7 ± 6.4	27.3 ± 4.0	37.0 ± 7.5
HEIGHT(cm)	128.5 ± 6.9	124.2 ± 5.7	129.3 ± 7.8	128.9 ± 6.5	131.7 ± 6.0
BMI(kg/m²)	18.2 ± 2.8	16.0 ± 1.1	20 ± 2.0	16.4 ± 1.3	21.2 ± 2.4
WEIST CIRCUMFERENCE (cm)	66.6 ± 9.2	59.8 ± 4.7	70.6 ± 7.7	61.1 ± 4.5	77.8 ± 7.0

Table 1: Description of the subjects by gender and BMI categories (mean ± SD).

Physical activity

Two-way ANOVA showed that there were no significant differences in the average daily total counts of PA, between the two BMI groups in each of the four consecutive days (p=0.549, p=0.662, p=0.703, p=0.848 for Thursday, Friday, Saturday and Sunday, respectively). But there were significant differences in the average daily total counts of PA, between two genders for the four consecutive days (p=0.001, p=0.004, p=0.186, p=0.088 respectively). Also there were no significant interaction effect between BMI groups and genders (p=0.767, p=0.761, p=0.973, p=0.835 respectively).

In addition there were no significant differences in the average minutes of moderate (p=0.184, p=0.672, p=0.563, p=0.834 for the four days respectively) and vigorous (p=0.920, p=0.836, p=0.877, p=0.729 respectively) PA between two BMI groups. In contrast there were significant differences in the average minutes of MPA in two from four days (p=0.054, p=0.264, p=0.272, p=0.087 for Thursday, Friday, Saturday and Sunday respectively) and in the average minutes of VPA (p=0.000, p=0.000, p=0.017, p=0.003 respectively) between two genders. Additionally significant differences existed between weekdays and weekend for average total PA counts ($F_{(1,87)}$=12.412, p=0.005), moderate ($F_{(1,87)}$=7.619, p=0.005) and vigorous ($F_{(1,87)}$=16.543, p=0.000) minutes of PA, for both BMI groups and for both genders, who were more active in weekdays than weekend. Specifically, only for VPA, there was significant interaction effect between gender and BMI factors. The results from this analysis are presented in Figure 2.

Physical fitness

Two-way ANOVA showed no significant differences in the four fitness tests parameters between the two BMI groups (p=0.834, p=0.369, p=0.097, p=0.260 for agility, long jump, balance and flexibility respectively). However boys obtained significant better performance than girls in both BMI groups in ASR and in SLJ (p = 0.000 and p=0.009 respectively). In addition there were no significant interaction effect between BMI groups and genders.

Achievement of the health-PA guidelines

Percentage frequency analysis showed that the percentage of NW children who met the international recommendation of 60 min MVPA was from 87.55%-96.9% and the percentage of OV/OB children ranged from 81.5%-96.3% for the four of the measured days (Figure 3).

Discussion

The results from this study suggests that no significant differences existed between NW and OV/OB boys and girls in the average daily counts of TPA or in the average daily minutes of MPA and VPA in early school age. Furthermore, there were no significant differences in scores of four fitness parameters tests, between the two BMI groups. However significant higher activity levels were observed in boys than in girls and significant higher activity levels in weekdays than in weekend in both BMI groups.

There has been considerable interest in the relation between PA and body composition in children but few researchers focused in 6-8-years olds. While it is generally accepted that PA decreases with age [11,16,24], pinpointing the age when the decrease starts and whether this reflects to body composition is important for targeted interventions. To our knowledge the only research in the same age is a recent UK study in 6-8-years olds which had use objective method (Actigraph LLC) of PA measurement and have found association of MVPA with OV/OB boys but not girls [25]. The use of a different model of accelerometer and the use of the specific cutpoint for classifying MVPA, as well as ethnically and socioeconomic criteria may explain these diverse findings. However our findings are in consistent with Thompson et al. [10], Treuth et al. [11] and in part with Mota et al. [8] who used a wide age range. No significant differences were found in objectively measured average daily total minutes of PA or in the average daily minutes of moderate, hard and very hard PA in the normal weight (≤85th percentile), at risk of overweight (>85th till ≤95th percentile) and overweight (>95th percentile) boys and girls 8-17 years old [10]. Similarly, Treuth et al. [11] reported no differences in TPA, MPA and VPA between normal and at risk/overweight boys and girls 7-19 years old. In the other hand Mota et al. [8] found no differences in TPA but significant differences only between non-obese and obese girls 8-15 years old in MVPA. Previous studies which found a negative relation between PA and BMI or body fat, used older children sample and focused specifically on associations of vigorous activity with body fat parameter [17,26-29]. This may have a biological explanation as spontaneous PA observed in young children covers the daily need for vigorous activity. Similarly latest studies in older children showed OV/OB children to be less active than NW children [5,19,30,31]. The contrast in findings from the present study may relate, in part, to the methodology used and the age groups examined. It seems that in that young age, Greek children, both OV and NW, have the time to play and make sport in the afternoon since they have not much homework and other learning obligations as older children do. Additionally, it seems that small cities still offer a safe environment for children's free play. However our finding reinforced by a recent study used questionnaires in 633, 10-12 years old Greek children reported that physical activity was unrelated to overweight [32].

Although health-related PA recommendations for children and adolescents have been established in at least 60 min of MVPA [33], few studies have looked at the relationship between the '60 min' guidelines and body composition. More than 87.55% of non-obese and 81.5% of OV/OB children in our study accumulated 60 or more minutes of MVPA per day. Similarly high compliance with guidelines (95.3% in boys, 77.5% in girls) showed a recent study in 6-12 years old French children [27] and in U.S. Hispanic 4-8 years old children (87%) [24]. Contrary UK studies in 3-5-years olds [34], 6-8-years olds

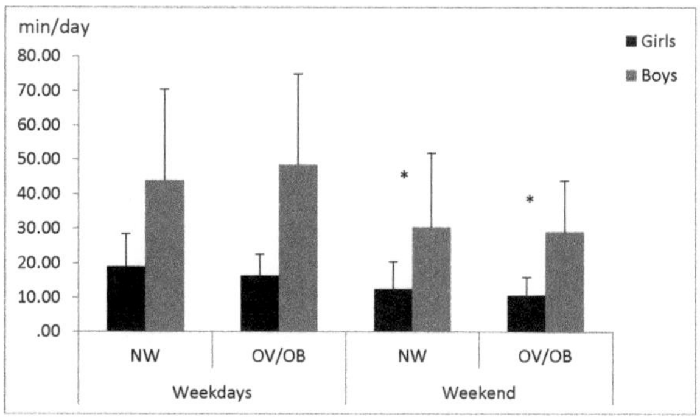

Figure 2: Vigorous PA (min/day) in weekdays and weekend (mean±SD), for both BMI groups and two genders.

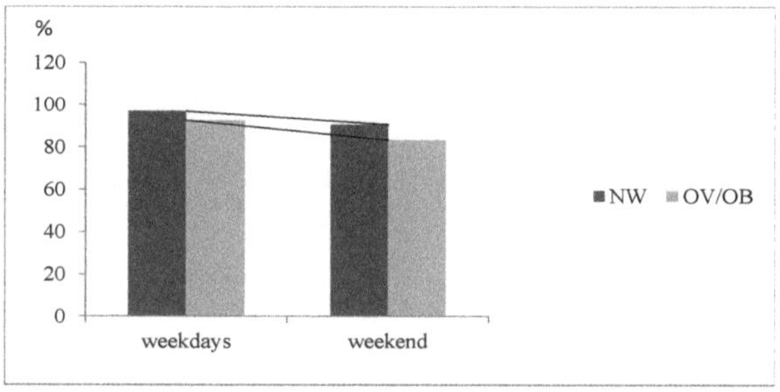

Figure 3: Compliance of NW and OV/OB groups with the international recommendation

and 11-12-years olds [35] which have used objective methods of PA measurement, have found low levels of PA with adherence to the 60 min/day recommendation of MVPA being achieved in <5% of their samples [25]. Low compliance (3% for under/normal weight; 2.6% for overweight/obese) with recommendation was noticed in Kenyan children 9-11-years old [36] in 9 years old children in Spain (37.5% for normal weight and 35% for overweight/obese) [31] and in 10-11 years old children from Malta (39% in boys and 10% in girls) [5]. The reduction of the proportion of children, normal and OV/OB, which meet the recommendation through ages, is clear as well as ethnically differences between studies. In our study it seems that the absence of a large number of obese children (only 8 in 89) combined with the intensity threshold used for vigorous intensity and the very good PA status of our cohort, affected the results on this parameter.

In this study we also examined the relation of overweight/obesity with selected fitness parameters. Most studies that have investigated differences in PF according to body fatness have focused on cardiorespiratory fitness. However we selected tests on agility, balance, flexibility and strength because as it is written before "activities of children aged 6 to 9 years are large anaerobic, and they help the child learn basic and more specialized motor skills" [37]. Additionally there is a subsidiary recommendation for activities which help children to enhance muscular strength and flexibility, at least twice a week [33]. We found no significant differences in flexibility test between the two BMI groups. These findings are in agreement with the findings of previous researchers [38-43]. On the balance test scores for the obese subjects in the present study were similar to those for their nonobese peers. Based on German BMI references (≥90 percentile overweight/obese) significant differences were found only between the obese and underweight 6-8 years old children [39]. Another study showed inferior scores for the obese subjects to those for their nonobese peers in balance but in an older sample [38], in contrast to Raudsepp et al. [44] who found no correlation between fatness and balance in prepubertal girls [44]. In the present study NW and OV/OB subjects had similar scores in weight-bearing activities, such as standing-broad jump and speed shuttle run. Other investigators have reported inferior performances for the obese subjects on these tests, compared with their non-obese counterparts [38,41,42], while Brunet et al. [43] reported significant differences, between the two BMI groups, in the scores of two tests only for children over 8 years old and Graf et al. [39] only between obese and normal/underweight children in SLJ. We must underline the significant better performance were observed in our study, in boys than in girls in SLJ and in ASR, in both BMI groups. Gender differences and better PA levels in boys probably explains these findings. However, it seems that the good level of PA for both BMI groups is a protecting factor to improve PF among children in that young age.

Our results corroborate previous observations consistently demonstrating that boys are more physically active than girls [8,11,16,17,24,26,28,29,45-47]. It was suggested that differences in gender roles (e.g. boys participating in higher energy expending roles or activities), and a higher motivation inherent in boys to participate in physical activity, may explain this sex difference [36].

Both sexes took part in significantly more PA on weekdays than weekends, highlighting the role the school environment plays in maintaining activity levels, and that more needs to be done to increase activity on weekends. These findings are in consistent with some previous studies [11,15,18,35,48] in contrast with another [31,49] whereas a study suggested similar activity pattern between weekdays and weekend [35]. Inconsistent results may exist due to geographical location, including environmental and socio-cultural factors.

Some limitations of the study should be recognized. Although accelerometry has been used to provide measures of intensity and duration of PA, current data cannot describe what the participants are doing while they are sedentary and cannot assess some activities like swimming and cycling. The study included primary-school children from one urban area only, which make difficult to generalize the findings. In addition, some limitations must be assumed when the current PA outcomes are compared with those of other studies because several factors such as type of monitor, length of the epoch and cut-off points selected. Furthermore, it is not possible to infer causal relationships using such a cross-sectional design. Therefore, longitudinal studies with more obese (>95th percentile) subjects should evaluate the effect.

Conclusion

This study pointed out an influence of gender and of the type of day on PA behavior of early schoolchildren. A high percentage of Greek 6-8 year olds (normal weight and overweight/obese) reached the recommended levels of daily MVPA. In contrast, overweight early schoolchildren appeared not to display different physical activity and fitness profiles compared to their peers. Therefore, if any, the effect of reduced physical activity levels on childhood obesity may be the result of a long term process, perhaps in combination with other factors. Early detection of weight status and physical performance, are important so that those in need of intervention can be targeted as early as possible.

References

1. Ng M, Fleming T, Robinson M, Thomson B, Graetz N, et al., (2014) Global, regional, and national prevalence of overweight and obesity in children and adults during 1980-2013: a systematic analysis for the Global Burden of Disease Study 2013. Lancet 384: 766-781.
2. Wijnhoven TMA, Joop M.A. Van Raaij JMA, Sjöberg A, Eldin N, Yngve A (2014)

WHO European Childhood Obesity Surveillance Initiative: School Nutrition Environment and Body Mass Index in Primary Schools. Int J Environ Res Public Health 11: 11261-11285.

3. Andreas AV (2011) National and cross-national comparisons of child and adolescent obesity: a greek national study. National Kapodistrian University: Greece.

4. Drenowatz C, Kobel S, Kettner S, Kesztyüs D, Steinacker JM (2014) Interaction of sedentary behaviour, sports participation and fitness with weight status in elementary school children. Eur J Sport Sci 14: 100-105.

5. Decelis A, Jago R, Fox KR (2014) Physical activity, screen time and obesity status in a nationally representative sample of Maltese youth with international comparisons. BMC Public Health 14: 664.

6. Gonzalez-Suarez CB, Caralipio N, Gambito E, Reyes JJ, Espino RV, Macatangay R (2013) The association of physical fitness with body mass index and waist circumference in Filipino preadolescents. Asia Pac J Public Health. 25:74-83.

7. Ara I, Moreno LA, Leiva MT, Gutin B, Casajús JA (2007) Adiposity, physical activity, and physical fitness among children from Aragón, Spain. Obesity (Silver Spring) 15: 1918-1924.

8. Jorge M, Paula S, Sandra G, Jose CR, Jose AD (2002) Differences of daily physical activity levels of children according to body mass index. Pediatric Exercise Science. 14: 442-452.

9. Nassis GP, Psarra G, and Sidossis LS (2005) Central and total adiposity are lower in overweight and obese children with high cardiorespiratory fitness. Eur J Clin Nutr 59: 137-141.

10. Thompson AM, Campagna PD, Rehman LA, Murphy RJ, Rasmussen RL, et al. (2005) Physical activity and body mass index in grade 3, 7, and 11 Nova Scotia students. Med Sci Sports Exerc 37: 1902-1908.

11. Treuth MS, Hou N, Young DR, Maynard LM (2005) Accelerometry-measured activity or sedentary time and overweight in rural boys and girls. Obes Res 13: 1606-1614.

12. Eston RG, Rowlands AV, Ingledew DK (1998) Validity of heart rate, pedometry, and accelerometry for predicting the energy cost of children's activities. J Appl Physiol (1985) 84: 362-371.

13. Kavouras SA, Sarras SE, Tsekouras YE, Sidossis LS (2008) Assessment of energy expenditure in children using the RT3 accelerometer. J Sports Sci 26: 959-966.

14. Ott AE, Pate RR, Trost SG, Ward DS, Saunders R (2000) The use of uniaxial and triaxial accelerometers to measure children's "free-play" physical activity. Pediatric Exercise Science 12: 360-370.

15. Gavarry O, Giacomoni M, Bernard T, Seymat M, Falgairette G (2003) Habitual physical activity in children and adolescents during school and free days. Med Sci Sports Exerc 35: 525-531.

16. Nyberg GA, Nordenfelt AM, Ekelund U, Marcus C (2009) Physical activity patterns measured by accelerometry in 6- to 10-yr-old children. Med Sci Sports Exerc 41: 1842-1848.

17. Ruiz JR, Rizzo NS, Hurtig-Wennlöf A, Ortega FB, Wärnberg J, et al. (2006) Relations of total physical activity and intensity to fitness and fatness in children: the European Youth Heart Study. Am J Clin Nutr 84: 299-303.

18. Nilsson A, Anderssen SA, Andersen LB, Froberg K, Riddoch C, et al. (2009) Between- and within-day variability in physical activity and inactivity in 9- and 15-year-old European children. Scand J Med Sci Sports 19: 10-18.

19. Kreuser F, Kromeyer-Hauschild K, Gollhofer A, Korsten-Reck U, Röttger K (2013) "Obese equals lazy?" analysis of the association between weight status and physical activity in children. J Obes 2013: 437017.

20. Cole TJ, Bellizzi MC, Flegal KM, Dietz WH (2000) Establishing a standard definition for child overweight and obesity worldwide: international survey. BMJ 320: 1240-1243.

21. Sung RY, Yu CC, Choi KC, McManus A, Li AM, et al. (2007) Waist circumference and body mass index in Chinese children: cutoff values for predicting cardiovascular risk factors. Int J Obes (Lond) 31: 550-558.

22. Rowlands AV, Thomas PW, Eston RG, Topping R (2004) Validation of the RT3 triaxial accelerometer for the assessment of physical activity. Med Sci Sports Exerc 36: 518-524.

23. [No Authors Listed] 1988 European test of physical fitness (EUROFIT), in Edigraf Editoriale Grafica.

24. Butte NF, Puyau MR, Adolph AL, Vohra FA, Zakeri I (2007) Physical activity in nonoverweight and overweight Hispanic children and adolescents. Med Sci Sports Exerc 39: 1257-1266.

25. Basterfield L, Jones AR, Parkinson KN, Reilly J, Pearce MS, et al. (2014) Physical activity, diet and BMI in children aged 6-8 years: a cross-sectional analysis. BMJ Open 4: e005001.

26. Abbott RA, Davies PS (2004) Habitual physical activity and physical activity intensity: their relation to body composition in 5.0-10.5-y-old children. Eur J Clin Nutr 58: 285-291.

27. Blaes A, Baquet G, Fabre C, Van Praagh E, Berthoin S (2011) Is there any relationship between physical activity level and patterns, and physical performance in children? Int J Behav Nutr Phys Act 8: 122.

28. Dencker M, Thorsson O, Karlsson MK, Lindén C, Eiberg S, et al. (2006) Daily physical activity related to body fat in children aged 8-11 years. J Pediatr 149: 38-42.

29. Wittmeier KD, Mollard RC, Kriellaars DJ (2008) Physical activity intensity and risk of overweight and adiposity in children. Obesity (Silver Spring) 16: 415-420.

30. Kwon S, Burns TL, Levy SM, Janz KF (2013) Which contributes more to childhood adiposity-high levels of sedentarism or low levels of moderate-through-vigorous physical activity? The Iowa Bone Development Study. J Pediatr 162: 1169-1174.

31. Laguna M, Ruiz JR, Gallardo C, García-Pastor T, Lara MT, et al. (2013) Obesity and physical activity patterns in children and adolescents. J Paediatr Child Health 49: 942-949.

32. Lagiou A, Parava M (2008) Correlates of childhood obesity in Athens, Greece. Public Health Nutr 11: 940-945.

33. Cavill N, Biddle S, and Sallis JF (2001), Health enhancing physical activity for young people: Statement of the United Kingdom Expert Consensus Conference. Pediatric Exercise Science 13: 12-25.

34. Reilly JJ, Coyle J, Kelly L, Burke G, Grant S, et al. (2003) An objective method for measurement of sedentary behavior in 3- to 4-year olds. Obes Res 11: 1155-1158.

35. Riddoch CJ, Bo Andersen L, Wedderkopp N, Harro M, Klasson-Heggebø L (2004) Physical activity levels and patterns of 9- and 15-yr-old European children. Med Sci Sports Exerc 36:86-92.

36. Muthuri SK, Wachira LM, Onywera VO, Tremblay MS (2014) Correlates of objectively measured overweight/obesity and physical activity in Kenyan school children: results from ISCOLE-Kenya. BMC Public Health 14: 436.

37. Strong WB, Malina RM, Blimkie CJ, Daniels SR, Dishman RK et al., (2005) Evidence based physical activity for school-age youth. J Pediatr 146: 732-737.

38. Deforche B, Lefevre J, De Bourdeaudhuij I, Hills AP, Duquet W, et al. (2003) Physical fitness and physical activity in obese and nonobese Flemish youth. Obes Res 11: 434-441.

39. Graf C, Koch B, Dordel S, Schindler-Marlow S, Icks A, et al. (2004) Physical activity, leisure habits and obesity in first-grade children. Eur J Cardiovasc Prev Rehabil 11: 284-290.

40. Kim J, Must A, Fitzmaurice GM, Gillman MW, Chomitz V, et al. (2005) Relationship of physical fitness to prevalence and incidence of overweight among schoolchildren. Obes Res 13: 1246-1254.

41. Tokmakidis SP, Kasambalis A, Christodoulos AD (2006) Fitness levels of Greek primary schoolchildren in relationship to overweight and obesity. Eur J Pediatr 165: 867-874.

42. Kamtsios S, (2007) Physical fitness, nutritional habits and daily locomotive action of 12-years children with different Body Mass Index. Inquiries in Sport and Physical Education, 5: 63-71.

43. Brunet M, Chaput JP, Tremblay A (2007) The association between low physical fitness and high body mass index or waist circumference is increasing with age in children: the 'Québec en Forme' Project. Int J Obes (Lond) 31: 637-643.

44. Raudsepp L, Jurimae T, (1996) Physical activity, fitness, and adiposity of prepubertal girls. Pediatric Exercise Science. 8: 259-267.

45. Trost SG, Kerr LM, Ward DS, Pate RR (2001) Physical activity and determinants of physical activity in obese and non-obese children. Int J Obes Relat Metab Disord 25: 822-829.

46. Vale S, Silva P, Santos R, Soares-Miranda L, Mota J (2010) Compliance with physical activity guidelines in preschool children. J Sports Sci 28: 603-608.

47. Eiberg S, Hasselstrom H, Grønfeldt V, Froberg K, Svensson J, Andersen LB (2005) Maximum oxygen uptake and objectively measured physical activity in Danish children 6-7 years of age: the Copenhagen school child intervention study. Br J Sports Med 39: 725-730.

48. Klasson-Heggebø L, Anderssen SA (2003) Gender and age differences in relation to the recommendations of physical activity among Norwegian children and youth.Scand J Med Sci Sports. 13: 293-298.

49. Trost SG, Pate RR, Freedson PS, Sallis JF, Taylor WC (2000) Using objective physical activity measures with youth: how many days of monitoring are needed? Med Sci Sports Exerc 32: 426-431.

Knee Objective Stability and Isokinetic Thigh Muscle Strength after Anterior Cruciate Ligament Reconstruction: A Randomized Six-Month Follow-Up Study

Matjaz Sajovic[1]* and Simona Pavlic Zaloznik[2]

[1]*Orthopaedics and Sports Trauma Surgery Department, General Teaching Hospital Celje, Slovenia*
[2]*UNIOR d.d. Unitur Spa and Rehabilitation Center Zreče, Cesta na Roglo 15, 3214 Zreče, Slovenia*

Abstract

Purpose: The most frequently used grafts for intra-articular anterior cruciate ligament (ACL) reconstruction are the autologous patellar tendon (PT) or doubled semitendinosus and gracilis tendons (STG) autografts. There are still controversies about graft selection for primary ACL reconstruction.

Methods: A prospective, randomized study was conducted on 57 patients who underwent arthroscopically assisted ACL reconstruction between January 2010 and February 2011. In 29 patients ACL reconstruction was performed with hamstring tendon autograft (STG group), and in 28 patients the ACL reconstruction was performed with patellar tendon autograft (PT group). At 6 months follow-up, all patients have performed the isokinetic extensor and flexor muscles strength and KT-1000 measurements.

Results: At 6 months after surgery, we found significantly lower average isokinetic quadriceps peak torque in the PT group compared to the STG group at angular velocity of 60°/s. However, at the same time we did not find significant difference in flexor muscle power comparing both groups. The manual maximum KT-1000 arthrometer side-to-side difference was 1.7 ± 1.7 mm for the PT group and 1.9 ± 1.6 mm for the STG group (P=0.398). No significant correlation was found between the knee objective stability (KT-1000 measurements) and the isokinetic thigh muscle strength (extensors, Spearman's rho=0.057, P=0.671; flexors, Spearman's rho=0.094, P=0.489).

Conclusions: Both hamstring and patellar tendon autografts provided good objective stability at 6 months after surgery In addition, regardless of which graft was used, a considerable percentage of patients continue to have strength deficits. In our opinion, the ACL-reconstructed leg should have 85% or greater return to the strength of the normal leg as one criterion before release to full sports activities. We were particularly intrigued to find only half of the competitive athletes achieved this goal at 6 months after surgery.

Keywords: Anterior cruciate ligament (ACL) reconstruction; Hamstring tendons (STG); Patellar tendon (PT); Isokinetic muscle strength; Knee laxity; Randomized clinical study

Introduction

The anterior cruciate ligament (ACL) rupture is the most common serious injury of the knee. It is widely believed that knee injury with associated ACL tear may lead to functional instability. In the active sporting population, such instability has been found to be associated with muscle weakness, meniscal and chondral injuries as well as with the development of degenerative disease within the joint [1-3]. The goals of ACL reconstruction are to decrease symptoms, improve function, and return patients to their pre-injury level of activity in the short term. ACL reconstruction is a common procedure that usually allows predictable and timely return to function for the patient [2]. It is customary now to allow return to full activities 6 months after the procedure, with some surgeons advocating return to sports as early as 4 months [4].

Because of numerous biologic advantages, the most frequently used grafts for intra-articular ACL reconstruction are the autologous patellar tendon (PT) or doubled semitendinosus and gracilis tendon (STG). Patellar tendon autograft has been the gold standard in ACL reconstruction, but during the last fifteen years, the use of hamstring tendons autograft has increased [5]. Disadvantages of patellar tendon autograft are potential increase in patellofemoral pain, loss of sensation, patellar fracture, inferior patellar contracture, and risk of persistent quadriceps muscle weakness [1,6,7]. Disadvantages of hamstring tendons autograft include potential loss of sensation, hamstring muscle weakness, and slower healing of the graft attachment site [5,8,9]. Weak hamstring muscles and low co-activity in relation to quadriceps are associated with a risk of ACL re-injury, and hamstring weakness is associated with poorer knee function after ACL reconstruction. Many questions have been raised as a result of accelerated rehabilitation programs. One area of concern is that of muscle weakness of the involved extremity due to donor-site morbidity. Several investigators have shown significant thigh muscle weakness that is present beyond the 6 months postoperative time period when using the two common ACL substitutes [1,4] Second area of concern is objective stability of the reconstructed knee. Postoperative accelerated rehabilitation must prevent thigh muscle atrophy in the early postoperative period, but not compromise stability of the reconstructed knee.

Despite an abundance of literature on ACL reconstruction and its outcome, there is little data directly comparing isokinetic thigh muscle strength after ACL reconstruction using patellar tendon and hamstring tendons autograft. The purpose of this prospective randomized study was to evaluate and analyze objective stability and isokinetic strength of

***Corresponding author:** Matjaz Sajovic, Senior Orthopedic Surgeon, Deputy Head, Orthopaedics and Sports Trauma Surgery Department, General Teaching Hospital Celje, Oblakova 5, 3000 Celje, Slovenia
E-mail: matjaz.sajovic@triera.net

knee extensor and flexor muscles at 6 months after ACL reconstruction using two different autografts (PT versus STG) with identical fixation (interference screws) in patients undergoing the same accelerated rehabilitation program. The hypotheses of this study were: 1) there is significantly lower quadriceps muscle power in the PT group compared with the STG group 2) there is no significant difference in flexor muscle power comparing both groups 3) there is no significant differences in knee laxity measurements between the two study groups 4) there is no correlation between objective stability and thigh muscle strength.

Materials and Methods

Patient selection

In this randomized controlled study, the key indication for arthroscopically assisted ACL reconstruction was a clinical diagnosis of ACL rupture in a patient desiring to return to his or her pre-injury level of activity. Patients with multi-ligament injury, previous surgery, an abnormality seen radiographically, chondral lesions diagnosed by arthroscopy, or an abnormal contralateral knee, as well as those who did not wish to participate in a research program, were not included into the study. Also, patients who required at ACL reconstruction additional meniscus repair were excluded from the study. From September 2009, the patients who fulfilled the study inclusion criteria were automatically included into the hospital database for ACL reconstruction. From January 2010 to February 2011, fifty-seven patients were randomized to primary arthroscopically assisted ACL reconstruction with a hamstring tendon autograft (N=29) or a patellar tendon-bone autograft (N=28). All patients signed an informed consent form.

The comparison between the hamstring tendon (STG) and the patellar tendon (PT) groups in relation to preoperative and intraoperative parameters showed that both groups were comparable. None of the patients´ radiographs shoved evidence of knee joint osteoarthritis. There were no significant differences between the two groups regarding age, sex, preinjury activity level, preoperative Lysholm knee scores, interval from injury to surgery, and meniscal resection (Table 1). Meniscal resections were performed in 20 of 29 STG patients (68%) and in 19 of 28 PT patients (65%) (P=0.408).

All procedures were performed by the first author (M.S.). The operations were performed using general or spinal anesthesia and a bloodless field. Antibiotic prophylaxis was given before tourniquet inflation as a single dose of 2 g cephalothin. Both groups were operated on using a single-incision technique. A systematic arthroscopic examination was performed initially and then additional surgery was performed. The ACL remnants were cleared away and a lateral notchplasty were performed when necessary.

Variable	Hamstring tendon group	Patellar tendon group	*P*
Total no. of patients	29	28	
Mean age, year (range)	27 (17 -51)	25 (18 - 52)	
Gender (n)			
Male	24 (83%)	24 (85%)	
Female	5 (17%)	4 (15%)	
International Knee Documentation Committee (IKDC) Preinjury activity Level 1	17 (58%)	18 (64%)	
Mean preoperative Lysholm scores (range)	57 (9 - 81)	55 (14 - 77)	0.622
Subacute reconstruction	4 (13%)	4 (14%)	
Chronic reconstruction	25 (87%)	24 (86%)	
Meniscal resection	20 (68%)	19 (65%)	0.408
Partial resection (Less than 30%)	12 (60%)	11 (57%)	
Subtotal resection (More than 30%)	8 (40%)	8 (43%)	0.039

Table 1: Comparison of Randomized Groups.

Operative technique

Apart from the graft harvesting the surgical technique was identical. For the patients randomized to the patellar tendon group, a 10-mm graft was harvested via longitudinal incision as a free autograft. The defects of the patella and the proximal tibia were not bone grafted. The graft included a 25-mm trapezoidal patellar bone block and a 15-mm rectangular tibial bone block. The bone blocks were trimmed to pass through a 9-mm diameter gauge. For the patients in the STG group, the graft was harvested through a longitudinal incision at the site of the pes anserinus insertion. The sartorius fascia was split and the gracilis and semitendinosus tendons were harvest with a tendon striper. The tendons were cleaned and looped over the No. 2 Vicryl absorbable suture to create a quadruple graft and the graft was sized between 7 and 9 mm. The graft was pretensioned up to 20 pounds with the surgeon's hands.

The femoral tunnel was drilled through the anteromedial portal prior to tibial tunnel drilling. The femoral tunnel was drilled through the most medial anatomic footprint of the posterolateral bundle, while the tibial tunnel was drilled through the central part of the anatomic footprint. Drill guides were used to confirm the correct position of the tunnels. To drill the femoral entry point, the author used the "bull's eye" drill guide (Linvatec, Largo, FL.). Tunnel size in the patellar tendon group was made 1 mm larger than the bone block size. In the hamstring tendons group, tunnel size was matched to the cross-sectional size of the graft. A marking suture using No. 0 absorbable suture was set 2.5 cm from the femoral end of the graft to ensure good entry of the graft in the tunnel and to prevent the graft from twisting around the screw during insertion. The graft was inserted via the tibial tunnel into a blind femoral tunnel. The left thread or right threads round-head, cannulated interference screws (RCI, ART-MAM, Slovenia) was used for femoral graft fixation [9]. In right knees the screw with left thread was used and in left knees the screw with right thread was used. In right knee the left thread screw turns in left direction and pushes the transplant away from lateral wall of the intercondylar notch, and vice versa. This fact prevented graft impingement against the lateral wall of the intercondylar notch. Tibial anatomical joint line fixation was achieved by absorbable interference screw (Linvatec) in an outside-in direction at a knee flexion angle of approximately 10° and manual pretension of the graft.

Postoperative rehabilitation

After skin closure and wound dressing, a cold compression device (Aircast, Inc., Summit, New Jersey) was applied and used during the first postoperative week. All the patients went through the same aggressive rehabilitation program, which permitted immediate full weight-bearing and full range of motion without use of rehabilitation brace (Annexure 1). During the hospital stay (mean, 3 days), the focus was set on ROM, muscles control, and pain/swelling management. After 2 weeks, closed kinetic chain exercises and stationary bicycling were started. The rehabilitation program has been completed in the Spa and Rehabilitation Center. After 8 weeks, agility training and light jogging were permitted. After 10 weeks, increased agility workouts, maximum strength training, and sport-specific activities were started. The patients were permitted to go back to full sports participation after 6 months if the criteria of full range of motion, no effusion, and good knee stability and strength were met.

Evaluation

Follow-up measurements were performed at 3 and 6 months

postoperatively in the Spa and Rehabilitation Center by the same senior physical therapist, which was not directly involved in the patient's rehabilitation and not blinded to the type of surgery (Table 2). The isokinetic evaluation has been performed first and then followed with knee laxity measurements.

Isokinetic strength of the extensor and flexor muscle groups was measured with the isokinetic dynamometer En – Knee (Enraf – Nonius). The subjects were told not to participate in any strenuous activities the day before the test session. They were also asked to continue their activities of daily living as usual before test session. The testing protocol was standardized to ensure reproducibility and validity. They performed a 10-minute warm-up on stationary bicycle. The patients were instructed on use of the isokinetic machine and allowed to become fully accustomed to the device before testing. The subjects also performed practice trials before the measurements were taken (pre-test). If a subject reported pain in the leg during the test, which occurred in few cases, this particular test was cancelled and the measurement was repeated. The uninvolved leg was evaluated first, followed by the involved limb. The strength tests (Endurance and Power test) were chosen to reflect quadriceps and hamstring muscle power during knee extension and knee flexion, respectively (open kinetic chain exercises). The peak torque values of the isokinetic strength tests were measured and then expressed as the difference between the involved and uninvolved limb and as the hamstring to quadriceps (H:Q, hamstring divided by quadriceps) ratio.

Objective anterior AP knee laxity measurements were performed by using the KT-1000 arthrometer (MEDmetric, San Diego, CA) [10]. The laxity data were recorded as the side-to-side difference in anterior tibial translation.

Statistical analysis

On September 23, 2009, a hospital database with all pre and postoperative variables was established. Statistical analysis was performed by an independent expert, not involved in the study protocol. Median (range) values are presented, except for the absolute anterior KT-1000 arthrometer laxity measurements, for which mean (range) values are presented. Unpaired *t*-test was used for the normally distributed numerical data (KT-1000 arthrometer). A non-parametric analogue was used, where appropriate (Mann-Whitney test was used to compare the differences between the groups. Spearman's rank correlation coefficient was used to assess the association between objective stability and isokinetic thigh muscle strength. A *P* value less than 0.05 was considered statistically significant.

Results

All 57 patients in the study were available at 3 and 6 months follow-up evaluation. There were no infections, deep venous thrombosis, nerve injuries, or other operative complications in this series. The median length of hospital stay was three nights (range, 2 to 3) for the hamstring tendon group and four nights (range, 2 to 5) for the patellar tendon group. All patients were comfortable with postoperative rehabilitation protocol. Full extension was achieved during early postoperative period. There were no signs of arthrofibrosis or impingement syndrome, so further surgeries were not required.

Comparison of the isokinetic results among the two graft sources showed general similarities (Table 3). The average deficit of the Endurance test (3 months after ACL reconstruction) for extensor muscles in the STG group was 18.8%. The average peak torque of the Endurance test for flexor muscles of the involved leg in the STG group was almost 95% of the uninvolved leg. The average deficit of the Endurance test of extensor muscles in the PT group 3 months after ACL reconstruction was 21.5%, and deficit of flexor muscles was minimal (3.9%). Between the two groups we did not find any statistical significant difference.

Endurance test	Power test	Anterior tibial translation
3 months postoperatively	6 months postoperatively	6 months postoperatively
angular velocity of 180°/s	angular velocity of 60°/s	KT- 1000 arthrometer
ROM 20°- 90°	ROM 10°- 90°	manual maximum force
25 repetitions	6 repetitions	average of 3 measurements

Table 2: Isokinetic and knee laxity evaluations.

		Group STG		Group PT		*P* (STG/PT)
		Average deficit (%)	SD	Average deficit (%)	SD	
Endurance test 180°/s	Extensor muscles	18.8	14.6	21.5	17.6	0.527
	Flexor muscles	5.2	13.2	3.9	8.6	0.667
Power test 60°/s	Extensor muscles	14.0	9.7	26.7	10.3	0.001
	Flexor muscles	3.9	16.8	1.4	10.1	0.497

Table 3: Group average deficit (%) and standard deviations (SD) for isokinetic strength measures comparing involved and uninvolved leg at 180°/s and 60°/s velocity and the level of statistical significance.

Patients have performed isokinetic Power test at 6 months postoperatively. In the STG group, the average deficit of peak extensor torque was 14.0%. The average peak flexor torque of the involved leg in the STG group was 96% of peak flexor torque of the uninvolved leg. In the PT group, the average deficit of peak extensor torque was 26.7%, and the average deficit of peak flexor torque was minimal (1.4%). We have found a statistical significant difference between the two groups in the extensor muscles power, while we did not find any statistical significant difference in flexor muscles power.

The patients with the hamstring tendons autograft had lower H:Q ratio in the injured leg than the patients with the patellar tendon autograft (0.60 vs. 0.79, $P < 0.001$), but not in the uninjured leg (0.54 vs. 0.56, P=0.415).

There was no significant difference between the groups with respect to the objective stability of the reconstructed knee (Table 4). At 6 months′ follow-up, the manual maximum KT-1000 arthrometer side-to-side difference was 1.7 ± 1.7 mm for the patellar tendon group and 1.9 ± 1.6 mm for the hamstring tendon group (P=0.558).

No significant correlation was found between the knee objective stability (KT-1000 measurements) and the isokinetic thigh muscle strength (extensors, Spearman's rho=0.057, P=0.671; flexors, Spearman's rho=0.094, P=0.489). There was no correlation between the KT-1000 side to side difference measurements and the isokinetic extensor muscle strength in either group (STG group, P=0.853; PT group, P=0.341). However, a moderate correlation was found between the knee objective stability and the isokinetic flexor muscle strength in the PT group (Spearman's rho=0.616, $P < 0.001$), but not in STG group (Spearman's rho=0.232, P=0.227).

KT-1000 measurements at 6 months postoperatively Manual maximum difference (mm)				
Group STG		Group PT		Statistical significance (STG/PT)
Average (mm)	SD	Average (mm)	SD	
1.9	1.6	1.7	1.7	*P* = 0.558

Table 4: KT-1000 measurements with average differences, standard deviation (SD) and statistical significance.

Discussion

In a prospective randomized trial, we compared the use of the well-established and the most frequently used central third bone-patellar tendon-bone autograft (PT) with use of a doubled semitendinosus and gracilis tendon (STG) autograft. Apart from the graft, all other important factors for the clinical outcome, such as surgeon experience, fixation technique and the rehabilitation protocol, were identical. Numerous studies have recently been published comparing patellar and hamstring tendon autografts in arthroscopic ACL reconstruction [1-9,11-14]. The present study continues to provide ongoing data showing the similarities and differences in the clinical results between the two groups. The results of our study substantiate the similarities found in previous reports that document that good or excellent results may be obtained in the majority of ACL reconstructions when using either PT or STG autografts [4,11,13]. However, Ageberg et al. [5], Aune et al. [1], and Bizzini et al. [6] reported significantly better isokinetic results in the PT group.

Strength deficit, secondary to graft harvesting, has been one area cited as to why neither STG nor PT grafts have been the ideal solution for the ACL reconstruction. Many studies reported that the extensor muscle strength was significantly worse in the PT group [1,7,8,15] and the flexor muscle strength was worse in the STG group [1,5-7] With the increasing efforts to expedite the return not only of the athlete to the playing field, but also the worker back to productive employment, ACL rehabilitation programs have progressed substantially in the recent past. Studies in which more aggressive rehabilitation was permitted have demonstrated improved leg strength with both graft types during earlier rehabilitation period. Carter et al. [4] found no statistically significant differences between the groups in knee extension or flexion strength at angular velocity of 180°/s and 300°/s at 6 months postoperatively. Our isokinetic evaluation confirmed their results at angular velocity of 180°/s already at 3 months postoperatively. At 6 months postoperatively, we found significantly lower isokinetic quadriceps peak torque (percentage of the contralateral side) in the PT group compared with the STG group at angular velocity of 60°/s (Table 3). Regarding the fact that the measurements was performed at 6 months after ACL reconstruction the results were good as according to the literature the reduced extensor muscles strength (on average up to 10%) is a normal phenomenon after ACL reconstruction [6,8,16] and that it can improve for several years after the surgery [17].

Lautamies et al. [8] recorded, even 5 years after the ACL reconstruction, that the subjects in both groups (PT and STG) had significant weaker thigh muscle strength in the involved leg compared with the uninvolved one. The reasons for bad results could be in irreversible preoperative tight muscle atrophy, inadequate operative therapy or/and inappropriate postoperative rehabilitation. The thigh muscles strength reduction is also influenced by the time from injury to surgery. Due to the consequently unstable joint the functional ability of knee joint is reduced, which leads to long term weakness in the leg muscles and compensation with the healthy extremity [1]. In our clinic the waiting time for ACL reconstruction is very long and preoperative rehabilitation programs are inhomogeneous, therefore, the ignorance of this factor can be one of the reasons for the significant difference in extensor muscle strength in the PT group at 6 months postoperatively. However, we did not find significant differences in respect to the waiting time for operative procedure comparing both groups (Table 1). There was significantly lower quadriceps muscle power in the PT group but not in the STG group. The reason for the reduced thigh muscles strength can also be the fact that the injury itself and the operation initiate changes in the neurocentral sensory apparatus, which can lead to changes in the neuromuscular activation of thigh muscles in comparison with the uninjured population [18]. One of the problems of ACL reconstruction with use of the patellar tendon autograft is the presence of postoperative anterior knee pain [1] and the increased possibility of patellar dysfunction [12].

Our accelerated rehabilitation protocol is focused on immediate postoperative passive and active extension of the knee and muscles activation of the whole leg. Full weight-bearing without using the brace enables rapid restoration of physiological walk and thus prevents development of leg muscles atrophy. The early stages of rehabilitation takes place under the expert supervision of a surgeon and it includes 14-day rehabilitation in the Rehabilitation Centre, where patients are instructed carefully on the proper way of doing exercises and gradual increase of activities. In the late stage of rehabilitation there is less physiotherapy control, however, patients are motivated to participate in objective testing at 3 and 6 months after the surgery. The advantage of our research is in the fact that all subjects were operated by the same surgeon and the rehabilitation process was led by the same physiotherapist. This is relatively rare in researching and represents a priority over research where more experts are included [16]. Based on the results we can confirm the effectiveness of the whole rehabilitation protocol. Despite the fact that the accelerated rehabilitation protocol was identical for both groups the extensor muscle strength was significantly worse in the PT group.

Considering the flexor muscle strength, measured at 3 months and at 6 months after surgery, the average deficit between the involved and the uninvolved leg was less than 5% in both groups. This is a very good result, particularly in the STG group because previous research has found that the hamstring tendons harvest significantly reduces the flexor strength for approximately 1 to 2 years after surgery [5,1,6]. Aune et al. [1] reported a significant difference in measurements of flexor muscle strength to the benefit of PT group. The results are justified with the presence of pain in the back of the knee and the reduced possibility of compensation of other muscles, especially the m. biceps femoris. Bizzini et al. [6] came to the same results where the cause for the difference was the trauma of flexor muscles during the surgery. The findings of our research do not confirm this. Excellent results resulted from good surgery technique of an experienced surgeon as well as rehabilitation program focusing on due and proper stretching and strengthening of flexor muscles.

The hamstring muscles play a major role in preventing or decreasing anterior and rotatory displacement of the tibia relative to the femur. Because the hamstring muscles are ACL agonists, recovery of hamstring muscle strength is of importance after ACL reconstruction, and it may be argued that this is of particular importance after reconstruction with the hamstring tendons autograft. Ageberg et al. [5] based on the results of their study suggested that a high H:Q ratio may be an important factor for dynamic knee-joint stabilization and seems to be relevant to the patient after ACL reconstruction. We agree with that conclusion, but results of our study proved that a high H:Q ratio in PT group correlated with a low quadriceps muscle power of the patients.

Beyaz et al. [14] reported no significant difference between patients who underwent single and dual-bundle ACL reconstruction in terms of hamstring and quadriceps isokinetic muscle strength at any angular velocities. In this prospective, randomized study semitendinosus and gracilis tendons ware used as autograft for ACL reconstruction. Probably that is the reason why they did not get any statistically significant differences in correspondence to isokinetic thigh muscle strength.

Numerous studies reported that both hamstring and patellar tendon autografts provided good objective stability [1,7,11,13]. In our study, there was no significant difference between the groups with respect to the objective stability of the reconstructed knee. At 6 months follow-up, the KT-1000 arthrometer side-to-side difference was 1.7 ± 1.7 mm for the patellar tendon group and 1.9 ± 1.6 mm for the hamstring tendon group (P=0.558). However, Bizzini et al. [6] reported that the PT group reaching significantly better results.

No significant correlation was found between the knee objective stability (KT-1000 measurements) and the isokinetic thigh muscle strength (extensors, Spearman's rho=0.057, P=0.671; flexors, Spearman's rho=0.094, P=0.489).

The strength of this study is the RCT design, the high follow-up rate and the independent observer assessment. The main limitation of our study is relatively small number of the patients who were included in our research. In order to obtain more reliable results, well-controlled, prospective long-term studies comparing patellar tendon with hamstring tendons autograft are needed.

Our study results showed that an appreciable quantity of patients had not regained adequate strength to be released to full sports activities without concern. In our opinion, the ACL-reconstructed leg should have 85% or greater return to the strength of the normal leg as one criterion before release to full sports activities. We were particularly intrigued to find only half of the competitive athletes achieved this goal at 6 months after surgery.

Conclusion

The strength deficiencies found in our study concur with what has previously been shown in regard to ACL reconstruction. In addition, regardless of which graft is used, a considerable percentage of patients continue to have strength deficits. At 6 months after surgery, we found significantly lower isokinetic quadriceps peak torque in the PT group compared with the STG group at angular velocity of 60°/s. However, at the same time we did not find significant difference in flexor muscle power comparing both groups. We did not find significant differences in knee laxity measurements between the two study groups. No significant correlation was found between the knee objective stability and the isokinetic thigh muscle strength.

Acknowledgements

Special thanks to my wife Romana, who has helped in the paperwork.

References

1. Aune AK, Holm I, Risberg MA, Jensen HK, Steen H (2001) Four-strand hamstring tendon autograft compared with patellar tendon-bone autograft for anterior cruciate ligament reconstruction. A randomized study with two-year follow-up. Am J Sports Med 29: 722-728.
2. Sajovic M, Strahovnik A, Dernovsek MZ, Skaza K (2011) Quality of life and clinical outcome comparison of semitendinosus and gracilis tendon versus patellar tendon autografts for anterior cruciate ligament reconstruction: an 11-year follow-up of a randomized controlled trial. Am J Sports Med 39: 2161-2169.
3. Xergia SA, McClelland JA, Kvist J, Vasiliadis HS, Georgoulis AD (2011) The influence of graft choice on isokinetic muscle strength 4-24 months after anterior cruciate ligament reconstruction. Knee Surg Sports Traumatol Arthrosc 19: 768-780.
4. Carter TR, Edinger S (1999) Isokinetic evaluation of anterior cruciate ligament reconstruction: hamstring versus patellar tendon. Arthroscopy 15: 169-172.
5. Ageberg E, Roos HP, Silbernagel KG, Thomee R, Roos EM (2009) Knee extension and flexion muscle power after anterior cruciate ligament reconstruction with patellar tendon graft or hamstring tendon graft: a cross-sectional comparison 3 years post-surgery. Knee Surg Sports Traumatol Arthrosc 17: 162-169.
6. Bizzini M, Gorelick M, Munzinger U, Drobny T (2006) Joint Laxity and Isokinetic Thigh Muscle Strength Characteristics After Anterior Cruciate Ligament Reconstruction: Bone Patellar Tendon Bone Versus Quadrupled Hamstring Autografts. Clin J Sport Med 16: 4-9.
7. Maletis GB, Cameron SL, Tengan JJ, Burchette RJ (2007) A Prospective Randomized Study of Anterior Cruciate Ligament Reconstruction A Comparison of Patellar Tendon and Quadruple-Strand Semitendinosus/Gracilis Tendons Fixed With Bioabsorbable Interference Screws. Am J Sports Med 35: 384-394.
8. Lautamies R, Harilainen A, Kettunen J, Sandelin J, Kujala UM (2008) Isokinetic quadriceps and hamstring muscle strength and knee function 5 years after anterior cruciate ligament reconstruction: comparison between bone-patellar tendon-bone and hamstring tendon autografts. Knee Surg Sports Traumatol Arthrosc 16: 1009-1016.
9. Sajovic M, Vengust V, Komadina R, Tavcar R, Skaza K (2006) A prospective, randomized comparison of semitendinosus and gracilis tendon versus patellar tendon autografts for anterior cruciate ligament reconstruction: five-year follow-up. Am J Sports Med 34: 1933-1940.
10. Vauhnik R, Turk Z, Pilih IA (2005) Intra-rater reliability of using KT 2000 COMPUKT for measuring anterior tibial translation. Zdrav Vest 74: 285-288.
11. Aglietti P, Giron F, Buzzi R, Biddau F, Sasso F (2004) Anterior cruciate ligament reconstruction: bone-patellar tendon-bone compared with double semitendinosus and gracilis tendon grafts. A prospective, randomized clinical trial. J Bone Joint Surg Am 86-A: 2143-2155.
12. Anderson JL, Lamb SE, Barker KL, Davies S, Dodd CA, et al. (2002) Changes in muscle torque following anterior cruciate ligament reconstruction: a comparison between hamstrings and patella tendon graft procedures on 45 patients. Acta Orthop Scand 73: 546-552.
13. Beard DJ, Anderson JL, Davies S, Price AJ, Dodd CA (2001) Hamstrings vs. patella tendon for anterior cruciate ligament reconstruction: a randomised controlled trial. Knee 8: 45-50.
14. Beyaz S, Ã–zkoÃ§ G, AkpÄ±nar S, Demir Åž, Adam M, et al. (2012) Comparison of tunnel expansion and isometric muscle strength after ACL reconstruction with single- or dual-bundle hamstring allograft: a prospective, randomized study. Acta Orthop Traumatol Turc 46: 353-360.
15. Rosenberg TD, Franklin JL, Baldwin GN, Nelson KA (1992) Extensor mechanism function after patellar tendon graft harvest for anterior cruciate ligament reconstruction. Am J Sports Med 20: 519-525.
16. Dauty M, Tortellier L, Rochcongar P (2005) Isokinetic and anterior cruciate ligament reconstruction with hamstrings or patella tendon graft: analysis of literature. Int J Sports Med 26: 599-606.
17. Dvir Z (1994) Isokinetics, Muscle Testing, Interpretation and Clinical Applications. Churchill Livingstone, Edinburgh.
18. Williams GN, Chmielewski T, Rudolph K, Buchanan TS, Snyder-Mackler L (2001) Dynamic knee stability: current theory and implications for clinicians and scientists. J Orthop Sports Phys Ther 31: 546-566.

PERMISSIONS

 Every chapter published in this book has been scrutinized by our experts. Their significance has been extensively debated. The topics covered herein carry significant findings which will fuel the growth of the discipline. They may even be implemented as practical applications or may be referred to as a beginning point for another development.

The contributors of this book come from diverse backgrounds, making this book a truly international effort. This book will bring forth new frontiers with its revolutionizing research information and detailed analysis of the nascent developments around the world.

We would like to thank all the contributing authors for lending their expertise to make the book truly unique. They have played a crucial role in the development of this book. Without their invaluable contributions this book wouldn't have been possible. They have made vital efforts to compile up to date information on the varied aspects of this subject to make this book a valuable addition to the collection of many professionals and students.

This book was conceptualized with the vision of imparting up-to-date information and advanced data in this field. To ensure the same, a matchless editorial board was set up. Every individual on the board went through rigorous rounds of assessment to prove their worth. After which they invested a large part of their time researching and compiling the most relevant data for our readers.

The editorial board has been involved in producing this book since its inception. They have spent rigorous hours researching and exploring the diverse topics which have resulted in the successful publishing of this book. They have passed on their knowledge of decades through this book. To expedite this challenging task, the publisher supported the team at every step. A small team of assistant editors was also appointed to further simplify the editing procedure and attain best results for the readers.

Apart from the editorial board, the designing team has also invested a significant amount of their time in understanding the subject and creating the most relevant covers. They scrutinized every image to scout for the most suitable representation of the subject and create an appropriate cover for the book.

The publishing team has been an ardent support to the editorial, designing and production team. Their endless efforts to recruit the best for this project, has resulted in the accomplishment of this book. They are a veteran in the field of academics and their pool of knowledge is as vast as their experience in printing. Their expertise and guidance has proved useful at every step. Their uncompromising quality standards have made this book an exceptional effort. Their encouragement from time to time has been an inspiration for everyone.

The publisher and the editorial board hope that this book will prove to be a valuable piece of knowledge for researchers, students, practitioners and scholars across the globe.

LIST OF CONTRIBUTORS

JL Ziltener, L Allet, P Sclison and M Grosclaude
Geneva University Hospital, Geneva, Switzerland

Julien S Baker
Institute of Clinical Exercise and Health Science, University of the West of Scotland, Scotland

Lawrence D Hayes
Institute of Clinical Exercise and Health Science, University of the West of Scotland, Scotland
School of Human Sciences, London Metropolitan University, UK

Fraser E Houston
Center for Exercise Science, University of Florida, USA

Masumi Takada and Motohiko Satoh
Graduate School of Medicine, Aichi University of Medicine, Nagakute 480-1195, Japan

Hiroki Takada
Graduate School of Medicine, Aichi University of Medicine, Nagakute 480-1195, Japan
Graduate Schools of Engineering, University of Fukui, Fukui 910-8507, Japan

Masaru Miyao
Graduate School of Information Science, Nagoya University, Japan

Kazuki Yoshikawa and Yasuyuki Matsuura
Graduate Schools of Engineering, University of Fukui, Fukui 910-8507, Japan

Igor I Miroshnichenko, Svetlana A Sergeeva, Angelina I Platova and Lyudmila M Krasnykh
Mental Health Research Center of RAMS, Moscow, Russia

Senthil P Kumar
Associate Professor in Musculoskeletal and Manual Therapy, Dept of Physiotherapy, Kasturba Medical College, Manipal University, Mangalore, India

Vaishali Sisodia
Department of Physiotherapy, Career Institute of Medical Sciences, Bhopal, India

Ernest Jacob
Assistant Professor, Dr. M.V.Shetty College of Physiotherapy, Mangalore, India

Spanoudaki S, Maridaki M, Bogdanis GC and Baltopoulos P
Department of Sports Medicine & Biology of Physical Activity, Faculty of Physical Education and Sports Science, National & Kapodistrian University of Athens, 41 Ethnikis Antistasis, Dafni, Greece

Karatzanos E
Cardiopulmonary Exercise Testing and Rehabilitation Laboratory, Evgenidio Hospital, School of Medicine, National & Kapodistrian University of Athens, Greece, 20 Papadiamantopoulou Str., 115 28, Athens, Greece

Spanoudaki C
Neonatal Intensive Care Unit, General Hospital of Chania, Greece

Julien S Baker
Institute of Clinical Exercise and Health Science, University of the West of Scotland, Scotland

Lawrence D Hayes
Institute of Clinical Exercise and Health Science, University of the West of Scotland, Scotland
School of Human Sciences, London Metropolitan University, Scotland

Gordon F Bickerstaff
Department of Biology, University of the West of Scotland, Scotland

Masato Takahashi and Yukitoshi Tatsugi
Faculty of Physical Education, International Budo Univ, Japan

Tosihiko Kohno
Faculty of Nursing, Kameda College of Health Science, Japan

Ali Moshiri
Veterinary Surgeon, Division of Surgery and Radiology, School of Veterinary Medicine, Shiraz University, Shiraz, Iran

Ahmad Oryan
Comparative Pathologist, Department of Pathology, School of Veterinary Medicine, Shiraz University, Shiraz, Iran

Xuan Tran
University of West Florida, USA

Roland Walker, William J Nash, Rajiv S Patel and Sam Singh
Orthopaedic Department, Guy's Hospital, Great Maze Pond, London, UK

Fernando Naclerio
Centre of Sport Science and Human Performance, School of Science, University of Greenwich, UK
Institute of Sport, Exercise and Active Living (ISEAL), Victoria University, Melbourne, Australia

Ahmad Alkhatib
Centre of Sport Science and Human Performance, School of Science, University of Greenwich, UK

Alfonso Jimenez
School of Sports Science, European University of Madrid, Spain

Jing Liu
Department of Martial Arts, Shanghai University of Sport, Shanghai 200438, China
Department of Psychology, School of Kinesiology, University of Michigan, Ann Arbor, MI, 48109, USA

Peijie Chen and Ru Wang
Department of Sports Medicine, Shanghai University of Sport, Shanghai 200438, China

Yonghong Yuan
Department of Sports Leisure, Shanghai University of Sport, Shanghai 200438, China

Chunying Li
Department of Biochemistry & Molecular Biology, Wayne State University School of Medicine, Detroit, Michigan 48201, USA

Bergstrom HC, Housh TJ, Traylor DA, Lewis RW, Schmidt RJ and Johnson GO
Department of Nutrition and Health Sciences, University of Nebraska-Lincoln, USA

Zuniga JM
School of Allied Health, Western New Mexico University, USA

Camic CL
Department of Health & Physical Education, University of Wisconsin- Platteville, USA

Eugenia Gortsila, Apostolos Theos and Maria Maridaki
Department of Physical Education & Sports Science, National & Kapodistrian University of Athens, Greece

Goran Nesic
Faculty of Sport and Physical Education, University of Belgrade, Serbia

Vasilios I. Kalapotharakos, Michalis Mitrotasios, Konstantinos S. Spaneas and Savvas P. Tokmakidis
Department of Physical Education & Sport Science, Democritus University of Thrace, Komotini, Greece

George Ziogas
Sports Clinic, Thessaloniki, Greece

Evaggelos Manolopoulos
Department of Physical Education & Sport Science, Aristotle University of Thessaloniki, Serres, Greece

Lawrence D Hayes and Catherine E Baker
School of Human Sciences, London Metropolitan University, UK

Julien S Baker
Institute of Clinical Exercise and Health Science, University of the West of Scotland, UK

Gordon F Bickerstaff
Department of Biology, University of the West of Scotland, UK

Kalaskar AR and Kalaskar R
Government Dental College & Hospital, Nagpur, Maharashtra, India

Aaron Hermann and Maciej Henneberg
School of Medical Sciences, University of Adelaide, University of Adelaide, Adelaide, South Australia, Australia

A. Lee Dellon
Department of Plastic Surgery and Neurosurgery, Johns Hopkins University, USA

Zoran Milanovic and Nebojsa Trajkovic
Faculty of Sport and Physical Education, University of Nis, Nis, Serbia

Goran Sporis and Dario Novak
Faculty of Kinesiology, University of Zagreb, Zagreb, Croatia

Marko Erceg
Faculty of Kinesiology, University of Split, Split, Croatia

Fumio Aita
Edosaki Sohgoh High School, Inashiki, Japan

Shukoh Haga
Institute of Health and Sport Science, University of Tsukuba, Tsukuba, Japan

Shogo Sato, Takuya Sakurai, Junetsu Ogasawara, Takako Kizaki and Hideki Ohno
Department of Molecular Predictive Medicine and Sport Science, Kyorin University, School of Medicine, Mitaka, Japan

Kazuki Esaki
Faculty of Education, Shiga University, Ohtsu, Japan

Takafumi Hamaoka
Faculty of Sports and Health Science, Ritsumeikan University, Kusatsu, Japan

Masao Mizuno
Faculty of Education, Hokkaido University, Sapporo, Japan

Koji Toshinai
Faculty of Medicine, University of Miyazaki, Miyazaki, Japan

Hiromi Miyazaki
Division of Traumatology, National Defense Medical College Research Institute, Tokorozawa, Japan

Tohru Takemasa
Graduate School of Comprehensive Human Sciences, University of Tsukuba, Tsukuba, Japan

Noboru Hashimoto
Department of Judo Therapy, Faculty of Health Science, Tokyo Ariake University of Medical and Health Science, Kotoh-ku, Japan

Toshihito Katsumura
Department of Sports Medicine for Health Promotion, Tokyo Medical University, Shinjuku-ku, Japan

Dickinson J
Endurance Research Group, University of Kent, Chatham Maritime, UK

Hu J, Chester N and Whyte G
Research Institute for Sport and Exercise Sciences, Liverpool John Moores University, Liverpool, UK

Loosemore M
The Institute of Sport, Exercise and Health, University College London, London, UK

Yoko Tanabe
Nihon University, Tokyo, Japan

Graduate School of Sport Sciences, Waseda University, Saitama, Japan

Shin Asakawa
Japan Anti-Doping Agency, Tokyo, Japan

Yuko Arakida
Japanese Olympic Committee Tokyo, Japan

Ichiro Kono
University of Tsukuba, Ibaraki, Japan

Takao Akama
Faculty of Sport Sciences, Waseda University, Saitama, Japan

Harumi Hayashida
Faculty of Health Promotional Sciences, Tokoha University, Japan
Institute for Nanoscience & Nanotechnology, Waseda University, Japan

Mayura Shimura
Faculty of Health Sciences, Health Science University, Japan

Kaoru Sugama
Institute for Nanoscience & Nanotechnology, Waseda University, Japan
Division of Cell Regeneration and Transplantation, Department of Functional Morphology, Nihon University School of Medicine, Japan

Kazue Kanda
Institute for Nanoscience & Nanotechnology, Waseda University, Japan

Katsuhiko Suzuki
Faculty of Sport Sciences, Waseda University, Japan

Giovanni Messina, Giovanni Di Bernardo, Antonietta Messina, Carmine Dalia, Sergio Chieffi, Umberto Galderisi and Marcellino Monda
Department of Experimental Medicine, Section of Human Physiology and Clinical Unit of Dietetics and Sports Medicine, Second University of Naples, Naples, Italy

Baker JS, Buchan DS and Kilgore L
Institute for Clinical Exercise & Health Science, University of the West of Scotland, Hamilton, ML3 0JB, Scotland, UK

Wong DP
Human Performance Laboratory, Technological and Higher Education Institute of Hong Kong, Hong Kong, P.R. China

Davies B and Davies M
Health and Exercise Science Research Unit, School of Applied Sciences, University of South Wales, Pontypridd, CF37 1DL, Wales, UK

Cooper SM
Cardiff School of Sport, Cardiff Metropolitan University, Cardiff CF23 6XD, Wales, UK

George A
Biotropics Malaysia Berhad, Lot 21, Jalan U1/19, Section U1, Hicom-Glenmarie Industrial Park, 40150 Shah Alam, Selangor, Malaysia

Liske E
Departments of Life Sciences, Technical University of Braunschweig, Germany

Chen CK
Sports Science Unit, School of Medical Sciences, Universiti Sains Malaysia, Malaysia

Ismail SB
Department of Family Medicine, School of Medical Sciences, Universiti Sains Malaysia, Malaysia

Leon I Foster, Steve J Haake and Dave M James
The Centre for Sports Engineering Research, Faculty of Health and Wellbeing, Sheffield Hallam University, UK

Alan M Nevill
Faculty of Education, Health and Wellbeing, University of Wolverhampton, UK

Hein FM Lodewijkx
Faculty of Psychology and Educational Sciences, Open University of The Netherlands, Heerlen, The Netherlands

Haluk H. Oztekin and Bulent Zeren
Orthopaedic Surgeons, Private Clinic for Sports Traumatology and Orthopaedics, 1738 Sokak, No: 10, Karsiyaka, Izmir, Turkey

Elif Ozcan
Marmara University Faculty of Dentistry Department of Oral and Maxillofacial Surgery, Turkey

Guhan Dergin
Associate Professor, Marmara University Faculty of Dentistry Department of Oral and Maxillofacial Surgery, Turkey

O'Brien CP
Sports Surgery Clinic, Santry Demesne, Dublin, Ireland

Watson A
Raglan Sports Medicine, 4 Fitzwilliam Square East, Dublin, Ireland

Mark R McKean, Timothy B Stockwell and Brendan J Burkett
Faculty of Science, Health, Education and Engineering, University of Sunshine Coast, Queensland, Australia

Paschaleri Z, Arabatzi F, Papitsa A, Giagazoglou P and Kellis E
Aristotle University of Thessaloniki, Serres, Greece

Matjaz Sajovic
Orthopaedics and Sports Trauma Surgery Department, General Teaching Hospital Celje, Slovenia

Simona Pavlic Zaloznik
UNIOR d.d. Unitur Spa and Rehabilitation Center Zreče, Cesta na Roglo 15, 3214 Zreče, Slovenia

Index